ACUTE MEDICINE

3rd EDITION

ACUTE MEDICINE

3rd EDITION

DECLAN O'KANE, MD, FRCP, FAcadMEd

Consultant Physician
Royal Sussex County Hospital
University Hospitals Sussex

Scion

Third edition © Scion Publishing Limited, 2023

ISBN 9781914961038

Second edition published in 2018 (ISBN 9781907904912)
First edition published in 2015

A CIP catalogue record for this book is available from the British Library.

Scion Publishing Limited
The Old Hayloft, Vantage Business Park, Bloxham Road, Banbury OX16 9UX, UK
www.scionpublishing.com

Important Note from the Publisher

The information contained within this book was obtained by Scion Publishing Ltd from sources believed by us to be reliable. However, while every effort has been made to ensure its accuracy, no responsibility for loss or injury whatsoever occasioned to any person acting or refraining from action as a result of information contained herein can be accepted by the authors or publishers.

Readers are reminded that medicine is a constantly evolving science and while the authors and publishers have ensured that all dosages, applications and practices are based on current indications, there may be specific practices which differ between communities. You should always follow the guidelines laid down by the manufacturers of specific products and the relevant authorities in the country in which you are practising.

Although every effort has been made to ensure that all owners of copyright material have been acknowledged in this publication, we would be pleased to acknowledge in subsequent reprints or editions any omissions brought to our attention.

Registered names, trademarks, etc. used in this book, even when not marked as such, are not to be considered unprotected by law.

Feedback, errors and omissions

We are always pleased to receive feedback (good and bad) about our books – if you would like to comment, please email info@scionpublishing.com.

We've worked really hard with the editors and authors to ensure that everything in the book is correct. However, errors and ambiguities can still slip through in books as complex as this. If you spot anything you think might be wrong, please email us and we will look into it straight away. If an error has occurred, we will correct it for future printings and post a note about it on our website so that other readers of the book are alerted to this.

Thank you for your help.

Typeset by Medlar Publishing Solutions Pvt Ltd, India
Printed in the UK
Last digit is the print number: 10 9 8 7 6 5 4 3 2

Contents

17   Oncology. 415

18   Miscellaneous 423

19   Dermatology 431

Preface

I wrote this book for my own needs to reference the questions that come up when dealing with acutely unwell medical patients. I was conscious that the answers I often needed could frequently not otherwise be found quickly and readily. I hope this will be a useful text for others at all levels, especially the on-call Medical SpR. Emergency department doctors and others may also find it useful. It is a quick reference of 'what and why' that covers common and not so common emergencies. It is compact and facts can be found quickly. I am very aware of the frailties of human memory and decision-making. A simple checklist at hand can hopefully enhance safety and clinical care. Included at the back is a quick emergency drug reference where drug information is consolidated to avoid repetition. This does not replace the *British National Formulary* (*BNF*) which has now been released as a free app and is the best source of prescribing information. Despite great care, we may have errors of omission or fact. This is not a cookbook to slavishly follow, but a guide to help the reader to analyse a difficult situation with a framework and some salient facts. Lastly, this is a book by a generalist. It is not intended to replace experts. All difficult cases benefit from early expert help – this book should aid the dialogue and identify key issues. To some the information will be new, and to others it is simply a reminder. It needs to be compact and concise so let us not waste further words or space.

 ## Acknowledgments

I'd like to thank my wife and my two girls for their love, patience and support. This book is dedicated to the memory of my good friend, Jeremy Sherman FRCS. In my training I was fortunate to work for many wonderful hard-working clinicians. I am particularly indebted to Professor Jennifer Adgey CBE and the late Dr Seamus Coyle. I'd like to thank those who have read the manuscript and made helpful suggestions and additions including Dr Jacob F. de Wolff, Dr Andrew Solomon, Dr Pad Boovalingam, Dr Omar Kirresh, Dr Peter Rhead and Dr Christopher Miller, and Dr V Srinivasan and Dr Abdul Elmarimi for their kind help.

 ## Updates to the 3rd edition

For this new edition almost all subjects have been edited and updated. We have Covid-19 and many other updates. I am grateful to Dr Omar Kirresh who is now a fellow colleague of mine here in Brighton. I'd also like to thank Dr Matthew Palethorpe who provided superb and detailed feedback and suggestions, and Simon Daley for his advice on ACS. In addition, I'd like to thank Dr Andrew Leonard, a fantastic colleague and first class acute medicine physician, for his leadership over what have been challenging times for all. Any remaining errors are mine. Finally, many thanks to Jonathan Ray and Clare Boomer at Scion for their wonderful support and encouragement.

If you have any comments, questions or suggestions, please write to me at drokane@gmail.com. Errata will be available on the page for the book at www.scionpublishing.com, on the Resources tab.

Declan O'Kane, 2023

Disclaimer

Every effort has been made in preparing this publication to provide accurate and up to date information in accordance with accepted standards and practice at the time of publication. The author can make no warranties that the information contained herein is totally free from error, not least because clinical standards are constantly changing. The author therefore disclaims all liability for direct or consequential damages resulting from the use of material within this publication. Readers are recommended to check all drug doses, indications and C/I and interactions used with the *BNF* or drug data-sheet prior to use. If a reader is unsure what to do then they should seek support from their senior medical adviser. Patients should seek help from their own doctor/ healthcare provider.

 ## Decision-making for the medical registrar

The first medical registrar year is tough and stressful, but with the years it gets easier and more enjoyable: you recognise the same patterns and problems like a chess puzzle and the solutions become easier to resolve in seconds, and you can solve other people's puzzles for them. Sometimes, however, a problem is completely new so you need to sit down and work it out from first principles and/or ask for help from someone who may have encountered the situation before. Referrals will come thick and fast – regard these as compliments to your skills in problem-solving. Get help once you have thought (time allowing) it through yourself and presented your plan. If you are unhappy or concerned call for advice. Share diagnostic dilemmas and don't sit on them. Don't go home without resolving your concerns. As consultants we constantly discuss interesting and difficult cases. Good medical practice is about reflection and seeking feedback. Good luck.

Abbreviations

5-HIAA	5-hydroxyindoleacetic acid	APML	acute promyelocytic leukaemia
AAA	abdominal aortic aneurysm	APTT	activated partial thromboplastin time
ABC	airway, breathing and circulation	AR	aortic regurgitation
ABCDE	ABC + disability, exposure	ARB	angiotensin-II receptor blocker
ABG	arterial blood gas	ARDS	acute/adult respiratory distress syndrome
ABU	asymptomatic bacteriuria		
ACA	anterior cerebral artery	ARF	acute respiratory failure
ACE	angiotensin-converting enzyme	ART	antiretroviral therapy
		ARVC	arrhythmogenic right ventricular cardiomyopathy
ACEi	ACE inhibitor		
Ach	acetylcholine	AS	aortic stenosis
ACOMM	anterior communicating artery	ASD	atrial septal defect
ACS	acute coronary syndrome	ASO(T)	antistreptolysin O (titre)
ACTH	adrenocorticotrophic hormone	AST	aspartate aminotransferase
ADA	adenosine deaminase	ATN	acute tubular necrosis
ADEM	acute disseminated encephalomyelitis	AV	arteriovenous/atrioventricular
		AVM	arteriovenous malformation
ADLs	activities of daily living	AVNRT	atrioventricular nodal re-entrant tachycardia
ADR	adverse drug reaction		
AED	automated external defibrillators or anti-epilepsy drug	AVPU	awake, voice, pain, unresponsive
		AVRT	atrioventricular re-entrant tachycardia
AF	atrial fibrillation		
AFB	acid-fast bacilli (TB)	AXR	abdominal X-ray
AFLP	acute fatty liver of pregnancy	BAL	bronchoalveolar lavage
aHUS	atypical haemolytic uraemic syndrome	BBB	bundle branch block
		BD/bd	twice daily or 12-hourly
AIDP	acute inflammatory demyelinating polyneuropathy	BE	base excess
		BiPAP	bilevel positive airway pressure
AIDS	acquired immunodeficiency syndrome	BJP	Bence Jones protein
		BMS	bare metal stents
AKI	acute kidney injury	BNP	B-type natriuretic peptide
ALA	alanine aminotransferase	BP	blood pressure
ALF	acute liver failure	BUN	blood urea nitrogen
ALI	acute lung injury	BVM	bag–valve mask
ALP	alkaline phosphatase	CABG	coronary artery bypass grafting
ALS	advanced life support	CAD	coronary artery disease
ALT	alanine aminotransferase	CBG	capillary blood glucose
AMAN	acute motor axonal neuropathy	CC	chest compression
AMTS	abbreviated mental test score	CCB	calcium channel blocker
ANA	antinuclear antibody	CCF	congestive cardiac failure
ANCA	antineutrophil cytoplasmic antibody	CEA	carcinoembryonic antigen or carotid endarterectomy
ANP	atrial natriuretic peptide	CFU	colony-forming units
APKD	adult polycystic kidney disease	CHB	complete heart block
APLS	antiphospholipid syndrome	C/I	contraindications

CI-AKI	contrast-induced acute kidney injury
CIDP	chronic inflammatory demyelinating polyneuropathy
CIS	clinically isolated syndrome
CK	creatine kinase
CKD	chronic kidney disease
CLO test	*Campylobacter*-like organism test (rapid urease test)
CMP	cardiomyopathy
CMV	cytomegalovirus
CO	cardiac output
COPD	chronic obstructive pulmonary disease
CPAP	continuous positive airway pressure
CPR	cardiopulmonary resuscitation
CRH	corticotropin-releasing hormone
CRP	C-reactive protein
CRT	cardiac resynchronisation therapy
CSF	cerebrospinal fluid
CSM	carotid sinus massage
CSU	catheter sample urine
CTG	cardiotocogram
CTPA	computed tomography pulmonary angiogram
CVP	central venous pressure
CVST	cerebral venous sinus thrombosis
CXR	chest X-ray
DAPT	dual antiplatelet therapy
DBP	diastolic blood pressure
DCM	dilated cardiomyopathy
DCR	damage control resuscitation
DES	drug-eluting stents
DHEA	dehydroepiandrosterone
DI	diabetes insipidus
DIC	disseminated intravascular coagulation
DKA	diabetic ketoacidosis
DM	diabetes mellitus
DNACPR	do not attempt cardiopulmonary resuscitation
DOAC	direct oral anticoagulant (previously NOAC)
DOB	date of birth
DPG	2,3-diphosphoglycerate

DRESS	drug rash with eosinophilia and systemic symptoms
DSA	digital subtraction angiography
DVT	deep vein thrombosis
DWI	diffusion weighted imaging
EBV	Epstein–Barr virus
ECG	electrocardiogram
ECMO	extracorporeal membrane oxygenation
EEG	electroencephalogram
EF	ejection fraction
ELISA	enzyme-linked immunosorbent assay
EMA	endomysial antibodies
EMG	electromyography
EPAP	expiratory positive airway pressure
EPO	erythropoietin
EPS	electrophysiological study
ERCP	endoscopic retrograde cholangiopancreatography
ESBL	extended-spectrum beta-lactamases
ESR	erythrocyte sedimentation rate
EST	exercise stress test
ESWL	extracorporeal shock wave lithotripsy
EVD	external ventricular drainage
EWS	early warning score
FBC	full blood count
FEV	forced expiratory volume
FFP	fresh frozen plasma
FMF	familial Mediterranean fever
FSH	follicle-stimulating hormone
FVC	forced vital capacity
G5W	5% glucose (dextrose)
GBM	glomerular basement membrane
GBS	Guillain–Barré syndrome *or* Glasgow–Blatchford Score
GCA	giant cell arteritis
GCS	Glasgow Coma Score
GFR	glomerular filtration rate
GGT	gamma-glutamyl transpeptidase
GH	growth hormone
GHB	gamma-hydroxybutyric acid
GI	gastrointestinal
GN	glomerulonephritis

GORD	gastro-oesophageal reflux disease	ICH	intracerebral haemorrhage
GRACE	Global Registry of Acute Coronary Events	ICP	intracranial pressure
		ICS	intercostal space
GTN	glyceryl trinitrate	IGF-1	insulin-like growth factor 1
GTT	glucose tolerance test	IHD	ischaemic heart disease
GvHD	graft-versus-host disease	IJV	internal jugular vein
HAART	highly active antiretroviral therapy	IM	intramuscular route
		IMA	inferior mesenteric artery
HAP	hospital-acquired pneumonia	INR	international normalised ratio
HAS	human albumin solution	IP	incubation period
HBV	hepatitis B virus	IPAP	inspiratory positive airway pressure
HCM	hypertrophic cardiomyopathy		
HCV	hepatitis C virus	ITP	immune (idiopathic) thrombocytopenic purpura
HDU	high dependency unit		
HELLP	syndrome of haemolysis, elevated LFTs, low platelets	IVC	inferior vena cava
		IVDU	IV drug user
HF	heart failure	IVIg	intravenous immunoglobulin
HHS	hyperosmolar hyperglycaemic state	IVII	intravenous insulin infusion
		IVT	intravenous thrombolysis
HHT	hereditary haemorrhagic telangiectasia	IVU	intravenous urogram
		Ix	investigations
HIT(T)	heparin-induced thrombocytopenia ± thrombosis	JVP	jugular venous pressure
		KUB	kidneys, ureter, bladder
		LA	left atrium
HIV	human immunodeficiency virus	LAD	left axis deviation *or* left anterior descending
HOCM	hypertrophic cardiomyopathy		
HONK	hyperosmolar non-ketotic state	LAFB	left anterior fascicular block
HPTHM	hyperparathyroidism	LBBB	left bundle branch block
HR	heart rate (ventricular rate)	LCA	left coronary artery
HRCT	high resolution CT	LCHAD	long-chain 3-hydroxyacyl-coA dehydrogenase
HRS	hepatorenal syndrome		
HRT	hormone replacement therapy	LDH	lactate dehydrogenase
HSC	haemopoietic stem cell	LFT	liver function test
HSE	herpes simplex encephalitis	LIMA	left internal mammary artery
hsTn	high sensitivity troponin	LMN	lower motor neuron
HSV	*Herpes simplex* virus	LMWH	low molecular weight heparin
HTIG	human tetanus immunoglobulin	LOC	loss of consciousness
		LP	lumbar puncture
HTLV	human T cell lymphotropic virus	LPFB	left posterior fascicular block
		LTOT	long-term oxygen therapy
HUS	haemolytic uraemic syndrome	LV	left ventricle
IABP	intra-aortic balloon pump	LVAD	LV assist device
IAH	impaired awareness of hypoglycaemia	LVEDP	LV end-diastolic pressure
		LVEF	LV ejection fraction
IBD	inflammatory bowel disease	LVF	left ventricular failure
IBS	irritable bowel syndrome	LVH	left ventricular hypertrophy
ICA	internal carotid artery	LVOT	LV outflow tract
ICD	implantable cardioverter–defibrillator	MAHA	microangiopathic haemolytic anaemia
		MAOI	monoamine oxidase inhibitor

MAP	mean systemic arterial pressure
MAT	microscopic agglutination test *or* multifocal atrial tachycardia
MCA	middle cerebral artery
MCH	mean cell haemoglobin
MCV	mean cell volume
MDAC	multidose activated charcoal
MEN	multiple endocrine neoplasia
MERS	Middle Eastern respiratory syndrome
MG	myasthenia gravis
MGUS	monoclonal gammopathy of undetermined significance
MI	myocardial infarction
MIC	minimum inhibitory concentration
MLF	medial longitudinal fasciculus
MND	motor neurone disease
MODS	multiple organ dysfunction syndrome
MPO	myeloperoxidase
MR	mitral regurgitation
MRCP	magnetic resonance cholangiopancreatography
MRSA	meticillin-resistant *Staphylococcus aureus*
MS	multiple sclerosis *or* mitral stenosis
MSH	melanocyte-stimulating hormone
MSU	mid-stream urine *or* monosodium urate
MT	mechanical thrombectomy
MTP	massive transfusion protocol
MTS	mental test score
MUMS	migraine with unilateral motor symptoms
MVP	mitral valve prolapse
Mx	management
NAAT	nucleic acid amplification test
NAC	*N*-acetylcysteine
NBM	nil by mouth
NC	nasal cannula
NCS	nerve conduction studies
NCSE	non-convulsive status epilepticus
NDI	nephrogenic diabetes insipidus
NEAD	non-epileptic attack disorder
NEWS	National Early Warning Score
NG	nasogastric
NIH	National Institute for Health
NIPPV	non-invasive positive pressure ventilation
NIV	non-invasive ventilation
NMO	neuromyelitis optica
NMS	neuroleptic malignant syndrome
NOAC	new/novel oral anticoagulant (*see* DOAC)
NOS	nitric oxide synthase
NRTI	nucleoside reverse transcriptase inhibitors
NS	0.9% normal saline
NSAID	non-steroidal anti-inflammatory drug
NSTEMI	non-ST elevation MI
N&V	nausea and vomiting
NVE	native valve endocarditis
OCP	oral contraceptive pill
OD	overdose *or* once daily
OGD	oesophagogastroduodenoscopy
OGTT	oral glucose tolerance test
OPs	organophosphates
PA	pernicious anaemia *or* posterior–anterior
PAF	paroxysmal atrial fibrillation
PAN	polyarteritis nodosa
PAWP	pulmonary artery wedge pressure
PBC	primary biliary cirrhosis
PBG	porphobilinogen
PCA	posterior cerebral artery
PCC	prothrombin complex concentrates
PCI	percutaneous coronary intervention
PCOMM	posterior communicating artery
PCP	*Pneumocystis carinii* pneumonia
PCWP	pulmonary capillary wedge pressure
PE	pulmonary embolism
PEEP	positive end-expiratory pressure
PEFR	peak expiratory flow rate
PEG	percutaneous endoscopic gastrostomy *or* polyethylene glycol
PEJ	percutaneous endoscopic jejunostomy

PEP	post-exposure prophylaxis	RAST	radioallergosorbent test
PET	pre-eclamptic toxaemia *or* positron emission tomography	RBBB	right bundle branch block
		RBC	red blood cell
PFO	patent foramen ovale	RCA	right coronary artery
PFTs	pulmonary function tests	RCVS	reversible cerebral vasoconstriction syndrome
PICA	posterior inferior cerebellar artery	RF	respiratory failure *or* rheumatoid factor
PICC	peripherally inserted central catheter	RIF	right iliac fossa
PICH	primary intracerebral haemorrhage	ROSC	return of spontaneous circulation
PMC	primary motor cortex	RPGN	rapidly progressive glomerulonephritis
PML	progressive multifocal leucoencephalopathy	RR	respiratory rate
PMR	polymyalgia rheumatica	RRT	renal replacement therapy
PNH	paroxysmal nocturnal haemoglobinuria	RSV	respiratory syncytial virus
POCUS	point-of-care ultrasound	RTA	renal tubular acidosis *or* road traffic accident
POTS	postural orthostatic tachycardia syndrome	RV	right ventricle
		RVH	right ventricular hypertrophy
PPCI	primary percutaneous coronary intervention	Rx	treatment
		SACD	sub-acute combined cord degeneration
PPD	purified protein derivative	SAH	subarachnoid haemorrhage
PPE	plasma protein electrophoresis *or* personal protective equipment	SAN	sinoatrial node
		SARS	severe acute respiratory syndrome
PPI	proton pump inhibitor	SBO	small bowel obstruction
PPM	permanent pacemaker	SBP	systolic blood pressure *or* spontaneous bacterial peritonitis
PRES	posterior reversible encephalopathy syndrome		
PRL	prolactin level	SC	subcutaneous route *or* sickle cell
PSA	prostate-specific antigen		
PSC	primary sclerosing cholangitis	SCD	sudden cardiac death
PSM	pansystolic murmur	SDH	subdural haematoma
PT	prothrombin time	SE	status epilepticus *or* side-effect
PTH	parathyroid hormone	SIADH	syndrome of inappropriate ADH secretion
PTX	pneumothorax		
PUD	peptic ulcer disease	SIRS	systemic inflammatory response syndrome
PUO	pyrexia of unknown origin		
PVD	peripheral vascular disease	SJS	Stevens–Johnson syndrome
PVE	prosthetic valve endocarditis	SL	sublingual route
PVL	plasma viral load	SLE	systemic lupus erythematosus
Px	prevention or prophylaxis	SMA	superior mesenteric artery
QDS	four times a day or 6-hourly	SMX	sulfamethoxazole
RA	rheumatoid arthritis *or* right atrium	SOB	shortness of breath
		SOFA	sepsis-related organ failure assessment
RAA	renin–angiotensin–aldosterone		
RAD	right axis deviation	SOL	space-occupying lesion
RAS	renal artery stenosis *or* reticular activating system		

SPECT	single-photon emission computed tomography
SR	sinus rhythm
SSP	secondary spontaneous pneumothorax
STEMI	ST-elevation MI
STI	sexually transmitted infection
SUDEP	sudden unexpected death in epilepsy
SUND	sudden unexpected nocturnal death
SVC	superior vena cava
SVR	systemic vascular resistance
SVT	supraventricular tachycardia
T1DM	type 1 diabetes mellitus
T2DM	type 2 diabetes mellitus
TAB	temporal artery biopsy
TACI	total anterior circulation infarct
TACO	transfusion-associated circulatory overload
TB	tuberculosis
TCA	tricyclic antidepressant
TdP	torsades de pointes
TDS	three times a day
TEN	toxic epidermal necrolysis
TF	typhoid fever
TFTs	thyroid function tests
TIA	transient ischaemic attack
TIBC	total iron-binding capacity
TIMI	thrombolysis in MI
TIPS	transjugular intrahepatic portosystemic shunt
TLOC	transient loss of consciousness
TMP	trimethoprim
TNF	tumour necrosis factor
TOE	transoesophageal echocardiogram
tPA	tissue plasminogen activator
TPHA	*Treponema pallidum* serology
TPN	total parenteral nutrition
TPO	thyroid peroxidase
TRAb	TSH receptor antibodies
TRALI	transfusion-associated lung injury
TSH	thyroid-stimulating hormone

TSS	toxic shock syndrome
TTE	transthoracic echocardiogram
TTG	tissue transglutaminase
TTP	thrombotic thrombocytopenic purpura
TVR	target vessel revascularisation
UA	unstable angina
U&E	urea/creatinine and electrolytes
UFH	unfractionated heparin
ULN	upper limit of normal
UMN	upper motor neuron
URTI	upper respiratory tract infection
USS	ultrasound scan
UTI	urinary tract infection
VATS	video-assisted thoracoscopic surgery
VB	variceal bleed
VBG	venous blood gas
VDRL	Venereal Disease Research Laboratory
VEGF	vascular endothelial growth factor
VF	ventricular fibrillation
VIHE	valproate-induced hyperammonaemic encephalopathy
VKA	vitamin K antagonist
V/Q	ventilation/perfusion
VRE	vancomycin-resistant enterococcus
VRIII	variable rate IV insulin infusion
VSD	ventricular septal defect
VT	ventricular tachycardia
VTE	venous thromboembolism
vWF	von Willebrand factor
VZV	varicella zoster virus
WBI	whole bowel irrigation
WCC	white cell count
WG	Wegener's granulomatosis/ granulomatosis with polyangiitis
WPW	Wolff–Parkinson–White syndrome
ZIG	zoster immune globulin

01 Resuscitation

1.1 Introduction

Survival depends on the immediate initiation of chest compressions and early defibrillation if the rhythm is shockable.

- Ensure that you are up to date with BLS and ALS courses. There are 2021 UK and European resuscitation guidelines and much in common in the guidelines. The things that differ are due to a lack of evidence and so either way is defensible. Check out resuscitation videos available online (www.YouTube.com).
- It is difficult to perform trials on resuscitation and much is extrapolated from basic theory and laboratory and animal experiments. Guidelines are just that. Experienced clinicians who understand the evidence or lack of it can deviate to a degree.
- Resuscitating an unresponsive, pulseless apnoeic patient can be stressful. It is never as simple as a basic algorithm suggests. It is not uncommon to find yourself trying to cope with a collapsed patient wedged in a toilet cubicle. Such a patient is certifiable as dead and you cannot make that situation any worse. In a few cases, you can save a life and add years of quality. You may bring someone back to a very poor outcome with a catastrophic hypoxic brain injury. It is not easy. Do your best. Try to do what the patient would want, if known.
- What is the rhythm – could it be VF? If so, do not hesitate to defibrillate. If there is **any** delay in defibrillation, then get good quality CPR going, at least using chest compressions.
- As soon as you arrive, use the ABCs to quickly determine the basics – check the **Airway** is not obstructed, look for **Breathing** whilst palpating a major pulse to assess the **Circulation**. Commence chest compressions as quickly as possible; hopefully, someone else will already have done so. Your concern is whether unresponsiveness is due to circulatory collapse or not. If unsure start CPR. It is less harmful to CPR a patient who turns out to have a pulse than to delay CPR in a pulseless patient. If possible, let someone else do CPR as you take stock and look at the bigger picture. This is a very useful reason for the ABCs – to buy you some thinking and information-gathering time.
- Once you have the defibrillator leads on, look at the rhythm and assess if it is shockable. If shockable then shock and treat for VT/VF. Go through the standard list of treatable causes, ensuring effective CPR continues.
- There is some new evidence that early Head Up CPR works and increases the probability of ROSC. This has not entered current guidelines.

1.2 Initiating resuscitation

- Is there a 'do not resuscitate' form in the notes? Check for an advanced directive or community DNACPR order. Time allowing, always look at the paramedics' patient care records.
- If not and you can't be sure, then start and continue resuscitation as long as is reasonable. See DNACPR ▶ Section 15.9. Reassess and take senior advice especially in a young or hypothermic or overdosed or suspected PE post lysis patient. Stop when continuing is considered futile.

- Those without a DNACPR should have attempted resuscitation but guidance states that "if the healthcare team is as certain as it can be that a person is dying as an inevitable result of underlying disease or a catastrophic health event, and CPR would not re-start the heart and breathing for a sustained period, CPR should not be attempted" (*Decisions Relating to CPR* 3e (BMA, Resus Council (UK), RCN) 2016). Prior to cardiac arrest, there should be reasonable attempts to discuss DNACPR with family if death is predictable.
- Emphasis should be on cardiac arrest anticipation and prevention where possible. In an unstable patient have a defibrillator on hand. If a patient is *in extremis* and pre-arrest, then get help before the patient is pulseless. Using the ABC assessment gives you time to think of your plan. Delegate roles.
- If leading the arrest, ask others to get venous/intraosseous access and notes and obs. What is the ceiling of care? Contact your senior if this is not clear. Send away excess staff if there are demands elsewhere. They may be more productive seeing other sick patients and preventing cardiac arrests elsewhere.
- Stop once you all feel that continuing is futile. Thank everyone. Is everyone okay? Complete paperwork and record all in the patient notes. Offer to talk with family. Do a self-debrief: anything you would do differently or better? Seek feedback and add to your PDP.
- **Favourable outcome:** witnessed arrest; in-hospital; early effective CPR; shockable rhythm; early defibrillation; hypothermia (e.g. submerged in icy water). Keep CPR pauses <5 seconds and only when ROSC seems likely. Aim to have defibrillator <3 min, in hospital much sooner.

1.3 ▶ Basic life support: UK guidelines 2021

- **Diagnosis of cardiac arrest: cardiac arrest can be diagnosed in an** unresponsive person with absent or abnormal breathing. Slow, laboured breathing (agonal breathing) should be considered a sign of cardiac arrest.
- **Assess safety:** keep you, the victim, bystanders all safe. Move if needed.
- **Assess response:** shake shoulders and ask loudly: "Are you all right?". If responds then not cardiac arrest, continue assessment. If unresponsive, quickly continue assessment.

Airway management

- If a definitive airway has not already been secured prior to the arrest, a basic airway manoeuvre, use head tilt and chin lift.
- **Head tilt and chin lift:** place one hand on the patient's forehead, and the fingertips of your other hand under the point of the chin, then gently tilt the patient's head backwards, lifting the chin to open the airway.
- **Jaw thrust** is preferred if suspected cervical spine injury along with manual inline stabilisation of the head and neck by an assistant. Standing behind the patient and placing the index fingers under the angle of the mandible on either side. The mandible is then lifted forward through a steady upwards and forward pressure. If the airway remains obstructed and is life-threatening, then add a head tilt in small increments until the airway is open. Adequate airway opening takes priority over cervical spine precautions.
- **Ensure airway patent:** open the airway. Turn victim onto back. Place your hand on forehead and gently tilt head back; with your fingertips under the point of the

victim's chin, lift the chin to open the airway. If cervical injury suspected then use head-tilt/chin-lift.

- **Assess breathing:** look, listen and feel for normal breathing within 10 seconds. Slow, laboured breathing (agonal breathing) or seizure-like activity may be seen at the start of cardiac arrest. If unsure assume cardiac arrest and prepare to start CPR. If breathing normal it is not cardiac arrest. Call for help and Arrest Team.
- **AED:** in any unresponsive person with absent or abnormal breathing get an AED if available. If on your own, do not leave the victim, start CPR.
- **High-quality chest compressions:** if unresponsive and with absent or abnormal breathing, kneel by the patient and place the heel of one hand on the lower sternum. Place heel of other hand on top of the first hand. Interlock the fingers of your hands and ensure that pressure is not applied over the patient's ribs. Keep arms straight. Do not apply any pressure over the upper abdomen or the bottom end of the bony sternum. Position your shoulders vertically above the patient's chest and press down on the sternum to a depth of 5–6 cm. After each compression, release all the pressure on the chest without losing contact between your hands and the sternum; repeat at a rate of 100–120 per min. Do not lean on the chest. Ensure patient is on a firm surface.
- **Rescue breaths:** after 30 compressions open the airway again using head tilt and chin lift and give 2 rescue breaths. Pinch the soft part of the nose closed, using the index finger and thumb of your hand on the forehead. Allow the mouth to open but maintain chin lift. Take a normal breath and place your lips around victim's mouth, making sure that you have a good seal. Blow steadily into the mouth over 1 second, watching for the chest to rise; this is an effective rescue breath. Maintain head tilt and chin lift, take your mouth away from the victim and watch for the chest to fall as air comes out. Take another normal breath and blow into the victim's mouth once more to achieve a total of two effective rescue breaths. Do not interrupt compressions by more than 10 seconds to deliver two breaths. Then return your hands without delay to the correct position on the sternum and give a further 30 chest compressions. Continue with compressions and rescue breaths in a ratio of 30:2. If you are untrained or unable to do rescue breaths, give chest compression only CPR at a rate of at least 100–120 per min.

Airway adjuncts

- These are simple devices inserted into either the mouth (oropharyngeal airway) or nose (nasopharyngeal airway) to maintain a patent airway. They prevent airway obstruction by displacing the base of the tongue from the posterior pharyngeal wall and breaking contact between the tongue and soft palate. The are used with basic airway manoeuvres and can be used with bag–valve–mask ventilation.
- **Oropharyngeal airway:** an oropharyngeal (Guedel) airway is a curved plastic tube that sits in the mouth and lies over the tongue, preventing it from displacing backwards. The size is measured from the incisors to the angle of the jaw. A size 3 or 4 airway is optimal.
- **Nasopharyngeal airway:** is inserted through the nostril that lies within the nasopharynx, preventing soft palate obstruction of the airway. Avoid if a suspected basal skull fracture. Typically in adults, a 6 mm diameter tube is used for women, and 7 mm diameter for men.

- **Suction:** useful to remove liquids (e.g. blood, gastric contents, saliva) that can obstruct the upper airway. Use a wide bore rigid sucker which is available on most resuscitation trolleys.

Bag–valve mask

- Managing a BVM is a vital technique as it can provide 100% oxygen to a non-breathing patient. It is the fallback position when any other airway intervention fails.
- It is less possible if difficult seal due to facial injury or heavy beard or when there is obesity or no teeth. Ensure optimal position.
- It may be used with an oropharyngeal or nasopharyngeal airway (unless fear of a basal skull fracture). It can be done one-handed but a two-person technique for BVM ventilation is preferable but avoid overinflation.
- Deliver each breath over 1 second and give a volume that corresponds to normal chest movement; this represents a compromise between giving an adequate volume, minimising the risk of gastric inflation, and allowing adequate time for chest compressions.
- Give 2 ventilations to every 30 compressions. Once intubated, ventilate the lungs at a rate of about 10 breaths/min.

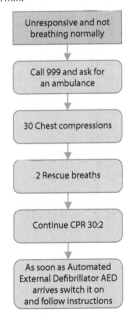

Basic life support algorithm.
Reproduced with permission from the Resuscitation Council (UK) 2021.

- **If an AED arrives:** switch it on. Attach the electrode pads on the patient's bare chest. If more than one rescuer is present, CPR should be continued while electrode pads are being attached to the chest. Follow the spoken/visual directions. Ensure that nobody is touching the patient while the AED is analysing the rhythm. If a shock is indicated, deliver shock but ensure that nobody is touching the patient, push shock button as directed (fully automatic AEDs will deliver the shock automatically), immediately restart CPR at a ratio of 30:2. Continue as directed by the voice/visual prompts. If no shock is indicated, immediately resume CPR. Continue as directed by the voice/visual prompts.

- **Continue CPR:** do not interrupt resuscitation until you become exhausted or the patient is definitely waking up, moving, opening eyes and breathing normally. It is rare for CPR alone to restart the heart. Unless you are certain the person has recovered, continue CPR.
- **Recovery position:** if certain the patient is breathing normally but still unresponsive, place in the recovery position. Remove the patient's glasses, if worn, kneel beside the patient and make sure that both legs are straight. Place the arm nearest to you out at right angles to his body, elbow bent with the hand palm-up. Bring the far arm across the chest and hold the back of the hand against the patient's cheek nearest to you. With your other hand, grasp the far leg just above the knee and pull it up, keeping the foot on the ground. Keeping his hand pressed against cheek, pull on the far leg to roll the patient towards you on to side. Adjust the upper leg so that both the hip and knee are bent at right angles. Tilt the head back to make sure that the airway remains open. If necessary, adjust the hand under the cheek to keep the head tilted and facing downwards to allow liquid material to drain from the mouth. Check breathing regularly. Be prepared to restart CPR immediately if the patient deteriorates or stops breathing normally.
- **American guidance 2015** for the single rescuer is to initiate chest compressions before giving rescue breaths (C–A–B for chest compression (100–120 per min)–airway–breathing rather than A–B–C) to reduce delay to first compression. The single rescuer should begin CPR with 30 compressions then 2 breaths. All lay rescuers should, at a minimum, provide chest compressions for victims of cardiac arrest.

1.4 ▶ Advanced life support: UK guidelines 2021

> **Minimise all interruptions to chest compression (CCs) to <5 seconds when attempting defibrillation or tracheal intubation by preplanning and coordination.**

- Peri-arrest ultrasound can help identify reversible causes. Extracorporeal life support techniques may be used as a rescue therapy in selected patients where standard ALS measures are not successful.
- **Extracorporeal cardiopulmonary resuscitation:** an external pump and oxygenator is used during cardiac arrest. These machines are able to provide the functions of both the heart and lungs during an arrest. May improve survival in select groups of patients (e.g. witnessed arrest, immediate high-quality CPR, little comorbidity). Availability is rare. May help to facilitate specific interventions (coronary angiography and PCI, pulmonary thrombectomy for massive pulmonary embolism, rewarming after hypothermic cardiac arrest).
- **Mechanical chest compression devices: more widespread.** Trials have shown no benefit over normal CPR. May cause more trauma. Consider for prolonged CPR, e.g. during PCI or when rescuer safety may be compromised (e.g. in the back of a moving ambulance).

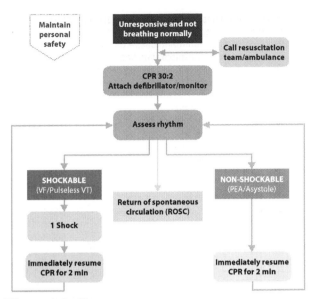

Advanced life support algorithm.
Reproduced with permission from the Resuscitation Council (UK) 2021.

Any ECG with a slow or wide rhythm: consider hyperkalaemia.

1.5 Shockable rhythms (VF/pulseless VT)

Ventricular fibrillation

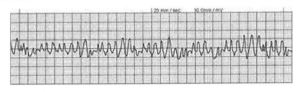

Pulseless VT (pVT)

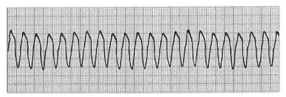

- **Confirm cardiac arrest:** signs of life and normal breathing. If trained to do so, check for breathing and pulse simultaneously. Call resuscitation team. Perform CPR while applying defibrillation/monitoring pads – one below the right clavicle and the other in the V6 position in the midaxillary line. Plan and communicate pausing CPR for rhythm analysis. Stop CPR; confirm VF/pVT from the ECG. This pause in CPR should be brief and no longer than 5 seconds. Resume CPR immediately; warn all rescuers other than the individual performing the CPR to "stand clear" and remove any O_2 delivery device as appropriate.
- **Prepare defibrillator:** the designated person selects energy on the defibrillator and presses the charge button. Use at least 150 J for the first shock, the same or a higher energy for subsequent shocks. If unsure of the correct energy level for a defibrillator, choose the highest available energy. Ensure the person performing CPR is the only person touching the patient. Once the defibrillator is charged and the safety check is complete, tell rescuer doing the compressions to "stand clear"; when clear, give the shock. After shock delivery immediately restart CPR using a ratio of 30:2, starting with chest compressions. Do not pause to reassess the rhythm or feel for a pulse. The total pause in CPR should be brief and no longer than 5 seconds.
- **Pad placement:** keep at least 8 cm from any PPM/ICD. Consider pads in the mid-axillary line on either side of the chest (at the V6 position of an ECG on the left and equivalent on the right). Alternative is the left electrode over the apex of the heart, and the right placed on the right upper back. Another is one pad over the precordium, and the other is placed just below the left scapula.
- **Continue CPR for 2 min;** the team leader prepares the team for the next pause in CPR. Pause briefly to check the monitor. If VF/pVT, repeat steps above and deliver a second shock. If VF/pVT persists, repeat steps above and deliver a third shock. Resume CPR immediately. Give **Adrenaline** 1 mg IV and **Amiodarone** 300 mg IV while performing a further 2 min CPR. Withhold adrenaline if there are signs of return of spontaneous circulation (ROSC) during CPR. Repeat this 2 min CPR – rhythm/pulse check – defibrillation sequence if VF/pVT persists. Give further **Adrenaline** 1 mg IV after alternate shocks (i.e. approximately every 3–5 min). If organised electrical activity compatible with a cardiac output is seen during a rhythm check, seek evidence of ROSC (check for signs of life, a central pulse and end-tidal CO_2 if available). If there is ROSC, start post-resuscitation care. If there are no signs of ROSC, continue CPR and switch to the non-shockable algorithm. If asystole is seen, continue CPR and switch to the non-shockable algorithm. Consider a further dose of **Amiodarone** 150 mg IV after 5 defibrillation attempts. **Lidocaine** 1 mg/kg may be used as an alternative. Do not give both.
- **Waveform capnography:** can detect ROSC without pausing CPR. It may help avoid a further adrenaline bolus after ROSC has been achieved. Several human studies have shown that there is a significant increase in end-tidal CO_2 when ROSC occurs. If ROSC is suspected during CPR withhold adrenaline.
- **Adrenaline** (epinephrine): regardless of the arrest rhythm, give further 1 mg doses of adrenaline every 3–5 min until ROSC is achieved; in practice, this will be about once every two cycles of the algorithm. If signs of life return during CPR (e.g. purposeful movement, normal breathing or coughing), or there is an increase in end-tidal CO_2, check the monitor; if an organised rhythm is present, check for a pulse. If a pulse is palpable, start post-resuscitation care. If no pulse is present, continue CPR.
- **Witnessed, monitored VF/pVT:** if a patient has a monitored and witnessed cardiac arrest in the catheter laboratory, coronary care unit, a critical care area or whilst monitored after cardiac surgery, and a manual defibrillator is rapidly available:

confirm cardiac arrest and shout for help. If the initial rhythm is VF/pVT, give up to three quick successive (stacked) shocks. Rapidly check for a rhythm change and, if appropriate, ROSC after each defibrillation attempt. Start CPR and continue for 2 min if the third shock is unsuccessful.

- **Precordial thump:** unlikely to cardiovert. Consider only when it can be used without delay whilst awaiting the arrival of a defibrillator in a monitored VF/pVT arrest. Using the ulnar edge of a tightly clenched fist, deliver a sharp impact to the lower half of the sternum from a height of about 20 cm.

> **Indications for 'stacked shocks' (3 shocks in sequence) in a cardiac arrest**
> 1. VF/VT occurring during cardiac catheterisation.
> 2. VF/VT occurring early after cardiac surgery.
> 3. VF/VT arrest and patient is already connected to a manual defibrillator.

There is little evidence to support the use of stacked shocks; in these select cases, they are more likely to achieve ROSC when compared with chest compressions.

1.6 ▶ Non-shockable rhythms (asystole/PEA)

- **Pulseless electrical activity** (PEA): cardiac arrest in the presence of electrical activity (other than VT) that would normally be associated with a palpable pulse. Often have some mechanical myocardial contractions, but not enough to produce a detectable pulse or BP. PEA can be caused by reversible conditions that can be treated if they are identified and corrected. Survival with asystole or PEA is unlikely unless a reversible cause can be found and treated effectively.
- **Asystole:** check the ECG for P waves as patient may respond to cardiac pacing when there is ventricular standstill with continuing P waves. There is no value in attempting to pace true asystole.
- **Treatment of PEA and asystole:** start CPR 30:2. Give **Adrenaline** 1 mg IV as soon as intravascular access is achieved. Continue CPR 30:2 until the airway is secured – then continue CCs without pausing during ventilation. Recheck the rhythm after 2 min: if electrical activity compatible with a pulse is seen, check for a pulse and/or signs of life and if a pulse and/or signs of life are present, start post-resuscitation care. If no pulse and/or no signs of life are present (PEA or asystole): continue CPR, recheck the rhythm after 2 min and proceed accordingly. Give further **Adrenaline** 1 mg IV every 3–5 min (during alternate 2 min loops of CPR). If VF/pVT at rhythm check, change to shockable side of algorithm.

1.7 ▶ Reversible causes of cardiac arrest

- **Hypoxia:** ensuring airway patent, adequate ventilation, maximal FiO_2 during CPR with BVM or intubation. Check for chest rise and bilateral breath sounds. Check ET tube is not misplaced in a bronchus or the oesophagus. The end-tidal capnograph waveform should confirm ET tube is in the trachea. ▶ Section 4.5.
- **Hypovolaemia:** PEA caused by hypovolaemia is usually due to severe haemorrhage. Clues may be trauma, GI bleeding or signs of ruptured AAA. Stop the haemorrhage and restore intravascular volume with fluid and blood products. Other causes include anaphylaxis and other causes of shock. Needs IV access ×2, IV fluids (normal saline (NS)). Blood if severe haemorrhage (O-neg). See Haemorrhagic shock ▶ Section 2.22.

- **Hyperkalaemia:** if suspect K⁺ >6.5 mmol/L or >6.0 and ECG changes give 10 ml 10% **Calcium chloride** (more irritant but higher calcium concentration than gluconate) IV or 30 ml of 10% **Calcium gluconate** into large vein. Then **10 U Insulin with 25 g Glucose** as 50 ml 50% Glucose or 125 ml of 20% or 250 ml of 10% glucose over 15 mins. Shift potassium into cells: give **50 mmol Sodium bicarbonate (50 ml 8.4% solution)** IV by rapid injection. Consider dialysis for refractory hyperkalaemic cardiac arrest. ▶Section 5.3.
- **Hypocalcaemia/calcium channel blocker toxicity:** 10 ml 10% calcium gluconate IV. ▶Section 5.6.
- **Hypoglycaemia:** ▶Section 5.2.
- **Hypothermia:** drowning, exposure. Rectal temperature. Rewarm. Hypothermic cardiac arrest patients should receive continuous CPR during transfer. Stop only when patient rewarmed, and subsequent resuscitation fails. If VF persists after three shocks, delay further attempts until the core temperature is >30°C. Withhold adrenaline/amiodarone until core temperature >30°C and give every 6–10 minutes if the core temperature is 30–34°C. Consider ECMO and cardiopulmonary bypass. ▶Section 15.6.
- **Hyperthermia:** cool. Oxygen. Lie flat. Malignant hyperthermia. IV fluids. Treat high K⁺. Give **Dantrolene** 2.5 mg/kg initially, and 10 mg/kg as required. Active cooling if needed, e.g. water immersion.
- **Thrombosis: coronary:** chest pain prior to arrest, IHD, VF, pulseless VT, post-resuscitation 12-lead ECG ST-elevation/LBBB. STEMI then consider PCI <120 mins. CPR continued if felt non-futile. NSTEMI take advice. Even if ROSC not been achieved, consider primary PCI if STEMI/new LBBB continuing CPR. For ACS ▶Section 3.7.
- **Thrombosis: pulmonary embolism:** low ETCO₂ readings (<1.7 kPa or 13 mmHg) while performing high-quality CPR may support a diagnosis of PE, although it is a non-specific sign. If PE suspected consider immediate thrombolysis if unstable or cardiac arrest. Assess if appropriate to continue CPR for 60–90 minutes and take senior advice. Consider giving **Alteplase** 50 mg IV bolus if cardiac arrest. If no ROSC or improvement after 15 minutes then consider further **Alteplase** 50 mg IV bolus and CPR. In a stable patient or with ROSC then **Alteplase** 10 mg IV over 1–2 mins followed by an infusion of 90 mg over 2 hours (if <65kg then give 1.5 mg/kg). Consider CPR for 60–90 mins before stopping. In some, surgical or mechanical thrombectomy can considered. ECMO can be considered. For PE ▶Section 4.17.
- **Tension pneumothorax:** trauma-associated or ventilated patient. A helpful clue may be subcutaneous emphysema. Bilateral tension PTX can occur. Clinical/USS diagnosis. Do not wait for CXR. Insert needle in 2nd interspace on affected resonant side (trachea pushed away) or the 5th intercostal space for needle decompression. Listen for 'hiss' as needle enters. BP should improve. Insert chest drain. If cardiac arrest, then examine (resonant and trachea pushed away) and ultrasound. Consider bilateral thoracotomies ▶Section 4.12.
- **Tamponade:** signs (raised JVP, low BP) obscured by the arrest itself. Suspected if penetrating chest trauma, anticoagulants, recent MI or cardiac intervention. May need resuscitative thoracotomy or needle pericardiocentesis. Ultrasound is diagnostic. ▶Section 3.20.
- **Toxins:** look for evidence of drugs taken and treat accordingly. Local anaesthetic or lipophilic drug cardiotoxicity consider 100 ml IV bolus of 20% intralipid emulsion in a 70 kg adult followed by an infusion and continue good quality CPR. See intralipid in toxicology chapter (▶Sections 14.6 & 14.8).

1.8   Resuscitation issues

- **Mechanical chest compression** if having to transport patient or to relieve other members of the team during prolonged arrests.
- **Ultrasound imaging:** focused echo/USS can help diagnose reversible causes of cardiac arrest. Challenging to perform during CPR. A sub-xiphoid probe position is recommended. Placement of the probe just before compressions are paused for a planned rhythm assessment enables a well-trained operator to obtain views within 10 seconds. Can diagnose tamponade, PE, hypovolaemia, PTX. Absence of any cardiac motion is highly predictive of death.
- **Blood gas values:** during cardiac arrest bear little relationship to the tissue acid–base state. Analysis of central venous blood may provide a better estimation of tissue pH.
- **Oxygen during defibrillation:** remove O_2 mask or nasal cannulae at least 1 m away during defibrillation. Leave the ventilation bag connected to the tracheal tube or other airway adjunct or disconnect the ventilation bag from the tracheal tube and move it at least 1 m from the patient's chest during defibrillation.
- **Airway management and ventilation:** options are no airway and no ventilation (compression-only CPR), compression-only CPR with the airway held open (with or without supplementary O_2), mouth-to-mouth breaths, mouth-to-mask, bag-mask ventilation with simple airway adjuncts, supraglottic airways (SGAs), and tracheal intubation (inserted with the aid of direct laryngoscopy or video laryngoscopy, or via an SGA). Patients who remain comatose post-resuscitation will usually require intubation. Personnel skilled in advanced airway management should attempt laryngoscopy and intubation without stopping chest compressions; a brief pause in chest compressions may be required as the tube is passed through the vocal cords, but this pause should be less than 5 seconds. In the absence of these, use bag-mask ventilation and/or an SGA until appropriately experienced and equipped personnel are present.

Alternative airway devices

- **Cuffed ET tube** is the optimal method of managing the airway during cardiac arrest. However, it is not without its difficulties in insertion. It should be attempted only by trained personnel able to carry out the procedure with a high level of skill and confidence. No intubation attempt should interrupt CPR for more than 5 seconds. Use an alternative airway technique if tracheal intubation is not possible. After intubation, tube placement must be confirmed, and tube secured adequately.
- **Video laryngoscopy:** used increasingly as it enables a better view of the larynx and increases success rate of intubation. May be useful during CPR.
- **Confirmation of correct placement of ET tube:** end-tidal CO_2 detectors that include a waveform graphical display (capnographs, see below). If not available, observe chest expansion bilaterally, listen over lung fields bilaterally in the axillae (breath sounds should be equal and adequate) and over the epigastrium (breath sounds should not be heard).
- **Laryngeal mask airway (LMA):** easy to insert for those trained. Easier to use than BVM. If gas leakage is excessive, chest compression will have to be interrupted to enable ventilation and airway protection.
- **Others:** several other alternative airway devices have been used for airway management during CPR. These include the classic laryngeal mask airway, the laryngeal tube (LT) and the i-gel, and the LMA supreme (LMAS).
- **Emergency Front of Neck Airway (eFONA)** when *cannot intubate or cannot oxygenate.* See ▶ Section 2.7.

1.9 Drugs for cardiac arrest

Amiodarone and lidocaine improve survival to hospital admission but long term are no better than placebo. Drugs are advised by guidelines but the key is high quality uninterrupted CPR and early defibrillation where indicated.

- **Adrenaline** (epinephrine): no evidence for improved survival to hospital discharge, only improved short-term survival, but with neurological damage.
- **Vascular access during CPR:** get vascular access if possible. Peripheral venous cannulation is quicker, easier to perform and safer. Once drugs given then give a 20 ml flush and elevate the limb for 10–20 sec to facilitate drug delivery to the central circulation.
- **Intraosseous route:** if no IV access then consider intraosseous (IO) route. Plasma concentrations comparable with IV injection. Sternal IO route comparable with IV adrenaline. Several IO devices are available using humerus, proximal or distal tibia, and sternum. Use per local experience and skills and kit.
- **Extracorporeal cardiopulmonary resuscitation** (ECCPR): should be considered as rescue therapy for those patients in whom initial ALS measures are unsuccessful and/or to facilitate specific interventions (e.g. angiography and PCI or pulmonary thrombectomy for massive PE). Requires vascular access and a circuit with a pump and oxygenator and can provide a circulation of oxygenated blood to restore tissue perfusion. Can be a bridge to allow treatment of reversible underlying conditions. Can improve survival when there is a reversible cause for cardiac arrest (e.g. ACS/PE, severe hypothermia, poisoning). Useful if cardiac arrest is witnessed, the individual receives immediate high-quality CPR, and ECPR is implemented early (e.g. within 1 h of collapse) including when instituted by emergency physicians and intensivists.
- **Duration of resuscitation attempt:** if resuscitation is unsuccessful, the team leader should discuss stopping CPR with the team. Requires a careful assessment of the likelihood of success. It is reasonable to continue if the patient remains in VF/pVT, or there is a potentially reversible cause that can be treated. The use of mechanical compression devices and ECPR techniques make prolonged attempts at resuscitation feasible in selected patients. It is generally accepted that asystole for more than 20 min in the absence of a reversible cause and with ongoing ALS constitutes a reasonable ground for stopping further resuscitation attempts. Guidance is that resuscitation may be discontinued if all of the following apply: (1) 15 min or more has passed since the onset of collapse, (2) no bystander CPR was given before arrival of the ambulance, (3) there is no suspicion of drowning, hypothermia, poisoning/overdose or pregnancy, (4) asystole is present for more than 30 sec on the ECG monitor screen.
- Do not interrupt CPR unless definite signs of recovery. Keep pauses as short as possible. Plan and coordinate interruptions so they are as short as possible. Compression-only CPR where unable/unwilling to give rescue breaths.

1.10 Special cases in resuscitation

- **Post-cardiac surgery cardiac catheterisation:** cardiac arrest where CPR is difficult. Give three quick consecutive 'stacked' (repeated) shocks before starting CCs. Consider re-sternotomy (reopening the sternal wound) to exclude tamponade. Internal defibrillation with paddles. Direct cardiac compression can be given to the heart. Use 20 J in cardiac arrest but only 5 J if supported on cardiopulmonary bypass.

- **Post drowning:** immediately start CPR and high FiO_2; ROSC prior to the hospital suggests better prognosis. Look for and treat high K^+ with freshwater drowning. Look for and manage compounding issues, e.g. associated hypothermia/exposure, drug overdose or suicide attempt. Duration of hypoxia is the most critical survival factor.
- **Post electrocution:** extensive burns can affect face, neck and airway. CPR because patient may be in VF or asystole with early intubation if possible. Asystole is seen after DC shock and VF after AC shock (mains supply). Check for secondary spinal injury or other trauma. Muscle paralysis can cause respiratory failure (FVC <1.5 L). Fluid resuscitation as tissue/muscle damage. Ensure good diuresis, watch for AKI and check CK and K^+.
- **Cardiac arrest in pregnancy:** see ▶ Section 16.2.

1.11 ▶ Return of spontaneous circulation (ROSC)

- **ROSC:** diagnose if palpable central pulse or sudden increase in end-tidal CO_2 trace. (Continuous quantitative waveform capnography for monitoring of ET tube placement is a useful marker that identifies ROSC.) If signs of ROSC then complete assessment: ABC. O_2/ventilation. You bring the patient back from death so the immediate questions are why the cardiac arrest and anticipate possible complications. Get an ECG, ABG, U&E, troponin. Again ask why. Get a 12-lead ECG. Is it STEMI needing primary PCI/thrombolysis, acute PE needing thrombolysis, hyperkalaemia needing calcium and insulin/glucose?
- **Stabilise: ABC:** give 100% O_2 until sure that sats are 94–98%. Check FBC, U&E, ABG, CXR, 12-lead ECG, Mg^{2+}, Ca^{2+}, troponin, lactate. Of these the ECG is the most useful as a large MI should be evident. If STEMI then PPCI is the next approach if stable.
- **Comatose patients** should be intubated and mechanically ventilated. Use waveform capnography to ensure trachea intubated. Target PCO_2 to 4.5–6.0 kPa. Use a lung protective strategy with tidal volume 6–8 ml/kg ideal body weight.
- **Look for cause:** if hypotensive or evidence of myocardial ischaemia then consider coronary angiography. If normal consider CT head and/or CTPA. Less evidence for immediate coronary angiography if no ST elevation.
- **Induced hypothermia** may be neuroprotective. **Targeted temperature management** for OOH cardiac arrest or those in hospital with any rhythm who are unresponsive after ROSC. Involves cooling to 32–36°C for 12–24 h or longer post-ROSC. Avoid fever (>37.7°C) for at least 72 h after ROSC in patients who remain in coma. Do not use pre-hospital IV cool fluids to initiate hypothermia.
- **Glycaemic control:** aim for glucose control of 7.8–10 mmol/L. Use VRIII if needed. Avoid hypoglycaemia which can cause or exacerbate brain injury.
- **Coagulopathy:** check APTT, FBC, PT, platelets, fibrinogen if any doubt.
- **Hypotension:** target MAP >65 mmHg or SBP >100 mmHg. Choice of inotrope and/or vasopressor (▶ Section 2.17 on inotropes). Fluids: 1–2 L of NS or Ringer's lactate. Other vasopressors are listed later.
- **Post-arrest myocardial dysfunction:** may be due to underlying STEMI. A period of hypoperfusion can result in impaired pump function for up to 72 h. Support with **dobutamine** and intra-aortic balloon pump if required.
- **Coronary angiography/PCI** recommended for patients with ST elevation or new LBBB. See ACS STEMI (▶ Section 3.7).
- **Low BP/shock** may be partly driven by a SIRS-type mechanism with a drop in systemic vascular resistance and in these cases **Noradrenaline** infusion may be useful – take expert advice (and ▶ Section 2.17 on inotropes). This is best delivered within an ITU setting with access to invasive monitoring. Target MAP >65 mmHg.

- **Arrhythmias:** see below for management of tachy-/bradyarrhythmias.
- **Seizures and myoclonic jerks:** can be seen post-ROSC in up to 10% of patients. These can be managed conservatively but if significant and frequent then may consider anticonvulsants. Levetiracetam and sodium valproate are preferred instead of phenytoin for the treatment of seizures [2021 guideline].
- **Electrolytes:** keep potassium between 4.0 and 4.5 mmol/L. Monitor BM and avoid tight glucose control, particularly hypoglycaemia.

1.12 ▶ Bradycardia management: be prepared to pace

Hyperkalaemia can cause a broad complex slow rhythm, so always consider the diagnosis and consider IV Calcium and check K.

- **Introduction.** Be prepared to pace. Avoid atropine post cardiac transplants. Denervated hearts do not respond to vagal blockade by atropine. It may cause paradoxical sinus arrest or high-grade AV block.
- **Causes:** physiological (sleep, in athletes), cardiac (AV block or sinus node disease), non-cardiac causes (vasovagal, hypothermia, hypothyroidism, high K), **drugs** (beta-blockers, diltiazem, digoxin, amiodarone).

Management: if shock/syncope/myocardial ischaemia/heart failure
- **Atropine** 500 mcg IV stat. Can give up to 5 × 0.5 mg (3 mg) more doses. Avoid post heart transplant as either no effect or paradoxical complete AV block or sinus arrest.
- **Isoprenaline** infusion 5 mcg/min IV.
- **Adrenaline** infusion 2–10 mcg/min.
- **Dopamine** infusion 2–10 mcg/kg per minute. Bradycardia, ▶ Section 3.16.
- **Pacing:** transcutaneous pacing and transvenous pacing.

Alternative drugs
- **Beta-blocker or CCB toxicity.** Can give **Glucagon** 5–10 mg IV over 1–2 min (*BNF*) then infusion 50 mcg/kg/h. Can also consider **High dose insulin therapy** 1 unit/kg given with IV Dextrose. See local policy.
- **Digibind** if life-threatening bradycardia/arrhythmias due to digoxin toxicity unresponsive to atropine.
- **Glycopyrronium bromide** 200–400 mcg can be used instead of atropine.
- **Aminophylline** 100–200 mg slow IV if bradycardia due to inferior MI, cardiac transplant or spinal cord injury.

Risk of asystole after satisfactory response to Atropine 500 mcg IV
- Recent asystole or Mobitz II AV block.
- Complete heart block with broad QRS or ventricular pause >3 sec.
- If any of these, continue drug management or consider pacing.

Transcutaneous pacing: ▶ also see Section 3.10
- Pace any compromising bradycardia. Life-threatening features: shock/syncope or myocardial ischaemia or heart failure. Usual causes are acute MI, sinus node dysfunction, age-related conduction disease. Treat initially with atropine.
- Transcutaneous pacing should be started immediately for patients who are unstable, particularly those with high-degree (Mobitz type II second-degree or third-degree) block. If transcutaneous pacing is ineffective (e.g. inconsistent capture), prepare for transvenous pacing.

- Pads are placed on the patient's chest either in anterolateral position or preferably the anterior–posterior (AP) position. The pacer pad placement 'sandwiches' the heart anteroposteriorly. Begin at 10 mA. Increase by increments of 10 until capture is noted at 60–80 bpm.
- It is important to ensure that the electrical pulses achieve ventricular contraction by measuring pulse and BP or arterial line.
- Consider sedation, as it can be quite uncomfortable especially with currents >50 mA. Set current as 1.25× what was required for capture.
- Both electrical and mechanical capture must occur to benefit the patient. Pulses are difficult to palpate due to excessive muscular response. It is safe to touch patients (e.g. to perform CPR) during pacing.
- **Reference: Adult bradycardia algorithm.** Resuscitation Council UK (2021).

1.13 ▶ Tachycardia management: be prepared to shock

- **Basics:** ABCDE O_2 if SpO_2 <94%. Obtain IV access. Monitor ECG, BP, SpO_2, record 12-lead ECG. Identify and treat reversible causes, e.g. electrolyte abnormalities, hypovolaemia causing sinus tachycardia.
- **Unstable:** life-threatening features: shock/syncope or myocardial ischaemia or heart failure. Consider synchronised DC shock up to 3 attempts. Sedation or anaesthesia if conscious. If unsuccessful: **Amiodarone** 300 mg IV over 10–20 min. Repeat synchronised DC shock.
- **Stable and broad QRS:** irregular: could be AF + BBB. Consider **Amiodarone** if uncertain. Also polymorphic VT (e.g. torsades de pointes). **Magnesium sulfate** 8 mmol (2 g) in 100 ml NS over 10 min.
- **Stable and broad QRS:** regular: VT (or uncertain rhythm): **Amiodarone** 300 mg IV over 10–60 min. If previous certain diagnosis of SVT with bundle branch block/aberrant conduction: treat as for regular narrow complex tachycardia. If ineffective: synchronised DC shock up to 3 attempts. Sedation or anaesthesia if conscious.
- **Stable and narrow QRS:** regular: vagal manoeuvres. If ineffective: give **Adenosine** (if no pre-excitation) 6 mg rapid IV bolus. If unsuccessful, give 12 mg then 18 mg. Monitor ECG.
- **Stable and narrow QRS:** irregular: probable atrial fibrillation. Control rate with beta-blocker. Consider **Digoxin** or **Amiodarone** if in heart failure. Anticoagulate if duration >48 h.
- **Reference: Adult tachycardia algorithm.** Resuscitation Council UK (2021).

1.14 ▶ Emergency DC cardioversion

- **Indication:** DC cardioversion (if we treat VF it is called defibrillation) should be considered in all fast and unstable tachyarrhythmias. Usually the ventricular rate is >150/min. Consider cardioversion if there is ischaemic chest pain, pulmonary oedema, syncope or shock due to the arrhythmia. Cardioversion not harmful to a fetus. Not cardioverting may be very harmful to fetus.
- **Contraindications: these are relative.** For elective DCC digitalis toxicity is a concern as it can cause ventricular arrhythmias – usually 1 or 2 doses omitted if elective. DCC does not reverse sinus tachycardia or multifocal atrial tachycardia. Concerns about non-anticoagulated AF of duration >48 h and embolic/stroke risk need to be weighed against the need for improving haemodynamics. Ideally a TOE to identify left atrial appendage thrombus should be done. This may not be practical or feasible or available in the emergency situation. Take expert advice. In these cases

some form of rate control rather than rhythm control may be tried, but DC cardioversion is quick and often effective. If DCC done then start anticoagulation immediately unless contraindicated.

- **Sedation:** enlist help of anaesthetist to protect airway. If conscious needs sedation, e.g. **Midazolam** 2.5 mg slow IV (max 7.5 mg) is the sedation of choice and provides amnesia and sedation. **Flumazenil** 200 mcg over 1–2 mins may be repeated at 100 mcg/min (max 1 mg) and airway control and BVM should be available for oversedation. Written consent if possible. Use pulse oximetry and ECG monitoring via the pads. Remove nitrate patches. Ensure good IV access. Remove O_2 at shock.

- **DC cardioversion:** place pads on the chest (anterior–posterior may be preferred for AF). Some start at 50 J for an SVT if no urgency. Broad complex or AF use a biphasic shock of 120–150 J or monophasic 200 J; for atrial flutter or SVT, use 70–120 J. Ensure that the defibrillator is 'synced' with the R wave of the QRS complexes. There is a sync button which does this and a bright dot appears on the R wave – this avoids shocking on a T wave and inducing VF. Give 3 successive shocks if there is no immediate cardioversion, giving up to full energy available. Ensure you warn all before giving the shock. If no success, consider repeating after **Amiodarone** 150–300 mg slow IV over 20 min. Post procedure recovery position as tolerated until wakes up.

- **Elective cardioversion for AF:** those on warfarin should have evidence of levels of INR within the therapeutic window for the past 4 weeks prior to the procedure. Evidently in the emergency situation this is waived, but therapeutic LMWH should be given if not anticoagulated and continued for 4 weeks post procedure, irrespective of outcome. In some cases a TOE showing absence of thrombus in the left atrial appendage can suggest that elective cardioversion can proceed without pre-existing anticoagulation, but start anticoagulation. Take advice if unsure.

- **Complications:** skin soreness like a burn over the pads, arrhythmias, stroke (DC cardioversion – cardioembolism) especially in AF which is not anticoagulated, failed cardioversion is seen in many with AF. DCC more successful in VT and atrial flutter and SVT, mild troponin rises.

1.15 Emergency pericardiocentesis

- **Relative contraindications** need to be balanced with urgency and risks of inaction. Include uncorrected bleeding disorders, e.g. low plts, raised INR. A long needle is passed using a sub-xiphoid approach under strict asepsis and local anaesthesia, with echo/ultrasound control, aspirating with needle at 30° to skin with the patient sitting up at 45° angle, aiming for tip of the left shoulder. Connect a 20–50 ml syringe to the spinal needle, and aspirate 5 ml of IV NS into the syringe. While advancing the needle, the occasional injection of up to 1 ml of NS helps to keep the needle lumen patent.

- The Seldinger technique is used and a wire is passed; once the pericardial space is entered then a floppy soft-tipped guide-wire is passed into the space and around the heart. A pig tailed or soft straight multiperforated sterile drainage catheter is inserted over the wire and the wire removed. Allows drainage and filling and improved BP.

- **Take senior advice** if available and transfer patient to cardiology centre as soon as possible. Drainage of large pericardial effusions, especially if chronic ones, should be slow. Risk is acute ventricular dilation or pulmonary oedema.

- **Complications:** PTX, myocardial damage or coronary vessels, arrhythmias, pulmonary oedema.

1.16   Implantable cardioverter defibrillator (ICD)

- **About: ICDs** often function as a pacemaker but also deliver low-energy synchronised cardioversion and high-energy defibrillation shocks that successfully terminate 99% of ventricular fibrillation attacks.
- Indications are as follows (patient on chronic, best medical therapy and have a reasonable expectation of survival with good functional status for >1 y).
- An ICD can be combined with cardiac resynchronisation therapy (CRT-D) or pacemaker (CRT-P) options were needed.

Indications for ICD: NICE 2014
- Have survived a cardiac arrest by VT or VF.
- Spontaneous sustained VT with syncope or significant compromise.
- Sustained VT but no syncope or cardiac arrest but has EF <35% and symptoms no worse than dyspnoea on minimal exertion (may need CRT).
- Familial cardiac condition with a high risk of sudden death, such as long QT syndrome, HOCM, Brugada syndrome, ARVD or have undergone surgical repair of congenital heart disease.

Managing ICD problems: discuss with Cardiology
- **Cardiac arrest with ICD:** these patients are at high risk of cardiac arrest. If ICD senses a shockable rhythm it will fire a 40 J shock internally which may cause pectoral muscle contraction. Shocks to rescuers doing CPR are minimal, especially if wearing gloves. It produces a maximum of 8 possible discharges. Shock pads to avoid the ICD, e.g. antero–posterior: left precordium to below left scapula.
- **Patients with ICDs receiving shocks:** those who have received shocks need a full assessment of their clinical status and device function. Shocks are a red flag for clinical events. Even if inappropriate there is a related increased mortality. Shocks are unpleasant, causing psychological distress, anxiety and decreased quality of life. Catheter ablation of arrhythmias may be needed. Specialist assessment is needed.
- **Ongoing SVT/AF/VT with haemodynamic compromise:** ignore presence of the ICD and treat. Consider external DC shock, IV amiodarone and/or beta-blockers (if haemodynamically tolerated). To shock avoid placement of paddles in the skin area over the ICD pocket. If possible, attempt an anterior–posterior electrode position.
- **Repetitive ICD shocks without a tachyarrhythmia or due to tachyarrhythmia** (atrial or ventricular) that is haemodynamically well tolerated by the patient. A magnet over the device inhibits further shock delivery until patient can be seen by technicians.
- **Contact with the patient during ICD discharge** is harmless but gloves (1–2) decrease conductivity and attenuate potential discomfort.
- **ICD and end of life care:** following discussions with patient and those important to the patient it may be appropriate to deactivate an ICD. This will involve some form filling to record the decision making. It is deactivated by placing and taping a circular magnet over the ICD. The ICD should be removed prior to cremation.

1.17 Adult choking algorithm

- **Choking.** Whilst eating patient clutches neck/chest and unable to speak. If mild airway obstruction then encourage coughing, but do nothing else. If severe then progresses from wheeze/stridor to unconscious. If conscious stand to the side and slightly behind the patient. Support chest with one hand and lean the victim well forwards so that when the obstructing object is dislodged it comes out of the mouth rather than goes further down the airway.
- **Back blows:** give up to 5 sharp blows between shoulder blades with heel of your other hand.
- **Abdominal thrusts:** if no relief then give up to five abdominal thrusts – stand behind the patient and put both arms round the upper part of his abdomen. Lean the victim forwards. Lock clenched fists between the umbilicus and the bottom end of the sternum and pull sharply inwards and upwards up to five times. Continue alternating five back blows with five abdominal thrusts.
- **Collapse/unconscious:** help the patient carefully to the ground. Call ambulance immediately. Begin CPR without feeling for a carotid pulse in the unconscious choking victim.
- **Following successful treatment** for choking, foreign material may nevertheless remain in the upper or lower respiratory tract and cause complications later. Patients with a persistent cough, difficulty swallowing, or with the sensation of an object being still stuck in the throat should therefore be referred for an immediate ENT opinion.

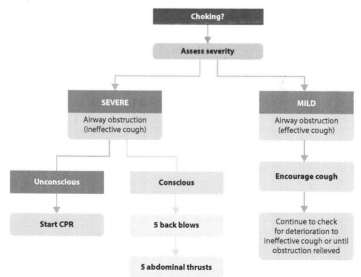

Adult choking algorithm.
Reproduced with permission from the Resuscitation Council (UK) 2021.

02 The acutely ill patient

.1 Levels of care

Introduction: Clinicians need to assess patients' clinical and nursing needs to ensure they are in the right place. Equipment, medical staff and the ratio of skilled nursing staff to patients is fundamental for the optimal level of care and observation. That is one of the main advantages of escalating care. If a patient needs organ support – cardiac, renal, pulmonary, etc. there may be a need to move the patient to a level of care that is appropriate, which may mean moving them to the medical assessment unit or to an HDU or ITU bed. Involve critical care outreach as early as possible who can often quickly see that the patient needs moving and will know who to call.

- **Level 0:** normal ward care in acute hospital. Nursing may be 15:1.
- **Level 1** (MAU/AAU/Respiratory Unit): step down. Support from critical care outreach. Tracheostomy, CVP line, chest drain, VRIII, PCA, post-op.
- **Level 2** (HDU): 2:1 nursing. Frequent monitoring. Support for a single failing organ system/post-op care. Step down. Hourly monitoring, FiO_2 >0.5.
- **Level 3** (ITU): 1:1 nursing, advanced respiratory support with invasive ventilation together with support of at least 2 organ systems. Complex patients with multi-organ failure.

Other critical services that may be needed at tertiary or specialist centres

- Extracorporeal membrane oxygenation (ECMO): severe respiratory failure.
- Mechanical support of the circulation: LVAD/IABP for cardiac failure.
- Liver dialysis (molecular adsorbent recirculation system (MARS)).

.2 National early warning scores

- Studies show that those needing ITU have had major derangements in SaO_2, HR, respiratory rate and BP in the hours before, with delayed or unsatisfactory responses. Early warning scores provide a 'track-and-trigger' system to identify and respond to deteriorating patients.
- The RCP developed the NEWS 2nd version in December 2017. It is recommended that escalation communication can be improved using the SBARR protocol (see ▶ Section 2.6).
- Sick patients are sliding metaphorically along an icy slope to the edge of the cliff and can be saved if caught earlier. Cardiac arrest patients have fallen. Their chance of survival is then so much worse. Far better to treat earlier.
- NEWS2 is an aid to, but not a substitute for a competent experienced clinical assessment. It looks at 6 parameters: resp rate, O_2 sat, systolic BP, pulse rate, level of consciousness or new confusion, temperature. Early trigger can enable earlier review and assessment of critically ill patients through medical emergency teams (MET) and involve critical care outreach earlier.

2.3 Clinical risk and response to NEWS2 score

Response must consider ceilings of care/treatment escalation plans
- **Score 1–4:** assessment by a competent registered nurse or equivalent to decide whether a change to frequency of clinical monitoring or an escalation of clinical care is required.

- **Score 3 (low)** in a single parameter is unusual. Urgent review by a clinician competent in assessment of acute illness (ward-based doctor) to determine cause and decide on the frequency of subsequent monitoring and whether an escalation of care is required.
- **Score 5–6 (medium):** urgent review by a ward-based doctor or acute team nurse, who should urgently decide whether escalation of care to a critical care outreach team is required.
- **Score ≥7 (high):** medical emergency team (MET) assessment by a clinical team/ critical care outreach team with critical care competencies. May need moved to HDU or above or re-establishment of ceilings of care.
- **Common medical scenarios needing ITU:** respiratory failure, exacerbation of COPD, acute severe asthma, severe pneumonia (often complicated by sepsis/septic shock), meningococcal infection, status epilepticus, severe DKA/HHS, coma.
- **Medical emergency team** should attend all arrests; threatened airway; RR <5/min or >36/min; pulse <40 or >140/min; SBP <90 mmHg; fall in GCS; prolonged seizure; other emergency undefined here.
- **Reference:** Royal College of Physicians (2017) National Early Warning Score (NEWS): *Report of a working party.*

2.4 ▶ Assessment and escalation

- While assessing ABCDE get help from nursing or other medical staff, work quickly to get and maintain IV access, and send bloods, ABG and ECG and arrange a CXR, depending on the assessment. It is helpful if one can be doing the tasks and the other can be thinking about what is going on and what needs to be done.
- In all emergencies, one or more people need to be leading and thinking of the underlying diagnosis and management.
- **Important signs of impending demise:** tachy-/bradycardia, increased RR, low/ falling BP, cold peripheries, oliguria/anuria, fall in GCS, new confusion, cyanosis, distress, silent chest.

Focus	Assessment, warning signs and actions
Airway	**Ideal:** normal speech, no added airway noises. **Warning:** GCS <9, paradoxical chest movements, wheeze, snoring, drooling, grunting, stridor. **Actions:** chin lift, jaw thrust, remove foreign bodies, oropharyngeal airway, suction visible debris, recovery position, intubation, treat any suspected anaphylaxis
Breathing	**Ideal:** talks in full sentences, comfortable, RR 12–20. SaO$_2$ >94–98%. **Warning:** RR <8 or >20 and tired. Wheeze, reduced chest expansion one side – dull or resonant, silent chest, accessory muscles, cyanosis, tracheal deviation. **Possible actions:** O$_2$ 15 L/min unless COPD. Urgent portable CXR and ABG, **Salbutamol** 2.5 mg neb for wheeze, **Furosemide** 50 mg IV, **GTN** SL or IV for pulmonary oedema, chest drain for PTX, CPAP, NIV, cough assist device, ventilation, IV antibiotics
Circulation	**Ideal:** cap refill <2 sec. HR 50–90 bpm. SBP 120–140 mmHg. Urine output 40 ml/h. Normal heart sounds, no murmurs. **Warning:** cold shut down, delayed cap return, obtunded, peripheral cyanosis, SBP <90 mmHg or >220 mmHg, raised JVP, urine output <40 ml/h. **Possible actions:** repeated 250 ml NS fluid bolus. IV antibiotics. ECG, echo, PCI/thrombolysis (ACS/PE), LMWH (PE), inotropes, balloon pump. Transfusion if bleeding and/or correct coagulopathy

Disability	**Ideal:** normal GCS, orientated. **Warning:** low GCS, confused, comatose, pupil signs, Cheyne–Stokes. Check plantars. Use **A**lert, **V**oice, **P**ain, and **U**nresponsive. **Possible actions:** glucose if CBG low or hypoglycaemia suspected. **Naloxone** for opiates. IV antibiotics, **Aciclovir** for CNS infection.
Exposure	**Ideal:** full examination. **Warning:** top to toe exam. Meningism, peritonitis, hypothermia, fractures, spinal injury, palpate, check hips, bruising, pain. Saddle anaesthesia and PR if cauda injury suspected. **Actions:** cautious rewarming, watch observations, bloods
End of life	Some are dying and the appropriate action should be a communication with patient and/or family and DNR discussions and a personalised care plan for the dying. HDU and ITU are inappropriate and patients need good holistic compassionate care with families and loved ones
DEFGH	**D**on't **E**ver **F**orget **G**lucose or **H**eroin (opiates) if comatose

.5 ▶ Getting senior help and calling for advice

- **Seeking help** from seniors, peers or other disciplines is a key skill at all levels. Pre-call organisation is crucial. It depends on what time is available. If *in extremis* get the notes, observations and call quickly whilst others continue to manage the patient or do CPR. If more time, get the notes and make a quick summary list of clinical details as listed below.
- **Get lab results**, imaging and pathology and make a summary note. Check notes, drug chart, fluid balance and observations charts and bring all of this to the phone with you. Know SaO_2, BP, HR, FiO_2, IV drugs and infusions.
- **Premorbid state/patient wishes:** these may be known. Do your best to establish these before escalating and respect the patient's wishes. Is there a treatment escalation plan?
- **Introduce yourself and grade.** Use SBARR; see ▶ Section 2.6. State from the start why you are calling. This frames the information for the recipient. "I have a patient who may need stroke thrombolysis...". Then present the details.
- **Before you call think of your plan if you can, but don't delay.** I encourage those who can to have their own plan which they are ringing to run it past me. They may say that they plan to do A and B, and I may say A is good but do C rather than B. It's a good learning experience as soon they will be the person being rung.

.6 ▶ Phone protocols and SBARR

- **Advice:** the person who initiates the call should usually be the one to regain contact if communication breaks down or you will both be ringing engaged numbers. This should be an agreed protocol. You may also be the recipient of bleeps/calls. Those calling will have different skills and experiences. If unsure or it doesn't sound right then you must go and see for yourself. If you can try to prioritise the call then do so. Give an estimate of how long it will take you to attend. If you need an ECG or NEWS2 or bloods or venous access or O_2 then this can be done before you arrive. Consider analgesia or GTN for chest pain.
- **Communication:** much depends on attitude. Even as a senior consultant who can hold his own there have been colleagues I would avoid ringing as their rudeness would

grate so much as to really affect my ability to work productively for several hours! This is unacceptable and can cost lives. One can challenge and probe professionally, but a patient always comes first, and all conversations should centre on that. Recording calls might help. Please don't be that person. Everyone can have a bad moment but repeated unprofessionalism or worse is unacceptable and should be escalated. It often suggests a clinician who may be struggling and needs help or a new career.

SBARR communication tool (kindness and politeness on both sides is key)

- **Introduction:** identify self, specialty and grade and role.
- **Situation:** give name, age, sex of patient. Issue to resolve or request? E.g. *"patient new weakness, it may be a stroke for thrombolysis"*.
- **Background:** clinical context. Give current presentation and relevant past history. Have notes and observation and drug charts to hand.
- **Assessment:** latest observations, examination and NEWS2.
- **Recommendation:** details the actions required and any queries.
- **Read back/Response:** review actions. Check all understood correctly.

2.7 Advanced airways management

Methods for airway support

> The primary goal of airway management is the maintenance of alveolar oxygenation. This needs good airways management. Three routes: nasal/oral and in some a tracheostomy.

- **Oropharyngeal airway:** insert Guedel pointed up until you reach the soft palate and then rotated 180° from pointing up to pointing down during insertion over tongue. Guedel is J-shaped and is passed between teeth into oropharynx. It can be useful to apply a jaw thrust as you insert the oropharyngeal airway. Too large or too small will obstruct the airway further. Measure from the tip of the oropharyngeal airway at the corner of the mouth and the distal end of the oropharyngeal airway at the tragus. Often used when BVM ventilation being used. In a semi-comatose patient, a nasopharyngeal airway is better tolerated.
- **Nasopharyngeal airway:** used in semi-comatose patient who is making satisfactory attempts at breathing. Can place patient in the recovery position with O_2 and a nasopharyngeal airway and monitor closely. The main contraindication is basal skull fracture (major trauma, CSF, coma, should be seen on CT). General advice is to choose the size of nasopharyngeal airway to match the width of the patient's little finger or nares. Average height females require a size 6 Portex and males a size 7. Lubricate the end with KY jelly. They go straight back into the nasal cavity and turn downward towards the posterior pharynx. Insert into largest nares. Attach a safety pin at the nose end to prevent further tube movement into airway.
- **Laryngeal mask airway:** the supraglottic airway. Classic laryngeal mask airway (LMA) may be preferred over an ET tube because of the ease and speed of deployment. For those familiar with its use. Deflated and pushed in and then inflated.
- **Endotracheal intubation:** a bridging measure to allow treatment/recovery. Elective intubation is much safer than emergency intubation. Ensure adequate preparation. Ensure pre-oxygenated with 100% O_2 before commencing. Intubation

must only be by appropriately trained personnel. Rapid sequence induction (RSI) will require sedation with an induction agent, e.g. propofol, which is commonly used but can drop BP. Used with neuromuscular blocker such as suxamethonium. Analgesia may also be given.

- **Elective tracheostomy:** preferred in those needing ongoing airways protection. Better tolerated and more comfortable than ET tube. Less sedation is required. Less dead space to ventilate and airways resistance is reduced. It avoids many of the upper airways complications of an ET tube. Those with tracheostomies are sometimes managed in step-down units outside an HDU/ITU facility. Ensure nursing and medical staff are trained in their use.

Can't intubate or oxygenate (CICO) scenario: eFONA

- **CICO:** despite attempts to ventilate with BVM or failure to pass ET tube and sats <75% in an apnoeic patient, delivery of O_2 through an eFONA should be considered. Follow local pathways – often ENT team. This may help in securing of a patent airway via the anterior neck to facilitate emergency alveolar oxygenation. It is final life-saving step in airway management to reverse hypoxia and prevent resulting brain injury, cardiac arrest, and death. The 'can't intubate, can't oxygenate' (CICO) situation occurs after attempts to manage the airway with a facemask, a supraglottic airway device, and an ET tube have all failed.
- **Technique:** trained individuals only. Declare CICO. Get help. Ensure neuromuscular blockade. Oxygenate. High flow nasal O_2. Size 10 scalpel. Bougie. 6 mm cuffed tube. Patient: head extended no rotation. Right-handed operator on left of patient (left hander reverse approach). Laryngeal handshake left hand, local cricothyroid membrane. Stretch skin, fix trachea, left thumb and middle fingers. Stab membrane transverse with right hand. Then keep scalpel perpendicular to patient and twist scalpel so that sharp edge points to patient's feet. Swap hands, hold scalpel with left and get bougie in right hand. Hold near angle tip. Insert and rotate to 10 cm. Place tube. Railroad size 6 tube over bougie directed down to lungs until cuff disappears. Hold tube and remove bougie. Inflate cuff to 20 cmH$_2$O. Check placement using end-tidal CO$_2$. Auscultate both lungs, axilla and stomach. Get senior anaesthetic and ENT help.

2.8 ▶ Tracheostomy/laryngectomy emergencies

> **In a post-laryngectomy patient if you are unsure of the anatomy give high flow oxygen to both mouth/nose and over tracheostomy stoma until details are clear.**

- **About:** a tracheostomy allows a tube inserted directly into the trachea to let air enter lungs by normal breathing or by mechanically ventilation. It provides a way to get air to alveoli. It can relieve upper airway obstruction, provide airway protection, and enable weaning from mechanical ventilation.
- **Early post-insertion complications** include haemorrhage, loss of the airway, blockage or complete or partial tracheostomy tube displacement.
- **Long-term complications** include tracheomalacia, tracheal stenosis. The tube should be kept clean and secure. Key information is whether the patient has a patent upper airway, meaning that it is anatomically possible for the upper airway to connect to the trachea and thus allow ventilation by this route.

- **Total laryngectomy:** post surgery patients have a tracheostomy stoma and do not have a patent upper airway and cannot breathe through the nose or mouth so a face mask/nasal O_2/NIV is of no value. Those with a partial laryngectomy have a stoma and may have a patent upper airway. Give O_2 to the stoma and facemask if unsure what surgery has been done. If stoma is blocked, try to clear it. There should be a tube in the stoma which should not be removed except as a last resort by expert staff. Call arrest team and ENT for anaesthetic support urgently if airway compromised.
- **Stoma:** assess patency, ABCDE approach as ever, consider passing suction catheter to see where blockage is and remove any debris. The following equipment should be available immediately. BVM, O_2 with facemasks (non-rebreathing type) and tracheostomy masks, working suction and suction catheters, intubation equipment (including bougie) and a range of endotracheal tubes, laryngeal mask airway (LMA) device, dilating tracheostomy forceps, spare tracheostomy inner-tube appropriate for tracheostomy in place (i.e. dedicated to the patient and their tracheostomy). Staff should be competent in management of tracheostomy and complications.
- **Reference:** Tracheostomy Safety Project website, www.tracheostomy.org.uk

2.9 Assessment and managing fluid balance

- **Basics:** you do not need to provide perfect replacement if the patient has functioning kidneys and normal adrenal cortical function. They cannot, however, manage if they are not provided with basic fluids and electrolytes and the patient is profoundly volume- and electrolyte-depleted due to drugs, disease or surgery. You must provide these.
- **Assess hydration.** Clinical context is key when reviewing clinical signs. Patients on a general ward can have very poorly recorded I/O charts. Weight changes if reliable and recorded are useful as 1L = 1 kg. Rapid changes in weight are losses or gains of water usually with electrolytes. Seek experienced help if unsure as it can be difficult. Challenging when complex, e.g. where there is ongoing organ failure (e.g. cardiac/renal/liver) or sepsis, pyrexia and drains losing fluids. If patient/lungs seem 'dry' consider fluid challenge and reassess. If 'wet' then pulmonary oedema is critical and needs IV furosemide. If unsure get help. Peripheral oedema can be managed more gradually.
- **Check notes:** cause of admission, history, procedures, drugs, diuretics, observations, pyrexia, BP, HR, urine output, output of drains, all of which should be stored within the fluid balance chart. What has preceded the assessment? Surgery, new drugs given?
- **Look for evidence:** do not hang your diagnosis on one sign or parameter: the fluid balance chart may be badly completed, even weights can be wrong, a raised JVP might suggest RV infarction or a PE and a need for filling rather than overload, a CVP line may be blocked or erroneously measured, a BP might be recorded in an arm with atherosclerotic arteries and be misleadingly low so check other side. Healthy scepticism and a second opinion always wise, especially when the appearance of a patient and signs do not match.
- **Fluid loss:** significant circulatory fluid losses may be hidden in ascites, intestinal lumen or generalised oedema. Sepsis and anaphylaxis and inflammation increase fluid in the interstitium and this depletes the circulating volume. Urine output is a crude measure of renal perfusion. Oliguria/anuria where there is no evidence of

renal obstruction suggests renal water and sodium retention and even incipient AKI. Using the JVP is not without its limitations and potential complications. The physiological response to volume loss is the release of ADH and free water retention. There is sodium retention through the RAA mechanism. Stress/surgery and pain also cause cortisol and ADH release. The hypovolaemic patient is typically vasoconstricted with cold peripheries, mild tachycardia and dry mucous membranes, typically oliguric with a low urinary sodium.

- **Dehydration (dry):** sunken eyes, dry mouth and reduced skin turgor, thirst. With time becomes obtunded. Low BP, postural drop, thready pulse, raised HR. Reduced body weight. Low urine output. Low urinary Na. Raised Hb, raised urea, AKI, high Na if free water loss. Causes, e.g. vomiting, diarrhoea, obstructed fluid-filled bowel, polyuria, sweating, fistulae. CVP low. Fluid balance chart shows net loss (if accurate and all I/O recorded). Management is appropriate fluid replacement. Is it just water depletion or salt too and other electrolytes? Stop diuretics. Manage stomas or other losses.

- **Overhydration (wet):** raised JVP, gravitational oedema, ascites, anasarca, breathless if pulmonary oedema and effusions. BP normal or elevated, tachycardia if CCF. Increased body weight. Normal/increased urine output and urine Na. Bloods normal. High BNP. Check oedema not due to very low albumin; low Na possible. Evident cause, e.g. increased intake, liver/cardiac/renal failure/nephrotic syndrome. CVP raised. Fluid balance chart shows net gain (if accurate and all I/O recorded). Fluid restriction, diuretics, match losses + 500 ml orally if possible. Prioritise – fluid around the legs and ankles is disabling and needs gradually treated but untreated fluid/oedema in the brain and lungs is lethal.

- **Euvolaemic:** warm, well-filled. BP and HR normal. Body weight unchanged. Normal urine output. Normal I/O. Bloods normal.

- **Osmosis:** water moves to dilute any solvent. If the interstitium and blood is hypertonic then water moves into the vascular space. If the blood is hypotonic it moves into cells and can cause swelling and in the brain, cerebral oedema (Hyponatraemia, ▶Section 5.10).

Assessment

- **Gastrointestinal losses:** net loss into GI tract per day is saliva 1 L, gastric 2 L, bile 1 L, pancreatic 1.5 L and small bowel secretions 2–3 L, putting the total to be at most 8.5 L. Gastric fluid is acidic with a pH of about 2. All of these fluids contain Na and K so match with normal saline + KCl. Bowel infections can greatly increase output. Cholera can cause a severe loss of fluid and electrolytes and needs aggressive rehydration in severe cases. For those who can take oral fluids, replace fluid losses with a solution containing salt and sugar.

- **Stoma loss:** normal ileostomy loss up to 1 L/day and colostomy about 500 ml/day. An output greater than this can result in electrolyte and water imbalance. Colostomies tend to be in the left iliac fossa and ileostomy in the right iliac fossa. Ileostomy output is more irritant to skin so have a spout. Excess output often managed with high doses of loperamide once infection excluded.

- **Replacing losses: general GI losses:** replace with equivalent volumes of oral rehydration (if mild and able to drink) and/or IV NS and treat cause.

- **Significant diarrhoeal losses:** often lose significant amounts of K (e.g. 40 mmol/L) causing hypokalaemia which may well worsen any ileus and other problems. Potassium should be monitored. Replace with oral rehydration (if mild and able to drink) and/or IV NS with potassium, and treat cause.

- **Fistulae and overactive ileostomies:** loss of Cl⁻ and HCO_3^-. Replace with oral rehydration and/or IV NS, and treat cause.
- **Systemic sepsis with 3rd space losses:** replace with oral rehydration (if mild and able to drink) and/or IV NS, and treat cause.
- **Pyrexia, sweating, insensible losses:** replace with oral rehydration (if mild and able to drink) and/or IV NS with Na/K, and treat cause.
- **Enteral replacement:** encourage normal oral intake if possible. Ensure adequate access and able to hold beaker or use straw or other handheld devices. Good nursing/healthcare assistance if unable to swallow. Unable/unsafe to swallow: consider NG tube. Longer-term PEG/RIG tube placement. IV fluids only when above routes are unsatisfactory.

Choice of fluids

- **5% glucose (G5W):** a way to give water. Glucose is metabolised. It is isotonic and provides enough calories to prevent protein breakdown. Used to replace free water loss, e.g. hypernatraemia. 1 L contains 50 g glucose and no electrolytes. 170 kcal/litre. It can worsen cellular oedema and so avoided for example in stroke and cerebral oedema.
- **0.9% NaCl (normal saline NS):** crystalloid. NaCl which is 154 mmol/L. First line for hypovolaemia. pH is 4.5–7. It is high in sodium and chloride and acidic with a pH of 5.5. Isotonic. High volumes cause a hyperchloraemic metabolic acidosis. Short half-life. Approximately 25% remains in vascular space.
- **Glucose-saline:** 0.18% NaCl (1/5th of the concentration of NS) and 4% glucose. Short half-life and remains in the vascular space for only minutes.
- **Hartmann's** (lactated Ringer's): crystalloid. Contains NaCl, KCl, $CaCl_2$ and sodium lactate. For hypovolaemia. Distributes throughout extracellular space. Rapidly lost from the intravascular space. Na^+ 131 mmol/L, K^+ 5 mmol/L and Ca^{++} (2 mmol/L). Lactate 29 mmol/L can help buffer acidosis. Cl⁻ 111 mmol/L lower than NS.
- **Plasmalyte (PL148):** 'balanced' crystalloid solution. Mimics human plasma in its content, osmolality, pH. Can buffer capacity with acetate, gluconate, lactate which are converted to HCO_3^-, CO_2, water. Use for hypovolaemic shock. Contains Mg^{2+}.
- **Gelofusine:** colloid formed from gelatin. Remains for longer within intravascular compartment. May cause histamine release and rash and bronchospasm. No evidence superior to crystalloids.

2.10 ▶ Fluid replacement regimens

- **About:** these are usually for people having no oral or enteral intake e.g. peri-/post-operative, those nauseated or with oesophageal/gastric or bowel obstruction or unable to swallow e.g. stroke patients without an NG tube. They should only be used transiently, and feeding should be started as early as possible. If on IV fluids, then check electrolytes at least daily.
- Avoid excessive fluid replacement in those with cardiac failure or renal failure and take expert advice if unsure. In an uncomplicated average patient requiring fluid replacement, titrate Na, H_2O, and K^+ added by weight, U&E result, record fluid balance input and output, clinical examination and comorbidities.
- **Normal daily fluid and electrolyte requirements:** 25–30 ml/kg/d water = 1 mmol/kg/day sodium, potassium, chloride, 50–100 g/d glucose (1 L 5% glucose = 50 g glucose). Reassess and monitor the patient. Stop IV fluids when no longer needed. Can be given as 1 L NS and 2 L G5W at rate of 1 L/10 h. Traditional 3 L/d may

be excessive. Nasogastric fluids or enteral feeding are preferable when maintenance needs are more than 3 days.

- **NB:** *NS (0.9% saline) and G5W (5% glucose) are used as simple shorthand here but must be written out in full in clinical practice.*
- **Potassium** replacement: 60–100 mmol/d. Omit or reduce in the first 1–2 days post-surgery or where there is significant trauma/burns/blood transfusions as tissue damage will release K. Those on potassium infusions need regular testing. Target 3.5–5 mmol/L (4–5 mmol/L on the CCU). Take advice if unsure. See Hypokalaemia (▶Section 5.4) or Hyperkalaemia (▶Section 5.3) if situation requires. Most potassium-containing fluids come prepared, e.g. with NS or G5W.

> **Potassium must never be given quickly IV due to risks of cardiac arrest. Ward areas may give infusions of up to 10 mmol/h e.g. 40 mmol/L in 500–1000 ml over 4 h for severe hypokalaemia. Critical care areas can give 20 mmol/h with close ECG/K monitoring. All must be given by infusion pump and ECG and bloods closely monitored for hyperkalaemia.**

2.11 ▶ Venous access: choosing a venous cannula

- Flow is proportional to radius R^4 (Poiseuille's law). A small increase in radius can greatly improve flow. A pink 20G cannula is unsuitable to resuscitate a patient needing volume. Ideally one or more grey 16G would be used. Smaller G is larger cannula.
- Flow rates can double with pressure on the bag of up to 300 mmHg. Flow is also inversely proportional to length and so long lumen central lines are inappropriate for rapid volume replacement. Central lines have higher risk of infection and complications than peripheral.

Choices of cannula
- Blue 22G: can give 1 L in 22 min. For thin fragile veins/infants.
- Pink 20G: can give 1 L in 15 min: smallest in adults. IV drugs and IV fluids routine use.
- Green 18G: can give 1 L in 10 min. Standard in adults. Blood transfusions and IV fluids. Unwell then insert 2 if possible or 16G/14G.
- Grey 16G: can give 1 L in 6 min. For rapid IV infusion, hypovolaemic shock, ruptured AAA, haemorrhagic shock.
- Brown or orange 14G: can give 1 L in 3.5 min. For rapid blood transfusion e.g. PPH, ectopic pregnancy, AAA, haemorrhagic shock.

2.12 ▶ Acid–base balance and blood gas interpretation

- Introduction: we are all net producers of acid, which must be excreted by kidneys and by the lungs removing CO_2. To assess acid–base balance we can measure an ABG. Once primary respiratory cause excluded then VBG will give us pH and $[HCO_3^-]$ which may be enough. The pH depends on renal/respiratory function, diet, metabolic activity and buffering systems.

Arterial versus venous blood gas: venous lower pH, higher PCO_2, lower O_2
- ABG vs. VBG there is better correlation than is appreciated. VBG will suffice in many situations. VBGs carry less risk of vascular injury, nerve damage, and cause much

less pain to the patient, along with lower risk for accidental needlesticks compared to ABGs. VBGs show increased discordance from ABGs in hypotensive patients. Before you do the test, ask what I am testing for and why will it make a change to management?

- **Hypoxaemic patients or shocked get an ABG.** Arterial pH is venous + 0.03. Arterial PO_2 is higher and PCO_2 is lower. Differences between pH, HCO_3^-, BE are small and probably clinically unimportant. Arterial and venous pH correlate well even in shock and DKA. Arterial PO_2 is generally 5 kPa higher than venous PO_2. Levels correlate with O_2 saturation. A VBG may be needed if circulatory state so poor that ABG not possible.
- Venous PCO_2 <5.4 kPa excludes hypercarbia. VBG PCO_2 >6 kPa(45 mmHg) suggests true hypercapnia and can be used for COPD, DKA with O_2 saturations.
- Lactate: a normal venous lactate likely means the arterial lactate is normal.
- ABGs over VBG: helpful in hypotensive states or with complex acid–base disorders, severe acidosis, resp failure or those with an arterial line, or where venous gas is abnormal and raises questions and you may need more info.

Interpretations of blood gas/acid-base disturbances:

	pH 7.35–7.45	H+ 35–45 nmol/L	Primary disturbance	Secondary response
Metabolic acidosis	<7.35	>45	HCO_3^- <22 mmol/L	Normal/low PCO_2
Metabolic alkalosis	>7.45	<35	HCO_3^- >26 mmol/L	Normal/raised CO_2
Respiratory acidosis	<7.35	>45	PCO_2 >6.0 kPa (>45 mmHg)	Normal/raised HCO_3^-
Respiratory alkalosis	>7.45	<35	PCO_2 <4.5 kPa (<35 mmHg)	Normal or low HCO_3^-

- **Check the P_aO_2.** In an arterial sample this should be at least 10 kPa in a normal adult on room air. Ideally 11–13 kPa or 82.5–97.5 mmHg. If P_aO_2 <10 kPa, that is hypoxia and if <8 kPa, that is respiratory failure. Severe hypoxia is life-threatening and needs urgent management.
- **Check the P_aCO_2.** If this is elevated, it suggests hypercarbic respiratory failure. The patient is usually acidotic. If chronic respiratory acidosis, the HCO_3 is secondarily elevated due to renal retention. See Respiratory failure, ▶ Section 4.5. If CO_2 low in acute severe asthma it can suggest tiring and imminent respiratory arrest. It is also low in hyperventilation due to anxiety attacks.
- **Check the pH** – if <7.35 this is acidosis and >7.45 is alkalosis. Metabolic acidosis stimulates hyperventilation and a low PCO_2. HCO_3 is elevated with a compensated respiratory acidosis and low with metabolic acidosis.
- **Metabolic acidosis:** pH is low as is HCO_3. Check anion gap for unmeasured toxic anions leading to increased ventilation and the excretion of CO_2 from the lungs; this takes minutes. There is also bicarbonate retention in the kidneys; this takes hours to days. Also measure the **anion gap** (AG) which is [cations] – [anions] and is normally <12 mmol/L. Measure as [Na] – [Cl] – [HCO_3]. Normally, measured [cations (positive ions)] > [anions (negative ions)], so there is normally an 'anion gap'.
- **Osmolar gap:** you will need to measure the calculated and laboratory calculated osmolar gap when indicated – usually with a RAG metabolic acidosis.
- **Alveolar–arterial PO_2 gradient:** $P_AO_2–P_aO_2$. $P_AO_2 = (FiO_2 \times (76–47) – (P_aO_2/0.8)$. An increase suggests shunting. Normal = 4–10.

- **Base excess:** a calculated value. Normal −2 to +2. It is an estimate of 'metabolic' as opposed to 'respiratory' disturbance. A BE <−2 indicates metabolic acidosis; a BE >+2 indicates metabolic alkalosis. The more negative the worse. Less than −5 is a met acidosis and less than −10 is severely ill.
- **Pathophysiology:** the pH = −log10 [hydrogen ions]. pH varies from 0 (acidic) to 14 (highly alkaline), with neutrality being 7. Blood is alkaline with a pH of 7.35–7.45. Gastric acid pH = 1–2. Ketone bodies are water-soluble, fat-derived fuels that are used by many tissues for energy generation when there is limited glucose availability. The brain becomes especially dependent upon ketones for fuel when plasma glucose levels are inadequate. Henderson–Hasselbalch equation. Note PCO_2 dependent on lung function getting rid of CO_2. Hyperventilating lowers P_aCO_2, hypoventilation leads to a rise in P_aCO_2.

Typical blood gas abnormalities

- **Metabolic acidosis with raised AG:** pH <7.35 HCO_3 <22 mmol/L, AG >12 mmol/L. Clinical: Kussmaul breathing. Causes: AKI, lactic acidosis, diabetic or alcoholic ketoacidosis, methanol, CO, cyanide, metformin, paraldehyde, iron, ethylene glycol, salicylates. Measure osmolar gap to identify ethylene glycol, methanol, alcohol excess.
- **Metabolic acidosis with normal AG:** gap pH <7.35, HCO_3 <22 mmol/L, AG <12 mmol/L. Clinical: Kussmaul breathing. Causes: RTA, diarrhoea, small intestinal fistula, pancreatic alkali losses, carbonic anhydrase inhibitors, ureterenterostomy, rapid hydration with NaCl, Addison's disease.
- **Metabolic alkalosis:** primary issue is pH >7.45, HCO_3 >28 mmol/L, P_aCO_2 normal. Clinical: paraesthesia, tetany. Causes: antacids, dialysis, milk-alkali syndrome, pyloric stenosis/gastric outlet obstruction with vomiting, Bartter's syndrome, adrenogenital syndromes, Cushing's syndrome, Conn's syndrome.
- **Respiratory acidosis:** pH <7.35, PCO_2 >6 kPa (45 mmHg) normal or compensated rise HCO_3. Clinical: hypoventilation, drowsy, hypoxic. Causes: chest disease, e.g. asthma, COPD, hypoventilation, respiratory muscle weakness.
- **Respiratory alkalosis:** primary issue is P_aCO_2 <4.7 kPa, pH >7.45, normal HCO_3. Clinical: paraesthesia, tetany. Causes: hyperventilation (anxiety), asthma, CCF, hypoxia, PE, ventilation/perfusion mismatch, aspirin/salicylate overdose.

2.13 ▶ Assessment of shocked patient

- **Definition:** shock is a clinical syndrome with generalised tissue hypoxia due to reduced O_2 delivery or increased extraction. May be worsened by anaemia, reduced cardiac output, pyrexia, hypoxaemia. Low BP can be the first sign of a serious acute illness, e.g. MI, sepsis, haemorrhage, Addison's, anaphylaxis.
- **Clinical syndrome:** pale, sweating, cold, clammy, confused, obtunded, raised HR, SBP <90 mmHg. Tachypnoea, oliguric, raised JVP cardiogenic shock, PE, RV failure, tamponade. Warm peripheries, bounding pulse, hypo- or hyperthermia, sepsis, rash, erythema.

Pathophysiology of shock

- O_2 extraction increases, but anaerobic lactic acidosis can occur. Sepsis causes release of bacteria and other molecules with vasodilatation. Impaired cardiac output, capillary permeability and hypovolaemia. Reduced oxidative phosphorylation,

ATP and cell pump dysfunction. Release of cortisol, GH causes hyperglycaemia. Progressive downward spiral of multi-organ failure and death.

- **Clinical findings:** MAP <65 mmHg and SBP <90 mmHg. Urinary catheter: oliguric unless polyuria state, e.g. HHS/ DKA/hypercalcaemia.

Initial investigations

- **FBC:** low Hb if bleeding (normal initially), raised WCC/plts.
- **U&E:** AKI, dehydration, consider prerenal, renal, post-renal.
- **Troponin:** occlusive MI, type 2 MI/sepsis.
- **D-dimer:** DIC/DVT/PE non-specific. **Lactate** >4 mmol/L poor prognosis.
- **Echocardiogram:** assess LV, valves, wall motion, pericardial fluid/blood or vegetations.
- **CXR:** wide mediastinum – dissection; cardiomegaly – heart failure, effusion, consolidation, tension PTX, lobe collapse, malignancy, pulmonary oedema.
- **12-lead ECG:** arrhythmias, ischaemia, infarction, high K, cardiomyopathy.
- **Sepsis screen:** blood cultures, urinalysis, sputum, USS for fluid collection/liver abscess.
- **Arterial blood gases:** metabolic or respiratory acidosis, or both.
- **AXR** for acute abdomen, bowel obstruction or perforation suspected.
- **Supporting investigations: CTPA or V/Q scan:** exclude PE. CT may show lung and aortic pathology. **CT abdomen:** if suspected AAA, pancreatitis or suspected retroperitoneal bleeding or fluid collection or bowel obstruction or ischaemia. **Abdominal–pelvic USS:** renal obstruction, cholecystitis, jaundice, liver abscess or pelvic collection.
- **Coagulation screen:** DIC: low fibrinogen, platelets and raised APTT and raised PT. A ROTEM or TEG if available. Used in trauma or bleeding but can be useful in medical emergencies such as DIC.
- **Invasive monitoring:** intra-arterial BP monitoring useful for inotrope management. CVP and pulmonary artery (capillary) wedge pressure (PAWP) to diagnose and monitor therapy but not without risk.
- **Urgent endoscopy:** for diagnosis and therapy of suspected upper GI bleed.

2.14   Immediate actions in a shocked patient

- **Immediately:** get good IV access, e.g. ×2 antecubital fossa green/brown/grey cannula, good access to monitoring, e.g. intra-arterial lines on HDU, O_2 to give sats 94–98%. Get ECG, CXR, send FBC, U&E, LFT, lactate and cultures and consider troponin and D-dimer.
- **Cross-match if haemorrhage.** If low BP and unsure if volume depleted give 500 ml NS IV over 10–20 min and see if HR and BP improves. Get help if patient expiring, even summoning arrest team if periarrest. If no bleeding, inpatient, no MI on ECG then think PE or sepsis. But keep reviewing. You may rationally treat multiple aetiologies, e.g. sepsis and PE until the diagnosis is confirmed. (NS = 0.9% saline and G5W = 5% glucose).
- **Major haemorrhage:** blood loss >150 ml/min, loss of more than one blood volume in 24 hours, loss of 50% blood volume in 3 hours, activate the major haemorrhage protocol and request a shock pack from the transfusion lab (6 red blood cells, 4 FFP).
- **Good venous access is key.** A grey cannula (16) can give 1 L NS over 6 min and a brown or orange can give 1 L NS over 3.5 min – the lines of choice in volume loss. However, 2 green cannulas are far better than nothing and may be easier to site

than a larger-bore cannula in a shocked constricted patient. Central access takes time and flow is poor as long hub and there are risks. The femoral vein is always worth trying and, short-term, can give good access. Once you get access ensure it is protected so not pulled out in the melee of sorting out a sick patient.
- **An arterial line:** usually only possible in an HDU/ITU setting and useful if there is a plan to use inotropes and optimise fluid balance.

2.15   Quick review of different forms of shock

- **Cardiogenic shock** ▶ Section 2.16
- **Hypovolaemic shock:** ▶ Section 2.20
- **Distributive shock:** ▶ Sections 2.18 & 2.21
- **Haemorrhagic shock:** ▶ Section 2.22
- **Obstructive shock:** ▶ Section 2.23
- **Neurogenic shock:** ▶ Section 2.24

2.16   Heart failure and cardiogenic shock

- **About:** cardiac failure is almost always low cardiac output due to impaired systolic and diastolic cardiac function. Cardiogenic shock is a progression to hypotension and marked organ and tissue hypoperfusion. This may be compounded by pulmonary oedema with impaired oxygenation. 40% one-year mortality.
- **Definition:** cardiogenic shock goes a stage beyond with SBP <90 mmHg for 30+ and urine output <30 ml/h or cool extremities or depressed cardiac index (<2.2 L/min per square metre of body surface area) and an elevated pulmonary capillary wedge pressure >15 mmHg. It needs rapid action and senior help as mortality 70%. A bedside echo helps confirm the diagnosis and possible aetiology – valves, muscle, tamponade, signs of PE. Acute heart failure and cardiogenic shock differ by degrees of cardiac dysfunction/output.
- **Aetiology:** failure of the LV leads to forward failure and failure to perfuse organs. Backward failure due to rise in LA pressure, PA pressure, and then CVP. Increased pressure moves fluid into the interstitium and alveoli. There is perfusion without oxygenation (V/Q mismatch) and so hypoxia. Mitral stenosis especially with AF causes pulmonary oedema but LV function is normal. Chronic MR better tolerated as left atrium has dilated so lower LVEDP.

Diagnosis
- Severely impaired tissue perfusion and PCWP >18 mmHg.
- Cardiogenic shock when MAP <60 mmHg or SBP <90 mmHg.
- Systolic: reduced EF <40%.
- Diastolic: reduced LVEDV due to wall stiffness ('inflating a stiff balloon').

Causes of cardiogenic pulmonary oedema 'pump failure' and shock
- **Acute MI:** NSTEMI/STEMI with LV impairment due to left main stem or proximal LAD disease or acute MR/AR or VSD. Check 12-lead ECG. Urgent echo. Escalate for reperfusion with PPCI/thrombolysis. Check troponin/dimer.
- **Precipitants:** missed medications, e.g. diuretics, comorbidities, pneumonia, excess volume/alcohol, arrhythmias, ischaemia. PE with RV failure.
- **Cardiomyopathy or myocarditis:** potential recovery with supportive management. Viral, peripartum, toxic, genetic.

- **Valve failure/wall rupture:** aortic stenosis (murmur fades when severe), mitral stenosis (loud S1 and MDM and AF), severe aortic regurgitation (widening pulse pressure and loud EDM, endocarditis), severe mitral regurgitation (loud PSM, papillary muscle infarction or endocarditis). Acute VSD post MI. Aortic dissection with acute AR.
- **Arrhythmias:** fast AF, VT, CHB reducing cardiac output.
- **Cardiac tamponade:** impaired diastolic filling. Echo/pericardiocentesis.
- **Hypertensive crisis:** consider renal artery stenosis or phaeochromocytoma.
- **Neurogenic:** SAH, ICH, traumatic cord lesion.

Clinical
- BP normal or <90/60 mmHg. HTN causes pulmonary oedema. AF/VT.
- **Left HF:** severe dyspnoea, cyanosed, agitated, HR >100 low vol. pulse. Cold peripheries. Pink frothy sputum, oliguria. Triple rhythm, S3, pulsus alternans.
- **Right HF:** raised JVP, dependent oedema, ascites, hepatomegaly.
- **High output cardiac failure:** rare AV fistula, Paget's disease.
- **NYHA grade:** I. None II. Moderate exercise. III. Minimal exercise. IV. Symptoms at rest.

Investigations
- **FBC/U&E:** low Hb, AKI/CKD. Raised LFTs liver congestion.
- **ABG:** type 1 RF, lactate >2 mmol/L.
- **Biomarker:** raised troponin with NSTEMI/STEMI or myocarditis.
- **ECG:** arrhythmia, low voltage, ST elevation (consider PCI) ST depression – NSTEMI/UA. New LBBB, true post MI. RBBB may suggest PE or ASD. Low voltage QRS tamponade.
- **CXR:** pulmonary oedema, cardiomegaly and increased upper lobe venous markings, bat wing oedema, Kerley B lines, bilateral pleural effusion.
- **BNP/NT-proBNP:** BNP >500 pg/ml or NT-proBNP >2000 pg/ml suggests heart failure. BNP <100 pg/ml or NT-proBNP <300 pg/ml heart failure unlikely. Levels correlate with impaired LV function.
- **Echocardiogram:** LV/RV dysfunction, valves – acute MR, wall motion, tamponade or VSD. Severe aortic stenosis mean gradient >40 mmHg or area <1 cm^2.
- **Swan–Ganz:** may be attempted if diagnosis or management uncertain.
- **Cardiac catheterisation:** image coronary vessels looking for occluded vessel, culprit lesion, poor LV, severe AR, dilated root. Angioplasty, stenting.

Management: get early Cardiology and echo and HDU support
- **ABC.** Sitting patient up in a position of comfort reduces preload. O_2.
- **Analgesia: Diamorphine** 2.5 mg or **Morphine** 5 mg IV + **metoclopramide** 10 mg IV anti-emetic can relieve chest pain/dyspnoea/anxiety.
- **Loop diuretic: Furosemide** 50–100 mg IV when SBP >110 mmHg. Avoid if BP <90 mmHg. Modest doses venodilate + diuresis. Consider adding IV **Acetazolamide** 500 mg OD – can improve diuretic efficiency.
- **Consider Buccal glyceryl trinitrate** 2–5 mg and then **Glyceryl trinitrate** 50 mg in 50 ml IV infusion. Start 0.6–12 ml/h if SBP >100 mmHg.
- **CPAP:** 5–10 cmH$_2$O. Slowly increase to 10 cmH$_2$O. Check ABG 30 min and 1 h post-CPAP. When changing pressure turn flow up in 2 cmH$_2$O steps at 2–3 min intervals over the first 10–15 min. CPAP can improve oxygenation but may compromise venous return.

- **Arrhythmias:** fast AF then consider loading with **Digoxin** or **Amiodarone** via a large or central cannula. **Amiodarone** for VT with SBP >90 mmHg, otherwise DC shock if unstable tachyarrhythmia (low BP, angina, LVF).
- **Hypertension:** manage with IV nitrates/IV diuretics. If BP low consider stopping/ holding verapamil, diltiazem, alpha-blockers, class I antiarrhythmics.
- **Anticoagulate** with LMWH if patient in AF or LV thrombus.
- **Acute coronary syndrome:** ▶Section 3.7. If STEMI then reperfusion by PCI/ thrombolysis can improve LV function. Get senior help quickly and decisions on CCU and need for thrombolysis/PCI/CABG.
- **Valve failure/VSD:** discuss with Cardiology if candidate for urgent valve repair or replacement or VSD repair.
- **Cardiac tamponade:** globular heart on CXR. Urgent bedside echo if available. Consider needle pericardiocentesis.
- **Stop/avoid drugs** which can worsen heart failure, e.g. calcium channel blockers, antiarrhythmics, NSAIDs, COX-2 inhibitors, steroids.
- **Salbutamol** 2.5–5.0 mg neb stat for bronchospasm. Causes tachycardia.
- **Aminophylline** 250 mg IV over 30 min loading dose has been used and may help bronchospasm but rare now as concerns over arrhythmias. Get Senior approval.

Drugs that improve prognosis with stabilised HF (HFrEF) if EF <40%

- ACEi or ARB. Beta-blockers. Sacubitril/Valsartan (Entresto).
- Aldosterone antagonist. Dapagliflozin 10 mg OD (SGLT2 inhibitor).

Stabilised heart failure BP >90 mmHg

- **Maximise vasodilator therapy** once BP >110 mmHg (ACEi/ARB) before increasing diuretic therapy, e.g. **Ramipril** 1.25 mg; start lowest dose and titrate gradually up to full dose over several weeks + beta-blockers (once stable), e.g. bisoprolol/carvedilol. In those with EF <40%, reduces the risk of hospitalisation and the risk of premature death. If ACEi not tolerated due to hypotension, cough, consider AG2 receptor blockers. Monitor U&E for renal dysfunction and hyperkalaemia. C/I pregnancy and renal artery stenosis.
- **Angiotensin receptor antagonists:** if cannot tolerate ACEi. Up-titrate dose. Can cause high K$^+$. Monitor U&E. **Candesartan** 4–8 mg OD.
- **Aldosterone antagonists: Spironolactone** 25–50 mg OD/**Eplerenone** 25–50 mg OD: in NYHA III/IV failure (symptoms at rest or minimal exercise). Add to ACEi/ARB (87%) and a beta-blocker (75%). Spironolactone can cause high K$^+$ and worsening renal function. Eplerenone is a similar drug with proven benefits post-MI and in heart failure, but with less gynaecomastia.
- **Beta-blockers:** not if cardiogenic shock. Stabilised HF **Carvedilol** 12.5 mg OD up to 25–50 mg OD, **Bisoprolol** 1.25 mg to 2.5 mg to 5–10 mg OD, or **Metoprolol**. Start low and titrate dose up.
- **Loop diuretics: Furosemide** 40–80 mg OD or **Bumetanide** 1–2 mg OD (low K$^+$), combined with aldosterone antagonists. Monitor U&E.
- **Dapagliflozin** 10 mg OD (SGLT2 inhibitor) used for diabetes but now used for chronic heart failure, even if not diabetic. Reduces hospitalisations and death. Risk of diabetic ketoacidosis. May be useful for those with HFpEF and HFrEF. Some reported cases of Fournier's gangrene. May cause volume depletion and hypotension in elderly.
- **Nitrates:** (avoid if low BP) give SL **GTN** 400–800 mcg (2 sprays) and then consider IV **GTN** if SBP >100 mmHg. Titrate to symptoms/BP.

- **Potent thiazide diuretics: Metolazone** 2.5–10 mg OD. Given oral short-term (days only). Needs daily weight and hydration assessment. Really used short-term in hospital or community heart failure team.
- **Ivabradine** 2.5–5mg BD up to 7.5 mg BD: inhibits I_f channels in SAN. Antianginal. Reduces hospitalisation in SR with an EF <35%, a heart rate remaining >70/min, and persisting symptoms despite maximal standard treatment.
- **Hydralazine/oral nitrates** if ACE inhibitor/ARB not tolerated.
- **Digoxin:** for those with heart failure and AF. Reduces hospitalisations.
- **Non-pharmacological:** exercise rehabilitation programmes have been shown to improve functional capacity. Combine with salt restriction and weight loss and smoking cessation.
- **Revascularisation:** angiogram/revascularisation by PCI or CABG.
- **Implantable cardioverter–defibrillator** high risk for VF/VT.
- **Anticoagulation: warfarin/DOAC** if AF or thromboembolic event or cardioembolic source. Warfarin for AF and mitral stenosis. Heart failure increases risk of stroke.
- **Cardiac resynchronisation therapy** indicated if LVEF <35%, sinus rhythm, LBBB with a QRS >150 ms, and NYHA functional Class II–IV on guideline-directed medical therapy.
- **Surgery:** CABG, valve surgery (AVR/MV repair/replacement), repair LV aneurysms, ventricular assist devices. Transplantation end-stage cardiac failure in those suitable.
- **Those with anaemia and coronary heart disease** aim for a Hb of 90 g/L. Those with heart failure and anaemia may benefit from IV iron.
- **Reference:** European Society of Cardiology (2012) *ESC guidelines for the diagnosis and treatment of acute and chronic heart failure.*

Cardiogenic shock: prognosis is poor

- **Vasopressors:** consider if BP <90 mmHg. Target MAP >65–70 mmHg. **Noradrenaline** but it increases myocardial O_2 demand.
- **Inotropes: Dobutamine** inotrope of choice. Metaraminol increases inpatient mortality.
- **HDU/CCU/ITU** bed with cardiac monitoring, physiological monitoring, urinary catheter. Venous/arterial line. May be a role for CVP line.
- **Ultrafiltration:** veno-venous isolated ultrafiltration can remove fluid. Reserved for unresponsive/resistant to diuretics or severe renal failure.
- **Mechanical ventilation:** reduces work of breathing and O_2 demand. May reduce cardiac filling and cause hypotension.

Intra-aortic balloon pump (IABP)

- 25–50 ml elongated polyethylene helium-filled balloon inserted via the femoral artery. Placed distal to the left subclavian artery, but proximal to the renal arteries. Balloon inflates with diastole and deflates with early systole. The myocardial oxygen supply:demand ratio is improved, and CO may be increased by up to 40%. Improves oxygenation in cardiogenic shock due to myocardial damage or acute MR and acute LVF, refractory UA and ischaemic ventricular arrhythmias via the augmentation of the intrinsic 'Windkessel effect', whereby potential energy stored in the aortic root during systole is converted to kinetic energy with the elastic recoil of the aortic root.
- Most coronary perfusion is in diastole. Thrombogenic. Anticoagulated with heparin. Balloon inflates as systolic pressures fall with a second pressure rise in diastole which then falls off in presystole. The balloon can be set to assist every beat (1:1) or less often (1:2, 1:4, or 1:8). Oliguria may occur if the balloon lies too distal and occludes renal vessels. The balloon causes haemolysis. Never switch the balloon off

while *in situ*. **Contraindicated use:** aortic regurgitation (AR) and aortic dissection and aortic aneurysm.

Left ventricular assist devices

- **Impella device** is a catheter-based miniaturised ventricular assist device. Use a retrograde femoral artery access. Placed in the LV across the aortic valve. It pumps blood from LV to ascending aorta and helps to maintain a systemic circulation at an upper rate between 2.5 and 5.0 L/min. Causes sustained unloading of the LV increasing overall systemic CO. Used for AMI with cardiogenic shock and to facilitate high risk coronary angioplasty. Other indications include treatment of cardiomyopathy with acute decompensation, post-cardiotomy shock, off-pump coronary bypass surgery. Has complications. Lack of randomised controlled trial data supporting this observation.
- **Take expert advice** on transplant, ECMO or other LV assist devices.
- **VTE prophylaxis:** advocated because high risk of DVT/PE.

2.17 Vasopressors and inotropes

- **About:** aim to maintain core cerebral, coronary and renal perfusion, at the cost of skin and other less vital areas. Inotropes/vasopressors may improve the numbers. Little evidence they improve outcomes. Some may worsen it.
- **Vasopressors:** raise peripheral vascular resistance and MAP. May help sepsis-driven vasodilation. Noradrenaline, adrenaline, vasopressin.
- **Inotropes:** improve cardiac contractility which also increases myocardial O_2 demand, e.g. adrenaline, dobutamine. Use usually restricted to the ITU, CCU or HDU as needs intra-arterial BP monitoring. Often given by central line.
- **Cardiogenic shock:** despite much evidence ESC recommends **noradrenaline** as vasopressor and **dobutamine** as inotrope of choice.
- **Intra-aortic balloon pump:** may be used in cardiogenic shock. Anti-shock suits are sometimes used pre-hospital in hypovolaemia.
- **Septicaemic shock:** ensure adequate fluid replacement before using inotropes. **Noradrenaline** is main vasopressor as it causes vasoconstriction to maintain MAP ≥65 mmHg following adequate volume replacement.
- **Dobutamine** is main inotrope used. Is the main inotrope through its beta-1 agonist effects and vasodilates through its beta-2 agonist effects.
- **ADH/vasopressin** may be considered for salvage therapy. Steroid may be added for refractory hypotension for those who fail to respond.
- **Neurogenic shock/anaphylaxis:** noradrenaline as there is vasodilation.

2.18 Anaphylaxis and shock

- **About:** anaphylaxis is a severe, life-threatening, generalised or systemic hypersensitivity reaction, with significant disturbance of one or more of airway, breathing or circulation. It can recur, so monitor for 6–12 h as needed. Over 50% of the intravascular volume can shift to extravascular space which may include tissues around the airway or gut or other organs. New guidance focuses on early use of adrenaline (epinephrine) acutely and for ongoing management.
- **Aetiology:** it is not clear why one person with specific immunoglobulin E (IgE) to an allergen will have an anaphylactic reaction on exposure, another only a local reaction, and in a third individual no reaction at all. A pre-current episode and antigen exposure causes IgE antibody generation. Later re-exposure may produce

mast cell degranulation due to antigen cross-linking IgE-releasing histamine. Histamine activates receptors with massive release of cytokines/chemokines. Increases postcapillary venule permeability. Fluid moves into interstitium with laryngeal, pharyngeal, cutaneous oedema, bronchial or bronchospasm and/or low BP. Anaphylactoid reactions are identical but not IgE-mediated, e.g. opiates, radiocontrast, NSAIDs.

- **Causative agents:** drugs (e.g. penicillin), radiological contrast, insect bites/stings, eggs, fish, peanuts. Consider latex (e.g. gloves/tourniquets/BP cuffs) if occurs in healthcare/dental setting. Blood products. IVIg to those with selective IgA deficiency. NSAIDs, ACEi and Alteplase can cause angioedema/angioneurotic oedema. Aspiration of a hydatid cyst.
- **Clinical:** onset over minutes. Flushing, itching, urticaria, low BP. Chest pain, tachycardia, incontinence. Airway oedema/constriction – wheeze, stridor, hoarseness, staccato cough. Periorbital itching. Urticaria is not seen with C1 esterase deficiency. Abdominal pain, colic, diarrhoea, vomiting, angioedema. Face/lips swell, sneezing. Metallic taste, confusion.
- **Investigations:** FBC: high WCC/CRP if infection. Check **mast cell tryptase:** initial, after 1–2 h and 24 h/follow up. Normally <1 ng/ml; post-anaphylaxis >100 ng/ml. Normal levels do not exclude anaphylaxis and can be seen with food-induced allergy. **ECG:** SR, high HR, ST/T wave changes, new AF. Infection screen: blood/urine cultures. C1 esterase inhibitor deficiency is a rare cause of angioedema (no urticaria). Check C4/C1 inhibitor levels. Allergy testing: allergen skin testing; RAST identifies specific IgE.
- **Differential:** vasovagal syncope, sepsis, scombroid (high histamine in ingested fish), systemic mastocytosis (high tryptase), carcinoid syndrome (urine high HIAA). Panic attack, causes of syncope/presyncope, causes of breathlessness. Red man syndrome after IV vancomycin. Monosodium gluconate ingestion: skin warm and feels burning, headache, nausea, bronchospasm. No urticarial/angioedema or low BP.

Management: repeated IM adrenaline (epinephrine) is the main therapy

- **ABC:** monitor BP, HR, SaO$_2$ and ABG and ECG. Crash call Senior Anaesthetist and ENT (if stridor) for help if any concerns of airway obstruction and oedema or any stridor, severe bronchospasm or respiratory compromise.
- **Life-threatening features:** airway swelling/hoarseness stridor, rapid breathing, wheeze, resp distress, cyanosis, SpO$_2$ <92%, confusion, pale, clammy, low BP, faint, drowsy.
- **Outside hospital:** ABC. Lie patient flat, elevate legs though some may feel less breathless sitting. If pregnant place on left side. If life-threatening features (above) of anaphylaxis then remove syringe cap and give Epipen (Adrenaline 0.3 mg) into lateral thigh through clothes if needed. Hold for 10 seconds. Call 999 for an ambulance.
- **General:** give O$_2$. Stop any drug infusion, blood or blood product, remove bee sting. Lie patient flat with legs elevated as above if symptoms + low BP.
- **Start fluid challenge** 500–1000 ml NS over 20–60 min (20 ml/kg) and fluid replacement as needed to fill vascular space.
- **In hospital:** if life-threatening features give **Adrenaline [Epinephrine]** 0.5 ml of 1/1000 (0.5 mg) IM into anterolateral thigh using a blue/green needle in adults. Repeat in 5 mins if no improvement. Reduces histamine release. Causes skin vasoconstriction (reduces absorption of the bee sting or other allergen).

No improvement despite 2 appropriate doses of intramuscular adrenaline

- **Adrenaline infusion:** start peripheral low-dose IV adrenaline infusion: 1 mg (1 ml of 1:1000) adrenaline in 100 ml of NS. Start at 0.5–1.0 ml/kg/h. Titrate to clinical response. Prime and connect with an infusion pump via a dedicated line. DO NOT 'piggyback' on to another infusion line. DO NOT infuse on the same side as a BP cuff, as this will interfere with the infusion and risk extravasation. Continuous monitoring and observation is mandatory. High BP suggests adrenaline overdose. Arterial cannula for ABG/BP monitoring. Central venous access.
- **Fluids:** adult 500–1000 ml per bolus of glucose-free crystalloid (e.g. Hartmann's solution, Plasma-Lyte). Large volumes may be required (e.g. 3–5 L in adults).
- **If refractory to adrenaline infusion:** consider adding a second vasopressor in addition to adrenaline infusion: of **Noradrenaline, Vasopressin** or **Metaraminol.** Consider ECMO.
- **Second line: Glucagon** 5 mg slow IV in G5W (protect airway in case of vomiting), followed by IV infusion 50 mcg/kg/h for persisting low BP if bradycardia on a high dose of beta-blockers (directly activates adenylyl cyclase). Partial upper airway obstruction/stridor: nebulised **Adrenaline** (5 ml of 1mg/ml). **Salbutamol** 2.5–5 mg Neb for wheeze and dyspnoea which may be repeated.

In event of cardiac arrest

> **Cardiac arrest – follow ALS algorithm and start chest compressions early. Use IV or IO Adrenaline bolus as per cardiac arrest. Aggressive fluid resuscitation and consider prolonged resus/extracorporeal CPR.**

Not in current 2021 guidelines but may be considered

- **Steroids:** deprecated now as evidence lacking. Follow local guidance. Some may consider **Hydrocortisone** 200 mg IV stat dose and start oral steroids. Some may continue **Prednisolone** 40 mg PO OD for 3 d along with an antihistamine if asthma or allergic.
- **Histamine blocker: Chlorphenamine** 10 mg slow IV/IM (H_1). **Ranitidine** 50 mg IV over 5 min (H_2 blockade). Consider if urticaria and itch.

Angioedema

- Angioedema is common in the ED. Oedema of cutaneous and mucosal tissues such as lips, eyes, oral cavity, larynx, genitals, and gastrointestinal system. Laryngeal oedema causing airway obstruction is the main fear.
- Bradykinin is a potent vasodilatory mediator. Excess bradykinin leads to swelling of the mucosa and submucosa. Consider abdominal CT if GI symptoms.
- A clinical history of allergy or drug exposure can suggest an underlying diagnosis. If no obvious trigger identified, then measure complement C4. If C4 levels are low, further investigations should be initiated to look for evidence of C1 inhibitor deficiency. Angioedema associated with allergen exposure generally responds to ABC, slow IV/IM chlorphenamine and hydrocortisone, and admit and observe.
- **Hereditary angioedema (HAE):** autosomal dominant inherited C1 inhibitor deficiency causes increased local bradykinin levels, giving rise to local pain and swelling. Bowel oedema may cause abdominal pain and result in a laparotomy. Some may develop laryngeal obstruction at the dentist which can be fatal. Usually self-limiting, <48 hours. Can be seen in early adulthood. May not have urticaria.

Check for low C4 levels during attack. If low, then measure C1 inhibitor levels and function. Acute attacks can mimic anaphylaxis, but they need **Icatibant** (C1-esterase inhibitor concentrate) 30 mg for 1 dose, then 30 mg after 6 hours if required; maximum 3 doses per day. Consider fresh frozen plasma or C1 inhibitor concentrate (plasma-derived), and prophylaxis is with rituximab with or without chemotherapy and splenectomy.

- **Acquired C1 inhibitor deficiency:** rare and clinically same as HAE. Seen in older patients with autoimmune and B cell lymphoproliferative diseases. Develop antibodies to C1 inhibitor or activate C1. Treat underlying disorder. Check low C4 is seen during acute episodes. For treatments see above. Also include **Tranexamic acid, Danazol,** and **Icatibant.** Take expert advice.
- **Reference:** NICE Scenario: Angio-oedema without anaphylaxis (last revised September 2021), www.cks.nice.org.uk.

Consider discharge and follow-up

- Monitor for 6–12 h post full recovery to ensure no late biphasic reactions. Discharge with 2 **Epipens** each containing **Adrenaline** 0.3 mg for IM usage with instructions on how to self-administer a dose. The second is in case one injector fails or patient needs a second dose.
- **Education:** to use Epipen if anaphylaxis occurs with difficulty breathing or becoming faint. Give self-injection in the lateral thigh. It may be given through clothing, avoiding seams and pockets. Hold needle in place for 10 sec to ensure the adrenaline dose has been delivered completely. In an obese patient ensure injection given deep into muscle and not subcutaneously. Check the patient's injection technique regularly (see self-teach videos on www.YouTube.com).
- Long term patients should wear a medic-alert bracelet. All need a referral to a specialist for allergy clinic, immunology opinion and identification of cause and antigen avoidance. Skin testing is more rapid, cheaper and sensitive for allergy testing. Immunotherapy is useful in those with IgE-mediated disease.
- **Reference:** UK Resuscitation Guidelines 2021.

2.19 ▶ Toxic shock syndrome

Superantigens overstimulate B/T cells causing cytokine storm.

- **About:** toxic shock syndrome (TSS) is rare exotoxin-mediated illness due to streptococcal skin lesions or *Staphylococcus* postpartum and tampons.
- **Aetiology:** releases staphylococcal toxic shock syndrome toxin 1 (TSST-1) which acts as a super antigen that binds to MHC II and T-cell receptor, resulting in polyclonal T-cell activation and cytokine release (TNF, interleukin-1, M protein and gamma interferon). Huge immune response. Overstimulation of Th cells. *Streptococcus* group A beta haemolytic. High mortality due to Toxins A and B superantigens.
- **At risk:** can occur with no risks. Some are menstruating or postpartum, females using barrier contraceptives. Postoperative patients, varicella, or herpes zoster infection. Patients with chemical or thermal burns.
- **Clinical:** signs are initially subtle and then inexorable decline in healthy adult. Headache, high fever, nausea, vomiting, abdominal pain, severe muscle pain, tenderness. Profuse watery diarrhoea and erythroderma more likely staphylococcal.

SBP <90 mmHg and increased HR, warm peripheries possibly. Vaginal exam for retained tampon. Look for simple wound. There may be evidence of soft tissue infection and necrosis, e.g. necrotising fasciitis or pneumonia or bacteraemia. Later after 1–2 weeks: desquamation of the palms and soles.

- **Investigations:** FBC: raised neutrophils/WCC, low plts. U&E: high urea/creatinine, raised lactate/CRP/CK/AST. Low albumin/calcium. Clotting: coagulopathy – raised APTT but PT and fibrinogen normal unless DIC. Blood/urine/sputum dipstick and cultures. CXR: look for infection.
- **Complications:** AKI, rhabdomyolysis, liver failure, limb loss, circulatory collapse. DIC mortality is 5%.
- **Differentials:** severe group A *Strep.* infections (scarlet fever, necrotising fasciitis, toxic shock-like syndrome), Kawasaki syndrome, *Staph.* scalded skin syndrome, Rocky Mountain spotted fever, leptospirosis, meningococcaemia, Gram-neg. sepsis, viral syndromes (e.g. measles, adenoviral infection, enterovirus infections, dengue), allergic drug reactions.
- **Management:** ITU bed (non-contagious). ABC: O_2 94–98%. Invasive monitoring. Fluid resuscitation (5–10 L per d) IV crystalloids and colloids due to the extreme low BP and diffuse capillary leak. Wound decontamination: drain or debride the lesion, remove foreign material, irrigate copiously. Recent surgical wounds should be explored and irrigated even when signs of inflammation are absent. Inotropes, e.g. **Dobutamine** and/or **Noradrenaline** may be needed. Antibiotics: **Flucloxacillin** 2 g 6 h IV ± **Clindamycin** 1.2 g 6–12 h IV. **Vancomycin** 1–1.5 g 12 h IV may be needed. **IV Ig** 400 mg/kg has been used for streptococcal TSS to neutralise super antigens and opsonise streptococci. **Steroids:** consider **Hydrocortisone** 50 mg IV 6 h in those with refractory shock despite adequate antimicrobial therapy and resuscitation.
- **Reference:** see www.toxicshock.com.

2.20 Hypovolaemic shock

- **About:** primary water/salt loss. Hypovolaemia with decreased peripheral perfusion. Leads to multi-organ failure. Haemorrhagic shock ▶ Section 2.22.
- **Causes:** severe gastroenteritis, HHS, DKA, cholera, burns, overdiuresis, diabetes insipidus: cranial or nephrogenic, high Ca/low K, heat stroke, surgical drains and stomas losing excessive fluids, Addison's disease, major burns, erythroderma.
- **Clinical:** assess state of hydration. Reduced skin turgor, cold, clammy, cold peripheries. High HR, postural low BP, obtunded, reduced cap. return, oliguria, delirium and coma. Polyuria – exclude diabetes insipidus or DKA/HHS or high Ca/low K or post obstruction.
- **Investigations:** FBC: Hb initially normal and may fall. U&E/Ca: raised urea (GI bleed or AKI/CKD), raised creatinine (AKI/CKD), high K if AKI or haemolysis. APTT/PT: look for coagulopathy. ABG: hypoxia, met. acidosis, lactate >2.0 mmol/L. Cortisol/SynACTHen test.
- **Management:** needs IV access (2 green/grey cannulas antecubital fossa), baseline bloods, urinary catheter (urine Na low), physiological monitoring. Look for and manage cause. Watch for AKI. Consider HDU and invasive monitoring. Give **antibiotics** immediately if sepsis is possible. Volume replacement rate depends on the clinical state, age, cardiac status, renal function and suspected deficit: 1 L (20 ml/kg) crystalloid, e.g. NS IV over 15–30 min depending on BP, then 1 L over 1 h and replace in response to clinical change. Large volumes of NS can cause a

hyperchloraemic acidosis. If there is concern over volume overload then consider 200 ml NS fluid challenges and reassessment. Replace electrolytes as needed. Transfuse to ensure Hb >8 g/dl. Manage Na and K levels. Body weight can help manage fluid status. Determine if there is any steroid deficiency. If Addison's disease suspected at all give **Hydrocortisone** 100 mg IV/IM 6-hourly. Diabetes insipidus suspected – polyuria. Consider if cranial or nephrogenic. Treat with DDAVP as needed. Also see DKA and HHS ▶ Section 5.18 and 5.19.

2.21   Sepsis

Sepsis is life-threatening organ dysfunction caused by a dysregulated host response to infection.

- **Introduction:** new guidance came out in October 2021 from the Surviving Sepsis Campaign.
- **Septic shock** should be defined as a subset of sepsis in which particularly profound circulatory, cellular and metabolic abnormalities are associated with a greater risk of mortality than with sepsis alone. A quantitative definition of **septic shock is** sepsis not corrected by volume resuscitation that needs vasopressors to achieve a MAP >65 mmHg. Lactate >2 mmol/L (18mg/L). Mortality 40%.
- **Sepsis 3 started SOFA** (sequential [sepsis-related] organ failure assessment) to assess organ dysfunction; defined as an increase in the score of 2 or more points and is associated with an in-hospital mortality greater than 10%. From this came **qSOFA:** which was sepsis + 2/3 of GCS <15, RR ≥22/min, SBP ≤100 mmHg. Recommended now to use NEWS2 or SIRS.
- **Systemic Inflammatory Response Syndrome (SIRS):** Temp >38°C or <36°C, HR > 90/min, RR >20/min, WCC >12,000 or WCC <4000.
- **High risk:** age >75, frail, immunocompromised, pregnant women.
- **Pathophysiology:** infected causes induced by endo-/exotoxins. Release of cytokines (TNF, IL-1, IL-6) and iNOS relaxes vascular smooth muscle and bradykinin. This is opposed by IL-4 and IL-10 which reduce TNF-alpha, IL-1, IL-6 and IL-8. Result is low O_2, hypovolaemia, vasodilation, capillary leak. There is a fall in SVR with increased CO and SBP <90 mmHg and a fall in DBP and warm extremities with a good capillary refill. Non-vital organs are hypoperfused at the expense of heart, kidneys, liver and brain.
- **Clinical:** they may be more ill than they appear. Warm or cool peripheries (in other causes of shock the peripheries are cold), delirium, and be obtunded and agitated, deterioration can be rapid with rigors, fever or hypothermia, vomiting, diarrhoea. Low BP <90/60 mmHg, low volume central pulse, purpura (meningococci), macular rash (toxic shock syndrome).

Infective screening in sepsis
- Have a logical system and work top to toe in symptoms and signs.
- **General:** malaise, fever, night sweats, weight loss give idea of onset.
- **Neurology:** meningitis, encephalitis, abscess, vasculitis. Get CT/MRI/LP.
- **Respiratory:** chest signs for cough, fever, pneumonia, empyema, TB.
- **Urinary:** renal angle tenderness, urinary symptoms. Urinalysis.
- **Hepatobiliary:** RUQ pain, jaundice, pale stools, positive Murphy's sign.
- **Peritonism:** appendicitis, paralytic ileus, abdominal.
- **Endocarditis:** new murmurs, stigmata, recent cardiac operations/interventions.

- **Dermatology:** abscesses, boils – check perineum, cellulitis, and burns. TEN/necrotising fasciitis.
- **Gynaecology:** pelvic pain, STI, retained tampons.
- **Foreign bodies:** new heart valves, catheter, central line, hip replacement.
- **Immunosuppression:** neutropenia, myelodysplasia, haem. malignancy, HIV.
- **Sore throat:** tonsillitis/abscess, Lemierre's syndrome, mononucleosis.
- **Foreign travel:** viral illness (dengue, VHF), malaria, HIV conversion.
- **CNS infection:** headache, seizure, encephalopathy, focal signs, cold sores.
- **Joint pain/back/bone pain:** septic joint, prosthesis, osteomyelitis, brucellosis.
- **Post-operative:** chest infection, catheter-related sepsis, cannula-related sepsis, surgical site infection, intra-abdominal abscess, DVT.

Clinical assessment for symptoms and signs of septic sources

- **Non-infectious causes of SIRS:** pancreatitis, liver failure and cirrhosis, bowel ischaemia, infarction or perforation, any major surgery (general or obstetric), trauma and tissue damage, malignancy, transfusion reaction, GI bleed/haemorrhagic shock, drug reaction, systemic vasculitis, myocardial infarction, skin reactions (TEN, SJS), seizures.
- **Potential complications of SIRS:** DIC (low fibrinogen, delayed clotting times, low platelets), respiratory failure/ARDS (hypoxia), acute kidney injury, multi-organ failure, GI bleeding/stress ulcer, anaemia, coagulopathy, DVT and VTE, hyperglycaemia, electrolyte disturbances.
- **Final thoughts:** always ask about travel. Malaria, dengue, VHF fever.

> ### The top sepsis killers are:
> - *Neisseria meningitides* (meningitis/septicaemia)
> - *Staph. aureus* (boils, endocarditis, bone, joint, discitis)
> - *Strep. pneumoniae* (pneumonia, sepsis, meningitis)
> - *Strep. pyogenes* (cellulitis, pharyngitis).

Investigations

- **FBC:** low Hb, neutropenia. High WCC/platelets. Raised CRP/ESR.
- **Lactate** >2 mmol/L with sepsis and higher values suggest greater mortality.
- **VBG/ABG:** metabolic acidosis ± respiratory failure.
- **Base deficit** 0 to −10 moderately severe. Less than −10 severely ill.
- **Procalcitonin:** elevated with bacterial infection.
- **Infection screen: blood cultures:** aerobic/anaerobic before antibiotics. 2 blood cultures from 2 sites 20 min apart. Avoid skin contaminants; get ×3 blood cultures from different sites 20 min apart. No-touch technique. Ensure good skin decontamination and asepsis. In those >65 the commonest source is genitourinary then chest. Take before antibiotics. Not as part of cannula insertion which is notoriously unreliable with false positives.
- **Urine:** urinalysis and culture. **Thick/thin blood films** if malaria suspected.
- **Faeces:** culture if diarrhoea. **Effusions:** diagnostic tap pleural/ascitic fluid.
- **CXR:** pneumonia may show consolidation, effusion, empyema.
- **CT/MRI head + CSF:** LP if meningitis/encephalitis considered and safe.
- **Skin: take scrapings if any haemorrhagic lesions.** Swab any infected sites or infected lines or pressure sores or wounds.
- **Abdomen-pelvis USS/CT:** fluid/pus collections, chest, spine, abdomen, liver, pelvis. MRI is better for perianal disease.

Management: involve seniors early

- **Treatment goals:** MAP >65 mmHg, urine >0.5 ml/kg/hr, CVP 8–12 mmHg and S_VO_2 of >70% and normal lactate.
- **Basics**: ABC, high FiO_2, IV access/cultures, fluids, IV antibiotics, IV fluids, monitor urine. Consider ITU/HDU. Involve clinical outreach. Move to ITU <6 h if needed. Mechanical ventilation: reduces work of breathing. For selected patients. Use capillary refill time (normal adult = 3 sec) to guide resuscitation as an adjunct to other measures of perfusion.
- **Circulation:** get IV access. Central venous line may help if concerns of overfilling or cardiac failure. Intra-arterial BP monitoring if possible. Target MAP >65 mmHg. Watch FBC, U&E, lactate and ABG. Transfusion to get Hct >30%. Closely monitor urine output. Consider urinary catheter.
- **Fluids:** septic shock and lactate >4 mmol/L should receive 30 ml/kg of IV crystalloid (NS/Hartmann's solution/Ringer's lactate) in first 3 h (2 L in a 70 kg adult). Repeat 250 ml saline boluses titrated to response. May need 4–6 L of fluid in total within 24 h. Repeated assessment is key.
- **Vasopressors:** use **Noradrenaline [Norepinephrine]** if needed as the first line agent to keep MAP >65 mmHg. Target CVP >8 mmHg and SvO_2 >70%, or mixed venous O_2 saturation (SvO_2) >65%.
- **Antibiotics stat <1 h of arrival.** Stop if a non-infective aetiology becomes apparent. If no allergy and renal function normal then consider **Tazocin** 4.5 g 6 h IV ± **Gentamicin** 5 mg/kg IV. If penicillin allergic then **Meropenem** 1 g 8 h IV. Consider **Vancomycin** 1–1.5 g 12 h IV if patient at high risk for MRSA. **Ceftriaxone** 2 g 12 h IV if suspected meningococcaemia. Listeria considered IV **Amoxicillin** 2g 4 h. Delays increase mortality. **Haem malignancies:** consider IV antifungal agents.
- **Blood transfusion:** transfuse if Hb <7 g/dl or bleeding or myocardial ischaemia. Target 7.0–9.0 g/dl. Goals >9g/L in IHD. Give platelets if count is <10,000/mm³ or <20,000/mm³ with bleeding.
- **Surgical consult:** if abscesses or pus collections or necrotising fasciitis or acute abdomen or suspected perforation or intra-abdominal sepsis. Consider **Tazocin** 4.5 g 8 h IV.
- **Steroids: Hydrocortisone** 50 mg IV 6 h with refractory shock despite 1 h of antimicrobial therapy, fluid and inotropic resuscitation. Evidence is poor.
- **Non-infective SIRS:** fluids, O_2, critical care monitoring and focused therapies and interventions are key.
- **Blood glucose:** target glucose level 4.0–8.2 mmol/L. Caution as tight control can result in hypoglycaemia <4.0 mmol/L (72 mg/dl). Consider VRIII.
- **Human activated C protein** was previously advocated in selected severe sepsis cases in ITU. *In vivo* activated protein C (APC) has antithrombotic, antifibrinolytic and anti-inflammatory properties, and its use has been discontinued.
- **Other considerations:** analgesia, nutrition, pressure areas care.
- **Sodium bicarbonate** should not be used for most patients with pH ≥7.15.
- **VTE prophylaxis** is important. **Stress ulcer prophylaxis:** PPI or ranitidine.

Multi-organ dysfunction due to severe sepsis

- **Pulmonary:** acute lung injury and ARDS.
- **Cardiac:** myocardial dysfunction, arrhythmias.
- **GI tract:** breakdown in normal mucosal integrity. Large surface area is a large area for entry for gut bacteria. Entry of toxins and bacteria to the pulmonary and systemic circulations. Develop ileus, pancreatitis, ischaemic colitis and acalculous pancreatitis and GI haemorrhage.

- **Renal/hepatic:** AKI, and progressive kidney and liver failure.
- **Neurological:** delirium, progressive coma, cerebral venous thrombosis.
- **Reference:** Surviving sepsis campaign: international guidelines for management of sepsis and septic shock 2021. *Intensive Care Med* 2021;47:1181.

2.22 Haemorrhagic shock

- **About:** trauma is commonest cause of deaths in the young worldwide after HIV/ AIDS. Death is usually due to brain injury or exsanguination. Haemorrhagic shock causes 30–40% of trauma fatalities. In medicine – GI/GU bleed, retroperitoneal, pelvic/femur fracture. You do not exsanguinate from ICH. Target SBP >80 mmHg or palpable radial pulse or cerebration.
- **NB:** give blood over crystalloids. Replace blood with blood/blood products, permissive hypotension, prevent/treat hypothermia, acidosis and coagulopathy. Avoid excess crystalloids: reduced crystalloid use has improved mortality; it increases BP, dilutes clotting factors, destabilises clots and leads to further bleeding. No significant O_2-carrying capacity. Careful balance allowing clot stability at the price of tissue hypoperfusion.
- **Traumatic haemorrhage: Tranexamic acid** 1 g over 10 mins then 1 g over 8 hours and reassess. Massive transfusion may be needed in medical conditions such as gastrointestinal haemorrhage. All life-threatening bleeding becomes surgical once coagulopathy reversed if homeostasis cannot be achieved by other means.
- **Major haemorrhage is defined as loss requiring a >4-unit transfusion.** Young may cope with loss and can look better than expected but can then suddenly decompensate. Older patients may have signs blunted by beta-blockers or have hypertension where a BP of 110 mmHg is for them hypotension. These patients must be identified early so that appropriate fluid strategies are applied. BP is usually the physiological parameter that defines shock, but cardiac output is also important and determines tissue O_2 delivery. A bleeding patient with signs of shock already has a significant blood loss.

Clinical severity assessment score
- **Class 1:** <15% blood volume loss. Tachycardia. May be clinically silent.
- **Class 2:** 15–30% blood volume loss. Partial compensation. Postural BP drop. Vasoconstriction, urine output <30 ml/h. Prevent progression.
- **Class 3:** 30–40% blood volume loss. Decompensating shock with low BP. HR >120, tachypnoea, urine output <20 ml/h, confused.
- **Class 4:** 40% blood volume loss. Marked low BP, tachycardia and tachypnoea. Anuria, comatose. Multi-organ failure. Needs rapid intervention.

Sources of bleeding
- **Basics:** check FBC (normal in very acute blood loss), clotting profile. Reverse any coagulopathy/anticoagulation/low platelets. Bleeding risk in a shocked patient overrides short-term thrombotic risks even with metal heart valves or previous PE. See below.
- **Trauma:** direct compression and control of bleeding points. Retroperitoneal, long bone and pelvic fractures, haemothorax. Splenic. Pelvic binder for pelvic trauma can reduce bleeding. Traction for long bone fractures. Combat Action Tourniquet if compression alone fails to control limb blood loss. Emergency thoracotomy for penetrating chest trauma.

- **Ruptured spleen:** abdominal trauma. Increased risk with splenomegaly or glandular fever. Requires urgent laparotomy. Urgent USS or CT abdomen.
- **AAA:** pulsatile expansile aneurysmal mass + abdominal or back pain. Needs urgent resuscitation as above. FAST scan if AAA >4.5 cm diameter then consider CT and vascular referral and laparotomy. If clinical suspicion high then surgery may proceed on clinical suspicion alone. If stable CT abdomen.
- **Upper or lower GI bleed:** ▶ Section 6.4. Is it variceal or non-variceal bleeding? If patient is dying all GI bleeding is a surgical issue and laparotomy or interventional radiology needed to arrest bleeding. Lower GI bleed consider CTA and interventional radiology for embolisation.
- **Ectopic pregnancy:** fertile female, abdominal pain, missed period, positive β-hCG. Needs urgent laparotomy.
- **Retroperitoneal bleeding:** mass in abdomen, pelvis, bruising at umbilicus (Cullen's sign) or flanks (Grey Turner sign). Anticoagulated. USS/CT abdomen. Reverse anticoagulation.
- **Cryptic shock** is found in those with normal BP and pulse despite significant blood loss. BP is also directly related to blood loss. Where there is brain injury a higher SBP >90 mmHg is advocated. Avoid a coagulopathy and ensure haemostasis maintained using a ratio of 1 FFP to 1–2 units packed cells from the start. Platelets also given.
- **Reference:** Harris T., *et al*. (2012) Early fluid resuscitation in severe trauma. *BMJ*, **345**:e5752.

Management
- **ABC, give O_2. IV access ×2.** Use permissive hypotensive resuscitation (aim for SBP <80–100 mmHg) until haemorrhage is controlled. If there is concern for traumatic brain injury then higher SBP acceptable. Monitor base deficit and lactate levels to assess adequacy of resuscitation. Correct electrolytes, e.g. high K from large volume of packed RBCs, low Ca from citrated anticoagulants, and Na and Cl abnormalities from crystalloid resuscitation. Limiting the use of crystalloid avoids dilutional coagulopathy. Limiting the use of large volumes of NS IV may reduce further hyperchloraemic acidosis.
- Give blood products through warmer. ABC. O_2, start with 1 L NS over 10–20 min. If there is an immediate need for transfusion collect **emergency group O blood** from fridge.

When to call code red
- Loss of more than one blood volume within 24 h (around 70 ml/kg, >5 L in a 70 kg adult) or 50% of total blood volume lost in less than 3 h or bleeding in excess of 150 ml/min.
- Major trauma + 2 or more of penetrating injury, FAST scan positive for intra-abdominal fluid, HR > 120/min, SBP <90 mmHg or senior clinician suspicion of ongoing haemorrhage.
- Non-trauma and bleeding >150 ml/min, blood loss >1500 ml, loss of half circulating blood volume in less than 2 h, rapid blood loss and circulatory failure despite volume resuscitation.
- Aim is correct coagulation. Stop bleeding by physical/surgical means as needed. Call blood banks. Let them know patient name, gender, DOB or approximate age and hospital number if known, location. Give brief clinical details, on warfarin, heparin, DOAC, pregnant or not. Send runner to collect blood. Aim for Hb >10 g/dl.
- **Targets:** Hb >90 g/L, plts >50, fibrinogen >2 g/L. SBP 80–100 mmHg, pH> 7.2, temp >34°C.

Code red: follow local policy

- Constantly reassess status. Repeat bloods (FBC, PT, APTT, fibrinogen, U&E, calcium) every 30 min. Consider if immediate surgery indicated to stop bleeding. Alert surgeons/radiology registrar as needed. May need surgery. Give 10–30 ml 10% **Calcium gluconate** or 10 ml 10% **Calcium chloride** by slow IV injection if low ionised calcium level. Involve other options to control bleeding, e.g. surgery, laparotomy, thoracotomy or obstetrics or interventional radiology as indicated.
- **Tranexamic acid** 1 g IV in 100 ml NS stat over 10 min then 1 g over 8 h slow if less than 3 h from injury. Reduces clot breakdown which reduces mortality and reassess. Avoid for upper/lower GI bleeds.
- **Reverse anticoagulation:** warfarin with 4 factor PCC if needed. **Patients on DOAC and bleeding** ▶ Section 8.11. **Patients on Heparin** and bleeding ▶ Section 8.10. **Heparin:** short half-life. Protamine can lower BP so discuss with haematology.

If code red massive transfusion: packs vary so follow local guidance

- Pack A: 4 units packed red blood cells + Fibrinogen 6 g IV.
- Pack B: 4 units PRBCs + 4 units FFP.
- Pack C: 4 units PRBCs + 4 units Cryoprecipitate, 1 pool platelets.
- Pack D: 4 units PRBCs, 1 unit platelets, 4 units FFP, 4 units cryoprecipitate + 6 g of Fibrinogen.
- Continue as clinically indicated. Reassess situation constantly and if MTP ceases at any time then tell switchboard to stand down. Continue with further shock packs until stand down.

General: monitor Hb, lactate, ABG, FAST scan

- Give (warmed transfusions if possible) packed red cells, FFP, cryoprecipitate and platelets as needed. Some need 10–20 units of PRBCs in 24 h. Once bleeding controlled, a restrictive approach to blood product transfusion is preferred because of the risks and negative outcomes of transfusion, such as multiple organ failure, SIRS, TRALI, increased infection and increased mortality. Large volumes of plasma are needed to correct coagulopathy.
- Early administration is best and may limit consumptive coagulopathy and low platelets and need for blood/blood products. Point of care coagulation testing may help guide haemostatic therapy. Standard coagulation tests such as PT, APTT, INR, platelet count, and fibrinogen usually require 30–60 min for results to be available.
- **Obstetric haemorrhage:** manage as above but caution as patients hypercoagulable and also at risk of DVT/PE.
- **Bleeding and prosthetic metal heart valves:** worst case scenario is an old metal mitral ball and cage valve. Annual risk of thromboembolism of 30% if anticoagulation is stopped. Lowest risks are aortic or newer tilting-disc valves. Lower incidence, 12% per annum, of thromboembolism. In those with potentially life-threatening acute bleeds and metal valves anticoagulation must be stopped temporarily/completely reversed as the risk of death by exsanguination will be significantly higher. Take senior advice. In ischaemic stroke the advice from national guidelines for patients with metal valves is to switch to antiplatelets for a week and then restart anticoagulation. For those with haemorrhagic stroke the risks need to be finely balanced but again anticoagulation should be reversed completely acutely for at least 1–2 weeks.

2.23 ▶ Obstructive shock

- **About:** obstructed circulation impairs low pressure right atrial/ventricular filling and stenosis can block outflow.
- **Haemodynamics:** tamponade / PE / air embolism / tension PTX can restrict right-sided filling. Aortic valve stenosis or aortic dissection can obstruct LV output.
- **Causes:** PE, cardiac tamponade, air embolism, tension PTX. Valve disease.
- **Clinical:** raised JVP and 'a' wave. Muffled heart sounds with tamponade. Tension PTX: hyper-resonant, deviated trachea, subcutaneous emphysema. DVT/PE and breathlessness.
- **Management:** see individual causes. Get ABG. Dimer. Urgent bedside echo, CXR. 14-gauge IV cannula 2nd/3rd ICS or safety triangle for tension PTX and chest drain, LMWH/thrombolysis for PE. Pericardiocentesis for tamponade can be lifesaving. Give fluids/inotropes. See individual sections.

2.24 ▶ Neurogenic shock

- **About:** vasodilation due to loss of sympathetic tone below lesion.
- **Causes:** low cervical or high thoracic cord injury or spinal anaesthesia, Guillain–Barré syndrome, autonomic nervous system toxins, transverse myelitis, other neuropathies.
- **Aetiology:** loss of sympathetic tone. Fall in SVR. Bradycardia.
- **Clinical:** traumatic or medical cord injury. Quadriparesis or paraparesis, bradycardia, warm dry skin, priapism, sensory level, vasodilation, hypoventilation, orthostatic hypotension. Can last 4–5 weeks.
- **Management:** ABC, collar and CT head/neck if suspected spinal trauma. IV fluids. Consider Noradrenaline, Aminophylline, Atropine, Isoprenaline or pacing for bradycardia. Keep SBP >90 mmHg.

03 Cardiology

3.1 Anatomy and physiology

- **Heart: a 4-chamber muscular pump** forcing blood around pulmonary and systemic circulations. Forward flow direction from atria to ventricles to aortic/pulmonary arteries maintained by one-way valves. Heart size of a clenched fist enveloped in a layer of fibrous pericardium within the pericardial sac hanging by the major vessels. Sandwiched between the lungs. Lies behind/protected by the sternum. Inferior surface is the right ventricle (RV) and left ventricle (LV) and part of the right atrium (RA) posteriorly. It is in contact with the diaphragm. Posteriorly is the base of the heart formed by the left atrium in close contact to descending aorta and oesophagus. Atria are storage containers to quickly fill the ventricles aided by atrial kick. The ventricles act as pumps. On the left the LA receives oxygenated blood from the lungs via the four pulmonary veins. The LA and LV are separated by the semilunar mitral valve with anterior and posterior leaflets. The LV pumps blood into the aorta. It has a thick muscular wall. On the right side the RA receives deoxygenated blood from the systemic circulation from the inferior and superior vena cava. The RA and RV are separated by the tricuspid valve with three leaflets. Blood is ejected with systole across the pulmonary valve into the pulmonary artery.
- Right-sided pressures are low (25/10 mmHg). RV is thin-walled compared with the LV (120/80 mmHg). It tolerates increased load poorly. Right border of the heart is formed almost entirely by the RA. Left border of the heart is formed almost entirely by the LV with the LA appendage superiorly. The base or posterior surface is formed almost entirely by the LA which is closely opposed to the oesophagus (useful for TEE/TOE). Inferior or diaphragmatic surface of the heart is made up by the RA/LA. Anterior heart made up of RA/RV and LV from right to left.

Coronary arteries: first branches of the aorta

- **Left coronary artery (LCA):** arises from the left aortic sinus, forms the left main stem (LMS) and branches into the left anterior descending (LAD) artery which lies between RV and LV and runs towards apex. Left anterior descending (LAD) (anterior intraventricular): the LAD gives off the diagonal branches (D1 and D2) and septal branches. Supplies anterior 2/3rd of IV septum and a major portion of left ventricular walls. Circumflex artery (CX), which lies in the left AV groove between the LA and LV, supplies the vessels of the lateral wall of the left ventricle. CX gives off the posterior descending artery (PDA) (10% of patients have a left dominant circulation in which the CX also supplies) and the obtuse marginal branches.
- **Right coronary artery (RCA)** is the first branch of the aorta and arises from the anterior aortic sinus and runs in the AV groove between RA and RV. It gives off the acute marginal branch which runs along the margin of the RV above the diaphragm, sinus node branch in 60% (otherwise supplied by the CX) and AV node branch and continues as the posterior descending artery (RCA dominant) in over 65%, which supplies the inferior wall of the LV and inferior part of the septum.
- **Blood flow** in coronary arteries relates to coronary vasodilatation, which is mediated by adenosine, K^+, hypoxia, and β_2 stimulants and nitric oxide. Flow is *maximal in diastole* when the ventricle relaxes and wall tension is low and O_2

extraction is near maximal, so increased demand requires increased flow and any significantly partially obstructive lesion (>70%) will cause ischaemia.

- Myocardial cells extract up to 70% of O_2 from blood. Tachycardia reduces diastolic interval and increases O_2 demand, which may reveal occult ischaemia. Slowing a fast heart lengthens diastole which aids coronary perfusion. Intra-aortic balloon pumps improve coronary perfusion.
- **Physiology:** normal cardiac output (CO) is about 5 L/min. CO = stroke volume (70 ml) × heart rate (70/min). LV volume 100 ml. EF 70% stroke vol. 70ml. Normal ventricular performance measured as CO depends on adequate stretching of the myocytes and appropriate LV filling. In heart failure excess filling cannot be accommodated. The ability to move blood also depends on afterload made up of systemic vascular resistance (SVR). Blood pressure (BP) = CO × SVR. SVR is maintained by vasoconstrictors, e.g. angiotensin II and aldosterone. MAP mean arterial BP = (SBP−DBP)/3 + DBP.

3.2   Chest pain assessment

Immediate killers are acute MI, aortic dissection, tension PTX and pulmonary embolism. Acute diagnosis and management of these must be your first concern.

- Check ECG, CXR, troponin and dimer. Recent warning to consider ACS in younger patients with a history of Kawasaki disease who may have large coronary artery aneurysms.
- **Cardiac:** ACS pain is central and heavy, radiating to arms or jaw but may be atypical, even pleuritic or chest wall tenderness. Silent in diabetics and elderly. Elderly may present as a fall or confusion. Patient may be pale, sweaty and terrified looking ('angor animi') with a large STEMI.
- **Aorta:** could this be an aortic dissection? History of HTN, tearing pain into back. BP disparity in arms. The lower BP arm has a compromised ipsilateral subclavian. Unfolded aorta on CXR, aortic regurgitation. If so, need urgent CT aorta and avoid any anticoagulants.
- **Lungs:** pleuritic pain if lung infarcts. Wells score for PE + hypoxia or signs of DVT. Signs of chest infection, pain pleuritic? Get CXR to exclude PTX/consolidation/rib fracture. May need CTPA if concerned about PE.
- **Oesophagus:** has patient had an oesophageal stricture dilated or any procedure? Oesophageal perforation. GORD symptoms, oesophagitis.
- **Chest wall:** sternal fracture, rib fractures, Bornholm's disease. Early shingles.

Who to admit (NICE 2015): chest pain and admission?

- **Chest pain killers:** MI, PE, tension PTX, tamponade, aortic dissection, and ruptured oesophagus. Admit those with features suggesting a potentially life-threatening cause. Ischaemic CP is usually related to exertion. MI is like a large weight sitting on chest, but not in all: some women/elderly/diabetics may possibly only have dyspnoea. Pressure or pain in the lower chest or upper abdomen, sweating, dizziness, pre/syncope, upper back pressure, nausea, extreme fatigue.
- **Admit** RR >30 breaths/min, HR >130 bpm, SBP <90 mmHg, DBP <60 mmHg (unless this is normal for them), O_2 sats <92%, central cyanosis (if no history of chronic hypoxia). Altered level of consciousness, temp >38.5°C. Suspected ACS who have current chest pain or signs of complications (pulmonary oedema or

are pain-free but have had chest pain in the last 12 hours and have an abnormal electrocardiogram (ECG).

Management

- **Support:** ABC, O_2 if sats <94% or 28% Venturi at 4 L/min if risk of hypercarbic RF, target 88–92%. Get IV access, rest, telemetry.
- **Check 12-lead ECG:** STEMI or new LBBB: cardiology consult for primary PCI/ thrombolysis. Non-specific ST/T changes suggest NSTEMI. Saddle-shaped ST elevation throughout all leads except aVr suggests pericarditis. In PE, raised HR and S1Q3T3 may be seen but often non-specific.
- **Check FBC, U&E, troponin and D-dimer** (if indicated). Dimer not needed if high probability of PE. Doing dimers without a PE risk assessment is not recommended. Troponin may be elevated in aortic dissection, PE and myocarditis.
- **Check ABG** if breathless or low saturations.
- Portable **CXR** if breathless or low saturations. Look for oedema, mediastinal widening, consolidation, tension PTX, fibrosis, apical shadowing, mass.
- If chest pain suggestive of angina suspected give sublingual **2 sprays of GTN** (800 mcg) or **GTN** 500 mcg tablet SL if SBP >110 mmHg and reassess. If pain is severe then give **Diamorphine** 2.5–5 mg **IV or Morphine** 5–10 mg IV with an anti-emetic, usually **Metoclopramide** 10 mg slow IV.
- If ACS possible, then consider Aspirin 300 mg PO and follow local guidance, which should be for PPCI if there is a STEMI; for further management see ▶Section 3.7. If aortic dissection, then avoid anticoagulation and arrange CT chest ▶Section 3.17. If PE considered and no contraindication then anticoagulate ▶Section 4.17.
- For those with likely angina not needing admission consider same day cardiology assessment and start appropriate medications and give advice.

3.3 ▶ Chest pain differentials

- **Acute coronary syndrome:** central heavy 'weight on chest' chest pain with radiation into arms/jaw. Risk factors: smoker, HTN, lipids, diabetes. Sweating, distressed, pale. ECG diagnostic for STEMI. IV access. Trop. Consider urgent reperfusion if <12 h ▶Section 3.7. Oxygen only if hypoxia. Give ACS pain glyceryl trinitrate (GTN) and/or an opioid (e.g. IV Morphine/Diamorphine, given slowly over 5 min). Give Aspirin 300 mg (unless clear evidence that allergic). Do a 12-lead ECG. NB: palpable chest wall tenderness is reported in some cases of ACS and is not a reliable sign to exclude ACS. ▶Section 3.7.
- **Aortic dissection:** history of HTN. Widened mediastinum on CXR. Hypertensive but appears 'shocked'. BP different in arms. Inferior MI on ECG if right coronary artery obstructed at ostia (left main stem obstruction usually fatal). Get urgent CT aortogram or TOE. BP lowering. Proximal lesion move now to cardiothoracic centre for surgery. Treat pain. Avoid ACS management. Lower BP and ▶Section 3.17.
- **Pulmonary embolism:** clinical context: immobility, cancer, stroke. Wells score. Sudden pain plus breathlessness. Sometimes with syncope and dyspnoea. Collapse in toilet. Obvious increased RR. Hypoxic ABG. Fall in saturations. Look for risk factors. Look for DVT. Anticoagulate, consider thrombolysis with RV dysfunction or circulatory collapse. IV fluids support RV dysfunction. Needs CTPA/VQ scan. ▶Section 4.17.
- **Pneumothorax:** sudden breathlessness and pain. Clicking sound heard on auscultation, hyper-resonant, CXR diagnostic but can be subtle. If tension PTX

(acute breathless hypotensive) then insert a large-bore cannula through the second intercostal space in the mid-clavicular line, on the side of the PTX, though some now advocate a cannula in the safety triangle, ▶ Section 4.12.

- **Pneumonia:** unwell, cough, fever, pleurisy, high WCC, CXR changes. ▶ Section 4.14.
- **Oesophageal spasm:** sudden intense chest pain lasts minutes. With swallowing. Benign.
- **Oesophagitis:** food-related, reflux symptoms, eased by antacids. Middle aged. Obese.
- **Oesophageal perforation/rupture:** Boerhaave syndrome. Severe chest pain following oesophageal instrumentation or forceful vomiting. Toxic patient. Avoid NG tubes or endoscopy. NBM. IV fluids. Urgent CXR/CT and cardiothoracic surgical consult.
- **Costochondritis** (Tietze's syndrome): tenderness over costochondral joints, classically the 2nd costochondral joint. NB: chest wall tenderness seen with ACS pain too. Treat with NSAID and determine if there is a physical cause.
- **Chest wall pain/musculoskeletal:** localised defined tenderness. X-ray ribs and sternum. Trauma-related or metastases. Check ALP/X-ray. NSAIDs.
- **Takotsubo cardiomyopathy:** similar to ACS. Older females classically, chest pain, dyspnoea, palpitations, N&V, syncope. Cardiogenic shock. Reversible. See ▶ Section 3.23.
- **Acute sickling crisis:** sickle cell disease. May be hypoxic with pleuritic pain. ▶ Section 8.2.
- **Pericarditis:** possibly viral or recent MI and Dressler's syndrome. Eased by sitting forwards, audible rub, saddle-shaped ST elevation. Treat with NSAIDs/colchicine. ▶ Section 3.19.
- **Shingles:** may be unilateral dermatomal distribution, chest wall pain before the distinctive band of vesicles. Elderly, immunocompromised. ▶ Section 9.22.
- **Kawasaki disease:** young person with chest pain and myocardial ischaemia. History of KD with large often calcified coronary artery aneurysms which can thrombose.
- **Idiopathic:** despite investigations, cause unknown. The main need is to exclude sinister causes. Manage residual pain with analgesia.
- **Pleurisy/pneumonia:** can be secondary to infection – viral or bacterial and underlying lung consolidation or possible connective tissue disease, neoplastic or idiopathic. Always consider if the history matches a possible PE and pulmonary infarction. Listen for a pleural rub. Check FBC, ESR, CXR. Consider autoantibodies if the suggestion of RA or SLE. Non-sinister causes are managed conservatively with NSAID analgesia. ▶ Section 4.14.

3.4 ▶ Palpitations

- **Red flags** to consider admitting to CCU or getting cardiology consult if: palpitations precede syncope, palpitations with exercise, associated chest pain or dizziness, family history of arrhythmic death, structural heart disease, HCM, poor LV function, abnormal ECG – LBBB, ischaemia, LVH, long QTc, VT, TdP, 2nd/3rd degree heart block.
- **Assessment:** find out what they mean by palpitations. Medically it is abnormal awareness of heartbeat. Ask patient to tap out the palpitations if possible. Rate and regularity, frequency. When started. Determine clinical context. Duration. Any obvious precipitants or relieving factors. Caffeine taken, other drugs, e.g. alcohol, cocaine. Antihistamines and other drugs that can alter QTc.

- **Associated symptoms:** dyspnoea, presyncope, polyuria, chest pain or other symptoms? How did it stop – slowly or suddenly? If they can provoke it please attempt it during ECG monitoring. If they have palpitations now then get an ECG or at least feel pulse. A normal pulse and symptoms is reassuring. Some just more aware of normal heartbeat.
- **Causes:** if SVT occurs, treat it and send home.
- **Investigations:** FBC, U&E, troponin, TFT, 24 h to 7-d tape as available and depending on the frequency of the arrhythmia and likelihood of capture. Patient should hopefully have an episode with tape on. Infrequent episodes may need a cardio memo device implanted. Consider advise not to drive if palpitations would affect driving. During spell can ask to attend ED for an ECG which may be diagnostic.
- **Risk assessment:** markers for lethal arrhythmias are known heart disease, family history, syncope or presyncope, poor LV or associated symptoms. These patients are 'higher risk'. Consider admission for monitoring or investigations. Senior consult if unsure.
- **Avoid admitting** benign ectopics and supraventricular arrhythmias who, once managed acutely, can be given advice, and followed up in clinic.
- **Extrasystoles:** atrial/ventricular ectopics cause a strong beat after the compensatory pause. Treatment not needed if out of the context of risks mentioned. Can be reassured and discharged, reduce caffeine. Manage precipitants. Rarely needs treatment. May consider cardiology or ambulatory care; follow up. If severe consider **Metoprolol** 25 mg OD or **Atenolol** 25 mg OD as needed. ▶Section 3.11.
- **SVT (AVRT/AVNRT):** common, often benign. OP cardiology follow-up for consideration of meds/ablation. Discuss WPW with cardiologists. Admit WPW and pre-excited AF. ▶Section 3.14.
- **AF:** determine if rate or rhythm control and anticoagulated. ▶Section 3.15.
- **VT:** admit and assess. See treatment algorithm ▶Sections 3.12–3.13.
- **2nd/3rd degree HB/sinus pauses >3 secs:** cardiology consult for PPM. Stop rate-slowing drugs. ▶Section 3.16.

3.5 ▶ Syncope and transient loss of consciousness

- **Introduction:** syncope is a sudden transient loss of consciousness (TLOC) and postural tone with spontaneous recovery. TLOC leads to a fall if the patient is upright and unsupported. However, not all falls are due to TLOC and are dealt with elsewhere (Simple falls, ▶Section 15.2). Always consider PE, arrhythmias fast and slow, aortic stenosis/HOCM, autonomic dysfunction. Differential includes causes of transient hypotension as well as neurological diagnoses. Transient syncope suggests a global CNS issue such as an episode of cerebral hypoperfusion, a generalised seizure, acute hydrocephalus and others. Some causes remain unknown and labelled as a 'funny turn'. This leaves the opportunity for later making the correct diagnosis.
- **Normal physiology of standing:** standing requires prompt physiological adaptation to gravity. There is an instantaneous descent of about 500 ml of blood from the thorax to the lower abdomen, buttocks and legs. There can be up to a 25% shift of plasma volume out of the vasculature and into the interstitial tissue, which reduces venous return to the heart. The result is a transient decline in both arterial pressure and cardiac filling. This has the effect of reducing the pressure on the baroreceptors, triggering a compensatory sympathetic mediated increase in heart rate and systemic vasoconstriction. The assumption of upright posture results in

a 10–20 bpm increase in heart rate, a negligible change in systolic blood pressure, and approximately 5 mmHg increase in diastolic blood pressure. With age, diuretics, vasodilators, dehydration and any transient obstructive element there is much more likelihood of a simple transient failure of cerebral perfusion pressure. Following gravity to the floor quickly restores cerebral perfusion.

- **Discussion:** feeling as if about to faint or buzzing ears or vision blurring and constricting, suggests a low BP cause with reduced cerebral flow. Bruising to the face or other injury may suggest severe and sudden loss of consciousness with no time for protective reflexes. Try to get the history from patient and a witness of the episode even if you need to ring them. Was there chest pain, headache (SAH) or breathlessness before? What position – standing, sitting, lying? Doing what – coughing, micturition, exertion? What was head position – looking up? Patient getting out of a hot bath or standing up in church? Did patient use GTN? Grey colour suggests faint and low BP. Vasovagal usually recover quickly. What was BP/pulse in ambulance notes? Vasovagal syncope common and often exacerbated by antihypertensives/anti-anginals. How long until regain of consciousness – before or after ambulance? Is patient pregnant? – a very common cause of fainting. Not all that jerks is a potential seizure. Momentary cerebral hypoperfusion in vasovagal syncope can cause jerks lasting 5–10 sec. Urinary incontinence also seen with vasovagal syncope. Determine real level of consciousness – ask witness if patient was 'like a dead person' and one often finds that an 'unconscious' patient was not so and was even communicating to the witness throughout. Truly syncopal patients will usually go to ground unless held up or supported in some way. Sitting is an active process and patients will fall out of a chair or slump on a sofa. Those who are unable to go to ground to restore perfusion (even simple vasovagals) can end up with more severe presentation with fitting and hypoxic brain injury. Give driving advice. In the UK it is the doctor's responsibility to advise a patient with a potentially recurring cause of syncope not to drive and document it. Take senior advice where unsure. It is the patient's responsibility to inform the DVLA.
- **Secondary trauma:** exclude ICH, SDH and ruptured spleens and fractures. Non-displaced hip fracture may be missed and so not all will have classical leg shortening and external rotation. Repeated examination may be needed. Pain may not be noted until attempts to mobilise. Initial trauma surveys can miss things so have a low threshold to repeat examination and imaging if there is evidence or suspicion of possible problems. Do not get distracted by the secondary trauma and forget about the primary cause of syncope.
- **Post-syncope clues:** headache, drowsiness, rapid recovery over minutes (vasovagal), gradual recovery over several hours (seizure). Breathless (PE), weakness (stroke/seizure), abdominal pain (leaking AAA), sore tongue (seizure – bites side of tongue).
- **Note:** the difficulty is often in separating causes of reduced cerebral perfusion and seizure. Potentially malignant causes of reduced cerebral perfusion are rare but need urgent cardiological specialist assessment.

Causes of syncope/TLOC

- **Acute coronary syndrome:** a potential cause of syncope (cardiac transplant, elderly, diabetics may not have chest pain). ECG will show ST/T wave changes, ST elevation, CHB, other forms of heart block, LBBB, RBBB, hemiblocks, VT, etc. Paramedics may capture a non-sustained VT, or heart block, or ischaemic changes, or the cause was 'pump failure' and poor LV or even RV. *Beware the rush to overdiagnosing ACS and starting antithrombotics in simple collapses unless there was* *chest pain and ACS-type ECG changes, or a definite ischaemic arrhythmia.* Without these most do not have ACS but may have had head trauma/SAH or hip trauma on falling and they will bleed and develop ICH/SDH, etc. If unclear wait for early troponin. ▸ Section 3.7.

- **Arrhythmias:** brady- and tachyarrhythmias can cause syncope/presyncope and falls. Ensure ECG checked and any ambulance recordings reviewed. Particularly interested in sinus pauses >3 sec, CHB and VT, non-sustained VT, and ECG evidence of conduction tissue disease. Rarely, but importantly, ECG changes of Brugada syndrome, e.g. RBBB or HCM or RV dysplasia, long QT syndromes precipitating VT, WPW syndrome with short PR and delta wave and SVT or AF, ACS, high/low K^+. A 12-lead ECG is mandatory. Most malignant arrhythmias are VT due to IHD/cardiomyopathy and are associated with poor LV function. Ask about chest pain or palpitations prior. If you suspect an arrhythmia then keep for at least 24–48 h of telemetry, echo and OP 7-d tape and cardiology consult. If there are sufficient concerns (family history of sudden death, poor LV function, Brugada syndrome or cardiac arrest), then patient stays until decision made, e.g. some may need **ICD** insertion. May need 7-d tape or reveal device. If there is conduction disease or low HR look to see if it is drug-induced (e.g. beta-blockers, verapamil) and discuss if sufficient evidence for pacemaker with cardiologist. No driving until resolved and DVLA referral. ▸ Section 3.10.

- **Cardiac structural:** look for murmurs of obstructive lesions (which may disappear with very severe AS and low CO): if mean gradient >40 mmHg or area <1 cm², HCM, mitral stenosis or atrial myxoma, tamponade. Get echo and ECG, telemetry and cardiology consult.

- **Pregnancy:** a cause of low BP and predisposition to fainting. Always consider in fertile female. Rarely ectopic pregnancy can present with collapse and abdominal pain and shock.

- **Respiratory:** PE, cough syncope, severe pulmonary hypertension.

- **Vasovagal syncope:** very common. Vasodepressor (BP falls), cardio-inhibitory (HR falls). Get ECG, consider tilt table if repeated episodes despite simple measures and cause not apparent. Lying/sitting and standing BP. Review medications – GTN spray? Are they hypovolaemic from diuretics? Consider cough syncope, micturition syncope, syncope during/after large meal ± alcohol. Fasting, fear, heat. Note twitching and jerks and urinary incontinence may be seen and can be misdiagnosed as epilepsy. For a reliable diagnosis look for the 3 Ps – provocation (pain, fright, etc.), prodromal (dimmed vision and hearing for a few seconds) and posture (when standing).

- **Postural hypotension:** precipitated by dehydration, hypovolaemia, pigmentation (consider Addison's disease), autonomic dysfunction (e.g. diabetes, multiple system atrophy, amyloid), Parkinson's disease. Check medications for antihypertensives, nitrates, GTN spray, calcium antagonists, levodopa, tricyclic antidepressants, phenothiazine. Telemetry, ECG, look for and stop unneeded drugs. Orthostatic low BP can be proven with tilt table.

- **Postural orthostatic tachycardia syndrome (POTS):** mostly in young females. Orthostatic tachycardia but not hypotension. Symptoms of raised HR >130 bpm, exercise intolerance, presyncope, disabling fatigue, headache, and mental clouding. HR increase ≥30 bpm with prolonged standing, elevated upright plasma noradrenaline, and a low blood volume. Tilt table, echo. Hydration. Increase water and salt intake – NaCl tablets 1 g/tablet TDS with meals. Exercise, propranolol, verapamil, ivabradine, sinus node ablation/modification are used.

- **Carotid sinus hypersensitivity:** pressure on neck causes syncope. Tight collars, shaving, head turning. Consider CSM whilst monitored. Looking for symptomatic pauses >3 sec or fall in SBP of > 50 mmHg. May need pacemaker if pause. It may be wise to get a Doppler before CSM as bilateral internal carotid stenosis can cause syncope and mimic hypersensitivity, especially if recent TIA or stroke. CSM should be done 10 sec each side with cardiac monitoring and done when supine and standing.
- **Hypoglycaemia:** a diabetic on insulin or oral hypoglycaemic agents or Addison's disease or insulinoma. Recovered with glucose.
- **Subarachnoid haemorrhage:** worst ever/thunderclap headache and collapse and recovery. Needs CT/LP. ▶Section 11.22.
- **Pulmonary embolism:** breathlessness and collapse, raised HR, hypoxia. Elevated D-dimer. DVT. Risk factors. Consider treatment dose LMWH prior to CT–PA/VQ scan. Mechanism may be a saddle embolus which disintegrates quickly. ▶Section 4.17.
- **Complex seizure:** loss of consciousness, tongue biting especially side, slow to wake up, known epilepsy, incontinent, headache after. Get a CT head acutely. No driving and DVLA referral. Seizure advice. Referral to first fit clinic. ▶Section 11.15.
- **Aortic dissection:** tearing interscapular/chest pain plus syncope. Consider diagnosis. CXR, CT aorta/chest. Raised D-dimers. ▶Section 3.17.
- **Occult haemorrhage:** GI where melaena delayed, leaking AAA but pain usually. Hidden bleeding, e.g. retroperitoneal, psoas muscle particularly in those on warfarin. Coagulopathy. PV bleed in pregnancy. Patient low BP and syncopal. ▶Section 2.22.
- **Autonomic dysfunction:** autonomic dysfunction seen with Guillain–Barré syndrome, acute porphyria or transverse myelitis, amyloid and diabetes and rarer causes. Lose the ability to sweat, bowel and bladder dysfunctions. Bloating, N&V, abdominal pain and impotence. Constipation alternates with diarrhoea. HR fixed rate of 40–50 bpm with an inappropriate response. Pupils dilated, poorly reactive to light.
- **Addisonian crisis:** occasional subtle presentation with syncope. Low BP, low Na, pigmentation, autoimmune disease, recent abrupt cessation of steroids. Check U&E, cortisol. Short synACTHen test. Give IV **Hydrocortisone** 100 mg ▶Section 5.1.
- **Colloid cyst:** CT brain generally diagnostic, shows a cyst in IIIrd ventricle. Syncope is due to abrupt rises in ICP.
- **Subclavian steal:** arm movement or exercise precipitates pre/syncope or posterior circulation symptoms. MRA aorta/subclavians for stenosis.
- **Somnolescence:** patients simply falling asleep. Consider sleep apnoea. Epworth sleepiness scale: >10 suggest excessive sleepiness. Sleep studies. Alcohol, sedation, smoking, large neck (obstructive).
- **Pacemaker dysfunction:** if concerns get pacemaker interrogated and reprogrammed if needed. Often pacing activity only kicks in when needed so absence of activity does not always mean dysfunction.

Assessment

- **Answering referral:** how is the patient now? BP, HR, pulse, glucose. Unresponsive, no breaths – call arrest team. Are they protecting the airway especially if GCS <9? Any injury sustained? Describe the events of syncope – low BP, chest pain, breathlessness, confusion (see above).

- **On arrival and thoughts:** the history and witness report are key. Anything sounding like a seizure or TLOC/syncope, must advise no driving until full assessment and later discussion. Look for any sign of structural cardiac disease. Run through typical causes. General and cardiovascular and neurological exam. Main worry is malignant arrhythmias and alarm bells should ring if ECG abnormal, history of ACS or poor LV function or long QT syndrome, family history or Brugada. If concerned admit under cardiology and place on CCU for telemetry. Arrange CT head if any concerns of acute seizure, SAH, colloid cyst or any other cause of syncope. Assess any obvious secondary injury. Has there been a hip or other fracture? Is there head or scalp injury? Is intracerebral haemorrhage the cause of the syncope or the result of it? Refer accordingly. Always give driving advice to drivers post-syncope. If unsure acutely of cause and happy to discharge for expectant management then reasonable to advise not to drive until all results back and then you can make an assessment or suggest referral to DVLA. Very definite vasovagal syncope in the standing position is unlikely to occur whilst driving. Eliminate any precipitant. If there is a convincing vasovagal syncope story with precipitant and rapid recovery, limit any causes or precipitants and consider discharge.

Focused investigations on likely causality
- FBC, U&E, LFT. Short SynACTHen, TFT, troponin, D-dimer.
- 12-lead ECG: long QTc, Brugada, cardiomyopathy. 7-day tape: NSVT, sinus node disease, bradycardia.
- External loop: if more than one attack per week. Internal loop: infrequent attacks, useful, expensive. Look for non-sustained SVT, bifascicular block, RBBB/LAFB or RBBB/LPFB, HR <50 bpm. QRS >120 msec, abnormal QT, pre-excited QRS, RBBB with ST elevation V1–V3 (Brugada), ARVC.
- ECG with carotid sinus massage: consider in elderly but get ultrasound to exclude severe atheroma which could result in syncope or stroke.
- Tilt table: cardio-inhibitory/vasodepressor/POTS: often fails to guide therapy.
- CT brain, MRI brain, LP for SAH, EEG for epilepsy.
- Echocardiogram, electrophysiological studies, cardiac MRI.
- Genetic testing for rare disorder: Brugada, congenital long QT.
- Electrophysiological studies: look for induced arrhythmias.

Some guidance on whom to admit, monitor and investigate:
- Syncope supine or exercising, associated palpitations, family history of sudden cardiac death.

Managing symptomatic postural hypotension
- Weigh up need to stop/reduce BP-lowering meds. ACEi, ARB, beta-blockers, diuretics, calcium channel blockers, vasodilators, tamsulosin, MAOI, TCA, phenothiazines, dopamine, dopamine agonists.
- Identify cause – may be a systemic autonomic neuropathy or part of a neurodegenerative illness or neuropathy or amyloid.
- Echo, tilt table, 24-h tape, EST – exaggerated increase in HR with POTS and mild exercise. Head up tilt on bed, compression stockings, salt loading. If persisting consider drugs: **Fludrocortisone** 50–100 mcg OD, **Midodrine** 2.5–10 mg TDS (alpha-1 agonist), beta-blockers, **Paroxetine** 10–20 mg OD.
- PPM: for cardioinhibitory syncope disease and bradyarrhythmia. Pauses >3 sec. Correlated with symptoms.

3.6   Sudden cardiac death

- **About:** most sudden cardiac deaths (SCDs) are arrhythmogenic due to ACS/IHD. Without early defibrillation (internal or otherwise) survival is poor. Other rare causes are shown below. Divide into normal heart (echo/MRI/angiography) and those without.
- **Management:** if likely acute ACS then see below. Try to determine aetiology. Risk assessment. Echocardiogram. Genetic studies in some. Electrophysiological studies. Selected groups require consideration for an AICD. Higher risk: poor LV <35%, cardiac arrest (VF/VT) post-MI especially post-acute phase, family history of sudden cardiac death, inducible VT at EPS, dilated cardiomyopathy.

Sudden cardiac death and a macroscopically normal heart

- **Brugada syndrome:** idiopathic VF. 20% of SCD in structurally normal hearts, sudden unexpected nocturnal death (SUND) in SE Asian men, onset after age 40, 'coved' ST segment elevation in V1–V3. ECG changes may be dynamic and concealed. Placing V1/V2 in the 2nd rather than 4th space can help detect changes. Minority have sodium channel defect. Only an AICD has been proven to help. May have self-terminating VT/VF, waking up at night after agonal respiration. Drugs used to unmask disease include ajmaline, flecainide under expert guidance only. Also see www.brugadadrugs.org.

- **Long QT syndrome:** congenital and acquired long QT syndrome. Check family history Ca, Mg, drugs and other causes.
- **Pre-excitation syndrome:** WPW with AF and an irregular fast ventricular rate over accessory pathway. Resting ECG may show short PR interval and delta wave of pre-excitation unless the pathway is concealed.
- **Commotio cordis:** young adults with low-impact precordial trauma with a projectile object such as a baseball, hockey puck, fist, rubber bullet, or even a rugby ball. The blow must occur in the 20 millisecond vulnerable point of a T wave. Early CPR and defibrillation.

Sudden cardiac death, structurally abnormal heart

- **Arrhythmogenic RV cardiomyopathy (ARVC):** see ▶ Section 3.23.
- **Ischaemic heart disease:** ACS setting. May be arrhythmic or asystolic or LV wall rupture and tamponade. Usually due to atherosclerosis but rarely APLS, arteritis, coronary embolism, coronary artery anomalies. Ischaemic cardiomyopathy with poor LV function. ▶ Section 3.8.
- **Cardiomyopathy:** DCM, HCM. IHD with poor LV, hypertrophic cardiomyopathy, LV non-compaction. ▶ Section 3.23.
- **Valve disease:** aortic stenosis. Critical gradient, heart failure, chest pain, syncope. Mitral disease, mitral valve prolapse.
- **Myocarditis:** ventricular arrhythmias. ▶ Section 3.18.
- **Congenital heart disease:** coarctation of the aorta, transposition of great vessels, VSD, Fallot's, anomalous coronary arteries.

3.7   Acute coronary syndrome

- **About:** ACS must be considered in all those with chest pain and some without chest pain: new dyspnoea, shock, syncope. Atypical (non-chest pain) presentations commoner in diabetics, elderly and women. An ECG is the key test to diagnose ACS with new acute changes. The immediate risk is of VF, pump failure and death from cardiac arrest. Defibrillation must be immediately available. Those with ST elevation ACS have vessel occlusion and must be assessed urgently for primary PCI or thrombolysis. Patients with non-ST elevation ACS are older with more comorbidities. Their need and timing for PCI depends on ongoing or refractory chest pain, or heart failure or cardiogenic shock, or assessed to be high risk. Thrombolysis never indicated for NSTEMI.

- **Epidemiology:** in-hospital mortality lower than STEMI, same at 6 months but worse long term. Those at higher risk should be considered for appropriate medical therapy and revascularisation within 72 h of admission. 12% of patients with ACS die within 1 month and 20% within 6 months of the index event.
- **Caution:** there are many cases of ACS with pain that was pleuritic, stabbing and with chest wall tenderness. Chest pain in females can be misdiagnosed as non-cardiac. Take advice if unsure. Determine risk factors.

MI classification based on aetiology

- **Type 1:** spontaneous MI due to plaque erosion/rupture, dissection or fissure. Seen in those with atherosclerosis – unstable plaque ruptures releasing thrombogenic material. *In situ* thrombosis and occlusive MI.
- **Type 2:** MI due to increased demand other than occlusive CAD: anaemia, arrhythmia, PE, critical illness, resp failure, shock, severe HTN.
- **Type 3:** MI with sudden cardiac death with no biomarkers.
- **Type 4:** post PCI and stenting ECG changes and raised troponins.
- **Type 5:** post CABG. ECG changes and raised troponins.

Classification and pathophysiology

- **Unstable angina (UA):** increasing CP or at lower levels of exercise. ECG changes of ischaemia but a normal troponin.
- **Non-ST elevation ACS:** sub-occlusive flow lesion and thrombus: needs antithrombotics and antianginals to maintain patency. Myocardial damage may be found. Chest pain or equivalent + ECG changes + raised troponin. The distinction between NSTEMI and UA is retrospective when the hsTn I result is available later.
- **ST elevation** (or new LBBB) ACS: plaque rupture and occlusive thrombus: needs 'culprit' vessel opening (PCI/thrombolysis) + antithrombotics. Chest pain/equivalent + ST elevation/new LBBB + raised troponin.
- **Myocardial infarction (± ST elevation)** needs a rise and/or fall of cardiac troponin (cTn), with at least one value above the 99th centile upper reference limit (URL) and with at least one of the following: symptoms, ST elevation or other changes, new LBBB, Q waves on ECG, imaging supports myocardial loss, intracoronary thrombus on angiography or at post-mortem.
- **Exacerbating factors:** reduced coronary flow due to raised wall pressures, e.g. aortic stenosis, HCM, raised HR, e.g. AF, VT with shortened diastole will lower coronary blood flow. Raised myocardial work will reduce O_2 demand and ischaemia. Anaemia: target Hb is 9–10 g/dl in IHD. Treat severe hypertension. Reduce O_2 demands – sepsis, PE, low BP, shock.
- **Clinical:** present as cardiac arrest, chest pain, breathlessness. Take careful history of onset of symptoms and relation to exertion. Ischaemic chest pain at rest is ominous. Central chest pain may radiate to arms/jaw. Nausea, vomiting, breathlessness, sweating, palpitations. Signs of LVF – dyspnoea, increased HR, S3, bibasal

crepitations. Look for murmurs, MR, VSD, aortic stenosis, HOCM. ACS in elderly – falls, delirium and syncope. Epigastric symptoms (inferior MI). No chest pain – MI in elderly and diabetics. Pale, terrified, cold peripheries, pulmonary oedema and cardiogenic shock.

- **Differentials:** pulmonary embolism, aortic dissection, pericarditis, oesophageal spasm/reflux/rupture, biliary tract disease, peptic ulcer disease, pancreatitis, chest wall pain, pleurisy/pneumonia, sickling crisis, herpes zoster, Bornholm disease.
- **Poor prognosis:** ongoing and recurrent ischaemia, widespread ECG changes, raised CK/troponins, low BP. MR with ischaemia, pulmonary oedema, cardiogenic shock. Prognosis for all ACS patients can be assessed using GRACE score (see www.mdcalc.com/calc/1099/grace-acs-risk-mortality-calculator).
- **Kawasaki disease:** can present with an ACS and may be STEMI/NSTEMI. Management is usually medical and involves anticoagulation. PCI to aneurysmal arteries usually avoided due to risks of rupture. Use medical therapy including thrombolysis but avoid streptokinase if recent (<6 months) streptococcal pharyngitis. Take early expert help.

Rapid assessment

- Targeted history, good IV access, rapid exam and BP in both arms. Send bloods for troponin, FBC, U&E, glucose, lipids, immediate 12-lead ECG and determine if criteria for ST elevation ACS present. Repeat at 15 min intervals if ongoing symptoms and non-diagnostic. Echocardiogram can be invaluable as it will show wall movement abnormalities suggesting ischaemia/infarction especially if ECG ambiguous.
- Echocardiogram if available to assess LV function and regional wall abnormalities. May even pick up evidence of a dissection – intimal flap, acute aortic incompetence. Consider differentials – see chest pain, notably PE and aortic dissection, myo-/pericarditis which may have ECG changes. If not ST elevation ACS assess GRACE/TIMI score to direct therapy. There is some variability in anticoagulant or antithrombotic regimens between centres and specialists and so local guidance should be taken and followed.

Investigations

- **Bloods: FBC:** low Hb exacerbates ACS. **U&E:** renal function. **Glucose:** diabetes. Check lipids.
- **12-lead ECG:** STEMI changes: (a) normal ECG; (b) hyperacute T waves; (c) ST elevation; (d) Q waves and T wave inversion; (e) Q wave and T wave normalises; (f) ST elevation resolves, Q wave persists. Persisting ST elevation consider LV aneurysm. Always repeat ECG every 15 min if new chest pain. Compare with previous ECG. ECG splits patients with a suspicion of ACS in two categories requiring different therapeutic approaches:
  1. **ST elevation MI/ACS:** see section below for changes.
  2. **Non-ST elevation MI/ACS:** symmetrical T wave changes including inversion (in leads V1–V4 can suggest LAD stenosis). Transient ST elevation ± but usually dynamic ST depression. **Pseudonormalisation:** T waves which are usually inverted become upright with ischaemia. **Poor R wave progression:** usually transition of raised R wave height V1 to V6 is lost with anterior wall infarction.

(a)

(b)

(c)

(d)

(e)

(f)

- **CXR:** widened mediastinum consider aortic dissection. LVF.
- **NT-proBNP:** a natriuretic peptide. Elevated with heart failure.
- **CKMB:** cardio specific. Useful if issues with troponin assay.
- **Cardiac troponin T:** admission and 12 h: <0.01 mcg/L unstable angina, 0.01–1 mcg/L: unstable angina/myocyte necrosis. Some guidelines define this as MI and others (UA) >1 mcg/L: MI.
- **Cardiac troponin I:** at admission and 12 h <0.06 ng/ml: normal; 0.07–0.49 ng/ml: indeterminate, >0.50 ng/ml: consistent with myocardial necrosis.
- **High sensitivity troponin (hsTn):** more sensitive but less specific. Assess within clinical context. Higher 'normal' levels are now used in older patients. **Normal (no MI)** (hsTn T <14 ng/L). A result of <14 ng/L more than 6 h after symptoms rules out MI. **Possible MI** (hsTn T 14–30 ng/L). If the history does not suggest ACS and the patient is stable with a low risk of MI a second sample is suggested at 3 h after the first. A rise or fall in the hsTn T will point to an acute diagnosis and possible MI. The patient should be admitted if the change in level is >±7 ng/L. **Probable MI** (hsTn T >30 ng/L). Large changes suggest MI. Other causes of elevated levels include sepsis, dissection, PE, myo-/pericarditis, cardiac failure, renal failure, stroke. Evaluation should be combined with clinical common sense and with history and risks assessed, ECG, TIMI/GRACE score (*Br J Cardiol*, 2013;20(4)). **Other causes of high troponin:** AKI/CKD, CCF/LVF, hypertensive crisis, arrhythmias, PE, severe pulmonary hypertension, myocarditis, stroke/SAH, aortic dissection, aortic valve disease or HCM, cardiac contusion, ablation, pacing, cardioversion, hypothyroidism, apical ballooning syndrome, infiltrative diseases, e.g. amyloidosis/sarcoidosis, drug toxicity, burns, rhabdomyolysis, critically ill patients, especially with respiratory failure, or sepsis.
- **Echocardiogram:** assess LV function, valves and useful to detect tamponade, cardiomyopathy and effusions. Look for wall movement abnormalities suggesting ischaemia/infarction. Useful if ECG ambiguous.
- **Cardiac stress tests:** if pain settles and ECG changes equivocal and troponin negative then consider controlled different ways to cause transient measurable myocardial ischaemia. Objective evidence of ischaemia may be displayed on ECG, echo or by scintigraphy. Tests to assess hibernating myocardium whose viability will improve with revascularisation by PCI or CABG. Cardiac MRI or PET scan. Dobutamine stress echo, thallium. Most give a sensitivity of over 90% except stress echo (70%).
- **Immediate angiography in ST elevation MI/ACS:** primary PCI is indicated in those with STEMI presenting <12 h from symptoms as it allows opening of culprit vessel and opportunity for angioplasty and stenting or thrombus aspiration. It may also be needed in later presentation with shock or failure or ongoing ischaemia. It can help select those for CABG (see below). In non-ST elevation ACS PCI is suggested in higher risk patients to diagnose IHD, define disease, identify vessels for angioplasty and stenting or patients for CABG. Angiography for medium to high-risk non-ST elevation ACS or NSTEMI is done on an individualised assessment.

ECG changes in STEMI (get old ECGs)

- ST elevation in 2 anatomically contiguous leads
  - V2/V3 >1.5 mm women, >2 mm men >40y and >2.5 mm men <40y
  - V4R/V3R >1.0 mm in men <30y or 0.5 mm in all others
  - All other leads >1 mm
  - V7–9 >0.5mm

- New LBBB
- ST depression in V1–V4 with dominant R wave: post MI
- The presence of reciprocal ST-segment depression opposite the infarct territory increases the specificity for acute MI.

- De Winter T waves: STE equivalent. 2% of acute LAD occlusions. Often missed. There is ST depression and peaked T waves in the precordial leads. Discuss for PCI. More likely younger/male/dyslipidaemia.
- Wellens syndrome biphasic or deeply inverted T waves in V2–V3. Recent resolved chest pain. Suggests critical stenosis of the LAD.

Localisation of likely culprit lesion
- **Large anterior:** V1–V6/I/AVL/LBBB: proximal LAD or left main stem.
- **Septal:** V1/V2 alone: thrombus septal branch of LAD.
- **Anterior:** V3–V6: mid LAD after septal branch.
- **Lateral:** V5, V6, I, aVL: proximal left circumflex or high diagonal of LAD.
- **Inferior:** II, III, aVF: right coronary artery or LCx. Inferior MI pattern: check for STE V3/4R suggest RV infarct.
- **Posterior:** ST depression in V1–V4 dominant R wave upright T waves RCA/LCx. Place leads V7/V8/V9 over posterior left below scapula. The degree of ST elevation seen in V7–V9 only 0.5 mm of STE diagnoses posterior MI!

Assessing the ECG with LBBB and acute STEMI
- New LBBB and chest pain can occasionally be due to MI. Avoid inappropriate thrombolysis or PCI using the following criteria as well as reviewing old ECGs. Echo can help but takes time and LBBB itself causes altered wall motion.

Sgarbossa/Smith criteria for STEMI with LBBB
- ≥1 lead with positive QRS complex with concordant STE of ≥1 mm (yes +1).
- ≥1 lead from V1–V3 that has ≥1 mm of concordant ST depression (yes +1).
- ≥1 lead with ≥1 mm STE and proportionally excessive discordant ST elevation, as defined by STE ≥25% of the depth of the preceding S-wave (an ST/S ratio of ≤−0.25) (yes +1). Yes to any criteria is 80% sensitive and 99% specific in identifying AMI in known LBBB.

Barcelona algorithm (published 2020 but needs further validation)
- ST deviation >1 mm concordant with QRS polarity in any ECG lead, or
- ST deviation >1 mm discordant with QRS polarity; in any lead with maximal QRS (R or S wave) voltage <6 mm considered predictive of STEMI equivalent.

ECG differentials of ST elevation (correlate clinically)
- **High take-off:** 'early repolarisation'. ST looks elevated in V1, V2. No reciprocal changes elsewhere. Younger athletic or Afro Caribbean pts.
- **Transient apical ballooning syndrome:** Takotsubo cardiomyopathy. Anterior ST elevation. See ▶ Section 3.23 for takotsubo. Can mimic STEMI/NSTEMI.
- **Myo-/pericarditis:** concave saddle-shaped ST elevation all leads (not cavity leads aVr). See ▶ Section 3.19 for pericarditis/myocarditis.
- **Prinzmetal's variant angina:** transient ST elevation during angina due to vasospasm settles with antianginals. Can provoke arrhythmias even SCD. Coronary vessels normal/minimal disease. Needs nitrates/CCB.

- **LV aneurysm:** history of previous anterior MI. Diagnose on echo.
- **Brugada syndrome:** see Sudden cardiac death ▶Section 3.6.
- **Hyperkalaemia:** bizarre tall T wave and wide QRS. ▶Section 5.3.

Management of ST elevation MI

- **Ensure comfort.** Sit up. Nitrates: give GTN 2 sprays (400–800 mcg) SL or GTN 500 mcg tablet SL or buccal nitrate 2–5 mg 8 h unless BP low. Watch BP. Ongoing pain or pulmonary oedema consider IV GTN infusion as GTN 50 mg in 50 ml NS IV and run at 1–10 ml/h through syringe driver. Titrate to pain, dyspnoea and BP.
- **Beta blockade:** in all patients consider **Metoprolol** 5 mg IV over 5 min which may be repeated (max 15 mg); stop if SBP <100 mmHg or HR <60 bpm. Later metoprolol 50 mg TDS PO for 48 h and then maintenance dose or **Atenolol** 50 mg OD PO or bisoprolol 2.5–5 mg OD. Titrate up doses. Avoid if asthmatic, low BP, LVF, HR <60, 2nd- or 3rd-degree heart block. Unable to take beta-blockers try **Diltiazem** 60–90 mg BD PO (up to 360 mg/d). All patients with ACS should be on long-term beta-blocker.
- **Opiate analgesia:** can reduce myocardial ischaemia. Give morphine (2.5–5 mg) until symptomatic relief has been achieved with an anti-emetic e.g. **Metoclopramide** 10 mg IV or **Ondansetron** 4–8 mg IV. Mild post-infarction chest discomfort is not uncommon on the second or third day, and a milder oral analgesic such as Co-codamol (paracetamol 500 mg + codeine phosphate usually 30 mg) or paracetamol alone. Avoid NSAIDs acutely.
- **Oxygen:** most do not need it. Treat hypoxaemia PO_2 <94% or dyspnoea and pulmonary oedema or low output cardiogenic shock. Give using a 35% mask or nasal cannula unless there is a contraindication. CPAP may be of value in severely hypoxic patients (arterial PO_2 <8.0 kPa/60 mmHg, despite 100% oxygen at flow rate of 8–10 L/min). Discuss with duty SpR/anaesthetist as mechanical ventilation may be more appropriate. Avoid ABG in patients in whom thrombolytic or glycoprotein IIb/IIIa inhibitors are being employed or contemplated. Monitor saturations.
- **Aspirin** 300 mg stat chew tablet and then 75 mg OD: give to all. For every 1000 patients treated, aspirin started within 24 hours of onset of infarct symptoms prevents around 40 vascular events in the first month and about 40 more over the next 2 years. If dyspepsia, consider PPI cover.
- **Second antiplatelet:** given in STEMI 12 months: Clopidogrel 600 mg loading dose pre-PCI otherwise 300 mg in STEMI followed by 75–150 mg OD for a week and then 75 mg OD. Ticagrelor (avoid in asthma / COPD / bradycardia) 180 mg then 90 mg BD. **Prasugrel** 60 mg stat then 10 mg OD for up to 15 months used instead of Clopidogrel with STEMI, NSTEMI for PCI, stent thrombosis on clopidogrel, ACS with diabetes mellitus, high risk stent thrombosis (NICE 2014, NG317). Prasugrel contraindicated in the following: previous TIA, CVA, ICH, weight <60 kg, age ≥75, patients for thrombolysis, patients on anticoagulation, severe hepatic impairment, propensity to bleeding (anaemia, GI bleed, etc.).
- **Consider for reperfusion strategies.** If PCI available then do within 90 minutes. If PCI can be done within 2 hours, then PCI. If time to PCI more than 2 hours, then thrombolysis within 30 minutes. Even if thrombolytics given consider move to PCI site.
- **ACS and hyperglycaemia:** all patients admitted to hospital should be closely monitored for hyperglycaemia. Those with a blood-glucose concentration greater than 11.0 mmol/L should receive insulin via a VRII.

Reperfusion strategies in STEMI (PCI/thrombolysis)

- Consider if ECG shows STEMI or new LBBB as defined above or resuscitated VF arrest with ST elevation / new LBBB.

- PCI/thrombolysis not generally advocated beyond 12 h from symptoms onset if asymptomatic or haemodynamically stable. Consider if 12–24 hours and ongoing ischaemia or cardiogenic shock.
- A bedside echo looking for regional wall motion abnormalities (RWMAs) can help the decision-making when ECG changes may be considered non-acute or conflicting, e.g. old MI, LVH, digoxin.

Primary percutaneous coronary intervention for STEMI

- **Primary PCI:** preferable over thrombolysis if it can be done in <2 hours. PCI offers superior vessel patency and perfusion (TIMI 3 flow) with less reinfarction, less risk of ICH, and improved survival regardless of lesion location or patient age. STEMI patients with symptom onset.
- **Contrast-induced nephropathy (CIN)** may be seen at 1–2 days. Creatinine settles in 7 days. Ensure hydrated. N-Acetyl-l-cysteine has no advantage.
- **PCI superior to lysis:** severe HF or cardiogenic shock, Killip class III/IV or TIMI risk score ≥5 represent high-risk groups where PCI is preferred despite a potential time delay, C/I to fibrinolytic therapy, recent PCI or prior CABG. Needs a skilled interventional cardiologist and ensure catheterisation laboratory with surgical backup are available. Allows angioplasty and stenting of culprit lesion with reperfusion and salvage of viable myocardium and assessment for CABG. Patients usually receive a combination of antiplatelet and anticoagulants prior to and during PCI as detailed above. Multivessel PCI at the time of primary PCI or as a staged procedure is now recommended for STEMI.
- **Primary PCI and additional anticoagulants** may be needed for patients undergoing primary PCI with radial access, heparin (UFH) should also be given. If femoral access is needed, bivalirudin should be considered instead (unlicensed). A bailout glycoprotein IIb/IIIa inhibitor may be given if indicated during the PCI. UFH should still be administered to patients who are on anticoagulant therapy already but stopped immediately on completion of the procedure. Dose is usually 70–100 IU/kg aiming for an ACT of 250–330 s.
- **GPIIb/IIIa inhibitor Abciximab:** GPIIb/IIIa inhibitor is used occasionally if there is clear evidence of thrombus or complex PCI. (0.25 mg/kg IV bolus followed by infusion of 0.125 mcg/kg/min up to a maximum of 10 mcg/min for 12 hours). Tirofiban: 25 mcg/kg bolus over 3 minutes followed by continuous infusion of 0.15 mcg/kg/min) has been evaluated in a number of trials involving patients with STEMI and is an alternative to abciximab.
- **Stenting:** bare metal stents (BMS) use mechanical force to hold open vessel but also induce intimal proliferation. They reduce mortality in acute MI. In those with stable disease they reduce angina but with no effect on death, MI or hospitalisation or costs. They are routinely used and need a minimum 3 months Clopidogrel 75 mg as well as Aspirin 75 mg. BMS preferred in those who cannot tolerate long-term dual antiplatelet therapy. Drug-eluting stents (DES) are BMS coated with a drug to suppress intimal proliferation. They need 12 months dual antiplatelet therapy (DAPT). There is a risk of stent thrombosis associated with the use of both DES and BMS, but seemingly more so with DES. The length of DAPT should be documented by the interventionist and depends on the stent type, the lesion/s and the indication – in the setting of ACS or not. DES have a small reduction in target vessel revascularisation (TVR) rates so only used in higher risk patients (diabetes/high risk lesions) and where the target artery to be treated has less than a 3 mm calibre, or the lesion is longer than 15 mm. DES and BMS show no difference in mortality or MI

rates or stent thrombosis. Avoid DES if raised bleed risk with prolonged DAPT for 12 months (NICE 2003, TA71: Ischaemic heart disease – coronary artery stents).

- **PCI and CKD:** be aware of impact of contrast media on renal function. If approaching ESRF liaise with nephrology as dialysis support may be required.
- **Post procedure:** monitor for signs of bleeding, especially from sites of vascular access. Unexpected low BP may be due to occult blood loss related to retroperitoneal bleeds, haemopericardium or GI bleeds and these conditions need to be considered. Groin complications are not uncommon and imaging with ultrasound may be indicated to exclude false aneurysms, etc. CT scanning may be necessary. Similar assessment should follow elective angiographic procedures. Vascular complications from radial procedures are unusual but patients must still be assessed carefully.
- **Emergency CABG** is high-risk but may be considered if severe left main disease or refractory ischaemia and failed PCI or coronary anatomy that is not amenable to PCI. Consider for STEMI and papillary muscle rupture, severe ischaemic MR, VSD, ventricular aneurysm formation in the setting of intractable ventricular arrhythmias, or ventricular free wall rupture.
- **Discharge:** many patients can be discharged within 2–3 days after treatment with primary PCI if they do not have evidence of heart failure and have not demonstrated any significant arrhythmias.

PCI after cardiac arrest in unconscious pt for STEMI

- Indications are ST elevation on ECG after resuscitation and chest pain preceding cardiac arrest. About 50% of patients are treated by PCI. Benefit is predominantly confined to those with ST elevation (M Godin, European Society of Cardiology, 2012).
- MIRACLE2 score is a practical risk score for early accurate prediction of poor neurological outcome after OOHCA, which is simple to use. Age >80, or adrenaline use are associated with worst outcome.
- Administering DAPT may need NG tube access in the catheter lab but should not significantly delay PCI. It may be done on ITU.
- Ventilated patients are cared for on ITU and are usually cooled to reduce the risk of brain injury. The responsible interventionist should continue to provide cardiology input. If unavailable, the CCU consultant on call should be involved.

Cardiac thrombolysis for STEMI: within 12 h of onset of symptoms

- **Indications:** STEMI but unsuitable for PCI (or PCI not available). Consider for those who seek medical attention <1 h after the onset of symptoms to abort the infarction. Or those with allergy to radiographic contrast material.
- **Aim for door to needle time <30 min.** Acute STEMI <12 h of onset of symptoms. If ST elevation persists for 60–90 min post-fibrinolysis then consider PCI. Readministration of fibrinolytic is not recommended.
- **Absolute contraindications** to cardiac thrombolysis: active bleeding or bleeding diathesis (excluding menses), significant closed head or facial trauma within 3 months, suspected aortic dissection, previous ICH, ischaemic stroke <2–3 months, structural cerebral vascular lesion, acute pancreatitis, known malignant brain tumour. Recent LP. Oesophageal varices. Warfarin INR (unless INR <2) or other anticoagulants.
- **Relative contraindications** to cardiac thrombolysis: non-compressible vascular puncture, recent major surgery <3 months, traumatic or prolonged CPR >10 min, recent internal bleeding <4 weeks, active peptic ulcer, chronic severe poorly

controlled HTN, BP >180–200/120 mmHg (treat it with labetalol, GTN, atenolol and review) pregnancy.

Thrombolytic agents
- **Streptokinase:** 1.5 MU in 100 ml NS (0.9% saline) over 1 h. SE low BP, fluid challenge but no need to stop. Alteplase preferred for anterior infarction or cardiogenic shock if no PCI. Streptokinase not reused because antibodies are formed which reduce efficacy. Anaphylaxis, ▶Section 2.18. **Hydrocortisone** 200 mg IV and Chlorphenamine 10 mg IV. ICH 0.4%. Patency 51%.
- **Tenecteplase:** 30–50 mg IV over 10 sec. <60 kg: 30 mg, 60–69 kg: 35 mg, 70–79 kg: 40 mg, 80–89 kg: 45 mg, >90 kg or greater: 50 mg. Risks ICH 0.7%. Patency 80%.
- **Alteplase:** 15 mg IV, 50 mg/30 min + 35 mg/60 min. ICH 0.7%. Patency 80%.
- **Reteplase:** 2 × 10 unit boluses given 30 min apart. ICH 0.8%. Patency 80%.

Post thrombolysis management
- **Post thrombolysis anticoagulation:** Alteplase, Reteplase, Tenecteplase need IV heparin for 24–48 h and then LMWH for 4–8 days or discharge. IV heparin is not needed following Streptokinase. Patients who appear to have had successful lysis should still be considered for angiography, ideally within a few hours of admission.
- **If there is bleeding on/after thrombolysis:** ▶Section 8.12. Advice on agents: Alteplase / Reteplase / Tenecteplase preferred over Streptokinase in anterior MI or new LBBB or those who have previously had Streptokinase where PPCI is not possible. ICH risk additional 4/1000 patients. Bleed risks are 0.5–1.0%.
- **If bleeding is serious and life-threatening** give **Tranexamic acid** 1g IV over 15 mins whilst awaiting coagulation indices. When thrombin time and INR are prolonged but fibrinogen >1 g/L give 15 ml/kg of FFP and 1 adult therapeutic dose (ATD ~ 330 ml) of cryoprecipitate. When thrombin time is prolonged and fibrinogen is low (<1 g/L), give 1 ATD of cryoprecipitate.

Those with STEMI not receiving lysis or PCI
- If it is decided that reperfusion therapy is not appropriate on admission, give aspirin as for usual STEMI management and enoxaparin or fondaparinux.
- Angiography before hospital discharge should be considered if there are no major contraindications (comorbidity, frailty, etc.), similar to patients after successful lysis (see below).

Risk assessment
- Exercise stress testing is used to risk-stratify patients except in those with severe aortic stenosis, LBBB, ongoing typical chest pain, haemodynamic instability, dynamic ST changes, severe LV outflow obstruction and hypertrophic cardiomyopathy, poor mobility.
- Risks of coronary angiography: death 1 in 1000 (0.1%), MI 1 in 1000 (0.1%), stroke 1 in 1000 (0.1%), arterial complications 1 in 500 (0.2%).
- Risk of PCI (angioplasty and stenting): death 0.7%, MI (usually minor) <1%, stroke <1%, emergency CABG 1 in 200 (0.5%), significant arterial complications 1 in 200 (0.5%).

TIMI score: risk assess all NSTEMI/ACS patients for early angiography
- TIMI risk score (0–7): age >65 y +1, >3 risk factors for CAD +1; known CAD (stenosis >50%) +1, aspirin use in past 7 days +1; severe angina (>2 episodes/24 h) +1, ST changes >0.5 mm +1; cardiac marker +1. Use the TIMI score to risk stratify NSTEMI

patients for an early angiography strategy: TIMI >4 is associated with 20% risk at 14 days of all-cause mortality, new or recurrent MI, or severe recurrent ischaemia requiring angiography and urgent revascularisation. TIMI 0–2 is low risk and the remainder are higher risk.

- Look for other markers of high risk: persistent/recurrent angina, ST depression >2 mm, deep negative T waves. Signs of heart failure or low BP EF <0.4, sustained VT, positive stress test, diabetes mellitus, renal impairment, reduced LV function, previous CABG or recent PCI <6/12.
- If hsTn I levels remain normal, with a normal ECG, early discharge should be considered. In some where concerns lie, pre-discharge treadmill testing or a functional test should be considered. If troponin elevated, then angiography may be undertaken prior to discharge. Angiography within 24 hours if GRACE score >140. The GRACE risk score can be assessed online (www.mdcalc.com/calc/1099/grace-acs-risk-mortality-calculator).

Management of NSTEMI / unstable angina

- **CCU:** if significant ECG changes. Give O_2 if sats <94% or shocked/LVF. Monitor for arrhythmias. Analgesia as needed. Look for complications. Thrombolytic therapy is of no benefit in UA / NSTEMI and may be associated with increased hazard. **Aspirin** 300 mg PO then 75 mg daily.
- **Dual antiplatelet:** if elevated troponin then start **Ticagrelor** 180 mg loading dose followed by 90 mg BD dose 12 months (plus **Aspirin** 75 mg daily lifelong), or **Clopidogrel** 300 mg stat and then 75 mg OD. Because of the potential need for surgical revascularisation, it may be worth considering deferring clopidogrel or ticagrelor in selected very high-risk patients who could be listed for angiography alone in the first instance. They could then potentially undergo surgical revascularisation sooner. If they are selected for PCI they could be subsequently loaded with the appropriate antiplatelet. Clopidogrel and especially ticagrelor should ideally be stopped for 5 days prior to CABG, dependent on the preferences of the individual surgeon.
- **Anticoagulation therapy:** choices are **Fondaparinux** 2.5 mg OD or **Enoxaparin** 1 mg/kg SC OD if renal failure; should be administered in medium and high-risk patients for the first 48 hours and then stopped if pain-free. Patients with NSTEMI requiring full anticoagulation (PE/metal valves) should have **Enoxaparin** 1 mg/kg SC BD unless otherwise anticoagulated. Oral anticoagulation may be held while enoxaparin given.
- **ACS and hyperglycaemia:** all patients admitted to hospital should be closely monitored for hyperglycaemia. Those with a blood glucose concentration greater than 11.0 mmol/L should receive insulin via a VRII.

Ongoing management of acute ACS (STEMI and NSTEMI / UA)

- **Antithrombotics: Rivaroxaban** 2.5 mg BD and aspirin considered for some.
- **Beta blockade:** see STEMI above.
- **Nitrates:** see STEMI above.
- **Opiates:** persisting chest pain see STEMI above.
- **Nicorandil** (5–30 mg BD) is an ATP-dependent potassium channel activator that has an uncertain role to play in the management of UA. Its action is similar to that of nitrates. No role in those on nitrates.
- **ACE inhibitors and ARB** reduce the progressive LV dilatation and reduction in LV performance seen following MI. Studies have also suggested a reduction in late

cardiac failure, MI and death. Start **Ramipril** 2.5 mg especially if large MI or LV failure or diabetes.
- **VTE:** DVT, PE. Usually on Fondaparinux or equivalent. Prevent with early mobilisation, antiplatelets, LMWH and TED stockings where appropriate.
- **Lipid lowering:** Atorvastatin or Simvastatin to get LDL <1.4 mmol/L.

Managing complications of myocardial infarction

- **Cardiac failure or cardiogenic shock: Morphine** 5 mg IV + **Furosemide** 50–100 mg IV. ▸Section 2.16. Get an echo if possible.
- **Myocardial rupture:** post MI or traumatic catheter-related perforation due to intervention. Causes tamponade and usually death. In days 3–5 with myocardial softening post STEMI, causes PEA. Recently documented with takotsubo cardiomyopathy or regional ventricular ballooning syndrome.
- **Acute mitral regurgitation:** day 2–7 post MI. Partial rupture – loud PSM, S3, low BP and CCF. Complete rupture of papillary muscle can cause rapid death, usually in first week. Surgery is high risk. Echo to confirm. Rupture of free wall causes tamponade and SCD. Discuss with tertiary cardiology centre.
- **Ventricular septal rupture and VSD:** VSD in 3%. Q wave MI affecting septum. Low BP, PSM at the left sternal edge. Less SOB than acute MR and less pulmonary oedema on CXR. Urgent echo and surgical referral, and IABP as a bridge to surgical closure. Discuss with tertiary centre.
- **LV aneurysm:** after 2–3 months presenting with dyspnoea, low BP and a dyskinetic parasternal pulsation and ST elevation. Take advice. Echocardiography. Some may need surgery. Rupture is main concern as well as thromboembolism and arrhythmias.
- **Intracardiac thrombus and cardioembolism:** from akinetic cardiac apex, left atrial or LV aneurysm. Causes stroke, ischaemic limb, mesenteric ischaemia. Tends to be acute and needs anticoagulation. Warfarin should be continued for at least 3 months and then reassessed.
- **Psychosocial:** depression, sexual impotence, employment issues.
- **Pericarditis:** early at the time of the MI. Late (Dressler's syndrome), widespread saddle-shaped ST elevation. Care with anticoagulation as bleeding into pericardial sac is a concern.
- **Tachyarrhythmias:** AF, sinus tachycardia, ventricular ectopics, idioventricular rhythm (do not treat if not compromised), VT, VF (particularly VF/VT amenable to early defibrillation, which is key).
- **Idioventricular rhythm:** seen post MI often post reperfusion. Broad complex 'slow VT' <120/min. Monitor and may not need treatment if stable.
- **Bradyarrhythmias:** sinus bradycardia, heart block; may need pacing if haemodynamically compromised and both bundle branches taken out.
- **Pacing in acute MI:** indications: asystole, CHB + anterior wall MI, alternating BBB, bifascicular block (new RBBB with left anterior fascicular block (LAFB)/left posterior fascicular block (LPFB) + long PR = trifascicular, Mobitz II block, Mobitz I with anterior or inferior wall MI, with wide QRS escape rhythm (a junctional escape which is narrow QRS and rate 50–60/min and SBP >100 mmHg may be monitored), symptomatic low HR despite atropine or chronotropes, new RBBB with anterior wall MI, new LBBB with anterior wall MI. Take expert advice if patient stable. Some may wait and insert a permanent system if they can wait for a formal insertion but they need to be haemodynamically stable. Pacing may be used to overdrive VT. Pacing wires go into the right ventricular apex and right atrial appendage. These routes are

low pressure (venous) and just easier access than left-sided chambers. ECG will show paced LBBB morphology.

- **LV dysfunction:** heart failure, cardiogenic shock; poor prognosis. Needs echocardiogram. Survival relates to LV function. Killip score can give a quick estimation of in-hospital mortality. Killip class I, no CHF (2–5%); Killip class II, S3, rales/creps (10–15%); Killip class III, overt pulmonary oedema (20–30%); Killip class IV, cardiogenic shock (50–60%).
- **Acute pulmonary oedema: Furosemide** 50–100 mg IV ± **Diamorphine** 2.5–5 mg IV or **Morphine** 5–10 mg IV with an anti-emetic, **Metoclopramide** 10 mg IV. Consider nitrates, e.g. GTN infusion. Revascularisation. ACEi: all patients with ACS and either heart failure, HTN or diabetes should be on long-term ACEi. Consider **Ramipril** 1.25 mg OD and up-titrate. Those with MI should be commenced on long-term ACEi within the first 36 h. Patients with MI complicated by LV dysfunction or heart failure should be commenced on long-term AT2 receptor blocker therapy if intolerant of ACEi therapy. **Eplerenone** 25–50 mg OD. MI complicated by LV dysfunction (EF <0.40). **Furosemide** 50–100 mg IV then 20–80 mg/day orally may be considered if severe pulmonary oedema in conjunction with ACEi and nitrates and revascularisation. Echocardiogram. Monitor K^+. Avoid low K^+ post MI. NIPPV: patients with an ACS with acute cardiogenic pulmonary oedema and hypoxia should be considered for NIPPV. Most evidence favours CPAP (2.5–10 cm/H_2O). Beta-blockers: **Bisoprolol** 1.25 mg starting dose is agent of choice in stabilised heart failure.
- **Cardiogenic shock:** See ▶ Section 2.16. Get an echo and make sure it is not RV failure: IV fluids: can help if evidence clinically, ECG or echo of RV failure possibly due to inferior MI with low BP and raised JVP. Occasionally intra-aortic balloon pumping or PCI or CABG or valve repair/replacement can help.

Secondary prevention and ongoing care for all ACS

- **Dual antiplatelets: Aspirin** 75 mg OD long term. **Clopidogrel** 75 mg or alternative as above, continue for 1 year after STEMI / NSTEMI. Minimum dual antiplatelet: BMS 3 months, DES 12 months. Stopping before 12 months must be discussed with interventional cardiologist.
- **Triple therapy:** Rivaroxaban with aspirin alone or aspirin and clopidogrel is also recommended as an option for preventing atherothrombotic events following an ACS with elevated cardiac biomarkers.
- **ACEi: Ramipril** 1.25–5 mg PO 12 hourly or **Enalapril** 10 mg PO 12 hourly for all non-hypotensive patients can help reduce ventricular remodelling in the first 4–6 weeks. Continue long term if impaired LV function.
- **Nitrates:** for chest pain or pulmonary oedema. IV nitrate or buccal nitrate 2–5 mg 8 hourly.
- **Beta-blockers:** long term, e.g. **Metoprolol** or **Bisoprolol** 2.5–5 mg PO OD especially with impaired LV function.
- **Ivabradine** (5–7.5 mg BD) is a sinus node blocking agent which may be an alternative rate-controlling agent especially where a β-blocker is contra-indicated or not tolerated. Can be used with LV dysfunction.
- **Lifestyle modifications:** smoking cessation services and diet/weight management and exercise support.
- **Diabetic control:** aim for glycaemic control for HbA1c <7%.
- **Vaccination:** annual influenza and pneumococcal vaccination recommended.
- **Antihypertensive:** aim for BP <140/90 mmHg.

- **Statins: Atorvastatin** 80 mg at night for at least 3 months. Reduces cholesterol and mortality. Aim to get total cholesterol <4 mmol/L and LDL-C <2 mmol/L.
- **Anticoagulation:** Warfarin/DOAC for AF, warfarin for LV thrombus, PE, DVT.
- **AICD:** if VT/VF >48 h after the initial MI then AICD should be inserted before discharge. For those with poor LV then clinical trials support a waiting period of 40 days post MI before AICD insertion. They may need electrophysiological study depending on local guidance.
- **Coronary artery bypass:** those with three vessel complex coronary disease derive a mortality benefit with surgery, diabetics especially. LIMA to LAD graft is suspected to be superior to saphenous vein to LAD.

3.8 ▶ Stable angina

- **Based on NICE guidance (2011, updated 2016, CG126). Diagnose stable angina** based on clinical assessment alone or clinical assessment plus diagnostic testing (i.e. anatomical testing for obstructive CAD and/or functional testing for myocardial ischaemia). Take detailed history and risk factors.
- **Anginal pain** is often a constricting discomfort front of chest, or neck, shoulders, jaw, or arms precipitated by physical exertion, relieved by rest or GTN < 5 min.
- If all 3 features are present the chest pain or discomfort is classified as **typical angina.** If 2 of 3 features are present the chest discomfort is classified as **atypical angina.** If only 1 of 3 features is present the chest discomfort is classified as **non-anginal chest pain.**

Medical management of stable angina

- **Antiplatelet: Aspirin** 75 mg taking into account the risk of bleeding and comorbidities.
- **Nitrates** should be prescribed. **Isosorbide mononitrate** 20–60 mg PO BD.
- **Weight loss/lipid control:** statin, e.g. **Atorvastatin** 20–80 mg or **Simvastatin**.
- **Beta-blockers: Bisoprolol** 1.25–10 mg OD, **Atenolol** 25–100 mg OD.
- **CCBs: Nifedipine** 5–10 mg TDS, **Amlodipine** 2.5–10 mg OD, **Nicardipine**.
- **ACEi** for stable angina and diabetes.
- **Nicorandil** 10–30 mg PO BD in those who cannot take nitrates.
- **Ivabradine:** inhibits if channels in SAN. Antianginal. Safe in heart failure.
- **Ranolazine:** a sodium channel inhibitor, is licensed as adjunctive therapy in patients who are inadequately controlled or intolerant of first-line antianginal drugs. The dose is initially 375 mg BD increasing to a maximum of 750 mg BD. Its use is mainly in patients with chronic stable angina.
- Optimising HbA1c and diabetic control.
- Referral. Consider referring for potential revascularisation (coronary artery bypass graft (CABG) or percutaneous coronary intervention (PCI)) for people with stable angina whose symptoms are not satisfactorily controlled with optimal medical treatment. CABG is preferred in those aged over 65, diabetes and complex three vessel or left main stem disease.

3.9 ▶ Arrhythmias

ECG interpretation of arrhythmias

- Heart rate = 300/R to R interval squares. ECG is a graph:
  - X axis (horizontal) is time at 25 mm/s; each small square is 40 ms
  - Y axis (vertical) is millivolts at 1 mV = 1 cm; each small square is 0.1 mV.

- Normal PR 120–200 ms (3–5 small squares).
- Normal QRS is <120 ms (3 small squares).
- QT (measured from the start of the QRS to the end of the T wave); correct for rate (QTc) to 60 beats/min using the equation:

$$QTc = (QT)/(\text{square root of } RR), \text{ where } RR \text{ is the RR interval in seconds.}$$

- Normal between 0.35 and 0.43 s (9–11 small squares).
- Irregular: measure RR interval and it changes beat to beat.
- Broad complex QRS >3 small squares.

3.10 ▶ Transvenous pacemakers

Pacemaker code

Chamber paced	Chamber sensed	Mode
Atria (A)	Atria (A)	Inhibits (I)
Ventricle (V)	Ventricle (V)	Dual (D)
Both (D)	Both (D)	

- **Introduction:** used to treat any symptomatic or persistent non-reversible compromising bradycardia if atropine and other measures, e.g. transcutaneous pacing, fail to help. Temporary wires used much less now. Preferable to put in a clean permanent system than a temporary wire which in an emergency is often less than sterile. Usually the tip of the wire is inserted into apex of the RV as that is the easiest ventricle to pace using the venous system. If needed an atrial lead is placed in right atrial appendage. The pacemaker paces and also senses so that it does not try to pace over an intrinsic beat causing R on T arrhythmias. New leadless RV pacemakers are now available. Placed via femoral vein. May have a higher risk of battery failure. The pacemaker code has 3 characteristics. A RV wire means the RV contracts then LV like LBBB, so V1 has LBBB morphology.
- **Types:** commonest is DDD (two leads R atrial appendage and RV on CXR) but also single lead are usually VVI (used when no P waves). If AV conduction normal and the problem is above ventricles, then an AAI may be considered. If there is LBBB and poor LV then either a DDD for heart block or a biventricular pacing (lead in RV apex and lateral LV (via the coronary sinus)) to improve function is needed.
- **Pacemaker syndrome:** seen with VVI pacing with presyncope, syncope, light-headedness, fatigue, exercise intolerance, malaise, lethargy, dyspnoea, headache, chest pain. Can be due to AV dissociation and atria contracting against closed M/T valves. Consider atrial lead. Less seen with DDD.
- **Pacemaker-mediated tachycardia:** seen with DDD and due to inappropriate sensing of retrograde P waves. Pacemaker settings need altered.
- **MRI** is generally contraindicated with a pacemaker, but newer devices which are MRI-compatible are being developed. Check online websites with model.
- **Magnet response:** application of a magnet starts magnet mode. This is fixed pacing at 70–80/min. This can be used to deactivate shocks in an ICD.
- Pacemakers should be removed before cremation.

Indications for a permanent pacemaker
- **Absolute:** sick sinus syndrome, symptomatic sinus bradycardia, tachy–brady syndrome. AF with sinus node dysfunction, complete AV block (3rd-degree block).

Chronotropic incompetence (inability to increase the heart rate to match a level of exercise). Prolonged QT syndrome, cardiac resynchronisation therapy with biventricular pacing.
- **Relative:** cardiomyopathy (hypertrophic or dilated). Severe refractory neurocardiogenic syncope.

3.11 Tachyarrhythmias

Rhythm	P wave (leads II/V1) QRS form and regularity	Onset	Notes
Sinus tachycardia	ECG: normal P wave before QRS Normal QRS width unless BBB Regular >100/min. Max HR: 220−age for men, 210−age for females. AV node limits ventricular rate	Gradual onset/end	Exercise related, hyperthyroid, etc.
Atrial fibrillation	Absent P wave Normal QRS width unless BBB Irregular random R to R interval Rate as for sinus tachycardia	Sudden Chronic, paroxysmal	See text
Atrial flutter	No P waves but saw-shaped flutter waves in inferior leads seen with CSM. Normal width regular rate is a divisor of 300, e.g. 75/100/150	Sudden/ paroxysmal	See text
SVT	Variable rate often >140/min to max HR. Normal width regular. Rate 150−200/min. Faster if conducts down accessory pathway bypassing AVN	Sudden stop − CSM, adenosine	Adenosine, ablation
Torsades de pointes (VT)	Dissociated P and QRS Broad changing axis, regular rate >120 Regular rate >120	Sudden	Long QT related
Idioventricular	Dissociated P and QRS. Broad fixed axis. Regular <120/min	Sudden	Post MI Benign
VT	Dissociated. Broad fixed axis Regular >100/min	Sudden	See text
Ventricular fibrillation	Dissociated. Random width, random irregular	Sudden	Cardiac arrest

Risk assessment and management
- **Slow ventricular rate:** look for sinus bradycardia, 2nd degree heart block, slow AF, complete heart block and width of QRS. If rate has caused the associated low BP and circulatory collapse, see Bradycardia, ▶ Section 1.12.
- **Irregular broad complex rhythm:** consider fast AF with aberrant conduction. Consider IV **amiodarone** or beta-blocker. If WPW suspected avoid IV digoxin or verapamil. If unwell consider low voltage DC cardioversion, ▶ Section 1.14.
- **Regular broad complex >120/min:** VT or aberrantly conducted SVT/flutter. If unsure always assume and treat as VT. Treat with IV **Amiodarone** 150−300 mg over 20−60 min. Consider carotid massage if safe (aged <50 and no suggestion of TIA/stroke/bruit) and/or adenosine if you think it's aberrantly conducted SVT. DC cardiovert if falling BP. **Avoid IV verapamil.** Consider IV NaHCO₃ for Amitriptyline OD.
- **Narrow complex regular AVRT or AVNRT or atrial flutter 2:1, 3:1 or 4:1 block:** can settle spontaneously. Usually benign unless in context of other cardiac disease.

See SVT, ▶ Section 3.14. IV **adenosine** or IV **metoprolol**. If unstable consider DC cardioversion. If AVRT+WPW avoid digoxin or verapamil.

- **Narrow complex irregular** fast AF: consider IV **amiodarone** or IV **metoprolol** or IV **digoxin**. If unstable consider DC cardioversion. Assess need for anticoagulation.

Differential of a narrow complex tachycardia

- **Regular:** sinus tachycardia, paroxysmal SVT, atrial flutter with 2/3/4:1 block, atrial tachycardia with conduction, AVRT (orthodromic) (WPW), AVNRT.
- **Irregular:** atrial fibrillation, atrial flutter with variable block, atrial tachycardia with variable block, multifocal atrial tachycardia.

3.12 ▶ Monomorphic ventricular tachycardia

Assume all new wide complex tachycardias are VT. Consider IV amiodarone unless long QT suspected. If unstable cardiovert.

- **About:** all fast unstable rhythms should be considered for urgent DC cardioversion. Most broad complex regular tachycardias are VT especially if IHD/structural heart disease. Some are aberrantly conducted SVT/atrial flutter. VT may be tolerated and then suddenly decompensate. Ensure immediate access to defibrillator. There are some rare benign forms of VT and some aberrantly conducted SVTs that mimic VT but this is for experts in the cold light of day. Assume it's a VT with possible fatal consequences until proven otherwise. A prolonged QT predisposes to both monomorphic and polymorphic VT.
- **Aetiology:** can originate in left or right ventricle. Often due to underlying myocardial damage and development of re-entrant tachycardia as well as some increased automaticity. Electrical waves form 'rotors' that give rise to rapidly rotating spiral waves. Inherited channelopathies such as Brugada and prolonged QT syndromes. Cardiomyopathies such as arrhythmogenic RV cardiomyopathy are being increasingly identified. In Brugada syndrome, the primary cause is abnormal conduction in the epicardium of the RVOT.
- **Types:** sustained (>30 sec) and non-sustained (<30 sec and more benign).
- **ECG:** >3 beats broad regular QRS complex >3 small squares (120 ms) wide and rate over 100/min. There is complete AV dissociation and P waves can be found as atrial activity continues. Idioventricular is a slow VT at 100–120/min seen post MI and usually benign. LBBB and RAD morphology and no other cardiac disease may suggest RV cardiomyopathy.
- **Causes of VT:** all cardiac disease: IHD especially with LV dysfunction, dilated or hypertrophic cardiomyopathy, arrhythmogenic RV cardiomyopathy (ARVC), myocarditis, sarcoidosis, haemochromatosis. Drug-induced, e.g. TCA overdose, digoxin, anti-arrhythmics, low or high K, low Mg, low Ca, cocaine, phaeochromocytoma. Channelopathies: Brugada syndrome, long QT syndromes, drugs causing long QT. Others: chest trauma, congenital disorders. Note that NSVT may be found in 3% of normal people with no heart disease.
- **Clinical:** *some tolerate VT well without hypotension but can quickly decompensate,* others develop angina, pulmonary oedema, cardiac arrest. Status depends on LV function, rate, coronary perfusion and comorbidities. Others develop palpitations, dyspnoea, acute pulmonary oedema, hypotension, angina, observe cannon 'a' wave in JVP (AV dissociation).

- **Ventricular ectopics:** these are mostly benign and do not need treatment unless severely symptomatic. Reassurance is the usual approach.
- **Investigations:** bloods: check FBC, U&E, cardiac troponin, Mg, Ca. Serial ECGs: ensure capture 12-lead of the arrhythmia if possible. Echocardiogram: for LV systolic and diastolic function and structural disease. Coronary angiogram to look for treatable coronary artery disease. Electrophysiology studies: provoke arrhythmias, mapping.
- **ECG differential of VT:** (accelerated) idioventricular rhythm (HR 100–120/min) seen post MI, monomorphic VT: regular wide complex, polymorphic VT (torsades de pointes) seen with long QT, SVT/atrial flutter or atrial tachycardia with aberrant conduction, WPW syndrome with retrograde conduction of an AVNRT/atrial flutter, motion artefact, pacemaker syndromes (consider turning off pacemaker with a magnet).
- **Evidence towards an ECG diagnosis of VT rather than SVT with aberrant conduction:** fusion beats, capture (narrow) beats, ischaemic heart disease, structural heart disease, no RS wave in V1–V6, AV dissociation (cannon 'a' waves), RBBB pattern >140 ms, LBBB pattern >160 ms, extreme LAD, extreme R to R regularity.
- **Management:** if pulseless then ALS algorithm ▶ Section 1.4. If unstable (low BP/chest pain/dyspnoea) then administer synchronised; DC cardioversion, ▶ Section 1.14, ABC, get IV access, give O_2 as per BTS guidelines. Treat any ACS. If STEMI suspected needs PCI/thrombolysis. Monitor. Defibrillator. **Correct electrolytes.** Keep K 4–5 mmol/L. Stop any drugs that prolong QT. Torsades or low Mg suspected (alcohol/diuretics): **Magnesium sulfate** 2 g (8 mmol) in 100 ml NS IV over 10 min. Persisting VT: commence **Amiodarone** 300 mg IV over 10–30 min then 900 mg/24 h. Use large vein or central line. **Lidocaine** 50–100 mg IV may also be considered. Most anti-arrhythmics are negatively inotropic and even proarrhythmic so use with caution. There are several forms of idiopathic VT with a more benign course seen in younger adults. Some of these respond to Adenosine or Verapamil. These treatments are the preserve of cardiologists. Until proven otherwise treat all VT as potentially life-threatening. DC shock if unstable.
- **Prevention:** refer cardiac electrophysiologist. Needs echocardiogram, angiography and electrophysiological studies and Holter monitoring and cardiac MRI. Treatment of underlying cause, e.g. treat IHD – drugs, PCI, CABG. Consider **sotalol** usually when LV function is good, **amiodarone** when LV function is impaired. Assess for need for ICD implantation.
- **Catheter ablation** can significantly reduce the frequency of recurrent VT and ICD discharge in patients with ventricular arrhythmias and prior MI.

3.13 ▶ Torsades de pointes

- **About:** torsades de pointes (TdP) is a polymorphic VT. Axis constantly changes. Due to an acquired or inherited long QT syndrome.
- **Aetiology:** caused by early after-depolarisations that arise during an abnormally prolonged action potential owing to a delayed repolarisation process in the setting of genetic long QT syndromes, LQT1, LQT2, and LQT3. Some drugs cause a long QTc >500 ms. It does not correlate with risk. QT is long if >450 ms in males and >460 ms in females. Avoid Amiodarone and other drugs that increase QT. May be seen with Brugada syndrome.

- **Drug causes of long QT** (check all in *BNF*): amiodarone, erythromycin, terfenadine, TCA, quinidine. Methadone, class I and III anti-arrhythmics, lithium, phenothiazine. Low K, low Mg, low Ca, congenital syndromes.
- **Congenital long QT syndromes:** genetically driven. Long QT channelopathies. Beta blockade advocated. Some may require ICD.
- **Investigations:** check FBC, U&E, troponin, Mg, Ca. Serial ECGs and ensure capture 12-lead of the arrhythmia if possible to show coved ST elevation in right precordial leads of Brugada. Echocardiogram for LV and valves or structural disease. Electrophysiology studies may be useful.
- **Management:** look for drug causes (see above) and stop any drugs which may be to blame (see *BNF*): avoid amiodarone or other drugs that lengthen QT. Correct any low K, low Mg or low Ca. Give IV **Magnesium sulfate** 2 g (8 mmol) in 100 ml NS over 10 min IV then 72 mmol over 24 h. If bradycardia then consider **Atropine** 0.5 mg IV stat repeat up to 3 mg to increase heart rate. Trancutaneous or transvenous pacing to get a rate of 100/min: temporary atrial or ventricular pacing increases ventricular rate and reduces the episodes of TDP. If unstable then consider long-term beta blockage or flecainide and if deteriorating, then DC cardioversion (▶Section 1.14). Quinidine may help Brugada syndrome.
- **Isoprenaline** to increase rate but not with congenital long QT syndromes.
- **ICD** for high-risk patients, i.e. QT >500 ms and high-risk genotypes with congenital long QT syndromes.

3.14 ▶ Supraventricular tachycardia

- **About:** SVT (classically excludes AF and flutter). Usually AVNRT or AVRT. A benign but troublesome arrhythmia not typically associated with cardiac death. Hospital admission if there is structural heart disease or severe symptoms. Seen in 3 in 1000, often young females but can occur at any age. The heart is usually structurally normal. The cure is ablation.
- **Differential of fast regular narrow tachycardia:** AVRT, AVNRT, sinus tachycardia, atrial tachycardia. Atrial flutter 2:1 or 3:1 block (vagal stimulation reveals flutter waves).
- **AVNRT:** circus re-entry pathways in or around the AV node. Two pathways: one fast conduction with long refractory period and one slow conduction and shorter refractory period. Usually anterograde (A to V) conduction is through the slow side and retrograde through the fast, then it is a slow–fast AVNRT (90%) and vice versa. Often induced by an ectopic atrial beat when the fast side is still refractory. Captures the slow path and conducts back along the fast pathway. Retrograde activated P waves seen in the QRS. Retrograde ventricular conduction is fast with slow–fast and so this is a short RP form as the atria is stimulated very quickly. Fast–slow are long RP forms. The rarest form is slow–slow.
- **AVRT:** accessory pathway joins atria and ventricles electrically. Seen with WPW syndrome or Lown–Ganong–Levine. Accessory pathways can conduct anterogradely or retrogradely. They are not always evident on the resting ECG and may be 'concealed'. Dangerous when patient develops AF and has an accessory pathway that allows rapid anterograde conduction.
- **Clinical:** palpitations, dizziness, light-headed even syncope, mild low BP but not cardiac arrest unless coexisting cardiac disease. Post palpitation polyuria due to release of ANP. SVT may cause heart failure if poor LV or other structural heart disease, e.g. mitral stenosis.

Electrocardiogram – record and keep

- **AVRT:** if SR pre-excited delta wave + short PR. Tall R wave in V1 suggests type A WPW.
- **AVRT:** orthodromic A to V activation via AV node. AVRT 180–220/min. P waves buried in QRS.
- **WPW:** if AF occurs in WPW it can lead to very rapid conduction down accessory pathway with wide irregular QRS complexes. Dangerous. DC shock.
- **AVRT:** antidromic A to V conduction across accessory pathway and back via AV node. Rate 200–300/min. Wide QRS. Can mimic VT.
- **AVNRT slow–fast:** (common) P waves are often hidden and embedded in the QRS complexes or cause pseudo 'r' (v1) or 's' waves (inf leads).
- **AVNRT fast–slow:** (rare) late negative P wave the QRS and T wave.
- **AVNRT slow–slow:** AVNRT with P wave before QRS complex.
- Abrupt termination occurs retrograde P wave ± brief asystole or low HR.

- **Investigations:** bloods: FBC, U&E, TFTs, CXR, CRP. Echo: exclude structural disease and assess LV function. Troponin only if IHD suspected, e.g. chest pain and ECG changes. Electrophysiology studies as precursor to ablation and other therapies.

Management (also see ▶ Section 1.13, Tachycardia)

- ABCs rarely indicated. If the patient is stable, then consider the modified Valsalva manoeuvres. Patient blows into 10 ml syringe for 15 sec to push back plunger, then lie patient immediately flat supine with legs elevated at 45° for 15 sec and then sit back up and observe for 30 sec for response. This should give increased vagal response. If this fails then consider CSM if age <50 and no history of TIA/stroke or audible bruit. Massage over right carotid sinus.
- **Adenosine** if SVT then give 6/12/12 mg into a large vein + saline flush. Heart transplant/Dipyridamole start at 3 mg. Excellent at terminating AVRT/AVNRT or slowing atrial flutter. Warn patient they will feel dreadful for a few seconds. Avoid in those with asthma.
- **Metoprolol** 5 mg slow IV over 10 min (up to 15 mg) or other beta-blocker is very reasonable if not asthmatic otherwise.
- **Verapamil** 5–10 mg slow IV is useful assuming LV function normal and the rhythm is narrow complex.
- **Amiodarone** 150–300 mg IV over 20–60 min is another possibility but would not be recommended for long-term therapy. If unwell as the management for any tachycardia if low BP or unwell consider rapid DC cardioversion (▶ Section 1.14). Most patients can go home following resumption of sinus rhythm for outpatient cardiology referral to discuss ablation therapy usually of the fast pathway for AVNRT or the accessory pathway in AVRT or drug therapy to prevent further arrhythmias. Exclude thyrotoxicosis.

3.15 ▶ Atrial fibrillation

- **About:** uncoordinated atrial activation with atrial mechanical dysfunction. Major risk of cardioembolism causing ischaemic stroke. Assess with risk score. Smart watches and devices may detect AF in 70% of users.
- **Aetiology:** atrial fibrosis, loss of atrial muscle mass. Increased automaticity or multiple re-entrant wavelets. Atrial 'rate' of AF is 400–600/min but it is the ventricular response that matters. Ventricular rate held in check by AV node at <200/min slows with age and conduction disease. An accessory bundle (WPW) can allow faster rates to conduct AV causing VF.
- **Haemodynamics:** increased HR shortens diastole and limits LV filling and coronary perfusion. LV filling already compromised by loss of atrial systole. Rate control with

drugs, treat failure and DC shock if needed. Impaired LV function or mitral stenosis much worse.
- **Clinical:** asymptomatic. Palpitations, dyspnoea, chest discomfort. Cardioembolic stroke, mesenteric/limb emboli, dyspnoea, fatigue, worsening heart failure, syncope, dizziness. Low BP with fast/slow AF, murmurs, signs of thyroid disease, hypertension.
- **Causes of atrial fibrillation:** ischaemic, valvular, rheumatic, hypertensive heart disease, cardiomyopathy, post cardiac surgery, thyrotoxicosis, alcohol acute binge ('holiday heart') or chronic, sick sinus syndrome, congenital heart disease, pulmonary embolism, pneumonia, sarcoidosis, amyloidosis, haemochromatosis, lone AF (idiopathic), pericarditis, myocarditis. Large meal (parasympathetic surge) 20%. Lone AF age <65, low risk of stroke <1% annually.
- **Classification of atrial fibrillation:** persistent: lasts >7 d. Paroxysmal: 2+ episodes self-terminating lasting <7 d. Permanent: lasts >1 year and fails to cardiovert. Lone AF: aged <60 y, no HTN, normal echo, no risk factors.

Investigations
- **Bloods:** FBC low Hb, raised WCC with sepsis, CRP, U&E, Mg, Ca, K, TFT – thyrotoxicosis, LFTs alcohol, haemochromatosis.
- **CXR:** cardiomegaly, pulmonary oedema, infection, post-surgery, effusion.
- **Troponin:** elevated with ACS or myocarditis and minor rise with DC shock or type 2 MI (not due to occlusive thrombus).
- **ECG:** absent 'P' waves – no organised atrial activity, fibrillatory waves that vary in amplitude, shape, and timing, random RR interval, QRS complexes which are irregularly irregular. **Aberrantly conducted AF** – wide complex and fast but irregular. **Pre-excited AF:** QRS 160–300/min and slurred up- or downstroke of delta waves seen giving wide complex appearance but very irregular; the irregularity means that it is not VT. Dangerous if it conducts to ventricles at 1:1 and can precipitate VT/VF. This depends on character of the accessory pathway. If there are RR intervals <260 ms this is considered unsafe and needs inpatient cardiology review for ablation. If unstable simply DC cardiovert.
- **Capturing PAF:** 24-h tape if suspected asymptomatic PAF. Loop recorder ECG in those with symptomatic episodes more than 24 h apart. 7-day tape.
- **Transthoracic echocardiogram:** assess LV function, valve disease, LA size. Anticoagulation rarely depends on the echo.
- **Transoesophageal echocardiogram:** closer inspection of valves, mitral disease, ASD, endocarditis, LA appendage thrombus may be seen and can help assess risk of thromboembolism.
- **Coronary angiography:** if IHD suspected.

Atrial fibrillation anticoagulation risk assessment (NICE 2022)
- **Stroke risk: CHA$_2$DS$_2$VaSc score:** **C**CF history (+1), **H**ypertension (+1), **A**ge: 65–74 (+1), >75 (+2), **D**iabetes (+1), **S**troke/TIA or thromboembolism (+2), **S**ex: female (+1), **Vasc**ular disease or CAD, MI, PAD, or aortic plaque (+1). Adjusted annual stroke risk by score: (0) 0%, (1) 1.3%, (2) 2.2%, (3) 3.3%, (4) 4.0%, (5) 6.7%, (6) 9.8%, (7) 9.6%, (8) 6.7%, (9) 15.2%. Discuss with patient. Offer anticoagulation if CHA$_2$DS$_2$VASc score 2 or more, and men with a CHA$_2$DS$_2$VASc score of 1 and more.
- **ORBIT bleeding risk score:** Hb <13 g/dl males and <12 g/dl females, or Hct <40% for males and <36% for females + 2 points. Age >74 y +1, bleeding history +2, GFR <60 ml/min/1.73 m^2 +1, on antiplatelet agents +1. Low 0–2: 2.4%, medium 3: 4.7%, High 4–7: 8.1% risks of bleed per 100 patient-years.

Management

- **AF and compromised.** AF can be a response to an infective, inflammatory or metabolic/toxic cause. Treatment must balance to focus on treating the underlying cause as well as using rate control drugs. Look for a cause. If fast AF is causing compromise: low BP, LVF, angina then consider DC cardioversion (▶ Section 1.14) which may be done without anticoagulation but start treatment dose LMWH (NICE 2014). If not severely compromised, consider one of several choices: **Amiodarone** 150–300 mg IV 30–60 min via a large-bore cannula or preferably a central line. Any deterioration then emergency DC cardioversion. Further amiodarone infusions require a central line. Alternatives include **Digoxin** loading or a **beta-blocker.** Consider cardioversion if arrhythmia <48 h and start rate control if AF duration >48 h or is uncertain. Anticoagulate both. Consider **Bisoprolol** 2.5 mg PO, **Atenolol** or **Metoprolol** (avoid sotalol) especially if angina or hypertension. Digoxin can be loaded (check not on it already) useful especially if in LVF as **Digoxin** 500 mcg PO/slow IV over 1 h and then 250–500 mcg PO/slow IV 6 h later. Digoxin slows resting rate and is an inotrope and best for those with CCF or a sedentary life. Reduce dose with renal failure. Rhythm control AF >48 h must wait until anticoagulated for a minimum of 3 weeks.
- **ABC, O_2** as needed. IV fluids if dry. Avoid/cautious if LVF or fluid overloaded. Start treatment dose LMWH or a DOAC in all with AF after assessing risks/benefits. Look for cause: infection, thyrotoxicosis, ACS, PE, sepsis, MI/ACS, pulmonary oedema, PE, alcohol excess or withdrawal.
- **AF and well:** ventricular rate 60–120/min and BP/HR well. Find cause. Anticoagulate (as above). Decide rhythm vs. rate control strategy.
- **Rate control:** consider oral beta-blocker or rate-limiting CCB. Digoxin if sedentary lifestyle. Avoid amiodarone long term as side-effects significant.
- **Rhythm control:** regain SR through cardioversion see below.
- **Anticoagulation and cardioversion:** you can electrically or chemically cardiovert immediately if you can be certain that AF duration is <48 h and age <65 and no HTN, DM, CCF or stroke/TIA one can cardiovert. If AF duration >48 hours and a TOE shows that there is no LA appendage thrombus then cardiovert and DOAC for a month. If AF duration >48 h and clot seen on TOE then DOAC for a month and then cardiovert or repeat TOE. Cardioversion can be electrical or chemical, e.g. IV **Amiodarone** infusion or Dronedarone. **Flecainide** can be used if LV function normal and no significant IHD.
- **Rhythm control preferred:** if unstable and SR would improve symptoms. Overall prognosis, however, is the same.
- **Catheter ablation** more effective and may improve quality of life – risk for cardiac perforation, pericardial tamponade and atrio-oesophageal fistula formation, and a 1% risk for stroke. Small risk for pulmonary vein stenosis.

Specific scenarios

- **Heavy alcohol binge ('holiday heart syndrome')** causing AF and other atrial arrhythmias. Echo usually normal. AST/ALT of 2:1. Elevated GGT. May have low Mg/thiamine. Cardioversion recommended. Reduce alcohol intake. Can cause LVF, arrhythmias, pneumonia and thromboembolism and even death. May need Pabrinex and Chlordiazepoxide. Assess CHA_2DS_2-VASc scores and bleed risk for anticoagulation.

- **Pre-excited AF and WPW syndrome:** IV Procainamide or IV Amiodarone or Sotalol or Flecainide if no structural disease. If unstable then immediate DC shock. *Avoid Digoxin, Verapamil and Diltiazem. They can precipitate VF.*
- **Prevention and management of postoperative AF:** with cardiothoracic surgery reduce postoperative AF by offering either amiodarone, a standard beta-blocker (not sotalol), a rate-limiting calcium antagonist. Continue any pre-existing beta blockade. Postop offer a rhythm-based strategy. For postop AF, use appropriate antithrombotic therapy and correct identifiable precipitants (U&E, low SpO_2) (NICE 2014).
- **Atrial flutter** also needs rate control and risk assessed and anticoagulation. Beta blockade or diltiazem or digoxin for rate control. Cardioversion should be considered with same assessment and anticoagulation as for AF. Amiodarone is useful for rapid rate control.
- **Anticoagulation:** consider in all with AF, atrial flutter or PAF. Determine **CHA$_2$DS$_2$VaSc score** and **HAS-BLED/ORBIT score** and assess risk/benefits of anticoagulation. Control BP, review need for aspirin or NSAIDs, stop/reduce alcohol. Do not avoid anticoagulation purely on 'risk of falls' without assessing or look to reduce falls risk where possible. Anticoagulate CHA$_2$DS$_2$VaSc >1 in men and >2 in women. If non-valvular AF (those with severe MS or AS or with a metal valve must have warfarin or LMWH) then consider warfarin or a DOAC (apixaban, dabigatran or rivaroxaban, etc.). High CHA$_2$DS$_2$VaSc score needs urgent commencement on LMWH or a DOAC or warfarin. If anticoagulation contraindicated or not acceptable then consider cardiology referral for left atrial appendage occlusion.
- **Bridging anticoagulation:** interruptions in anticoagulation can increase embolic risk. It is common to give LMWH bridging in the perioperative period but this may lead to risk of bleeding. A recent study has looked at this. The study **excluded** those with mechanical heart valves, stroke/TIA/systemic embolisation within 12 weeks, major bleeding within 6 weeks, renal insufficiency, low platelets or planned cardiac, brain or spinal surgery. The conclusion was that bridging is not warranted for most AF patients with CHA$_2$DS$_2$VaSc scores of <4, for low-risk procedures. This study must be interpreted along with local expert guidance balancing the risk of peri-procedure bleeding and embolic risk (*N Engl J Med* 2015;373:823).

3.16 Causes of bradycardia

Also see Bradycardia algorithm, ▶ Section 1.12.

Rhythm	ECG appearance and comments
Sinus	ECG: normal rate 60–100. Normal 1:1 AV. Regular/sinus arrhythmia. Normal.
Sinus bradycardia	ECG: normal P wave rate but <60/min. P:QRS ratio: 1:1. QRS: regular/sinus arrhythmia. Intrinsic rate is 100/min. Vagal tone reduces heart rate to 70/min or <50/min when sleeping. High vagal tone, e.g. post vasovagal syncope 'faint', cholestatic jaundice. Excess beta blockade, conduction tissue disease, hypothyroidism, raised intracranial pressure.
Slow AF	ECG: absent P waves, irregularly irregular QRS. Slow AF: irregular QRS complex, absent P wave. Natural rate 100/min. Slower rates are due to digoxin/beta-blockers or AV nodal disease.

Rhythm	ECG appearance and comments
Tachy–brady syndrome	ECG: AF or A flutter or paroxysmal atrial tachy-bradycardia or sinus arrest P:QRS ratio: 1:1 unless flutter. Regular QRS unless AF. Dysfunction of the sinus node – sinus pauses with AF, flutter or atrial tachycardias. Bradycardia is controlled by pacemaker and drugs (or ablation) NICE (2005) has recommended dual-chamber pacemakers for symptomatic bradycardia due to sick sinus syndrome without AV block.
Sinus arrest	Normal P missing for >3 sec. P:QRS ratio: 1:1 but may be ectopics. Irregular if recurrent. Sinus pauses/arrest: normal P QRS T wave then no P wave for 3 sec or longer. Stop exacerbating drugs. May need to be paced if symptomatic.
1st-degree	Normal P wave P:QRS ratio: 1:1 Normal but PR is delayed PR >0.2 sec 1st-degree: long PR >200–220 msec; each P wave followed by a delayed QRS complex. Overall HR unaffected. Rarely needs intervention. Review meds.
2nd-degree Mobitz I	Normal P wave. Lengthening PR until a P wave fails to be followed by a QRS complex. Normal. P wave and lengthening PR until a P wave fails to be followed by a QRS complex: Wenckebach phenomenon is due to a block at AV nodal level. May be physiological or seen at rest or sleeping, or in athletes. Pacing rarely needed.
2nd-degree Mobitz II	Normal P wave. P wave not followed by QRS. Normal QRS is intermittently dropped. Damage is infranodal and is a more significant arrhythmia with lower threshold to pace than Mobitz I. Pace if permanent or intermittent, regardless of the type or the site of the block, with symptomatic bradycardia. Consider pacing in setting of acute MI. Risk of asystole.
2nd-degree with 2:1 or 3:1 AV block	Normal. P wave not followed by QRS every 2nd or 3rd beat. Regular with dropped beat. 2nd-degree with 2:1 or 3:1 block: every 2nd or 3rd beat does not conduct to ventricles. AV node disease or below. Pace if symptomatic or acute MI.
3rd-degree Complete heart block	Normal P wave at 60–100/min or no P wave as AF. Wide and slower means lower origin and more unstable QRS rate is 30–40/min depending on the level. Regular but slow. Complete failure of communication between atria and ventricles. Ventricles' intrinsic rate is 30–40/min depending on the level (lower is slower). Cannon 'a' waves are seen with complete heart block. Nearly always requires pacing. Risk of syncope and even asystole.

- **About:** BP more important than HR. An extreme athlete can have a resting HR of 30–40 bpm. Second-degree heart block can suggest impending CHB/asystole.
- **Clinical:** pre/syncope, pale, shocked, low BP, HR <60 bpm. Obtunded. Some patients, e.g. bed-bound elderly, can tolerate CHB quite well. Stokes–Adams attacks are due to short periods of asystole or very slow CHB.
- **Investigations:** U&E, FBC, TFTs, troponin if ACS. ECG, echocardiogram to assess LV.
- **Management:** ABC O$_2$, IV fluids, IV access, ECG monitor. If BP <90/60 mmHg and HR <60 bpm see Bradycardia, ▶Section 1.12.

3.17 ▶ Aortic dissection

- **Discussion:** aortic wall consists of inner intima, media and adventitia. Dissection involves separation of the media and intima often with intramural bleeding and haematoma which can dissect distally or sometimes proximally (into pericardium) powered by the hammering pulsatile force of aortic flow. If dissection suspected, then arrange urgent CT aorta and if type A dissection found you must reduce the

BP whilst getting the patient to a cardiothoracic centre immediately. The mortality of untreated type A dissections is approximately 1% per hour in the first 24 h and within first 10 d, peaking with an overall in-hospital mortality of 58%, and 26% for those who undergo surgery. A negative D-dimer result may be useful to help rule out acute aortic dissection (and PE) in low-risk patients (*Ann Emerg Med* 2015;66:368).

- **Aetiology:** blood tracks under the intima and into the media. Bleeding from lumen or vasa vasorum causes intramural thrombus. The intima can tear distally and on CT or other imaging there can be a 'true lumen' and 'false lumen'. May be connective tissue disease (see below). Blunt thoracic trauma causes a tear in the arterial wall. Intima tears within a few cms of the aortic valve, usually on the right lateral wall of the aortic arch where shear stresses are high. Distal dissections occur beyond left subclavian artery. Obstruction of RCA more common. Occlusion of LCA usually instantly fatal. Dissection can therefore be accompanied by STEMI.
- **Causes:** HTN, atherosclerosis, Marfan syndrome, Ehlers–Danlos syndrome, Turner syndrome, cystic medial degeneration, Loeys–Dietz aneurysm syndrome, trauma – sudden deceleration, cocaine, phaeochromocytoma, heavy weightlifting. Pregnancy 3rd trimester, coarctation of the aorta, bicuspid aortic valve, aortitis – Takayasu's arteritis. Syphilis, aortic valve replacement, familial – autosomal dominant. Iatrogenic aortic manipulation (including angiography and stenting) and IABP.
- **Stanford classification:** Stanford type A (60%) – any involvement of ascending aorta. Mortality 80% in first 48 h and related to time to surgery. High risk rupture, tamponade, acute MI, stroke, acute AR and cardiogenic shock, innominate compromised (60–70%): involves proximal aorta and arch. Requires urgent surgery. Most tears are seen in upper right lateral wall of the ascending aorta. Stanford type B (30–40%): not involving aorta, distal to left subclavian artery and may extend down as far as the iliac vessels and have better outcome; management is medical.

Clinical

- **Chest/back pain:** sudden anterior (root and ascending aorta) or interscapular (descending aorta) chest wall pain or even abdominal pain. Some pain may radiate into the back. Syncopal or presyncopal episode with tearing/stabbing/ sharp interscapular pain. Aortic regurgitation: dissection can shear the aortic valve. Look for new early diastolic murmur suggesting AR and associated with acute LVF. History: Marfan's or EDS, bicuspid valve or hypertension. May be shocked if there is blood loss or tamponade.
- **Aortic arch syndrome:** dissection may shear off vessels in the proximal aorta (right brachiocephalic gives off right subclavian and carotid, left common carotid and left subclavian). Causes stroke. Reduced pulsation or reduced BP because the arm supplied by the subclavian/brachiocephalic artery is obstructed. Coronary artery: left main stem = sudden death with LV infarction; right coronary artery: inferior MI with chest pain. Right brachiocephalic: ischaemia of right subclavian, right common carotid and right vertebral. Devastating if complete with a right TACI with right hemiparesis or posterior circulation signs and right arm ischaemia and low BP. Left subclavian: ataxia (vertebral) and arm ischaemia and low BP left arm and posterior circulation symptoms and signs. Left common carotid: left TACI stroke with right hemiparesis. Anterior spinal artery: paraplegia affecting legs with preserved dorsal columns. Coeliac axis: ischaemic bowel. Renal artery: anuria, haematuria and AKI.
- **Differential:** chest pain (▶Section 3.3) ACS, PE and oesophageal and lung causes.

Investigations

- **Bloods:** U&E, FBC, LFTs, troponin, group and cross-match. Raised D-dimer with dissection (exclude PE/dissection with urgent CTPA/aorta).
- **CXR:** unfolded aorta, wide mediastinum (>6–8 cm), left pleural effusion may be exudate from an inflamed aorta. Widening mediastinum 80% of acute dissection. Left apical cap, deviation of the oesophagus, deviation of the trachea to the right, depression of the left mainstem bronchus, loss of the paratracheal stripe.
- **ECG:** arrhythmias. Inferior MI if RCA involved. Long-standing LVH. Can be normal.
- **CT aorta** is diagnostic. Spiral CT shows double lumen: one false lumen and one true lumen of dissection. Defines the operative anatomy and involvement of branch vessels. False lumen can have a greater cross-sectional area. False lumen beaks are often filled with low attenuation thrombus. Outer wall calcification is present in true lumen. The 'beak sign' is the cross-sectional imaging manifestation of the wedge of haematoma that cleaves a space for the propagating false lumen and that is present microscopically in all dissections. Contrast leak indicates aortic rupture. May be picked up incidentally on CTPA.
- **Echo:** transthoracic suprasternal views may be useful. Transoesophageal echo gives excellent views of aorta and valve and shows function. TOE can augment CT findings if time allows. It can show dissection flap, true and false lumen, thrombosis in false lumen and pericardial effusion.
- **Complications:** death from aortic rupture, ischaemic stroke – TACI-like presentation if brachiocephalic occluded. Subclavian obstruction may cause a possible posterior circulation event but collateral opposite vertebral. Cardiac tamponade (blood) – drainage can precipitate more bleeding and death. Acute aortic regurgitation and LVF, spinal cord infarction. Mesenteric/renal ischaemia. Left pleural haemothorax – ominous sign on CXR, sudden death, distal limb ischaemia.

Management (type A surgical repair, type B medical management)

- **ABC:** O$_2$. Good IV access ×2. If haemorrhage or tamponade death is usually immediate. Group and cross-match for perioperative blood loss. Acute dissection of the ascending aorta is highly lethal with a cumulative mortality rate of 1–2% per hour so rapid stabilisation and transfer are needed. ECG/CXR to exclude differentials for acute chest pain. Inadvertent anticoagulation or thrombolysis (before PCI not uncommon as mistaken for inf. STEMI) should be avoided as can cause haemorrhage or delay surgery. If suspicious discuss with Radiology for CT aortogram.
- **Analgesia: Morphine** 5–10 mg IV. Lower BP target MAP = 60–75 mmHg.
- **Labetalol** 20 mg IV stat in Type A which may be repeated. Labetalol is an anti-impulse agent and helps reduce the pulsatile driving pressure of dp/dt. Give bolus dose then infusion. Also consider nitroprusside (lower than normal dose). Dissection driven by pulsatile driving pressure of dp/dt BP. Lower BP target MAP = 60–75 mmHg and pulse pressure with **Nitroprusside** (lower than normal dose) and **Labetalol** IV in type A. Use beta-blockers with caution if acute AR as they may block a compensatory tachycardia.
- **Cardiac tamponade:** avoid emergency pericardiocentesis of an acute type A aortic dissection complicated by cardiac tamponade as it can result in sudden deterioration, but proceed urgently to surgical repair of the aorta with intra-operative drainage of the haemopericardium.
- **Cardiothoracic surgery on bypass cooled to 22°C** for type A involves replacement of proximal aorta by a tube graft – may require resection and

replacement of the aortic valve and sewing in of coronary vessels and repair of the coronary sinus.

- **Endovascular treatment:** percutaneous or minimal access endoluminal repair may be possible. Involves 'fenestrating' (perforating) the intimal flap so that blood can return from the false to the true lumen (so decompressing the former), or implanting a stent graft placed from the femoral artery.
- **Long-term management:** type B dissection lower BP acutely and long-term on oral medication aim for both type A and B. Beta-blocker-based therapy preferred and/or ACEi. Lifelong imaging of the entire aorta by either CT or MRI is advocated. Uncomplicated type B dissection has an in-hospital mortality rate of 10%.
- **Reference:** Braverman (2010) Acute aortic dissection: clinician update. *Circulation*, **122**:184.

3.18 ▶ Acute myocarditis

- **About:** serious acquired dilated weak heart, fatal arrhythmias, heart failure. Prognosis generally good. Most recover. 30% develop a dilated cardiomyopathy.
- **Aetiology:** inflamed myocardium with reduced function. Results in end-stage cardiac failure, thromboembolism and arrhythmias.
- **Causes:** idiopathic: all investigations negative; 50% presumably viral but unproven. Viral infection: parvovirus B19 and HHV6, Coxsackie A (mild), Coxsackie B (severe) and influenza; echovirus; adenovirus; HIV; CMV. Non-viral infection: Chagas disease (*Trypanosoma cruzi*), toxoplasmosis. Rickettsial: scrub typhus, Rocky Mountain spotted fever, Q fever, Lyme disease causes temporary conduction block. Bacterial: leptospirosis, diphtheria, TB, brucella. Drugs and toxins: doxorubicin, trastuzumab, cyclophosphamide, penicillin, phenytoin, methyldopa, cocaine abuse. Heavy metals: arsenic, cobalt, mercury exposure. Miscellaneous: radiation, peripartum cardiomyopathy, post cardiac transplant rejection. Inflammatory: sarcoidosis, Kawasaki disease, SLE, granulomatosis with polyangiitis (WG), thyrotoxicosis, rheumatoid arthritis, rheumatic fever. Giant cell myocarditis: rare usually fatal form of myocarditis. Ventricular arrhythmias and severe cardiac failure.
- **Clinical:** fatigue, dyspnoea, heart failure, chest pain, LVF, AF, VT or sudden cardiac death, MR, S4. Enquire viral illness, drug usage.

Investigations

- **Bloods:** FBC: raised WCC, CRP and ESR. Others: check ANA, dsDNA, ASO titres, TFTs. HIV test. BNP, troponin.
- **ECG:** AF, ST/T wave changes even mimicking STEMI/NSTEMI; those with Q waves or LBBB are a poor prognostic group; ectopics, VT, VF, heart block.
- **CXR:** cardiomegaly, pulmonary oedema.
- **Cardiac biomarkers:** raised CK, CKMB, troponin in proportion to damage.
- **Echo:** transthoracic to assess LV and RV dysfunction, enlarged chambers, thrombus, pericardial effusion, and valve regurgitation.
- **Cardiac MR (CMR):** non-invasive and valuable clinical tool for the diagnosis of myocarditis. Changes seen on T2-weighted oedema imaging.
- **Transvenous endomyocardial biopsy:** gold standard for diagnosis. It may show lymphocytic infiltration and myocyte necrosis. Giant cell myocarditis.
- **FDG-PET scan:** increased myocardial FDG uptake in the setting of myocardial inflammation.

- **Serology and PCR:** influenza, Coxsackie, parvovirus, Covid, dengue, Zika serology.
- **Coronary angiography:** if IHD/ACS suspected.
- **Complications:** some develop a dilated cardiomyopathy and end-stage heart failure which may improve. VT/VF. Heart block, sudden cardiac death, thromboembolism.

Management (get early expert cardiac input, admit CCU)

- **Acute:** afterload reduction and diuresis. Bed rest, treat heart failure and arrhythmias as usual. CCU with telemetry depending on presentation and severity. Inotropes. LV assist devices. IABP. Access to defibrillation. Avoid exercise during acute period and convalescence. Avoid NSAIDs.
- **Immune-mediated disease: Prednisolone** 1 mg/kg/day up to 90 days for cardiac sarcoidosis, giant cell myocarditis, autoimmune rheumatic disease.
- **Standard heart failure regime** including beta-blockers, diuretics, ACEi or angiotensin-II receptor blockers (ARBs) should be initiated.
- **Intra-aortic balloon pumping or LV assist device.** May augment cardiac output whilst awaiting improvement, treatment or transplant.
- **VTE prophylaxis** and full anticoagulation, if AF or LA / LV thrombus.
- **IV immunoglobulin** (400 mg/kg per day) for 5 days may help preserve LVEF in adult acute fulminant myocarditis. Needs expert input as evidence changes.
- **Others:** antiprotozoal therapy for Chagas disease. Withdraw toxic medications.
- **Heart transplant** in those with dilated CMP, giant cell myocarditis, end-stage cardiac failure. Cardiogenic shock and heart failure, see ▶ Section 2.16.
- **Reference:** Lampejo T, *et al.* (2021) Acute myocarditis: aetiology, diagnosis and management. *Clin Med (Lond),* 21:e505.

3.19 Acute pericarditis

Caution with anticoagulants as there is a risk of haemopericardium.

- **About:** seen in 5% of CCU chest pain admissions. TB seen in developing world. Otherwise 90% are idiopathic or viral. May be found in association with acute myocarditis and both have similar aetiologies.

Causes of pericarditis

- **Idiopathic** or unknown is commonest (presumably viral).
- **Viral:** parvovirus B19, echovirus, Coxsackie B, influenza, CMV, EBV, adenovirus, HBV, HCV, H1N1, HIV (may cause *Staph. aureus* effusion).
- **Bacterial/fungal:** TB may go on to constrictive pericarditis. Raised ESR/JVP, dyspnoea, fever, weight loss. *Coxiella burnetii*, pneumococcus, meningococcal. Pyogenic post-op pericarditis or post pneumonia. Fungal: histoplasmosis.
- **Inflammatory:** post myocardial injury (Dressler's syndrome), autoimmune disorder (SLE/RA/Behçet's), drug-induced lupus (hydralazine, procainamide), familial Mediterranean fever, rheumatic fever (with associated pancarditis and murmurs, rash, joint aches).
- **Malignancy:** lymphoma, carcinoma of bronchus/breast, melanoma, leukaemia.
- **Miscellaneous:** metabolic (uraemia – ESRF – needs dialysis), hypothyroid/myxoedema (large chronic effusion but rarely compromising).

Clinical

- Fever, malaise, myalgia, post-viral syndrome. Pleuritic-type chest pain eased by sitting forwards, worse lying flat and on inspiration. Pain referred to shoulder or scapula. Auscultation friction rub (very useful sign worth looking for) with a systolic (ventricular filling) and atrial systolic component.
- **Diagnostic criteria:** diagnosis of acute pericarditis requires the presence of any two of (1) pericarditic chest pain; (2) pericardial rub; (3) saddle-shaped ST-elevation and/or PR-depression; (4) non-trivial new or worsening pericardial effusion.
- **Differential:** ACS, aortic dissection, PE, oesophageal disease, musculoskeletal.

Investigations

- **Bloods:** FBC: raised WCC, ESR and CRP – infective/inflammatory causes. U&E: AKI or CKD uraemic pericarditis. TFT: TSH >10 mU/L low FT_4 hypothyroidism.
- **CXR/tuberculin testing:** if TB suspected. HIV test.
- **ECG:** saddle-shaped ST elevation and PR depression in all leads except aVr or V1 which look into the cavity of the heart where there is therefore an inverted lead, showing ST depression. Spodick's sign is downsloping of TP segment. Eventually ST and PR normalise and there is T wave inversion, which then normalises. May be AF or other atrial arrhythmias. ECG may be low voltage if effusion.
- **CXR:** usually normal. If enlarged heart look for an effusion.
- **Cardiac MR** can identify the presence of pericardial inflammation and any myopericarditis. This can help diagnosis and ensure appropriate treatment initiated earlier.
- **Echocardiogram:** to look for pericardial fluid, LV function (as ever very important), tamponade. Pericardial effusion may be classified into 3 groups according to diastolic distance between the pericardium and the ventricle: (1) <10 mm, (2) moderate 10–20 mm, (3) severe >20 mm. The incidence of cardiac tamponade secondary to severe pericardial effusion is about 3%. RV dysfunction seems to be the greatest predictor of mortality and cardiac transplantation. CK and troponin: elevated in 50% if there is an associated myopericarditis. Diagnostic pericardiocentesis: exclude TB and diagnose malignancy where appropriate.

Management

- **Acute treatment:** NSAIDs are the main treatment (consider adding PPI), e.g. **Indometacin** 50 mg 8 h or **Ibuprofen** 400–600 mg 8 h (+ PPI) until CRP/ESR normalises, usually in 10–14 d. Combine this with **Colchicine** 500 mcg BD for 3 months for patients weighing >70 kg or 500 mcg OD if weight ≤70 kg reduces symptoms by day 3 and incidence of recurrence from 55% to 24% at 18 months, as well as risk of subsequent hospitalisation. Avoid colchicine in pregnancy or breastfeeding. Check for interactions. Steroids are associated with an increased risk of recurrence and are usually avoided. Most can be managed with ambulatory care – see criteria below. Physical exertion is avoided in the acute phase and in up to 6 months in athletes. Repeat echo where needed. Therapeutic pericardiocentesis if evidence of tamponade but this is uncommon. Where diagnosis is unclear and pain continues and risk of IHD high then angiography may be required to exclude ACS. Patients should be given clear advice on re-admission if there are new or ongoing symptoms.
- **Risk assessment:** many can be managed as outpatient. Admit if fever >38°C, gradual onset, large effusion >20 mm or tamponade, immunosuppression, anticoagulation treatment, troponin negative, traumatic aetiology, myopericarditis,

no anti-inflammatory response after 1 week. Weigh up risks of low dose VTE and haemorrhage into pericardium. Pericarditis may be seen post pneumonia and may require IV antibiotics depending on the likely organism. Any suggestion of a purulent or malignant effusion will need urgent consideration for drainage following imaging.

- **Recurrent pericarditis:** consider further colchicine and reassessment. Some may develop a constrictive pericarditis. Pericardiotomy might also be performed if constrictive pericarditis has developed.
- **Effusion:** any concerns get an echocardiogram. Main worry is tamponade. See section below on pericardial effusion; if there is any effusion take expert advice.
- **Reference:** Acute pericarditis: Update on diagnosis and management (2020) *Clin Med (Lond)*, 20:48–51.

3.20 Pericardial effusion/tamponade

- **About:** also see pericarditis above (▶Section 3.19). Reverse all anticoagulants if suspected spontaneous or post interventional/trauma-related bleeding into pericardial space. Tamponade is uncommon even with large pericardial effusions – prevent with elective drainage. Small effusions are often found at routine echocardiogram.
- **NB:** look for tachycardia, low BP, narrow pulse pressure, and elevated neck veins, distant heart sounds with recent pericarditis, thoracic malignancy, chest trauma, coagulopathy or recent cardiac procedure. Pericardiocentesis can be life-saving and indicated in effusions >20mm deep.
- **Aetiology:** fluid/blood collects in the pericardial space. Normally pericardial space holds less than 50 ml of fluid. Chronic accumulation over months can produce up to 1000 ml without significant compromise as pericardial sac stretches, unless there is chronic scarring or thickening. In cardiac tamponade, the pericardial pressure may reach 15–20 mmHg, leading to an equalisation of pressures into the cardiac chambers and to a huge decrease in the systemic venous return. Acute accumulations of even 100 ml may be enough to cause haemodynamic collapse as increased volume and pressure leads the right atrium and then the right ventricle to collapse in diastole. Beck's triad can be detected with low BP, reduced heart sounds and raised JVP with prominent *x* descent and absent *y* descent. Slow collections tolerated well. If diastolic cardiac filling compromised then tamponade. Absence of pericardium is not problematic at all.
- **Causes of effusion: (see pericarditis)** idiopathic, viral, hypothyroid, SLE, amyloid, scleroderma, HIV, drugs: isoniazid, phenytoin, hydralazine, procainamide. Causes more likely to produce tamponade are neoplastic disease, idiopathic pericarditis, renal disease, tuberculosis, bleeding – warfarin, DOAC, heparin, DIC, trauma, uraemia, post MI and ventricular rupture, type A aortic dissection proximally. Post procedure – cardiac catheterisation or pacemaker insertion, transseptal catheter.
- **Clinical** (signs of effusion and likely causes): asymptomatic if small, pericarditis-type symptoms. Cough, fever, malaise and systemic symptoms. Muffled heart sounds. Right heart failure with peripheral oedema and hepatomegaly. Cachexia and weight loss may suggest malignancy, TB or HIV. **Acute tamponade:** low HR due to pericardial stretch followed by a fall in BP. Pulsus paradoxus: radial pulse impalpable during inspiration (marked fall in BP >10 mmHg). JVP: markedly raised (RA pressure) which rises with inspiration. Kussmaul's sign and loss of *y* descent. Heart sounds are quiet and area of cardiac dullness increases.
- **Differential:** ACS, aortic dissection, PE, oesophageal disease.

Investigations
- **FBC:** raised WCC, high ESR, high CRP if inflammatory/infective. **U&E:** uraemia.
- **Coagulation screen** if on anticoagulants.
- **ECG:** low voltage QRS complexes, AF, evidence of pericarditis or recent MI. Electrical alternans. CXR: shows cardiac enlargement (cardiomegaly or effusion need echo to differentiate) or may show underlying neighbouring malignancy. Large effusions present as globular cardiomegaly with sharp margins. If the effusion develops during catheterisation, it may also be identified by the development of lucent lines in the cardiopericardial silhouette or so-called epicardial halo sign or fat pad sign. Straightening and immobility of the left heart border.
- **CXR** may show globular heart, TB or lung malignancy.
- **Echocardiogram:** pericardial effusion – measure diastolic distance between the pericardium and the ventricle: (1) <10 mm, (2) moderate 10–20 mm, (3) severe >20 mm. The incidence of cardiac tamponade secondary to severe pericardial effusion is about 3%. Tamponade: diastolic collapse of RA and free wall of RV are signs of incipient circulatory compromise. RV collapse is the most specific echo finding. Also look for fall in mitral inflow velocity or aortic velocity by 25% with inspiration. Invasive monitoring would show a fall in aortic pressure and rise in RA pressure. Echo can be used to guide pericardiocentesis. Cardiac MRI is useful for detecting pericardial effusion and loculated pericardial effusion and thickening.
- **Cardiac troponin I/T:** usually negative except where there is an associated myopericarditis or ACS. Check clotting: if coagulopathy or warfarin and haemopericardium suspected. Diagnostic pericardiocentesis ± pericardial biopsy if TB or malignancy suspected. Exudate suggests an infective/inflammatory or malignant process. Measure pericardial effusion adenosine deaminase for TB, tumour marker measurement (CEA, cytokeratin 19 fragment) and cytology for neoplasms, and culture and PCR for infections. Protein, LDH, Hb, WCC, viral, bacterial, TB cultures. Others: tuberculin skin test, blood cultures, complement levels, ANA, ESR if SLE suspected.

Management
- **Not compromised** and infection not suspected then diagnosis can be made by other methods and pericardiocentesis not indicated. Treat underlying causes, e.g. thyroxine for hypothyroid, dialysis for uraemia. Need for anticoagulation should be assessed and balanced with risk of bleeding into pericardial space.
- **Effusions >1 cm** depth need repeat echo in 7 d and ongoing follow-up. Elective pericardiocentesis is relatively safe and easy with either echocardiography or fluoroscopy guided pericardiocentesis. Some advocate drainage of large effusions to prevent possible evolution of cardiac tamponade where the effusion >20 mm depth unresponsive to medical therapy after 4–6 weeks. Other indications include evidence of RA or RV collapse, and any significant chronic (>3 months) effusion. Pericardiocentesis often does not aid diagnosis but may prevent tamponade. Not all effusions need to be drained and can be followed by serial echocardiography.
- **Compromised:** ABCs. O_2. Good IV access. Avoid diuretics and volume depletion. Give 0.5–1.0 L NS to ensure filling pressures. Volume resuscitation and catecholamines are temporary but the only remaining effective treatment in tamponade is urgent needle pericardiocentesis, except where a type A proximal aortic dissection is suspected which can cause circulatory collapse – needs cardiothoracic advice. If anticoagulated suspect bleeding into pericardial space – stop and reverse any coagulopathy.

- **Volume loading:** may be beneficial and repeated trials of 250–500 ml of crystalloid should be assessed for improvement of haemodynamics. Catecholamines and IV **Nitroprusside** to reduce afterload and/or IV **Dobutamine** may also be of benefit in some patients. **Emergency pericardiocentesis:** consider transfer to tertiary centre if stable or summon local expertise. If high risk of recurrence consider cardiothoracic referral for pericardial fenestration to prevent any further build-up of fluid. It may be attempted in cardiac arrest in those at risk with PEA (see Emergency Pericardiocentesis Video. *New Engl J Med* (2012) 366:e17).
- **References:** Bodson *et al.* (2011) Cardiac tamponade. *Curr Opin Crit Care*, **17:**416. Maisch *et al.* (2004) Guidelines on the diagnosis and management of pericardial diseases: executive summary. *Eur Heart J*, **25:**587. Imazio *et al.* (2009) *Nat Rev Cardiol*, **6:**743.

3.21 ▶ Severe accelerated (malignant) hypertension

- **About:** uncommon now due to primary care screening and treatment. BP causes end-organ damage over years. Acute rises should be gradually reduced in most cases. Evidence-base for hypertensive emergency management lacking. Follow local guidance. A BP >200 mmHg in elderly not uncommon. Same in a younger person may well be an emergency from both cause and effect.
- **Aetiology:** untreated/undiagnosed essential hypertension; failure to take medication. Phaeochromocytoma or other secondary cause. Acute cocaine, severe anxiety, pain, acute urinary retention, pre-eclampsia. Acute stroke. There is accelerated microvascular damage with necrosis in the walls of small arteries and arterioles (fibrinoid necrosis) and by intravascular thrombosis.
- **Clinical:** asymptomatic to mild malaise, mild headache, anxiety, distress. Breathless with pulmonary oedema, microangiopathic haemolytic anaemia. Renal failure, stroke (ischaemic or haemorrhagic). Fundoscopy – retinal haemorrhages and papilloedema, confusion. Delirium – encephalopathy, look for clues in history and examine. Phaeochromocytoma, renal bruits, radiofemoral delay. Renal masses, examine drug chart – NSAID, ciclosporin.
- **Malignant hypertension:** high BP + retinal haemorrhages + papilloedema + nephropathy or chest pain. Beware watershed cerebral infarction with rapid lowering.

Investigations
- **Bloods:** FBC, U&E (CKD, low K with Conn's syndrome).
- **ECG:** AF, LVH, LAD, LBBB, ST/T wave changes. R + S >35 mm.
- **CXR:** cardiomegaly, rib notching with coarctation of the aorta.
- **Echocardiogram:** LVH, diastolic dysfunction, assess LV (exclude coarctation).
- **Renal USS:** small kidneys with CKD, polycystic kidneys, difference in size with RAS. Adrenal hyperplasia or tumour mass.
- **Urine** for proteinuria, cocaine, amphetamines, urinary catecholamines, dexamethasone suppression, renin/aldosterone levels.
- **CT/MRI head:** if new neurology, e.g. haemorrhage or infarct, tumour or posterior reversible encephalopathy syndrome.

Secondary causes of hypertension
- **Simple causes:** pain, agitation, delirium, hypercarbia, hypoxia, hypervolaemia, bladder distension, stroke. Treat and exclude these first.

- **Essential hypertension:** older patients. Often well tolerated. See SBP up to 220 mmHg in well patient. Lower cautiously. Exclude simple causes.
- **Conn's syndrome:** U&E low K, renin/aldosterone levels. Adrenal imaging. Adenoma or hyperplasia. Consider aldosterone antagonists.
- **Cushing's syndrome:** raised urinary free cortisol, dexamethasone suppression, cushingoid appearance, striae, weight gain, hirsutism. Low ACTH high cortisol suggests non pituitary source. Needs adrenal/pituitary imaging.
- **Drugs:** OCP, ciclosporin, alcohol, NSAIDs, amphetamines.
- **Cocaine-induced HTN:** IV GTN. CCBs, Diazepam. Avoid beta-blockers.
- **Aortic coarctation:** 0.25%. CXR changes, echo, MRA, CT aorta. Hypertension upper body. May need surgery, hypertension often persists.
- **Renal artery stenosis:** 0.5%. USS for size disparity, MRA, flash oedema, renal bruit, AKI with ACEi.
- **Polycystic kidney disease:** USS, family Hx, HTN. Berry aneurysms/SAH.
- **Pre-eclampsia:** pregnancy >20 weeks, proteinuria, etc. ▶Section 16.6.
- **Phaeochromocytoma:** elevated urine catecholamines, metanephrines and plasma catecholamines. Tumour seen on CT abdomen. 10% are extra-adrenal (in sympathetic chain from neck to bladder), 10% malignant and bilateral.

Indications for emergency BP reduction

- Ensure simple causes are looked for and treated. Acute BP lowering is not risk-free and risks vs. benefits need to be evaluated. A rapid fall can cause myocardial/cerebral hypoperfusion. In many 'new' cases in older patients BP has been chronically high for a long time, just unmeasured or unrecognised, or recognised but undertreated or non-compliant.
- A BP of over 220/120 mmHg in an 80-year-old who is asymptomatic is often essential hypertension and needs gradual reduction with oral agents. The same BP in a 35-year-old with proteinuria or LVH or neurology is much more concerning and needs admission and control. Context matters. Impending end-organ damage matters. Acute ICH is predominantly a problem of chronic HTN not acute rises. CT scan if any neurology. MRI if PRES.

Management

- **NICE 2019:** if BP >180/120 refer for same-day specialist review if retinal haemorrhage or papilloedema (accelerated hypertension) or life-threatening symptoms or suspected phaeochromocytoma.
- **NICE 2019:** if BP >180/120 then assess for target organ damage as soon as possible. Consider starting drug treatment immediately. If no target organ damage then review in clinic in 7 d.
- **Urgent:** suspected phaeochromocytoma, eclampsia (inform obstetricians) or encephalopathy, grade III/VI retinopathy, or severe pulmonary oedema consider CCU/ITU and urgent treatment. Inform renal if in renal failure.
- **General measures:** quiet room, 15–30 min NEWS monitoring. Environment can help reduce BP. Get patient out of the busy ED. No smoking, no coffee. Ensure relief of pain, agitation, treat urinary retention. Commence an oral agent. If well and no organ damage follow-up within days may be reasonable if it responds to treatment. Aim to lower BP in a slow controlled manner over hours and days to acceptable levels (e.g. to <180/110 mmHg) using slow onset oral agents. Target a gradual reduction to a normal BP over days rather than minutes or hours unless complicated.

Urgent reduction

- **General measures + oral drugs** – lower BP over hours unless urgent indications. No evidence base for which drugs to use. If patient well and renal function OK then suggest **Amlodipine** 5 mg PO or **Atenolol** 25 mg PO (caution if suspect phaeochromocytoma) or **Ramipril** 2.5 mg PO (caution if suspect RAS). Set a target that is perhaps 10–20% lower than the current BP, e.g. 180/110 mmHg. But immediate aim is not to achieve a BP of 120/80 mmHg. If precipitated by stopping usual BP meds and no adverse effects with these then consider re-introduction slowly, perhaps one by one until controlled.
- **Emergency BP reduction:** severe cases as described above or, if BP sustained at >220/120 mmHg despite other measures, then consider (if no history of bronchospasm/asthma) **Labetalol** 20–40 mg slow IV over 5 min which is easy to give as a bolus or infusion. An alternative, especially if angina or pulmonary oedema, is **IV GTN**. The nitric oxide donor **Nitroprusside** IV can also be considered. Treat BP in ischaemic stroke if sustained BP >220/120 mmHg, or patient is for thrombolysis or there is acute intracerebral haemorrhage. Reduce BP slowly.
- **Additional steps:** if agitation or delirium or aggression is a driver to the BP consider oral or IM sedation. Use **Lorazepam** 0.5–2 mg or **Haloperidol** 0.5–2 mg PO/IM. Beta-blockers avoided if phaeochromocytoma suspected. Give **Furosemide** 50 mg IV ± GTN 2 sprays (800 mcg) for pulmonary oedema.
- **Manage AKI and exclude renal causes:** check urine – blood, protein and nephritis and renal parenchymal causes (see AKI, ▶ Section 10.4). Consider a urinary catheter if you really need to assess urine output or exclude obstruction. Always double check (especially in older confused patient) that you haven't missed urinary retention or untreated pain with its usual pressor response. Patients can be significantly volume depleted and may need volume expansion once BP is controlled with IV NS.

Life-threatening symptoms needing urgent management

- **Acute pulmonary oedema: ACEi**, IV **Furosemide**, IV **nitrates.**
- **Acute MI:** IV **nitrates** + start small dose ACEi.
- **Acute aortic dissection:** BP target <120/80 mmHg if tolerated especially for proximal dissection. Use **Labetalol** 20–40 mg slow IV stat then infusion.
- **Acute intracerebral haemorrhage:** gradually lower by 10–20% over several hours, e.g. **Labetalol** 20–40 mg slow IV stat.
- **Hypertensive encephalopathy:** (headache, confusion, seizures, symptoms + papilloedema) use IV **Labetalol** 20–40 mg IV though no real preference.
- **Scleroderma crises** respond to ACEi (e.g. lisinopril) and/or angiotensin II receptor blockade (e.g. losartan).
- **Stroke thrombolysis:** lower BP to <185/110 mmHg if safe to do so within the thrombolysis time frame. A rapid drop in BP and cerebral blood flow might cause watershed infarcts and do more harm than thrombolysis benefits. Likely to be more at risk if significant cerebral atherosclerosis. Consider **Labetalol** 20–40 mg slow IV.
- **Phaeochromocytoma:** ensure alpha blockade before beta-blockers. If acute need to treat then **Phentolamine** 2–5 mg IV bolus. If stable then **Phenoxybenzamine** 20–80 mg/d initially in divided doses followed by propranolol 120–240 mg/d. Alternatively start **Doxazosin** 2–4 mg/d in divided doses. Also consider **IV Nitrates, calcium antagonists** and **diazepam.** There can be a huge fall in circulating catecholamines once the tumour is removed and sudden fall in SVR needing rapid volume replacement.

Ongoing long-term BP management algorithm

- **Age <55:** Step 1: ACEi/ARB. Step 2: add CCB or thiazide. Step 3: add CCB + thiazide. Step 4: low dose spironolactone/beta-blocker/alpha-blocker.
- **Age >55 or Afro-Caribbean:** Step 1: CCB. Step 2: CCB/thiazide + ACEi/ARB. Step 3: CCB + thiazide + ACEi/ARB. Step 4: add low dose spironolactone/beta-blocker/alpha-blocker.
- **BP targets:** age <80 clinic BP <140/90 mmHg; age >80 clinic BP <150/90 mmHg. Ambulatory BP target is above minus 5 mmHg.
- **Reference:** NICE (2019) *Hypertension in adults: diagnosis and treatment.*

3.22 ▶ Infective endocarditis

- **About:** infection of cardiac valves/endocardium. Underlying structural cardiac defects. Rheumatic heart disease less common so now seen in older patients and those with prosthetic valves. Mortality 15–20%.
- **Pathology:** infective vegetations form on heart valves containing fibrin, platelets and microorganisms. High pressure jet of blood on endocardium or valve. Vegetations can embolise. Rheumatic heart disease, congenital heart disease or other lesions. Seen with aortic sclerosis, and bicuspid aortic valves. IV drug user has a ×30 greater risk of *Staph. aureus* of tricuspid valve. Mitral valve prolapse ×10 risk and now commonest valve lesion affected.
- **Aetiology: Pacemaker endocarditis:** early cases caused by *Staph. aureus* and late cases by *Staph. epidermidis.* **Native valve endocarditis (NVE):** *Strep. viridans* 40%, *Staph. aureus* 20%, *Enterococcus* spp. 10%, others are streptococci, coagulase-negative staphylococci, Gram-negative bacilli, fungi.
- **Early onset prosthetic valve endocarditis (PVE):** (<60 d post-op): *Staph. epidermidis* 40%, *Staph. aureus* 9%, *Enterococci* 6%, Gram-negative bacilli 4%, fungi 11%, others. **IV drug users:** tricuspid valve endocarditis with *Staph. aureus/epidermidis.* **Bicuspid aortic valve:** aortic valve endocarditis.

Organisms causing endocarditis

- ***Staph. aureus:*** most common, more aggressive acute endocarditis-type disease of normal valves or may be post-operative, e.g. post pacemaker. Risks: central IV lines, IV drug users. Causes early and late prosthetic valve endocarditis and pacemaker endocarditis.
- ***Strep. viridans:*** a low virulence organism seen where there is a history of rheumatic fever. An oral commensal. Causes a subacute clinical picture.
- **Coagulase-negative staphylococcus:** causes early PVE. Occasionally pacemaker endocarditis. They may produce a biofilm on prosthetic surfaces, which also promotes adherence.
- **Fungal endocarditis:** prolonged antibiotics or parenteral nutrition. Often immunocompromised. Usually *Candida albicans* or *C. parapsilosis.*
- **HACEK group:** Gram-negative bacteria. Fastidious. *Haemophilus, Aggregatibacter, Cardiobacterium, Eikenella* and *Kingella* species. May be ill for months. Painful embolic lesion to an extremity.
- **Q fever endocarditis:** *Coxiella burnetii* is an example. May be no fever. Valvular heart disease and on immunosuppressive therapy. Vegetations rare on echo. Organism isolated from buffy coat cultures. Serological studies are reasonably specific.

Cardiac disease and risk of endocarditis

- **High risk:** previous endocarditis, aortic valve disease, rheumatic heart disease, prosthetic valves, mitral regurgitation or AR, VSD, ductus arteriosus, aortic coarctation, acyanotic congenital heart disease.
- **Medium risk:** aortic stenosis, mitral valve prolapse with MR (commonest cause), mitral stenosis, tricuspid disease, pulmonary stenosis. HOCM with LV outflow obstruction.
- **Low risk:** secundum ASD, IHD, previous CABG, MVP without MR.

Clinical

- Fever, malaise, joint pains, stroke/TIA-like episodes if emboli.
- Peripheral emboli – gangrene/ischaemic bowel, finger clubbing is rare.
- Osler nodes – painful, tender nodules on the pulps of fingers.
- Janeway lesions – small (<5 mm) flat painless red spots on palms and soles.
- Roth spots – retinal haemorrhage and micro-infarction.
- New or changing murmurs. Splenomegaly. Splinter haemorrhages hands and feet – also seen in manual workers, labourers on the dominant hand.

Investigations

- **FBC:** anaemia, high WCC, ESR and CRP. U&E. Urinalysis – microscopic haematuria.
- **ECG:** new AV block, increased PR interval suggests aortic valve/root involvement.
- **CXR:** evidence of cardiomegaly, mitral stenosis.
- **Echo (transthoracic) findings:** mobile intracardiac mass (vegetation), root or valve abscess, partial dehiscence of prosthetic valve, new valve regurgitation.
- **Transoesophageal echo:** TOE indicated if transthoracic echo negative and suspicion or with prosthetic valve. A normal echo does not exclude the diagnosis.
- **Blood cultures:** at least 6 from multiple sites spaced in time before antibiotics started. Use fastidious care to avoid contaminants. Do not start antibiotics until this has been done unless the organism is known or the infection is proven and severe. Great care especially where common skin contaminants may easily be interpreted as pathogens (e.g. prosthetic heart valves) aids interpretation of cultures showing coagulase-negative *Staph*.
- **Complications:** valve failure with heart failure (and cardiogenic shock), septic emboli, e.g. stroke (avoid anticoagulation), glomerulonephritis, aortic root abscess, valvular abscess. Pericarditis, death, conduction defects.

Modified Duke criteria: 2 Major, or 1 Major + 2 minor, or 5 minor

2 Major criteria are:

(1) **Positive blood culture for typical IE organisms** (*Strep. viridans* or *bovis*, HACEK, *Staph. aureus*, enterococcus), from 2 separate blood culture (BC) or 2 +ve BC drawn >12 h apart, or 3 or a majority of 4 separate BC (first and last sample drawn 1 h apart) OR *Coxiella burnetii* detected by at least one positive BC or IgG antibody titre for Q fever phase 1 antigen >1:800.

(2) **Echocardiogram** with oscillating intracardiac mass on valve or supporting structures, in the path of regurgitant jets, or on implanted material in the absence of an alternative anatomic explanation, or abscess, or new partial dehiscence of prosthetic valve or new valvular regurgitation.

5 minor criteria are:

(1) **Risk:** predisposing heart condition or IV drug use.

(2) **Fever:** >38.0°C.

(3) **Vascular phenomena:** major arterial emboli, septic pulmonary infarcts, mycotic aneurysm, ICH, conjunctival haemorrhages, Janeway lesion.
(4) **Immune phenomena:** glomerulonephritis, Osler nodes, Roth spots, positive RF.
(5) **Positive blood culture:** not meeting major criterion.

Management

- **Involve cardiology and microbiology for advice.** Those with valve destruction and heart failure or abscess formation or vegetations and embolic concerns or failing antibiotics should be urgently discussed with tertiary cardiac surgeons. Vegetations and surface of valves relatively avascular so difficult to treat effectively with antibiotics. See Cardiogenic shock and heart failure, ▶Section 2.16.
- **Starting antibiotics:** if patient stable and endocarditis uncomplicated can wait 1–2 d to get multiple cultures before starting antibiotics. Complicated endocarditis should receive empirical antibiotic as soon as 3–6 sets of blood cultures taken from different sites over a day if possible. Review antibiotics as soon as aetiological agent is identified. Duration of therapy is usually 4–6 weeks but depends on the organism, microbiology advice and whether native or prosthetic valve. Trend now for some to have 2 weeks IV and then oral.

Antibiotic therapy for endocarditis (PA = penicillin allergy)

- **Organism unknown native valve:** amoxicillin ± low dose gentamicin.
- **Blind prosthetic:** vancomycin + rifampicin + low dose gentamicin.
- **Native valve Staph.:** flucloxacillin IV 4 weeks; PA: vancomycin + rifampicin.
- **Prosthetic Staph.:** flucloxacillin IV + rifampicin + low dose gentamicin.
- **Streptococcus:** benzylpenicillin IV OR vancomycin ± low dose gentamicin.
- **Enterococcal:** amoxicillin or benzylpenicillin IV + low dose gentamicin; PA: vancomycin + low dose gentamicin.
- **HACEK group:** amoxicillin or ceftriaxone ± low dose gentamicin.

3.23 Cardiomyopathy

- **Aetiology:** a generic term for diseases affecting the myocardium with altered function. Some are inherited (often autosomal dominant), some toxic – alcohol and other drugs and others post infectious and the remainder idiopathic. Ischaemic-induced damage is usually excluded. Can cause issues with contraction (systolic) or filling (diastolic) or both. In some there may be outflow obstruction.

Cardiomyopathies: cause heart failure, arrhythmias, emboli

- **Dilated:** may be post viral myocarditis. Impaired contraction. Heart becomes globular and flabby. Many are idiopathic, some genetic (with muscular dystrophies), some autoimmune. Also seen with HIV. Causes chest pain, embolism, heart failure and SCD. Males > females. Needs beta-blockers, ACEi and consider AICD.
- **Restrictive:** impaired filling due to stiff walls. Seen in diseases with deposition of material in myocardium, e.g. amyloid (check for myeloma).
- **Hypertrophic:** inherited defect of cardiac muscle proteins. A minority also have LVOT obstruction (HOCM). ECG shows deep T wave inversion and inferior Q waves can mimic IHD. Heart is stiff with a mainly diastolic dysfunction due to asymmetrical septal hypertrophy (ASH) often with systolic anterior movement of anterior mitral valve leaflet. Jerky pulse, LVH. Systolic murmurs from LVOT and MR. Variants with mainly apical hypertrophy. Exertional chest pain and dyspnoea. SCD is seen often with or after exercise. Rx beta blockade, verapamil, disopyramide. Amiodarone for

arrhythmias. Myomectomy/septal ablation for LVOT obstruction. Avoid digoxin and vasodilators. High risk need AICD.

- **Takotsubo:** transient anterior and apical ballooning seen on echo. Emotional stress. Post-menopausal women. ECG anterior leads show ST elevation V3–V6 then T wave inversion. Normal coronary angiogram. Impaired but reversible LV function resolves in 2 months. Treat with IABP, fluids, beta-blockers or calcium channel blockers.
- **Alcoholic:** chronic alcohol abuse 5–10 years. Usually dilated. Multifactorial. Alcohol and malnutrition. Can entirely resolve with abstention.
- **Arrhythmogenic RV** (ARVC): genetic disorder (AD) of desmosomal proteins. Fibrofatty infiltration of RV. Risk of monomorphic VT with LBBB and RAD or VF and SCD. ECG: precordial T wave inversion in right precordial leads and epsilon waves. Diagnosis/screening by cardiac MRI. Treat with beta-blockers, amiodarone, AICD.
- **Ventricular non-compaction:** imaging (echo then MRI) shows prominent trabeculae at the apex. In some there is a risk of arrhythmias and thromboembolisms which in some needs an AICD and anticoagulation. In many is benign.
- **Obliterative:** endocardial fibrosis and reduced ventricular cavity. Develops MR/TR. Eosinophilia seen. High mortality. Diagnosis: echo/MRI/biopsy. Associated with Churg–Strauss (eosinophilic granulomatosis with polyangiitis). Transplantation may be needed.

Causes and individual management

- Clinically present with symptoms of heart failure, thromboembolism (stroke), palpitations, chest pain or arrhythmias – AF, ectopics, VT or even VF and syncope and cardiac arrest. ECG and echocardiography can help identify an abnormality.
- A cause is often looked for but in many it is idiopathic. Cardiac MRI is the imaging of choice in many. Angiography may be needed to exclude IHD. Management is that of heart failure and arrhythmias. End-stage heart failure may require cardiac transplant (see Cardiogenic shock and heart failure, ▶ Section 2.16).

04 Respiratory

4.1 ▶ Pathophysiology

- **Lung anatomy and physiology:** 2 lungs, 1 trachea, 2 main bronchi, 3 lobes and 10 segmental bronchi on the right and 2 lobes and 8 segmental bronchi on left. Lungs are covered by visceral pleura which continue as parietal pleura over the lateral surfaces of the mediastinum creating a pleural space. Repeated branching to level of terminal bronchioles, leads to 300 million alveoli. Normal ventilation is driven by external intercostals and diaphragm creating a negative airways pressure. Active process vulnerable to fatigue and neuromuscular weakness. 21% O_2 at atmospheric pressure (760 mmHg or 101.3 kPa) reaches the alveoli. In a perfect system arterial PO_2 = alveolar PO_2 but due to AV shunting in lungs and cardiac venous drainage into pulmonary veins there is a normal 2.5 kPa (20 mmHg) difference. In some pathological states this is increased. Moist atmospheric air at 37°C has a PO_2 of 20 kPa (150 mmHg) and there is an increased A–a gradient. This is seen with impaired diffusion across the alveolar capillary membrane or V/Q shunting. Hypoventilation and type 2 RF has a normal A–a gradient. PCO_2 is a useful guide of alveolar ventilation and rises with any hypoventilatory state. The alveolar–arterial difference in PCO_2 is only 1 mmHg.
- **Oxygen transport:** blood transports O_2 bound to Hb. O_2 carriage is not directly proportional to the partial pressure of O_2. The relationship is famously sigmoidal due to the cooperative sequential binding of four O_2 molecules with Hb. This enables it to load well when O_2 is plentiful and unload well when O_2 is scarce, giving it some advantage over the relationship being completely linear. The flat upper portion is alveoli and shows that the Hb is over 90% saturated even with reduced PO_2 down to 8 kPa (60 mmHg). Giving additional O_2 above 13 kPa (100 mmHg) adds little to O_2-carrying capacity. Where the graph is steepest this reflects the tissues with a PO_2 of 5 kPa (40 mmHg) and shows that increased metabolic demand is met with offloading of O_2 within a very small range of PO_2. It also shows that in giving appropriate O_2 even small increases can improve blood O_2 carriage markedly. Metabolic by-products, e.g. DPG, acidosis and high PCO_2 or temperature move the curve towards the right, which makes Hb release O_2 more readily.

Hypoxia PaO_2 <8 kPa (60 mmHg)
- Alveolar (A) – arterial (a) O_2 gradient = (FiO$_2$ %/100) * (P_{atm} – 47 mmHg (6.2 kPa) – ($PaCO_2$/0.8) – PaO_2).
- Normal A–a gradient: hypoventilation, FiO$_2$ <21% O_2, e.g. at altitude.
- Increased A–a gradient: diffusion defect or V/Q mismatching or shunting.

4.2 ▶ Oxygen therapy

- **Summary:** use a high concentration O_2 non-rebreathing mask in any hypoxic patients without chronic lung disease. Target 94–98% Scale 1 or 88–92% if Scale 2. Use a simple face mask / nasal specs for mild hypoxia, without chronic lung disease. Use 28% Venturi mask if known COPD or known type II respiratory failure. Use a tracheostomy mask if tracheostomy ± face mask until anatomy known.

- **Note:** BTS guidance Scale 1 SpO_2 of 94–98% and of Scale 2 88–92% with severe COPD. In the acutely ill patient where there is no concern of hypercarbic respiratory failure high concentration O_2 is best given as 15 L/min with a reservoir bag (FiO$_2$ of over 0.9). The ill patient should receive at least 60% O_2.
- **Risk of high FiO$_2$:** excessive O_2 leads to the formation of free radicals, absorption atelectasis and V/Q mismatches. It may conceal significant clinical deteriorations, e.g. patient with pneumonia saturating at 98% on 2 L O_2 via nasal route desaturates to 90% and improves to 98% when increased to FiO$_2$ of 0.4. This clinical worsening would have been hidden if given a non-rebreather at 15 L/min with saturations of 100%. Consider CXR to exclude a PTX, pulmonary oedema, or mucus airway plugging that could have been missed.
- **Titrate to O_2 saturation** of 94–98% and no more except with severe COPD where a target of 88–92% is advised. Exceptions where high FiO$_2$ needed (CO poisoning, PTX, decompression sickness).
- **Prescribe the desired saturation and not the delivery rate or flow or mask** which should be left to ward level policy. Desaturations and increases in FiO$_2$ to respond to falling desaturations should be escalated to medical staff and acted upon as needed. Where **COPD-related CO_2 retention** is likely it is recommended that treatment should be commenced using a 28% Venturi mask at 4 L/min in prehospital care or a 24–28% Venturi mask at 2–4 L/min in hospital settings, with target saturation of 88–92% pending urgent blood gas results. Monitoring with O_2 saturation probe will detect hypoxia but an ABG is needed to detect hypercapnia (CO_2 retainers). Hypercarbia is multifactorial and involves a mixture of vascular shunting (hypoxia vasoconstricts pulmonary arterioles) and hypoventilation in either or both depth and rate which should be clinically apparent. In chronic hypercarbia, hypoxia may be the main driver to respiration and a high FiO$_2$ may cause hypoventilation and CO_2 narcosis.
- **If peri-arrest and unable to maintain saturations:** BVM ventilation with 100% O_2 and urgently fast bleep anaesthetists or arrest team. Consider intubation and ventilation. Give humidified O_2 for patients who require high-flow O_2 for over 24 h or those who report respiratory discomfort due to dryness.
- **Hyperbaric O_2 therapy:** 100% O_2 at greater than atmospheric pressure. Concerns of O_2 toxicity and this must be borne in mind. Indications: CO poisoning, decompression sickness, air embolism, cyanide poisoning, gas gangrene, to improve wound healing (decubitus ulcers), refractory osteomyelitis, thermal burns, improves skin grafting success.

Measuring oxygenation

- Direct by arterial blood gas. Indirect by pulse oximetry. A photodiode uses light to determine the ratio of oxygenated Hb (940 nm) to deoxygenated Hb (660 nm). Measures pulsatile flow and subtracts background readings. Hb carries 1.3 ml of O_2 per gram. If resting CO approximately 5 L/min (HR 70 × cardiac output 70 ml) and Hb is 120 g/L then total carriage = $5 \times 120 \times 1.3$ ml/min = 780 ml O_2/min.
- **Pulse oximetry** (SpO$_2$): detects different red and infrared absorption profiles of oxyhaemoglobin and deoxyhaemoglobin to estimate arterial oxyhaemoglobin saturation (SaO$_2$). Measure only pulsatile absorption. Poor trace if poor perfusion. It will not detect carboxyhaemoglobin which it sees as oxyhaemoglobin. In those with methaemoglobinaemia, SpO$_2$ will tend towards 85%. Poor technique or severe tricuspid regurgitation (pulsatile venous flow) can lower SpO$_2$ reading. Less accurate below 80% saturation. A high bilirubin does not affect SpO$_2$.

Oxygen saturations (ABG is definitive test of blood O_2 carriage)
- **High sats but low PaO_2:** CO toxicity. ABG shows elevated COHb.
- **Low sats but normal PaO_2:** methaemoglobinaemia. Treat with IV methylene blue.

Oxygen delivery devices: mask types and their applied uses
- **Room air:** FiO_2: room air 21% O_2 and 78% N_2. Small increases in inspired O_2 produce large gains in tissue oxygenation. FiO_2 depends on amount of pure O_2 provided which is mixed with room air. This in turn depends on the rate and depth of breathing and mask design.
- **Nasal cannulae:** FiO_2 24–45% at 1–6 L/min: a nasal cannula (NC) is a thin tube with two small nozzles to go into the patient's nostrils. Provides O_2 at low flow rates, 1 L/min = 24%, 2 L/min = 28%, 3 L/min = 32%, 4 L/min = 36%, 5 L/min = 40%, 6 L/min = 44%. Well tolerated – some find this preferable to a facemask. No dead space. High flow rates (>6 L/min) cause nasal mucosal drying and nose bleeds. Indications: SaO_2 85–94% in non-critically ill patient. Reduce to minimum to keep SaO_2 over 94%.
- **Simple facemask:** FiO_2 24–65% at 2–12 L/min: fits over a patient's nose and mouth. Delivers O_2 as the patient breathes. Open side ports allow room air to enter and dilute the O_2 and allow exhaled CO_2 to leave. Connected to O_2 source by a narrow plastic tube. Mask held in place by an adjustable elastic band. Provides O_2 at low flow rates, 24% 1–2 L/min, 28% 2–4 L/min, 35–40% 5–6 L/min, 60% 8–10 L/min, 65% 12 L/min. Indications: SaO_2 85–94% in non-critically ill patient. Reduce to minimum to keep SaO_2 over 94%.
- **Non-rebreather with reservoir bag:** FiO_2 85–90% at 15 L/min: flow should be sufficient to keep reservoir bag inflated on inspiration. Similar to face mask but has 3 one-way valves with the 2 side ports which prevent 21% room air diluting the mix and allow exhaled air to leave the mask. A reservoir bag of O_2 helps and allows higher concentrations of O_2 for the patient to inhale. A flow rate of 15 L/min supplies up to 90% FiO_2 but requires tight-fitting mask. Used when high FiO_2 required, in critically ill patients. Titrated to SaO_2 94–98%.
- **Venturi mask** (max = 50% FiO_2) indications: COPD + CO_2 retention. Start at 28% mask. Monitor ABG. Variable fixed amounts. Delivery system with flow rate between 4 and 12 L/min, FiO_2 can be set specifically with different flow rate and air ports. FiO_2 can be 24% (2–4 L/min), 28% (4–6L/min), 35% (8–10 L/min), 40% (10–12 L/min) and 50% (12–14 L/min). External ports must remain open to entrain room air.
- **Bag–valve mask** (BVM) FiO_2 100% with high flow O_2 with intubation or nasopharyngeal or oropharyngeal airways: used for emergency ventilation until expected recovery or intubation attempted. It requires a good seal and a patent airway with usual airway opening techniques. The O_2 flow rate equals the minute volume of the patient so 100% O_2 is delivered. It can deliver O_2 to a spontaneously breathing patient. Can also be used to manually ventilate a patient via a mask or tube, or with an oral or nasopharyngeal airway. Indications: SaO_2 <85% or critically ill patient. Reduce flow to minimum to maintain BTS guidance.
- **High flow nasal O_2 therapy (Optiflow):** high flow equivalent to 5 cm H_2O. Give up to 60 L/min. Provides PEEP. Humidified warmed gas. Improves survival. Reduced need for intubation. Used for pneumonia, respiratory failure, COPD, post-extubation, pre-intubation oxygenation, sleep apnoea, acute heart failure, patients with do-not-intubate order. Available in critical care areas and certain AMUs and respiratory wards. Consider use in patients requiring high FiO_2 >40% after discussion with senior medical staff. HFNOT can be useful in preventing

postoperative respiratory failure. Cautions for its use are similar to those for non-invasive facemask positive pressure ventilation.

4.3 ▶ Acute breathlessness

- **About:** breathlessness can be cardiac, respiratory, metabolic or psychogenic.
- **Physiology:** stimulants to breathing are elevated PCO_2 or severe low PO_2, afferents from pulmonary vagal C-fibres.
- **Is breathlessness new:** PE, aspiration, CAP, pulmonary oedema or is it chronic recurrent, e.g. COPD/asthma/CCF? What are observations: RR, BP and HR, are they hypoxic? Context is important, e.g. post-op PE or LVF from excess fluids. Why are they in hospital? Exclude a metabolic acidosis, e.g. DKA.
- **Ask about chest pain, calf pain, haemoptysis.** Have a very low threshold for suspecting PE in an inpatient. If hypoxia or respiratory rate too fast or slow or if staff concerned get NEWS score and see immediately. Mildly breathless or *in extremis*? If *in extremis* hurry because it could be pre-arrest.
- **Start O$_2$ sats of 94–98%** unless there is COPD (28% O$_2$). Get ECG especially if chest pain, looking for VT/fast AF/sinus tachycardia or ST changes.
- **Get CXR especially if acute:** LVF, PTX, pneumonia, effusion, PE. If angina or LVF and BP >100 mmHg then GTN (2 × 400 mcg) sublingual or tablet.
- **If wheeze or known COPD/asthma** advise normal puffer, e.g. **Salbutamol** 100 mcg/puff progressing to **Salbutamol** 2.5–5.0 mg nebuliser if needed. Sudden breathlessness, especially if hypoxic or low BP in hospital, consider as PE if there is no obvious better alternative diagnosis.

Diagnostic clues

- **Sudden onset:** pulmonary oedema, PE, acute anaphylaxis and bronchoconstriction or airway oedema, acute PTX, aspiration pneumonia, hyperventilation syndrome, inhaled foreign body.
- **Gradual onset:** pulmonary oedema, non-cardiogenic pulmonary oedema (ARDS), COPD/bronchiectasis, acute asthma, pneumonia, small PTX, lymphangitis carcinomatosis.
- **Exacerbation of known cause:** exacerbation of COPD, bronchiectasis, asthma, CCF, pulmonary fibrosis, cystic fibrosis.
- **Breathlessness with normal CXR:** PE, early pneumonia, PCP, hyperventilation, COPD, small PTX (easily missed), Kussmaul breathing with DKA, any metabolic acidosis.
- **Post-operative/trauma: atelectasis,** rib fractures, hospital-acquired pneumonia, aspiration pneumonia, pulmonary embolus, PTX (esp. if on ventilator), pulmonary oedema. Anaesthesia may reduce normal lung protection and cause atelectasis and predispose to infection. Ensure pain controlled to allow deep breaths. Chest physiotherapy may help expectoration.

Clinical findings

- **Assess:** check O$_2$ sats, RR, temperature. Wheeze, pursed lips, prolonged expiration, tripod position of COPD. Asthma – check PEFR. Check HR: high HR, fast AF, VT. BP: low BP or JVP elevated (pulmonary oedema, PE, tamponade, SVC obstruction).
- **Auscultation:** murmurs, S3, S4, triple rhythm, systolic murmurs. Chest – dull at bases, stony dull effusion or consolidation. Air entry, breath sounds. Is much air moving? – always ask patient to breathe through mouth. Listen, compare both sides.

- **Chest pain:** ACS, PE, dissection, pericarditis. Legs: pedal oedema or ?DVT.
- **POCUS (point-of-care ultrasound):** increasing role to help differentiate pulmonary oedema and pneumonia, and pneumothorax and effusion, and PE and other causes.

Differentials for acute breathlessness

- **Acute severe asthma:** known asthmatic with increased wheeze, breathlessness and cough, reduced PEFR. Infection, pollution are triggers. Ask about previous episodes needing hospitalisation and even ITU. Difficult socioeconomic circumstances, alcohol and drug issues are all associated with poor outcomes (▶ Section 4.11).
- **Upper airway obstruction:** distress, breathless with stridor. Causes include laryngeal oedema, angioedema, inhaled foreign body, chemical burns, physical burns; inspect and remove if possible and consider Heimlich procedure if foreign body suspected. If intubation impossible then a cricothyrotomy may be needed – call ENT and anaesthetic fast bleep. Anaphylaxis or angioneurotic oedema of laryngeal mucosa: stridor or hoarseness may suggest histamine release, oedema and anaphylaxis. (▶ Section 2.18).
- **Pneumothorax (PTX):** breathless ± pain. Look for underlying lung disease or chest trauma. If chest examination shows reduced air entry, hyper-resonant quiet side may be a PTX – CXR diagnostic. Those with underlying lung disease are at higher risk and may need aspiration and a chest drain. 100% O_2 helps resorption but caution if COPD. (▶ Section 4.12).
- **Tension pneumothorax:** breathless and BP drops as RA filling compromised and signs and situation suggest tension PTX (ventilated patient or chest trauma). Immediate green/brown cannula in 2nd intercostal space mid-clavicular line or some now advocate safety triangle of affected side is called for. Should be an immediate hiss and escape of air. Give 100% O_2. Insert chest drain (▶ Section 4.12).
- **Pleural effusion:** breathless and stony dullness could be fluid. Get CXR. Usually significant size if symptomatic. Controlled drainage of effusion 1–2 L at a time. Risk of pulmonary oedema. Determine cause. (▶ Section 4.13).
- **Pulmonary embolism (PE):** *de novo* PE in high risk stroke, post op or those with fracture or immobile common in hospital. Breathless, low BP and increased RR. Increased JVP, RV heave, loud P2, signs of DVT, CXR often normal. Elevated D-dimer and risk factors. Anticoagulate and give IV fluids; thrombolysis in selected severe cases. Vigorous CPR may help. See VTE section. (▶ Section 4.17).
- **Exacerbation of COPD:** pre-existing COPD. Smoking history. Type 2 RF on ABG. Wheezy. Sputum. Consider NIV or if progressively acidotic then discuss ITU admission with intensivists. (▶ Section 4.10).
- **Acute LVF/pulmonary oedema:** acute dyspnoea, bibasal crackles, triple rhythm (S3/S4), worse lying flat. CXR diagnostic. ECG for STEMI needing PPCI. Echocardiogram when possible. (▶ Section 2.16).
- **Community-acquired pneumonia:** breathless, sputum, fever, dullness, reduced air entry, pleurisy, fever, Raised WCC/CRP. Consolidation on CXR may not be seen acutely. (▶ Section 4.14).
- **Aspiration pneumonia:** those with poor airways protection, stroke and coma and bulbar paralysis. (▶ Section 4.14).
- **Hospital-acquired pneumonia:** often post-operative atelectasis or debilitated. High mortality. Use local antibiotic protocols. Ensure post-op pain controlled to allow adequate deep breaths. (▶ Section 4.14).

- ***Pneumocystis* pneumonia:** seen with AIDS and immunocompromised patient, causes a more generalised alveolar shadowing (▶ Section 4.15).
- **Coronavirus pneumonias:** now with Covid-19 and variants. See Index for more information. History of contact or travel in high-risk areas with an acute fever and pneumonia (▶ Section 4.14).
- **Hypoventilating:** COPD, obesity, sedation, CO_2 narcosis, respiratory muscle weakness. May not be breathless. ABG show a type 2 RF.
- **Respiratory muscle weakness:** high cervical cord lesion, GBS, myopathy, MND, muscular dystrophies. Monitor FVC as well as ABG. Weakness of shoulder shrug is a bad sign. FVC <1.5 L is worrying. Monitor closely. Consider ITU for monitoring support and ventilation.
- **Metabolic acidosis:** Kussmaul breathing. DKA, salicylate toxicity. Get ABG.
- **Hyperventilation syndrome/panic attack:** setting of stress or anxiety. Normal exam, respiratory alkalosis on ABG. Breathe from bag. Sedation.
- **Fat embolism:** recent fracture, coma, sickle cell, skin rash. Agitated, hypoxia. (▶ Section 4.20).
- **ARDS:** non-cardiogenic pulmonary oedema. Sepsis, malignancy, lung injury, trauma, obstetric emergency. CXR changes in clinical context. Echo shows normal cardiac function. (▶ Section 4.9).
- **Aspiration pneumonia/pneumonitis:** suspect if NG tube may be misplaced and feed going into bronchus. Recent stroke or neurological disease (MND) or coma. Failure to protect airway due to sedation, alcohol, drugs, anaesthesia. CXR may show usually right middle or lower lobe changes. Mixed bacterial and chemical reaction produces a pneumonitis. A PEG tube does not prevent aspiration. (▶ Section 4.14).
- **Pulmonary haemorrhage:** bleeding within the alveoli and bronchioles. Goodpasture's syndrome, granulomatosis with polyangiitis (WG), CXR shows alveolar shadowing, renal failure.
- **Cheyne–Stokes breathing:** significant brain damage and brainstem compression. Alternating cycles of slow and then fast respirations in a profoundly comatose patient.
- **Burns victims:** initially suspect CO/cyanide inhalation and check baseline arterial gas (COHb) and O_2 saturations and administer 100% FiO_2. May be soot in mouth and abnormal voice and stridor. Intubate early before oedema.

Investigations

- **Bloods:** FBC, U&E, glucose, CRP. **ABG:** hypoxia ± hypercarbia. **Troponin:** ACS, myocarditis, myocardial injury. **D-dimer:** elevated with DVT/PE and other causes (sensitive but non-specific).
- **BNP normal is** BNP <100 pg/ml. NT-pro BNP is now preferred. If >400 pg/ml is abnormal and >2000 pg/ml requires urgent referral for cardiac echo.
- **ECG:** AF, STEMI, NSTEMI, tachyarrhythmias, S1Q3T3.
- **CXR:** pulmonary oedema, PTX, consolidation, pleural effusion.
- **Echocardiogram:** MI and poor LV, valve disease, tamponade.
- **CT pulmonary angiogram:** PE, unexpected other pathology.
- **V/Q scan:** for PE if normal CXR and no lung disease.
- **Pulmonary function tests** – obstruction/restrictive/diffusion defect.

Management

- **ABC and give O_2** as per BTS guidelines and reassess after ABG. If *in extremis*, cyanosed or severely hypoxic (SaO_2 <80%) then call cardiac arrest team. If airway obstructed by food or other objects then see choking algorithm. If suspected anaphylaxis with stridor give IV **Adrenaline** 0.5 mg IM and if cannot oxygenate or intubate then consider urgent ENT/Anaesthetics for Front of neck airway (FONA).

- **Common causes:** e.g. COPD, LVF, PE, asthma, chest infection. Signs of DVT? Look at hospital notes. Useful signs: raised JVP (CCF, PE, tamponade), loud systolic murmur, fast AF. New drugs or blood transfusion might suggest anaphylaxis and need for nebulisers, adrenaline and steroids.
- **Look for fever:** raised CRP, crackles on auscultation suggesting infection. If diagnosis still unclear or needs confirmation then CXR is useful, but may take some time to arrive and get information.
- **Treat as for cause found:** it can be useful to hedge bet and treat several causes at once whilst awaiting confirmatory tests or senior advice, e.g. IV antibiotic.
- **Furosemide** 50 mg IV if pulmonary oedema suspected and **Salbutamol** 2.5 mg neb. Look for new MI or valve disease.
- **If PE suspected** then follow PE diagnostic pathway. If *in extremis* consider thrombolysis. (▶ Section 4.17).
- **If chest pain and new LBBB or ST elevation** then give GTN 2 sprays (800 mcg) sublingual if SBP >110 mmHg. Pain persists **Diamorphine** 2.5–5 mg IV or **Morphine** 5 mg IV and take cardiac advice on urgent revascularisation (PCI/thrombolysis). (▶ Section 3.8).
- **If worsening hypoxia and acidosis** may require NIPPV or intubation and ventilation. Get help early if deteriorating. Consider a chest drain for PTX or massive pleural effusion.

4.4 Acute stridor

- **About:** 3 types of stridor high-pitched upper airway noise. **Inspiratory** laryngeal obstruction, **Expiratory** tracheobronchial obstruction. **Biphasic:** subglottic or glottic.
- **Red flags:** drooling, agitation, tripod position, cyanosis, decreased conscious level. Respiratory distress, silent chest, reduced HR and episodes of apnoea.
- **Acute causes:** *acute epiglottitis*: all ages commonly age 2–7, HiB, sore throat, drooling, distressed. *Peri-tonsillar abscess*: pain and swelling. *Croup, acute laryngitis*: hoarseness. *Anaphylaxis* pale, low BP. *Post-extubation laryngeal oedema, low calcium* and tetany, *vocal cord dysfunction. Foreign body inhalation* e.g. peanut seen in young and elderly, *neck space abscess, trauma* with oedema and bleeding, compression causing obstruction.
- **Chronic causes:** malignancy unless haemorrhage or acute oedema, subglottic stenosis, large goitre, laryngomalacia, recurrent – vocal cord dysfunction.
- **Clinical:** cyanosed, breathless, distressed, hoarse, foreign body sensation in throat. Loud (*volume of the stridor sound decreases as pt tired*) stridor, drooling if unable to swallow, feverish, toxic suggests infection. Allergic: rash, low BP, urticarial, anaphylaxis, known causative agent. Large goitre or mediastinal tumour.
- **Investigations:** no blood tests if epiglottitis until airway secure. Mast cell tryptase if anaphylaxis. **Lateral soft tissue neck film:** those with epiglottitis exhibit thickening and rounding of the epiglottis ('thumb sign'), with loss of the vallecular air space. The aryepiglottic folds are thickened, and the hypopharynx is distended. Consider CXR, fibreoptic nasal endoscopy can identify cause.

- **Management:** ABC, O_2 target 94–98% or Heliox 80:20 improves airflow and reduces stridor. Stabilise the patient. Refer ENT. No one plan as depends on likely diagnosis. Nil by mouth.

> **Acute epiglottitis avoid throat exam and get urgent senior ENT and anaesthetic assessment for intubation/front of neck airway (ENT) if needed in HDU/theatres.**

Suction secretions or clear any foreign body from airway if obvious or visible unless acute epiglottitis. Ensure close monitoring on HDU/ITU. May need examination under anaesthesia (EUA) and intubation in theatre where fibreoptic nasal endoscopy can be attempted, to try to visual the airway to confirm the diagnosis. **Steroids: Dexamethasone** 8 mg BD PO/IV or **Hydrocortisone** 200 mg IV stat then TDS. **Salbutamol** 5 mg neb if wheeze. **Adrenaline** 1 mg of 1 ml diluted in 10 ml 0.9% saline nebulised. Anaphylaxis, then follow anaphylaxis guidance. **Airway:** intubation may be necessary. If unable may require cricothyrotomy or tracheostomy to bypass laryngeal obstructions. **Antibiotics:** if infection, e.g. epiglottitis or bacterial tracheitis or abscess antibiotic therapy may be required, e.g. **Co-amoxiclav, Ceftriaxone. Other:** tumour: **Radiotherapy** if appropriate – discuss with oncologist. Laser/stenting for tracheal obstruction. Discuss with Respiratory team. Oropharyngeal abscess may be incised.
- **Reference:** Mohamad *et al.* (2012) Acute stridor – diagnostic challenges in different age groups presented to the emergency department. *Emergency Med*, **2**:125.

4.5 Acute respiratory failure (ARF)

- **Note:** concerned about RF then keep a low threshold for checking ABG.
- **Definition:** inadequate alveolar–arterial oxygenation such that PaO_2 <8 kPa (60 mmHg). Can be with low/normal $PaCO_2$ and with high $PaCO_2$.
- **Management:** give enough O_2 to target sats of 94–98%. Give high FiO_2 if cardiac arrest/peri-arrest, shock, patient *in extremis*, severe type 1 RF and/or prior to attempting intubation. Give controlled O_2 in type 2 RF 24–28% by Venturi. RF is seen in severe COPD when FEV_1 <1 L and in restrictive diseases when FVC <1 L. T2 hypercapnic RF can be due to a loss of drive or changes in lung ventilation and perfusion. Treat hypoventilation due to sedation, neuromuscular weakness (GBS/MND/muscular dystrophies), tiredness, pain, mucus plugs, atelectasis with V/Q changes (O_2 is a pulmonary vasodilator and hypoxia a constrictor). Those at risk of T2RF have severe COPD, polycythaemia/cor pulmonale, FEV_1 <1 L, home O_2, nebulisers, high HCO_3, normal respiratory rate. Aim for SaO_2 of 88–92%. Manage any hypoventilation with pain relief, chest physio, hydration. Consider NIV for T2RF with acidosis and raised CO_2; some need mechanical ventilation. Involve critical care and ITU team early.

Type 1 ARF PaO_2 <8 kPa (60 mmHg) PCO_2 <6 kPa (45 mmHg)
- Due to (1) ventilation/perfusion mismatch: increased A–a gradient, e.g. pneumonia; (2) impaired diffusion: increased A–a gradient, fibrosis/interstitial disease; (3) anatomical R–L AV shunt: perfusion of non-aerated lung. Increased A–a gradient, e.g. pulmonary AVM; (4) hypoventilation: normal A–a gradient, obesity/sedation, weakness; (5) breathing low pressure/FiO_2: normal A–a gradient, high altitude, aircraft. **Causes:** pneumonia, cardiogenic oedema, ARDS, pulmonary haemorrhage,

acute severe asthma, pulmonary fibrosis, cyanotic congenital lung disease, fat embolism, high altitude.

Type 2 ARF PaO_2 <8 kPa (60 mmHg) and PCO_2 >6 kPa (45 mmHg)

- It is usually due to alveolar hypoventilation due to neuromuscular weakness, sedation and lung disease as well as increased CO_2 production: malignant hyperthermia, severe thyrotoxicosis, fever, sepsis, shivering, overfeeding from parenteral nutrition, bicarbonate administration, CO_2 insufflation (laparoscopy). Ventilation/perfusion changes. **Typical causes:** hypercapnic RF in COPD, central hypoventilation, obesity-related hypoventilation, progressive coma, sedation, GBS, MG, poliomyelitis, muscular dystrophies, chest wall disorders, and all of the causes of type 1 when tired, hypoventilating with V:Q mismatch.
- **Clinical:** hypoxia leads to death. Hypercarbia leads to confusion, papilloedema, drowsiness, vasodilation and further hypoventilation and hypoxia until respiratory arrest. NB: Patients can move between types of RF. A hypoxic patient with pneumonia, heart failure or even severe asthma can tire and hypoventilate and retain CO_2 moving from type 1 to type 2. Patient may be breathless but not always (Covid). Cyanosis, drowsy, delirium, comatose and decreased respiratory effort. Cough, acute onset, smoker. Increased effort using accessory muscles, intercostal recession, tachycardia, tachypnoea. Look for PTX, PE, pneumonia, oedema, fibrosis, wheeze.

Investigations

- **FBC:** raised Hb suggests chronic hypoxia/smoking, low Hb anaemia.
- **U&E:** high urea, high creatinine, AKI or pulmonary–renal syndrome.
- **ABG/VBG:** PO_2 <8 kPa due to ARF. If increased PCO_2 then type 2. With ARF HCO_3 is normal, but with chronic RF kidneys preserve HCO_3 which rises and the pH will be less acidotic. The exception would be early type 1 RF with hyperventilation. In many cases hypercarbia and acidosis is detectable in a VBG and O_2 sats can guide oxygenation and this can reduce arterial stabs.
- **CXR:** pulmonary oedema, consolidation, alveolar haemorrhage, PTX, pleural effusion, collapse, tumour, bullae, fibrosis, emphysematous change. Often normal in PE.
- **ECG:** Look for raised HR, AF, LVH, ST changes, RVH, L/RBBB.
- **Echocardiography:** to exclude RV overload and PE and assess LV.
- **Pulmonary function tests (PFTs):** FVC correlates respiratory muscle strength. Reduced FEV/FVC obstructive lung disease.
- **Age-adjusted dimer/CTPA or V/Q scan:** suspected PE.

Management

- **ABC.** Controlled O_2 therapy to achieve PO_2 94–98% or 88–92% if COPD. An increased O_2 demand to hit the target SaO_2 needs to be escalated and patient reassessed as can signify a deteriorating patient.
- **Treat causes:** reverse/stop sedation, diuresis/nitrates for cardiogenic pulmonary oedema, bronchodilation (antibiotics, steroids, controlled O_2 for COPD), and anticoagulation for acute PE, chest drain for PTX. NIV in COPD with acidosis.
- **NIV:** consider if **COPD and PCO_2 >6 kPa and resp acidosis (pH <7.35).** Fails to improve then consider support from ITU/HDU for intubation.
- **Simple actions:** sit patients up or out of bed. Can aid lung ventilation by using lung bases and aiding expectoration of secretions aided by chest physio. Encourage

coughing. Prevent basal atelectasis and mucus plugging. Bronchoscopy for culture and remove obstructions.

- **Antibiotics:** tailor to the likely pathogen. Is it viral, bacterial, fungal? COPD exacerbation or community- or hospital-acquired pneumonia? Is the patient immunocompromised? Could it be PCP with undiagnosed HIV/AIDS?
- **Respiratory stimulants: doxapram** can be used to stimulate and increase breathing rate/depth and tried if NIV not available or tolerated.
- **Extracorporeal membrane oxygenation** (ECMO) for potentially reversible RF. It can be life-saving. Consider in those with persisting RF despite maximal therapy with a potentially reversible cause. Talk to local ECMO centre.

4.6 Non-invasive ventilation (NIV)

Before starting NIV or any form of positive pressure ventilation always get CXR to exclude pneumothorax.

- **About:** normal breathing physiology is negative pressure ventilation. External intercostal muscles and diaphragm contract. This increases thoracic volume, creates a negative airways pressure, and sucks air in to reach the alveoli. It was mimicked by the iron lungs used to treat polio victims. Normal lungs fill with a pressure of about 3 cmH$_2$O. However, generally we use **positive pressure ventilation** to push air in to inflate the lungs. This is done by non-invasive or mechanical ventilation. It is the most practical way to oxygenate lungs therapeutically. Positive airway pressure can be continuous (CPAP) throughout the respiratory cycle or varied with the cycle (e.g. BiPAP). The downside is that it can damage the lung through barotrauma and can reduce cardiac filling and so cardiac output.
- **Continuous positive airway pressure (CPAP): main use is for type 1 RF/ alveolar oedema.** CPAP is the application of continuous positive pressure whilst the patient continues to initiate and generate breaths. Prevents collapse of airways, recruiting more alveoli for gas exchange. The positive pressures are maintained even on expiration. Work of breathing is reduced. Can be accompanied by high FiO$_2$. It only takes 5 cm H$_2$O to inflate normal lungs. CPAP pressures used are 5–20 cmH$_2$O. Adjust FiO$_2$. Main use is *cardiogenic pulmonary oedema* at typical pressures of 5–15 cmH$_2$O. A trial can be given for 1–2 h to see improvement in O$_2$ sats, heart rate, etc. Primarily helps hypoxaemia rather than CO$_2$ retention and can help avoid intubation. Patient wears a tight-fitting mask which is essential to maintain the positive pressure. Outside of the acute setting it is useful for those with obstructive sleep apnoea because it acts as a 'pneumatic splint' maintaining a patent airway throughout the respiratory cycle.
- **NIV/BiPAP** can reduce work of breathing, improve ABG, avoid risks of intubation and invasive ventilation, improve outcomes (e.g. reduce mortality rates, decrease hospital length of stay), and decrease the cost of care. NIV improves oxygenation, increases minute volume and reduces *PaCO$_2$*. Bi-level positive airway pressure (BiPAP): indications are type 2 RF pH <7.35 *PaCO$_2$* >6 kPa after initial treatment. BiPAP switches between different pressures for inspiration and expiration. Needs a tight-fitting face mask and a ventilator capable of delivering an inspiratory (high pressure, e.g. 8 cmH$_2$O) and expiratory (lower pressure, e.g. 4 cmH$_2$O). Patients need to be conscious, cooperative and compliant and able to protect their airway.

- **Application:** NIV is used in respiratory failure related to COPD, neuromuscular disease and obesity. An effective seal is necessary. The patient needs to tolerate the mask and the feeling of breathing out against resistance – like trying to breathe with your head out of the window of a speeding car. Intolerable for some. Increased alveolar recruitment increases gas exchange, which reduces V/Q mismatches. Flow rate of O_2 is prescribed and administered via the port on the mask or, if available, into the disposable filter attached to the generator. Start with humidified O_2 2–4 L/min depending on the FiO_2 needed. NIV may be trialled in some conditions, e.g. asthma and pneumonia, but only if the patient is in ITU and can be intubated immediately if failing. It is not for hypoxic asthmatics or pneumonia or those with reversible lung pathology who are tiring and decompensating, unless there is immediate access to invasive ventilation if needed. NIV is not indicated in impaired consciousness, severe hypoxaemia or patients with copious respiratory secretions.

NIV protocol and settings

- See machine's instruction manual. In Spontaneous/Time (S/T) mode, the ventilator delivers pressure support breaths with PEEP. Spontaneous inspiratory effort triggers the ventilator to deliver inspiratory positive airway pressure (IPAP). It cycles to expiratory positive airway pressure (EPAP) during expiration. If the patient's breathing rate is lower than a prescribed rate, the ventilator triggers a pressure-controlled breath according to the IPAP prescribed. EPAP only to be altered by senior clinician as can cause hypoxia.
- The breath is ventilator-triggered, pressure-limited and time-cycled. The actual level of pressure support is equal to the difference between IPAP and EPAP. The monitor of the ventilator can display expired tidal volume, minute ventilation, peak inspiratory pressure, inspiratory time/total cycle time, and patient peak flow and % patient-triggered breaths.

Suggested indications and protocol for NIV

- **COPD:** hypoxia pH <7.35 and $PaCO_2$ >6 kPa (45 mmHg) persisting after bronchodilators and controlled O_2. EPAP of 3. IPAP 15. Up-titrate IPAP over 10–30 mins to IPAP 20–30 to achieve augmentation of chest/abdominal movements and slow HR. IPAP should not exceed 30. Back-up rate 16–20. IE ratio 1.2–1.3. Inspiration time 0.8–1.2 seconds.
- **Neuromuscular disease:** RR >20 if usual VC <1 L even if PCO_2 <6.5. Or pH <7.35 + PCO_2 >6.5. EPAP 3, IPAP 10, IE ratio 1:1, inspiration time 1.2–1.5 seconds.
- **Obesity hypoventilation:** pH <7.35, PCO_2 >6.5, RR >23. Or daytime PCO_2 >6 and somnolent. EPAP 3, IPAP15, IE ratio 1:1, inspiration time 1.2–1.5 seconds.

Contraindications to NIV

- Asthma/pneumonia. Relative: pH <7.15 or pH <7.25 and additional adverse features, GCS <8. Severe facial deformity, facial trauma or facial burns or fixed upper airways obstruction, impending respiratory arrest, inability to maintain sats 85–88% on NIV, COPD with RF $PaCO_2$ >6 kPa (45 mmHg), pH <7.25. Consider invasive mechanical ventilation. Cardiac/respiratory arrest, haemodynamic instability, moribund.
- Untreated PTX, delirium, vomiting, upper GI bleeding, bowel obstruction, facial trauma, unable to clear sputum, high risk of aspiration.

Protocol for managing NIV: see settings above

- **All patients:** sit patient up. Achieve position of comfort, explain procedure and consent verbally. Use smallest mask providing a proper fit. Full face mask. Aim sats 88–92% in all causes of hypercapnic RF. If high O_2 needed or desaturation consider ITU. Monitor for distress, coma, vomiting, excess secretions.
- **Repeat ABG at 2 h.** Red flags: pH <7.25 on optimal NIV consider ITU referral. RR >25 or new confusion. Seek and treat reversible causes of acute hypercapnic resp failure. The use of NIV should not delay escalation to IMV when this is more appropriate.
- Apply strapping to the mask once patient used to NIPPV. Tight enough to prevent leaks but allow entry of 1 or 2 fingers. Dressing on nasal bridge can help avoid pressure sores.
- **Measure success:** reduction in $PaCO_2$ or improved pH by +0.06 and/or correction of respiratory acidosis associated with a clinical improvement.
- **Failure:** signs of failing NIV and need for escalation include worsening acidosis or hypercapnia and/or falling GCS, especially if <9. Determine ceiling of therapy so that escalation if appropriate is rapid.
- **Difficulties:** include copious respiratory secretion with difficulty in clearance. Intubation and mechanical ventilation may be necessary depending on the ceiling of therapy which should have been ascertained.
- **Weaning off:** assess for weaning once there are signs of continued improvement or if NIV is not helping. For COPD a 3-d approach with decreasing time of NIV down to 16 h on day 2 and 12 h on day 3 with 6–8 h overnight adjusted to the patient's condition. Discontinue day 4 as appropriate. Re-check ABG 2 h after discontinuation of therapy. May use NIV overnight if nocturnal hypoventilation is present.

4.7 Invasive mechanical ventilation

- **Basics: involves similar concepts to NIV,** but requires intubation and ventilation, and oxygenation by placing of an endotracheal tube, laryngeal mask or tracheostomy. May require sedation and neuromuscular blockade. The settings usually allow timing to the patient's inspiratory effort. Air is pushed in and increases intra-alveolar pressure or lung tidal volume until a point where the lungs are allowed to deflate passively. Pressures generated can cause a PTX, reduce venous return or cause lung injury. Ventilators can be set basically using either volumes (tidal volume is preset and fixed and pressures vary) or pressure settings. Should be improved gas exchange and a decreased work of breathing.
- **Complications:** lung injury, difficulties in intubation, laryngeal injury, PTX, tension pneumothorax, pneumomediastinum, airway injury, alveolar damage, ventilator-associated pneumonia, weakness and atrophy of the diaphragm, reduced cardiac output, O_2 toxicity, acute lung injury (ALI) and acute respiratory distress syndrome (ARDS).
- **Monitoring effectiveness of mechanical ventilation:** use pulse oximetry, ABG, effort of breathing, tidal volume, respiratory rate, HR, BP, CXR findings.
- **Quantitative capnography:** end-tidal CO_2 of expired air is measured. It is the gold standard for confirming placement of ET tube. Low levels are detectable even during cardiac arrest. $EtCO_2$ 10–20 mmHg (1.3–2.6 kPa) suggest quality CPR. $EtCO_2$ >20 mmHg (2.6 kPa) associated with increased rate of ROSC. Continuous end-tidal CO_2 monitoring can confirm a tracheal intubation and absence should prompt removal of the tube and face mask ventilation before considering re-attempts at intubation. A good wave form indicating the presence of CO_2 ensures the ET tube is in the trachea. A persistently low level may indicate a poor prognosis.

- **Indications:** (1) protection of the airway and/or need to remove secretions; (2) GCS <9, airway obstruction, respiratory fatigue or drowsiness; (3) apnoea with cardiac/respiratory arrest; (4) hypoxaemia (PO_2 <8 kPa (60 mmHg)) despite high $FiO_2 \pm$ NIV; (5) SaO_2 <90% despite CPAP with FiO_2 >0.6; (6) control CO_2 (hyperventilate to lower PCO_2 for raised ICP); (7) control O_2/CO_2 (type 2 RF with acidosis); (8) respiratory rate >35/min or <10/min; (9) FVC <15 ml/kg or 1 L or <30% predicted; (10) tidal volume <5 ml/kg or inadequate inspiratory force <25 cmH$_2$O; (11) surgery to head and neck or involving muscular paralysis.
- **References:** BTS Standards of Care Committee (2002) NIV in acute respiratory failure. *Thorax*, 57:192. O'Driscoll *et al.* (2008) BTS guideline for emergency O_2 use in adult patients. *Thorax*, 63(Suppl 6):1. RCP (2008) Non-invasive ventilation in COPD: Management of acute type 2 respiratory failure.

4.8   Massive haemoptysis

Protect the airway by having patient lying on the side of the bleeding lung, to protect the unaffected lung.

- **About:** cough up 200–1000 ml blood per hour. Haemoptysis is common but massive life-threatening haemoptysis is rare. Death is from hypoxia.
- **Aetiology:** lungs perfused by the bronchial (120/80 mmHg) and pulmonary arteries (25/10 mmHg). 90% from the bronchial vessels. Embolise in severe haemorrhage. Tranexamic acid.
- **Causes:** primary lung cancer/pulmonary metastases (smoker, weight loss, clubbing). Pneumonia or bronchiectasis (cough + purulent sputum). Aspergillus, lung abscess (with pus). Pulmonary TB (weight loss, CXR changes), pulmonary oedema (bat wing alveolar oedema, Kerley B lines, cardiomegaly). Alveolar haemorrhage (WG/Goodpasture's alveolar shadowing and cavitation, raised CRP, haematuria). Hereditary haemorrhagic telangiectasia (HHT), pulmonary AV fistula, pulmonary artery aneurysms. Metastases, e.g. renal, testicular, gastrointestinal. HIV/TB, oral/facial telangiectasis (HHT).
- **Clinical:** distressed, breathless, cyanosed, clubbed, weight loss if tumour. Expectorating bright red frothy blood with oedema, hypoxic, low BP. Auscultation may hear gurgling from affected side. Upper zone blood may gravitate to lower lobes.
- **Investigations** (extensive test only if cause not evident): FBC: high WCC, ESR, CRP infective, inflammatory or malignancy. U&E, urinalysis (blood and protein): AKI – with granulomatosis with polyangiitis or Goodpasture's syndrome. Blood cross-match: if anaemic or bleeding is significant. Coagulation screen: APTT, PT, INR, platelets, fibrinogen. ECG: non-specific unless cardiac disease or acute PE. Echocardiogram. Sputum for culture, AFB and cytology. CXR: helps lateralise the cause and diagnose the lesion(s) causing the bleeding. CTPA: if PE considered also shows other pathology. D-dimer likely elevated regardless. Check ANCA/anti-GBM, ANA, RF, C3 and cryoglobulins. Echocardiogram if LVF, valve disease or PE suspected.
- **Management:** ABC O_2. Consider sedation in distressed patient. Positioning: lie on bleeding side down. Consider anaesthetic for optimal airways control/intubation as needed. Liaise early with cardiothoracic surgeons in terms of steps needed; they usually dictate care. Get IV access fluids, group and cross-match. Transfuse if needed. Reverse coagulopathy. Consider IV **Tranexamic acid. Adrenaline** 5–10 ml

(0.5–1 mg) of 1 in 10,000 nebulised may help. Intubation consider large-bore tube which may be single or double lumen. Flexible bronchoscopy or CT chest is the primary method for diagnosis and localisation of haemoptysis. Bronchoscopy difficult with acute bleeding in visualising the bleeding source. Case by case early expert assessment. Get help.

- **Active methods to stop bleeding** (tranexamic acid/reverse coagulopathy): bronchial artery angiography and embolisation may help. Discuss with interventional radiology (SE cord ischaemia/infarction if anterior spinal artery compromised). Bronchial balloon tamponade: where the bronchial balloon of a double-lumen tube, or a 4 French (1 Fr = 1/3 mm) 100 cm Fogarty embolectomy catheter, or Arndt endobronchial blocker, inserted via a single-lumen tube, can be inflated for 24 h before deflation and observation. There is a theoretical risk of mucosal ischaemia with this approach. Bronchial lavage: use of saline cooled in ice in 50 ml aliquots down the bronchoscope with volumes up to 1 L is well described and can arrest bleeding.
- **Topical procoagulants:** thrombin and fibrinogen concentrates have been topically instilled, with anecdotal success. Laser, diathermy or cryocautery: these are possible through a rigid bronchoscope and can be applied to, for example, a bleeding endobronchial tumour.
- **Surgical management** may be applicable if all else fails. In some, emergency pulmonary resection provides an effective treatment with acceptable morbidity and mortality in patients with massive haemoptysis. Palliation if a known malignancy and bleeding cannot be stopped. Give morphine/lorazepam.

4.9 ▶ Acute respiratory distress syndrome (ARDS)

- **About:** severe systemic disease develops acute hypoxia and multi-organ dysfunction. Due to trauma, sepsis, tissue damage, severe illnesses.
- **Aetiology:** type 1 RF with pulmonary oedema not due to cardiac dysfunction. Loss of type 2 pneumocytes. Pulmonary inflammation. Proteinaceous alveolar oedema and capillary leakage with flooding and collapse of alveoli. Stiff, poorly compliant lungs depleted of surfactant with severely impaired gas exchange.
- **Definition:** severity increases as the ratio of arterial PO_2/FiO_2 falls. Acute onset (within 1 week of known clinical insult). Bilateral opacities on CXR/CT unexplained by other pathology. Pulmonary artery wedge pressure (PAWP) <18 mmHg. Ratio PaO_2/FiO_2 mild <40 kPa, moderate <26.6 kPa, severe <13.3 kPa.
- **Clinical:** other severe illness and worsening hypoxia PaO_2 and CXR changes. Dyspnoea, cyanosis, basal inspiratory crackles, tachycardia.
- **Causes:** burns, smoke inhalation, pneumonia, pneumonitis from aspiration, high altitude, fat or air embolism, near-drowning, O_2 toxicity, sepsis, trauma, eclampsia, acute pancreatitis, heroin, barbiturates, transfusion-associated lung injury, malignancies, cardiopulmonary bypass.
- **Differentials:** cardiogenic pulmonary oedema, bilateral pneumonia (ventilator-associated or community-acquired), alveolar haemorrhage (vasculitis), acute interstitial pneumonia, acute eosinophilic pneumonia or hypersensitivity pneumonitis (need steroids).
- **Investigations:** ABG: PaO_2/FiO_2 40 kPa consistent with ARDS if obtained on PEEP or CPAP ≥5 cmH$_2$O. FBC: anaemia, increased neutrophils. U&E/LFT lactate: AKI may be seen, high lactate, deranged LFTs. CXR: bilateral opacities (oedema). Chest CT: not often needed but shows bilateral opacities, ground glass appearance. Echo: normal LV function. Right heart catheter: PAWP <15–18 mmHg. Blood cultures: sepsis.

Coagulopathy: DIC may develop with high APTT, PT and low platelets. Broncho-alveolar lavage may be useful if undefined infection.

- **Management:** determine and treat cause. Death due to multi-organ failure. Where mechanical ventilation is required, the use of low tidal volumes (<6 ml/kg ideal body weight) and airway pressures (plateau pressure <30 cmH_2O) recommended. For patients with moderate–severe ARDS (PF ratio <20 kPa), prone positioning is recommended for >12 h per day.
- High frequency oscillation is not recommended. Inhaled NO is not recommended. A conservative fluid management strategy is suggested. Mechanical ventilation with high positive end-expiratory pressure (PEEP) and the use of the neuromuscular blocking agent for 48 h suggested for those with PF ratios <27 and 20 kPa respectively. **ECMO** is suggested as an adjunct to protective mechanical ventilation for patients with very severe ARDS. Without adequate evidence, corticosteroids and extra-corporeal carbon dioxide removal (ECCOR) remain areas of research. **Complications:** PTX, ventilator-associated pneumonia, multiple organ failure, pulmonary fibrosis, RF. Death 30–50%.
- **Reference:** *Guidelines on the management of ARDS* (2018). FICM/ICS Guideline Development Group (see https://ficm.ac.uk)

4.10 Acute exacerbation of COPD

- **About:** COPD is a chronic illness punctuated with acute exacerbations, some infective. Community teams can help reduce hospital admissions. Post bronchodilation FEV_1 <80% predicted and FEV_1/FVC <70%. Not all smokers get COPD but unusual if <10 pack years. In-hospital mortality 4%.
- **Causes of worsening:** irritants, e.g. cigarette smoke, noxious particles and SO_2, NO_2, ozone. Viral: 50% rhinoviruses, coronaviruses, influenza, parainfluenza, adenovirus, RSV. Bacterial: *Haemophilus influenzae, Strep. pneumoniae, Moraxella catarrhalis, Pseudomonas aeruginosa, Chlamydophila pneumoniae.*
- **Clinical:** increased dyspnoea, expiratory wheeze, cough, sputum. Malaise, cachexia. Pursed lips breathing, barrel-chested, use of accessory muscles – tripod position. New cyanosis, peripheral oedema, nicotine staining. Bounding pulse, drowsy, tremor and headache can suggest CO_2 retention. Determine functional baseline, distance walked, guide of overall function and goals. Ask about pets and allergies, occupation, asbestos. Home O_2.

MRC Dyspnoea Scale should be used to grade the breathlessness
- Grade 0: breathlessness only with strenuous exercise.
- Grade 1: breathlessness hurrying on level or walking up a slight hill.
- Grade 2: walks slower than contemporaries on level ground due to dyspnoea.
- Grade 3: stops for breath after 100 m or a few minutes walking on the flat.
- Grade 4: too breathless to leave house; breathless dressing/undressing.

Classification of severity of airflow limitation in COPD
A postbronchodilator FEV_1/FVC ratio of <0.70 is considered diagnostic for COPD. GOLD system uses FEV_1 as severity. In those with FEV_1/FVC <0.70:
- GOLD 1 – mild: FEV_1 ≥80% predicted
- GOLD 2 – moderate: 50% ≤ FEV_1 <80% predicted
- GOLD 3 – severe: 30% ≤ FEV_1 <50% predicted
- GOLD 4 – very severe: FEV_1 <30% predicted.

Investigations

- **Bloods:** FBC: high WCC (eosinophils – better outcomes). CRP suggest infection. Steroids increase WCC. U&E: dehydrated with raised creatinine. Low Na if SIADH or Addison's.
- **CXR:** hyper-expanded lungs typical of emphysema. Patchy consolidation, PTX may be difficult to differentiate from bullae (get CT). Exclude lung malignancy (always suspect it). CT chest to assess emphysema or other diagnoses, e.g. PE/pneumonia.
- **ECG:** sinus tachycardia, AF, P pulmonale, RVH, ST/T wave changes.
- **ABG:** PO_2 <8 kPa (60 mmHg) and PCO_2 >6 kPa (45 mmHg), pH <7.35. High HCO_3 with chronic COPD. Compare with past admissions and previous ITU needs.
- **Theophylline level** on admission in people who are taking theophylline therapy.
- **Microbiology:** send a sputum sample for microscopy and culture if the sputum is purulent and take blood cultures if the person is pyrexia.
- **Pulmonary function tests:** when well determine FEV_1/FVC <0.7. Carbon monoxide transfer factor low in emphysema. Alpha-1antiproteinase if young and basal emphysema. Consider troponin and risk assess if PE considered for D-dimer: if suspicion this is ACS/PE. Exacerbations of COPD can be LVF or PE and these diagnoses should be sensibly considered.

Prognostic prediction: DECAF Score

- *Extended MRC Dyspnoea Scale (eMRCD)*: on a good day, within last 3 months: not too dyspnoeic to leave house 0; too dyspnoeic to leave house but independent with washing/dressing +1; too dyspnoeic to leave house and wash/dress +2; *eosinopenia*: eosinophils <0.05×10^9/L +1; *consolidation on chest X-ray*: +1; *acidaemia* pH <7.30 +1; *atrial fibrillation* +1. Low risk (0–1) consider early supported discharge or hospital at home.
- High risk (score 3–6) consider higher levels of care or addressing goals of care. Higher scores may correlate with increased length of stay.

Management

- **Don't always assume usual exacerbation.** Usually, it is the case but this could be PE, heart failure, lung cancer, PTX, pneumonia, upper airway obstruction, pleural effusion, recurrent aspiration. Get patient sitting up supported to allow use of accessory muscles to aid gas exchange. Breathing pattern may help. If expiratory phase not prolonged it may not be COPD. Chest physiotherapy may aid expectoration. IV fluids if too tired/breathless to drink.
- **Bronchodilators: salbutamol** 2.5–5 mg and **ipratropium bromide** 500 mcg nebs every 30 min then 4–6 hourly. Nebs driven by air if acidotic or hypercapnic.
- **Controlled oxygen** – concerns about hypercarbic respiratory failure give patients with COPD oxygen via a Venturi 24% mask at 2 L/min or Venturi 28% mask at a flow rate of 4 L/min or nasal cannula at a flow rate of 1–2 L/min (if a 24% mask is not available) to achieve O_2 saturation of 88–92% in most cases and PO_2 >8 kPa (60 mmHg) with <1.5 kPa rise in PCO_2. Repeat ABG 30 min after altering FiO_2. If the PCO_2 is normal then increase target O_2 saturation to 94–98% and repeat ABG after 30 min. The key is frequent reassessment. Rising PCO_2 and acidosis suggests respiratory support initially NIV.
- **Steroids:** usually commence **Prednisolone** 30–40 mg OD and continue for 5 d and then stop. **Hydrocortisone** 100–200 mg IV if *in extremis*. Consider osteoporosis prophylaxis for people requiring frequent courses of oral corticosteroids (3–4 courses per year).

- **Antibiotics: Amoxycillin** 500 mg 8 h PO for 5 d or if penicillin allergic **Doxycycline** 200 mg day one then 100 mg OD for 5 d or **Clarithromycin** 500 mg BD for 5 d. Save **Co-amoxiclav** 625 mg 8 h for 5 d for those with known resistance, severe attack or recent antibiotics. Use if infection suspected, e.g. fever, sputum, raised WCC or CRP. CXR changes suggesting infection. Those with history of bronchiectasis or pseudomonas may need **Tazocin** 4.5 g TDS IV or **Meropenem** 1 g TDS IV if penicillin allergic. There is some evidence that **Azithromycin** three times per week long-term may reduce the frequency of exacerbations and improve quality of life. Longer courses 5–10 d may be needed in some.
- **VTE prophylaxis:** standard UFH/LMWH and early mobilisation.
- **Aminophylline** 250 mg IV loading dose over 20 min if not on theophylline.
- **Roflumilast** 250–500 mcg OD is a phosphodiesterase-4 inhibitor licensed for COPD. It is used in patients with severe/very severe airflow limitation + frequent exacerbations that are not adequately controlled on long-acting bronchodilators.
- **NIV recommended** for acute hypercarbic exacerbation of COPD if respiratory acidosis pH <7.35 and PCO_2 >6 kPa (45 mmHg) despite controlled O_2 and bronchodilators and steroids and antibiotics for 1 h. See NIV protocol (▶Section 4.6).
- **Mechanical ventilation:** treat hospitalised exacerbations of COPD on ITU, including invasive ventilation when thought to be necessary.
- **Discharge:** measure spirometry before discharge. Consider home when patient confident they can manage, improving generally, pH >7.35, alert and orientated, no new focal abnormality on CXR, O_2 sats >88%, ability to cope at home, mobilising to toilet with minimum breathlessness, manage own personal ADLs, can cope with O_2 or nebulisers, no complicating comorbidities. Early supported discharge to support those who are not self-caring yet need additional help.
- **Prior to discharge:** offer long-acting muscarinic antagonists (LAMA), long-acting beta2 agonists (LABA). Optimise inhaler technique. LABA and inhaled corticosteroids (ICS) for those who are steroid-responsive. Tiotropium at night if early morning symptoms. Note: caution as antimuscarinics have risk of anticholinergic side-effects, e.g. in elderly. Consider mucolytic drug therapy for people with a chronic cough productive of sputum. Consider **Azithromycin** 250 mg 3 times a week if they do not smoke and have optimised non-drug management and inhaled therapies, relevant vaccinations and (if appropriate) have been referred for pulmonary rehabilitation and continue to have 1 or more of the following, particularly if they have significant daily sputum production (first exclude bronchiectasis by CT and TB): frequent (4 or more per year) exacerbations with sputum production, prolonged exacerbations with sputum production, exacerbations resulting in hospitalisation. Ensure QT and LFTs are normal before azithromycin. Review after 3 months.
- **Prevention:** prompt recognition and treatment of infection/exacerbation. Annual influenza vaccination. One-off pneumococcal vaccination if not given previously. Pulmonary rehabilitation (exercise, smoking cessation and nutritional advice). Long-term O_2 therapy (LTOT) for COPD if stable post-acute PO_2 <7.3 kPa or a PO_2 <8 kPa (60 mmHg) with secondary polycythaemia, pulmonary HTN or peripheral oedema. Requires 15+ h per day. Long-term O_2 therapy: keep SaO_2 >90% and PaO_2 >8 kPa. These patients become accustomed to worsening disease and hospital admissions.
- **End-stage COPD:** palliation and setting ceilings of care: it is becoming more common to ask patients with end-stage disease to discuss end of life plans with regard to interventions such as ventilation prior to this in the non-acute phase. Patient expectations need to be carefully balanced with the potential futility of some treatments.

- **Reference:** NICE (2021) Scenario: *Acute exacerbation of chronic obstructive pulmonary disease.*

4.11 Acute severe asthma

- **About:** assess severity, ensure appropriate treatment and rapid escalation. Close observation and early senior input and liaison with ITU are key. No asthmatic patient who gets to hospital breathing should die. If hypoxic give high FiO_2 (over 60%), steroids and nebulisers. Ensure accompanied at all times, e.g. in X-ray dept. Crash team if they are deteriorating. Senior medical and anaesthetic input early. Patients die daily in the UK from asthma.
- **Aetiology:** airway hyperactivity. Reversibility. Diurnal PEFR variation 20%. In some there is a potentially lethal mixture of tiredness and bronchoconstriction. Exacerbated by mucus plugging and V/Q mismatches. In fatal asthma, extensive mucus plugging of the airways is found at autopsy.
- **Higher risk:** lower admission threshold: age <18 years, poor compliance, isolated, depression, alcohol or drug misuse, physical or learning disability. Previous severe asthma attack, exacerbation despite adequate oral steroids before presentation, presentation in the afternoon or at night, recent nocturnal symptoms, recent hospital admission, pregnancy.

Clinical assessment and severity assessment of acute severe asthma

- **Acute severe:** any of these – unable to complete sentence in 1 breath, RR >25/min, HR >110 bpm, PEFR 33–50% best/predicted.
- **Life-threatening asthma:** acute severe asthma and any of these – silent chest, cyanosis, confusion, coma, exhaustion, arrhythmia, low BP, poor respiratory effort, unrecordable or PEFR or <33% predicted, SaO_2 <92% or PaO_2 <8 kPa (60 mmHg), $PaCO_2$ >4.6 kPa, pulsus paradoxus is an unreliable sign determining severity.
- **Near-fatal asthma:** life-threatening and $PaCO_2$ >6 kPa (45 mmHg), ventilation increased inflation pressures.

Investigations

- **Bloods:** ABG: hypoxia ± hypercarbia. FBC: raised WCC, CRP suggests infection. Eosinophilia: consider aspergillus, parasites, drugs, Churg–Strauss syndrome (eosinophilic granulomatosis with polyangiitis). U&E: ensure normal and check CRP. D-dimer if diagnosis unclear and needed.
- **ECG:** sinus tachycardia. Arrhythmias may be seen.
- **CXR:** (portable is safest) only needed if suspected PTX, consolidation, life-threatening asthma, failure to respond to treatment satisfactorily, requirement for ventilation.
- **PEFR:** difficult in acute severe asthma. Compare with best baseline. Acute severe 33–50%. Life-threatening <33% or too breathless to blow.
- **Spirometry:** done later if diagnosis unclear.

Management (liaise closely with ITU)

- **General:** high FiO_2 via O_2-driven nebuliser for sats 94–98%. Help patient to sit up if tired. Give bronchodilators and steroids. Needs support and time. It's the steroids that matter most. Reassurance, hydration, encourage slower and deeper respirations – a positive confident competent attitude from staff can help greatly because patient is working hard and *in extremis* and is often terrified. Ask ITU to review any patient not rapidly improving. Antibiotics only if clear evidence of

infection. Direct observation: patient must be accompanied at all times (e.g. in X-ray department) as rapid deterioration is possible.
- **Oxygen:** ABC O_2 to get target 94–98%. If sats <85% then give 15 L/min with non-rebreather mask. Get urgent help (patient is peri-arrest).
- **IV fluids:** avoid dehydration if patient too breathless/tired to drink and dry.
- **Salbutamol** (Albuterol/Ventolin) 5–10 mg OR **Terbutaline** 10 mg. Repeat every 20 min. Give with O_2 target 94–98% then reduce to 4-hourly.
- **Ipratropium bromide** (Atrovent) 500 mcg neb. 4–6-hourly.
- **Prednisolone** 40 mg PO or **Hydrocortisone** 100 mg TDS IV. Steroids for at least 5 d.

Further treatments if fails to improve (time to get senior consult and ITU)
- **Magnesium sulfate** 2 g (8 mmol) IV in 100 ml NS over 20 min.
- **Salbutamol IV.** Consider single bolus dose of IV salbutamol give 15 mcg/kg over 10 min. SE are elevated lactate, severe agitation and arrhythmias. Use with caution.
- **Aminophylline** loading dose 250–500 mg max 5 mg/kg IV over 20 min. Patient on aminophylline then 500 mcg/kg/h. See *BNF*. Monitor ECG. Macrolides/ciprofloxacin can cause toxicity. Watch serum levels.
- **Adrenaline** 0.5 mg IM may be repeated (not IV unless cardiac arrest) as for anaphylaxis may be used *in extremis* under senior supervision. Adrenaline infusions may be used in ITU.
- **Antibiotics:** exacerbations may be non-infectious or viral. Antibiotics if evidence of bacterial infection, e.g. consolidation, fever, purulent sputum, etc.

Ventilation/ITU referral for deteriorating acute severe asthma patient
- **Involve** ITU outreach and medical team early so aware of those with deteriorating PEF, look for worsening or persisting hypoxia, or hypercapnia, exhaustion, altered consciousness. If not improving, but cooperative, the intensivists may consider a trial of NIV but with a plan to immediately intubate if needed. FiO_2 1.0 IPAP 10 cmH_2O and EPAP 0–5 cmH_2O. Hypercapnia and failure to improve are indications to mechanically ventilate.
- Intubation in acute severe asthma is not an easy option as it can trigger laryngospasm and worsen bronchospasm. The decision to intubate a patient in the ED is multifactorial and must be weighed carefully. Ensure all reasonable medical treatments tried and given time if that is possible.
- Ketamine is one option to consider for preintubation sedation. It stimulates the release of catecholamines and might have a direct relaxation effect on bronchial smooth muscle, leading to bronchodilation. Propofol is an alternative. Both have bronchodilator effects. A neuromuscular blocking agent can be used for muscle paralysis.
- Poor respiratory effort or respiratory arrest. 1–3% require intubation. BVM ventilation is complicated due to severe airway obstruction. Expert rapid sequence induction is needed. When an asthmatic patient is ventilated, severe hyperinflation can result from breath stacking, placing the patient at risk for hypotension and barotrauma.

Other treatments
- **Pregnancy and labour:** (see ▶Section 16.17). Use prostaglandin F2α with extreme caution in women with asthma due to risk of inducing bronchoconstriction.
- **Allergic bronchopulmonary aspergillosis:** 1% of asthma patients, bronchiectasis on CT/CXR, eosinophilia. IgE >1000 ng/ml. Positive IgE RAST. Needs steroids and antifungals.

- **Eosinophilic granulomatosis with polyangiitis/Churg–Strauss syndrome:** chronic asthma, eosinophils, vasculitis, rash, neuropathy, nephropathy. p-ANCA (MPO). Needs immunosuppressive therapy.
- **Post recovery:** admit: if any feature of a life-threatening or near-fatal asthma attack or any feature of a severe asthma attack persisting after initial treatment.
- **Discharge:** those with PEFR >75% best or predicted within 2 h after initial treatment unless still have significant symptoms. If concerns about adherence, living alone/socially isolated, psychological problems, physical disability or learning difficulties, previous near-fatal asthma attack, asthma attack despite adequate dose steroid tablets pre-presentation, presentation at night, pregnancy, then consider admission.
- **Discharge medications:** give inhaled steroids (×2 normal dose), advise to return if worsens, see GP within 2 working days. Respiratory clinic in 4 weeks. Written asthma plan. Before discharge, trained staff should give asthma education on inhaler technique and PEFR record-keeping which can allow tailoring of therapy to guidelines to reduce morbidity and reduce relapse rates. Household to remove any precipitants, e.g. new pets before return and vacuum clean (high-filtration (HEPA) if possible) to minimise allergen exposure.
- **Reference:** NICE (2021) Scenario: *Acute exacerbation of asthma*.

4.12 Pneumothorax

- **About:** air in the pleural cavity. Those with secondary PTX are at higher risk and must be admitted for observation. Breathless and PTX needs active intervention. Primary pneumothorax occurs in those with normal lungs. Severe symptoms and haemodynamic collapse suggest tension PTX.
- **1° spontaneous PTX:** classically tall thin males age <40 without known lung disease but can be any sex. Commoner on the right side. Increased stresses on lung apices in tall people causes subpleural bleb formation, which can burst. Can recur within 1st year especially in tall adult (40% in 2 years). Commoner in smokers. Smoking cessation reduces recurrence.
- **2° spontaneous PTX** (age >40–50/traumatic, iatrogenic, chronic lung disease): trauma: especially penetrating chest trauma, iatrogenic trauma – pleural biopsy. Lung biopsy, central line insertion, high PEEP ventilation. Infection: lung abscess, PCP (AIDS), CF. Others: asthma, emphysema, idiopathic pulmonary fibrosis, sarcoidosis. Endometriosis/catamenial PTX – occurs within 72 h of menses. Oesophageal rupture. Lymphangioleiomyomatosis, lung carcinoma, histiocytosis X, eosinophilic granuloma, Marfan syndrome, and homocystinuria.
- **Tension PTX:** suspect post trauma, ventilation on ITU, or any patient with respiratory distress who then develops hypotension. Pleural space inflates like balloon needs deflated. Also asthma/COPD, a blocked or clamped or displaced chest drain. Patients receiving NIV or hyperbaric O_2 treatment.
- **Size:** measure horizontal gap (b on *figure* below) between lung margin and the chest wall at level of hilum: small <2 cm, large >2 cm rim (suggests >50% lung volume loss). For accurate PTX size calculations and to exclude bullae and other pathology get CT scan.
- **Clinical:** Small PTX: asymptomatic or mild dyspnoea in primary PTX. Larger PTX: causes mild to severe dyspnoea, cyanosis, pleurisy. Depends on size and lung function. Click or added sounds. Affected side hyper-resonant with reduced breath sounds. Tension PTX: See below under management.

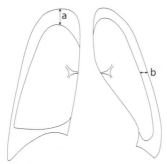

a = apex to cupola distance – American Guidelines
b = interpleural distance at level of the hilum – British Guidelines

Investigations

- **FBC, U&E, CRP:** raised WCC, infection, anaemia, inflammatory/infectious. **ABG:** if breathless and suspicion of RF. Look for hypoxia ± hypercarbia.
- **CXR:** departmental PA chest (± lateral) is the standard and shows an absence of lung markings between the ribs and a line demarcating the edge of the lung. Expiratory films no longer advocated. Lateral CXR or even CT may help if PTX suspected and PA chest not definitive. On a PA film measure the rim horizontal level of hilum. The BTS interpret PTX rim (b in *figure* above) as a large PTX.
- **Chest CT:** especially useful to differentiate complex bullae from PTX and to determine any underlying parenchymal pathology, to aid optimal drain position in complex cases and detect small pneumothoraces.
- **POCUS:** more sensitive and specific than CXR in detecting PTX: 'Absence of comet tails and/or sliding sign at >1 intercostal space'.
- **Other:** in selected cases HIV test in at-risk groups, ACE and calcium for sarcoidosis, bronchoscopy and lung biopsy, etc.

Management (large if >2 cm horizontal gap at hilum, small if <2 cm gap)

- **General points:** unless risk of hypercarbic RF give 10–15 L/min O_2. Helps resorb the nitrogen in the pleural cavity. Refer to a respiratory physician within 24 h of admission. Admit to chest ward with expertise. Manage where specialist medical/ nursing expertise is available.
- **Tension PTX:** give high flow O_2. Usually too ill to wait for CXR so proceed if progressive, severe respiratory distress, drum-like percussion on the affected side, hyper-expansion on affected side, tracheal shift away from affected side, progressive hypotension. Patient critical then immediate large-gauge IV cannula decompression in the 2nd ICS in MCL on the affected side sliding just over the lower rib. Alternative is the 5th ICS in the mid-axillary line. Identify space and mark it. Prepare the area as best one can. If time allows, wash hands, put on sterile gloves, clean area. There should be a 'hiss' as it decompresses, and BP should rise. Remove the inner metal needle of cannula and leave it to decompress. Then insert chest drain.
- **Primary small PTX:** monitor 4–6 h in A&E. Home if stable and not breathless for follow-up in 2–4 weeks with repeat CXR and assessment. Advise to return if symptoms. Give analgesia as needed. No diving/flying advice. Record it.

- **Primary large PTX and/or breathless,** then O_2 10 L/min. Aspirate with 16–18 G (grey/green) cannula up to 2.5 L with catheter in 2nd/3rd space at MCL. Repeat CXR. If rim <2 cm and less breathless then observe for 4–6 h and consider discharge and review in respiratory clinic in 4–6 weeks or sooner. If rim >2 cm after aspiration PTX or breathlessness not improved, then a small chest drain is inserted with size 8–14 Fr (15 Fr = 5 mm) and admit. Advise discharged patients to return by calling 999 if new SOB.
- **Secondary PTX:** all small and large are admitted and 10 L O_2 unless COPD. Large or symptomatic then chest drain (thoracostomy) with size 8–14 Fr. Smaller 1–2 cm rim of PTX and patient not breathless then aspirate with 16–18 G cannula up to 2.5 L and repeat CXR. If size now <1 cm then 10 L O_2 (unless O_2 sensitive) and observe for 24 h. If after aspirating PTX is still >1 cm then chest drain with size 14 Fr. All on positive pressure ventilation require chest drain insertion as positive pressure maintains the air leak.
- **PTX and pregnancy:** PTX recurrence commoner in pregnancy. Risks to the mother and fetus. Close cooperation between chest physicians, obstetricians and thoracic surgeons. May be managed by close observation if not dyspnoeic, no fetal distress and the PTX is small (<2 cm). Otherwise aspiration can be performed, chest drain insertion reserved for those with a persistent air leak. Risk of recurrence in subsequent pregnancies. Video-assisted thoracoscopic surgery (VATS) should be considered before next pregnancy.
- **PTX and AIDS/HIV infection:** admit. Chest drain and surgical referral. Treat for PCP/HIV. PCP causes necrotising alveolitis and subpleural necrotic thin-walled cysts and pneumatoceles. More air leaks, treatment failure, recurrence and higher hospital mortality. More aggressive intervention indicated.
- **PTX and cystic fibrosis:** early aggressive treatment/surgical referral. Procedures e.g. pleurodesis, do not affect the outcome of a subsequent lung transplantation.
- **Pleural aspiration for PTX:** (consider use of USS) infiltrate local anaesthetic down to the pleura, in the 2nd ICS in the mid-clavicular line (the axillary approach is an alternative). Using a cannula (14–16 Fr approx. 5 mm), enter the pleural cavity and withdraw the needle. Connect both the cannula and a 50 ml syringe (Luer lock) to a three-way tap, so that aspirated air can be voided. Aspiration should be discontinued if resistance is felt or the patient coughs excessively, or more than 2.5 L (that is, 50 ml removed 50 times) is aspirated. Repeat PA CXR in inspiration (an expiration film is unnecessary) in the X-ray department. If PTX is now only small, or resolved, the procedure has been successful. Note that failure to aspirate further may be due to the cannula being inadvertently withdrawn from the pleural cavity or becoming kinked. If this is suspected, another attempt at aspiration should be considered; aspiration should not be repeated unless there were technical difficulties. If this fails then a small-bore (<14 Fr (4.6 mm)) chest drain insertion is recommended (Chest drain, ▶ Section 21.3). Note no evidence that large drains are more effective except in trauma. Smaller drains (e.g. ≤16 Fr) easier to insert and better tolerated.
- Manage where specialist medical/nursing expertise is available. Failure of lung expansion may be due to extrathoracic placement, within a major fissure, obstructed or kinked tube. Other causes are ipsilateral bronchial obstruction, absence of suction, or 'trapped lung' due to pleural fibrosis. A large PTX >72 h with re-expansion can cause transient pulmonary oedema.

- **Pleurodesis:** can prevent recurrence. It incites an inflammatory response by pleura by instilling irritant into the pleural space leading to visceral and parietal pleura adhering.
- **Thoracic surgery:** decision by chest team and thoracic surgeons.
- **Discharge:** advise to return to hospital (999 if needed) if worsens/dyspnoea. Respiratory follow-up until full resolution. Tell/document no flying until CXR shows complete resolution. Most airlines suggest flying acceptable after 6 weeks of full resolution or a definitive surgical procedure. Risk is significant for a year and some may prefer to wait. Never scuba dive unless surgical bilateral pleurectomies and specialist approval.
- **Smoking cessation** reduces recurrence. It is key to management and prevention.
- **Reference:** Management of spontaneous pneumothorax: BTS pleural disease guideline. *Thorax*, 2010;65(Suppl 2):ii18.

4.13 Pleural effusion

- **About:** pleural effusions may be signs of local or systemic pathology. If large they can impair respiratory function. Exclude infection. Check a drug history. Small bilateral effusions often heart failure and may not need aspiration.
- **Aetiology:** a large collection of fluid within the pleural space may restrict lung function.
- **Clinical:** dyspnoea, pleurisy, fever, malaise, pneumonia, RA, SLE, heart failure, clubbing, malignancy. Assess symptoms. Depends on size, rate of accumulation and underlying cardiorespiratory function. Reduced wall movement, vocal resonance, and breath sounds. Stony dull to percussion, deviation of the trachea/mediastinum away if large.

Investigations

- **Bloods: FBC:** anaemia, high WCC infective, inflammatory, malignant cause. U&E CRP: AKI. Raised LFTs: albumin, raised CRP/ESR, raised ALP, ALT (metastases), PT.
- **CXR (PA is best):** needs 300 ml to be detectable. Hilar enlargement, cardiomegaly, pulmonary oedema, malignancy, TB, breast shadowing.
- **Echocardiogram or BNP/NT pro BNP:** useful to screen for heart failure.
- **Chest CT:** with contrast enhancement of the pleura and before complete drainage of pleural fluid. Indicated in all undiagnosed exudative pleural effusions to distinguish malignant from benign disease and pleural thickening. CT for complicated pleural infection when initial tube drainage has been unsuccessful, and surgery is to be considered.
- **Pleural USS:** to select aspiration site. Helpful if fluid loculated. Keep lateral.
- **Diagnostic tap aspirate 30–50 ml for** protein, glucose, LDH, Gram stain, cytology and culture. This can be done with a fine-bore (21 G) needle and a 50 ml syringe. Inspect appearance and send aspirate for cytology: protein, lactate, glucose, LDH. A low glucose (<3.3 mmol/L) suggests infection, tumour, RA, mesothelioma. Aspiration should be avoided for bilateral effusions in a clinical setting strongly suggestive of a transudate and CCF, unless there are atypical features or they fail to respond to therapy. Aspiration can be done on mechanical ventilation but with increased risk of a tension PTX if the lung is punctured.
- **Pleural fluid inspection:** bloody fluid is confirmed by measuring haematocrit. Gross blood usually due to malignancy, PE with infarction, trauma, benign asbestos

effusions or post-cardiac injury syndrome. Milky fluid suggests a chylothorax which may be due to damage to the thoracic duct. In this situation measure pleural fluid triglyceride and cholesterol levels.

- **Cytology:** malignant effusions show pleural fluid cytology in about 60% of cases. Immunocytochemistry can differentiate malignant cell types for oncology. Check amylase if oesophageal rupture or pancreatic disease suspected. Check pH where a value <7.2 with a suspected parapneumonic effusion indicates the need for tube drainage. Glucose: <1.6 mmol/L in RA.
- **Adenosine deaminase** (ADA) is raised in most TB pleural effusions.
- **Percutaneous pleural biopsy** under image guidance for pleural thickening.
- **Thoracoscopy:** exudate and pleural aspiration is inconclusive and malignancy is suspected.

Causes of pleural effusion by Light's criteria
- Exudate if pleural protein >50% serum protein.
- Exudate if pleural LDH >60% serum LDH.
- Exudate if pleural LDH >66% ULN for serum.
- **Transudate:** (low protein, low LDH). Failures: cardiac failure, nephrotic syndrome, liver failure. Others: myxoedema, low albumin, Meigs's syndrome: ovarian tumour and right pleural effusion.
- **Exudate:** (high protein, high LDH). Infection: pneumonia; tuberculosis; empyema. Cancer: (blood-stained) bronchogenic, mesothelioma, lung metastases, ovarian tumours. Cardiac/vascular: pulmonary infarct (bloody), post-MI; constrictive pericarditis. Gastro: pancreatitis, oesophageal rupture (both raised amylase). Connective tissue disease: SLE, RA, FMF. Drugs: methysergide, nitrofurantoin. Miscellaneous: radiotherapy; trauma; post-cardiac surgery; asbestosis (blood-stained); yellow nail syndrome.

Management
- **ABC** O_2 as per BTS guidelines. If an effusion is large causing compromise or associated with PTX then chest drain required usually with USS guidance. Caution when removing >1.5 L on a single occasion as may cause secondary oedema. Send excess volume for cytology if indicated. A diagnostic tap can be performed as suggested above. In a parapneumonic effusion, a pH of <7.2 indicates the need for tube drainage.
- **Outpatients:** if well, stable, managing and no significant breathlessness and mobile then refer to pleural effusion clinic. Advise to return if worse. Outpatient CT chest and pleural aspiration in outpatients.
- **References:** British Thoracic Society Pleural Disease Guideline Group (2010) *BTS Pleural Disease Guideline*. Kearon *et al.* (2016) Antithrombotic therapy for VTE disease: CHEST guideline and expert panel report. *Chest* (e-pub).

4.14   Pneumonia

- **About:** infection and acute inflammation of the air spaces and substance of the lung, which are normally sterile. Lobar is restricted to the whole of one lobe, exclude a bronchostenotic lesion. Bronchopneumonia affects lobules and bronchi. CURB-65 scoring for community-acquired pneumonias.

Types (there is much overlap)

- **Community-acquired (CAP):** symptoms, signs of consolidation. Often healthy young patients. At-risk groups: aspiration (stroke/MND), alcohol, diabetes, steroids, immunosuppression, smokers, COPD, nursing home residents.
- **Hospital-acquired (HAP) or institutional:** onset >2–3 days after admission. Acquired following admission. Often post-op or debilitated. High mortality. Excludes ventilator-associated pneumonia. These patients have significant comorbidities. Difficulty swallowing. Poor nutrition. More likely aerobic Gram-negative infections, e.g. *Klebsiella, Pseudomonas, E. coli*, anaerobes and *Staph. aureus* (ventilated). Elderly, immunosuppressed, respiratory disease, post-operative, ITU.
- **Aspiration pneumonia:** gastric acid pH <2.5 into lungs + foodstuff; a chemical pneumonitis. Often to right mid zone or apex of right lower lobe. May be a more subtle micro-aspiration syndrome especially where there is bulbar weakness.
- **Atypical pneumonias** due to *Mycoplasma pneumoniae, Chlamydophila pneumoniae*, or *Legionella pneumophila*. Dry cough, Headache, diarrhoea, vomiting, abdominal pain, myalgia, chest symptoms. Radiological changes and chest signs may be delayed.
- **Viral pneumonia:** influenza, adenovirus, RSV ± 2nd bacterial infection.
- **Risks:** young and elderly. Comorbidities – renal disease, HIV, diabetes, heart disease. Lung disease: COPD, cystic fibrosis, bronchiectasis, old TB, bronchostenotic lesion. Others: smoker, alcohol excess, IV drugs, steroids, dementia, stroke. Causative organisms: vary by study, age, location, comorbidities, exposure (see list below).
- **Pathology stages:** (1) congestion and vascular engorgement and alveolar bacteria; (2) red hepatisation – alveolar spaces full of polymorphs and fibrin and red cells; (3) grey hepatisation – RBC breakdown, fibrin and suppurative inflammation; (4) resolution – exudate removed by macrophages.
- **Clinical:** fever, sweats, rigors, dry cough initially, malaise, delirium (elderly and *Legionella*). Breathlessness, cyanosis, raised HR, low BP, pleuritic-type chest pain. Rusty sputum (*Pneumococcus*), yellow/green sputum, haemoptysis. Flare-up of herpes simplex (*Pneumococcus*), atypical diarrhoea. Myalgia, headache, reduced air entry and expansion and dullness to percussion. Raised vocal resonance, stony dull if effusion/empyema.
- **Complications:** lung abscess, exudative pleural effusion, parapneumonic effusion. Empyema, bacteraemia, sepsis, cerebral abscess, meningitis. ARDS, respiratory failure, cardiac failure, multi-organ failure, death.

Investigations

- **Send sputum/blood cultures:** help expectoration and send sputum samples for culture and sensitivity and blood cultures if pyrexial. Bloods: FBC: raised WCC. Low or mild increase with *Legionella* and atypicals. U&E: AKI. Low Na: *Legionella*. Elevated LFT: *Legionella*. Blood film: red cell agglutination suggests cold agglutinins and *Mycoplasma*. Raised procalcitonin levels with bacterial infection. ESR/CRP increased with pneumonia and fails to fall with abscess/empyema or wrong antibiotics.
- **Serology:** only those with CURB-65 >2; check urine – send in universal container/white top for *Legionella* and *Pneumococcus* antigens. Also, sputum/throat gargle (20 ml saline) for virology and mycoplasma PCR. If psittacosis suspected send for appropriate investigation. Consider HIV test if indicated.
- **CXR (PA ± lateral):** patchy consolidation with bronchopneumonia. Look for consolidation (lobar), masses, cavitation, parapneumonic effusion, PTX, bullae.

Changes lag behind clinical changes. CXR <4 h of presentation to hospital. Differentials of consolidation: alveolar blood, aspiration, lung infarction.
- **ABG:** type 1 or type 2 RF with V/Q mismatch and coexisting COPD.
- **Bronchoscopy:** in some cases to look for any bronchostenotic lesions or remove foreign bodies or mucus plugging or for sampling, e.g. PCP.
- **HRCT chest:** concerns of other related pathology or complications – abscess, empyema, tumour. Slow resolution look for empyema, underlying neoplasm or antibiotic resistance, or is it the wrong diagnosis?
- **Differentials of pneumonia:** PE, pulmonary oedema, ARDS, pulmonary haemorrhage. Cryptogenic organising pneumonia, lung cancer, acute extrinsic allergic alveolitis. Rare infections – anthrax, plague, tularaemia.
- **CURB-65 scoring defines severity and aids clinical management:** *Confusion*: MTS <8: +1, *Urea* (BUN) >7 mmol/L +1, *RR* >30/min +1, *BP* (<90/60 mmHg) +1, age >65 +1. **Risk score and response:** 0/1: low (<3% mortality risk), consider home-based care; **2:** intermediate (3–15% mortality risk), consider hospital-based care; **3–5:** high (>15% mortality risk), consider ITU outreach and HDU/ITU or defining level of care. CRB-65 (urea omitted) may be used in primary care to assess. Hospital assessment CRB-65 >0 especially >2. CURB-65 should only be used to assess severity in CAP. **Additional evidence of severity: WCC** >20 or <4 or 10% band forms. **CXR:** multilobe involvement. **Albumin** <35 g/L. **Microbiology:** positive blood culture. **Others:** stroke, COPD, cardiac disease, diabetes.

Microbial causes of pneumonia

- *Strep. pneumoniae* (39%): cold sore, rusty sputum, consolidation/cavities (serotype 3). Antigen in urine/serum.
- *Chlamydophila pneumoniae:* epidemics, high AST.
- *Mycoplasma pneumoniae* (10%): children and young adults. Autumnal, erythema nodosum and multiforme, myocarditis, pericarditis, meningoencephalitis, GBS, haemolytic anaemia, bullous myringitis, cold agglutinins in 50%, headache, otalgia, transverse myelitis, pancreatitis, lymphadenopathy, splenomegaly. Check IgM.
- *Legionella pneumoniae:* age >50 usually. Showers/air conditioning. Headache, malaise, myalgia, fever, dry cough, nausea and vomiting, diarrhoea, confusion, hepatitis, low sodium, low albumin, raised LFTs and CK. Delayed diagnosis worsens outcomes. Macrolides or fluoroquinolones. It is not passed person to person. *Legionella* antigen in urine. Direct fluorescent antibody stain sputum.
- *Moraxella catarrhalis:* (COPD) 2%.
- *Haemophilus influenzae* (5%): bronchopneumonia.
- *Staph. aureus:* winter. Post-influenza/viral pneumonia. CXR cavitation and abscess. Needs flucloxacillin.
- *Chlamydophila psittaci* (3%): sick bird. Malaise, low-grade fever, hepatosplenomegaly.
- *Coxiella burnetii* (1%): animal contact. Chronic influenzal illness with dry cough, conjunctivitis, hepatosplenomegaly, endocarditis. CXR: multiple segmental shadows.
- *Klebsiella pneumonia:* widespread consolidation and cavitation (upper lobes). High mortality. Bloody viscous sputum.
- *Pneumocystis pneumonia:* immunosuppressed, e.g. HIV, drug therapy.
- **Tuberculosis** not usually included as a cause of CAP but is a cause of pulmonary infection.

- **Viral pneumonia** (20%): influenza A and B, parainfluenza, measles, RSV in infants. Varicella can cause severe pneumonia with miliary nodular shadows, which may calcify. Direct fluorescent antibody stain sputum for viruses.

Management

- **ABC and O$_2$** to deliver sats of 94–98% or 88–92% if severe COPD. Check ABG. **IV fluids:** hydration important. Mobilise as tolerated. Sit out of bed if able. Antibiotics: give as shown below within 4 h for CAP patients who are admitted. Those with atypical pneumonias consider **Clarithromycin**, **Azithromyin** or **Doxycycline**. Prolonged courses may be needed. They can often be managed as outpatients.
- **Resp failure:** type 1 (and type 2) requires O$_2$. Usual care in COPD. Severe hypoxaemia needs ITU and invasive ventilation. Role for CPAP and NIV without COPD/pulmonary oedema undefined. Trials of NIV/CPAP in this situation should be short (1–2 h), and if no improvement admit to ITU if pH <7.26 or PO_2 <8 kPa or rising PCO_2 or breathless tiring patient.
- **Steroids:** a 7-d course, e.g. **Prednisolone** 20–60 mg/d for hospitalised CAP patients may reduce adverse outcomes and costs.
- **Others:** aspirate pleural effusions. Chest drain for empyema. Chest physiotherapy. VTE prophylaxis. Nutrition. Prevention: influenza and pneumococcal vaccination should be considered.

Differentials

- **Lung cancer:** lobar pneumonia due to underlying bronchostenotic lesion. Repeat CXR at 6 weeks. Fails to resolve needs CT/bronchoscopy. Suspect more so in smokers.
- **Tuberculosis:** if considered avoid drugs with anti-TB activity, e.g. fluoroquinolones. Send 3 sputum samples for smear and culture. Atypical presentation in HIV, immunocompromised and diabetics. Isolate especially if smear positive.
- **Heart failure:** raised BNP/NT proBNP and abnormal echo.
- **HIV:** low threshold to testing. Could this be PCP? (▶Section 4.15).
- **Asthma/exacerbation of COPD:** dyspnoea, cough, wheeze, smoking.
- **Fungal pneumonia:** histoplasmosis, cocciodioides, blastomycosis. Animal exposure, endemic areas, immunocompromised. Southwest USA or Mexico.
- **Organising pneumonia:** diagnosis of exclusion – usually diffuse bilateral patchy changes. May need lung biopsy and steroids.
- **Antimicrobial management of CAP:** mild (CURB-65 = 0/1): **Amoxicillin** 500 mg – 1 g 8 h PO or **Clarithromycin** 500 mg BD PO for 7 days. Moderate (CURB-65 >2): **Amoxicillin** 500 mg – 1 g 8 h IV/PO plus **Clarithromycin** 500 mg BD PO/IV for 7–10 days. De-escalate IV to PO when suitable. Severe: **Co-amoxiclav** 1.2 g TDS IV plus **Clarithromycin** 500 mg BD IV for 7–10 days. Alternatives include **Cefuroxime** 750 mg – 1.5 g TDS IV or **Meropenem** IV. Suspect *Staph. aureus* (measles, flu, immunocompromised, alcohol abuse, IVDU): **Flucloxacillin** 1–2 g QDS IV for 14–21 days. In all de-escalate IV to PO when suitable. MRSA suspected give **Vancomycin** 15–20 mg/kg TDS (max. per dose 2 g) IV.
- **Hospital-acquired pneumonia:** mild/moderate consider **Co-amoxiclav** 625 mg TDS PO or 1.2 g TDS IV. Alternatively, **Tazocin** 4.5 g 6–8 h IV, or **Meropenem** IV if penicillin allergic (severe/anaphylaxis). If evidence of aspiration, consider adding **Metronidazole**. Contact microbiology if MRSA-positive or if no improvement in 24 h.

- **Discharge:** not if in past 24 h they have had 2 or more of temp. >37.5°C, RR >24/min, HR >100/min, SBP <90 mmHg, O_2 sats <90% on room air, abnormal mental status, inability to eat without assistance.
- **Patient advice:** symptoms reduced by 1 week for fever, 4 weeks for chest pain and sputum production, 6 weeks for cough and breathlessness, 3 months for all but fatigue, and by 6 months most people will feel back to normal. Persisting symptoms beyond these should seek advice.
- **Palliation:** more than half of pneumonia-related deaths occur in those in their 80s and consider frailty and need for palliative discussions.
- **Reference:** NICE (2014) CG191: *Diagnosis and management of community and hospital-acquired pneumonia in adults.*

4.15 ▶ *Pneumocystis* pneumonia

- **About:** infection by fungus *P. jirovecii* (formerly *P. carinii*). Seen in untreated HIV infection (CD4 <200/mm³) or on immunosuppression, e.g. post-transplantation, methotrexate, long-term steroids.
- **Aetiology:** damages alveolar epithelium, impedes gas exchange. Type 1 RF.
- **Clinical:** slow insidious onset, progressive breathlessness, PTX, fever, dry cough, fine crackles. Desaturates on mild exertion. Look for signs of AIDS, e.g. oral candida, Kaposi's sarcoma, hairy leukoplakia, herpes zoster, etc.
- **Investigations:** bloods: **FBC:** low WCC. LDH >500 mg/dl is common but non-specific. **U&E: nephropathy ABG:** PaO_2 <8 kPa on air defined as severe PCP. Increased A–a O_2 gradient. Desaturation with exercise is useful but non-specific. **Rapid HIV test:** CD4 cell counts (usually <200/mm³) HIV viral load measurements. **CXR:** diffuse, bilateral, symmetrical interstitial infiltrates emanating from the hila in a butterfly pattern, cavitation, cysts, TB in AIDS, nodules or PTX. **HRCT:** characteristic ground-glass appearance, cysts, nodules, PTX. Can show filtrates when the CXR is normal. Diagnosis requires histopathologic or cytopathologic evidence of organisms in tissue from bronchoalveolar lavage (BAL) fluid, or induced sputum samples. **Beta-D-glucan test:** negative result makes PCP very unlikely.

Management

- **ABC,** O_2, antibiotics, steroids, HAART: take advice from HIV team/infectious diseases. ABC + high FiO_2 to deliver sats of 94–98%.
- **ITU referral:** if severe hypoxaemia. Watch for PTX which is seen with PCP.
- **Antibiotics (see current *BNF*):** *Mild to moderate* PaO_2 *>9.3 kPa on room air*: **Co-trimoxazole** oral 1920 mg TDS or 90 mg/kg/day in 3 divided doses (rounded to nearest 480 mg) for 21 days. Alternative **Clindamycin** oral 600 mg TDS + **Primaquine** oral 30 mg OD. Check G6PD. *Severe* PaO_2 *≤9.3 kPa on room air*: **Co-trimoxazole** IV infusion 120 mg/kg/day for 3 days then reduce to 90 mg/kg/day for 18 days. The total daily dose may be divided in 3–4 doses. Alternative: **Clindamycin** IV infusion 900 mg 8 h + **Primaquine** PO 30 mg OD. Check G6PD. Other drugs available. Get specialist advice.
- **Steroids:** if O_2 saturations <92% or PaO_2 ≤9.3 kPa on room air start steroids with treatment (<72 hours). **Prednisolone** 40 mg BD for 5 days, 40 mg OD for 5 days then 20 mg daily for 11 days, then stop. If IV required use **Methylprednisolone** at 75% of oral prednisolone dose.
- **Pneumothorax** is a common complication of severe disease and carries a poor prognosis. Get expert advice.

- **HAART:** should be initiated by local specialists within 2 weeks of diagnosis of PCP irrespective of CD4 count. Risk of immune reconstitution inflammatory syndrome which can be life-threatening. **Stop smoking:** advocated. PCP prevention: **Co-trimoxazole** 960 mg PO OD. **In pregnancy: diagnostics the same.** Take advice. Usually TMP-SMX plus folic acid first trimester.
- **Reference:** *Guidelines for Prevention and Treatment of Opportunistic Infections in HIV-Infected Adults and Adolescent* (last updated October 2022, see https://clinicalinfo.hiv.gov/en/guidelines/hiv-clinical-guidelines-adult-and-adolescent-opportunistic-infections/treatment-aids-associated).

4.16 Empyema

- **About:** pus in the pleural space usually post-bacterial pneumonia. It requires effective drainage and systemic antibiotics.
- **Aetiology:** parapneumonic effusion after bacterial pneumonia becomes infected. Associated with diabetes, alcohol abuse, IV drug use, GORD. Post trauma or a complicated lung abscess or thoracic surgery or infected draining catheter.
- **Clinical:** purulent cough, pyrexia, dyspnoea after recent pneumonia. Weight loss, pleurisy and fever, night sweats, clubbing.
- **Investigations:** bloods: FBC: raised WCC, raised CRP. U&E: AKI. CXR: pleural effusion, consolidation, mass, bronchiectasis. Pleural aspiration: shows a purulent or turbid/cloudy pleural fluid exudate which may be neutrophil-rich and viscous with raised protein, raised white cells. **Empyema:** glucose <2.2 mmol/L, pH <7.2. A pH >7.8 suggests *Proteus*. Ensure all pleural fluid analysed in blood gas machine has been heparinised. LDH: >1000 IU/L. Low pH (<7.30) causes are empyema, RA, malignancy, tuberculosis, lupus, oesophageal rupture. Blood cultures for aerobic and anaerobic bacteria performed. **Enhanced chest CT:** help locate drain optimally as cavities may become loculated. CT defines anatomy. Gas usually suggests an empyema.
- **Management:** ABC O_2 as per BTS guidelines. Ensure adequate nutrition in patients with pleural infection. Abstain from alcohol/smoking. Identify any immunocompromise. Ensure VTE prophylaxis as high risk and give LMWH.
- **Chest drain:** if diagnosis confirmed by aspiration then insert a drain large enough to drain the fluid. A small-bore catheter 10–14 Fr will be adequate for most cases of pleural infection. Occasionally viscid and difficult to drain but in many cases a small tube inserted by Seldinger method is adequate. The small catheters can be placed using either ultrasound or CT scans. Previously streptokinase to cause localised fibrinolysis has been used but less so now as data have not been positive. If parapneumonic effusion not confirmed by aspirate then do not drain but continue antibiotics and watch CRP and reassess and take advice. *Pleural procedures should not take place out of hours except in an emergency.*
- **IV antibiotics:** take microbiology advice – usually same antibiotics as pneumonia. Aminoglycosides are inactivated by low pH. May need to cover anaerobes and *Pseudomonas*. Get results of culture and adjust accordingly. Involve chest team and they may need to involve thoracic surgery (thoracotomy and decortication) in difficult cases. Decortication involves the removal of all fibrous tissue from the visceral pleura and parietal pleura, and the evacuation of all pus and debris from the pleural space.
- **Reference:** British Thoracic Society Pleural Disease Guideline Group (2010).

4.17 ▶ Pulmonary embolism/deep vein thrombosis

- **About:** deep vein thrombosis (DVT) and pulmonary embolism (PE) are all part of same disease. Reduce by early mobilisation and low dose LMWH or equivalent in those at increased risk. Untreated mortality is 30% (not all PEs are the same), which falls to 3–8% with treatment. However, data come from a time when only larger PEs were detectable. Can expect 500 per DGH per year. 65–90% emboli from legs. Several DOACs now licensed to treat DVT/PE. Many small DVTs and even PEs are potentially benign. Anticoagulation has bleed risks and these need to be balanced. PE is the commonest cause of death after day one in the trauma patient due to the prothrombotic response to trauma. High risk post knee and hip surgery.
- **Anticoagulation:** ensure patient anticoagulated. Give information booklet. An anticoagulant alert card (carry at all times). Verbal and written information on oral anticoagulation treatment, including: how to take, duration of treatment, adverse effects and advice, advise if pregnant or planning pregnancy, advise on dental treatment and sports and travel.
- **Aetiology:** thrombi originate in the proximal veins of the lower leg and pelvis. Consider thrombophilia in those under 45 without a clear precipitant. DVT can block pulmonary artery and/or embolise across a R/L shunt (e.g. PFO/ASD) to cause an embolic stroke. Most emboli go to lower lobes. 10% cause infarction. Autopsies show high incidence of undiagnosed VTE as a cause of death.
- **Major risk factors for PE include:** DVT, previous DVT or PE, active cancer, recent surgery, lower limb trauma, significant immobility (e.g. due to hospitalisation), pregnancy and, in particular, for 6 weeks postpartum. **Others:** COCP/HRT, known thrombophilias, long-distance travel, obesity, and age >60.
- **Clinical DVT:** pain, redness, swelling, dilated veins, increased circumference, can extend to the calf or the whole leg swollen if large proximal thrombosis. Thrombus usually starts distally extends proximally even to pelvic veins. Proximal clots are most likely to embolise.
- **Upper limb DVT:** 10% of DVT: risks: local cancer, pacemakers, central lines, thrombophilias, Paget–Schroetter syndrome. PE less likely. May be clinically silent post ITU.
- **Clinical PE:** <u>single small PE</u>: may be silent or subtle and non-specific, e.g. causing confusion especially in elderly. Peripheral PE causing severe pleuritic chest pain with infarction and anatomically. <u>Chronic PE</u>: repeated PE with progressive SOB and pulmonary HTN. <u>Medium-sized PE</u>: increased RR and HR, haemoptysis, pleuritic chest pain, pleural rub, collapse, low BP, syncope or presyncope. <u>Large PE</u>: there is acute right heart failure with marked dyspnoea, tachypnoea, presyncope or syncope. Urge to defecate (often collapse in toilet), chest pain, raised HR, JVP and loud P2 on auscultation, low BP. <u>Massive PE/saddle embolism</u>: PE to one or both pulmonary arteries – sudden cardiac death, obstructive shock.
- **Complications:** bleeding if thrombolysis, sudden death, pulmonary hypertension PAP >25 mmHg 6/12 after PE. Death due to progressive right heart failure. Post-thrombotic syndrome of the legs: chronic venous insufficiency seen in 50% of those who experience DVT or PE. Can lead to leg ulcers and oedema. Paradoxical embolism: with right/left shunts and stroke.
- **High risks:** previous DVT/PE, malignancy, hospital immobility, perioperative event, stroke, severe illness, spinal injury, GBS, trauma, HHS, localised trauma. Varicose veins ± phlebitis, post-MI, pregnancy, postpartum, pelvic tumour.

- **Medium/low risks:** thrombophilias, smoking, combined OCP, HRT, recent long-haul travel >6 h, obesity, blood transfusion, antiphospholipid syndrome, nephrotic syndrome, polycythaemia, sickle cell disease. Steroid usage.

DVT probability: Wells clinical scoring (see www.mdcalc.com)

Only apply test if after history and physical exam suggest DVT is a diagnostic possibility! It helps guide which test first. D-dimer if low risk. Doppler if high. Not validated for pregnant or postpartum women or IVDU with possible DVT so use with caution.

- Active cancer (treatment <6 months or palliative) +1
- Paralysis, paresis, recent cast immobilisation of leg +1
- Recently bedridden >3 d, or major surgery in last 3/12 +1
- Previously documented DVT +1
- Calf swelling >3 cm other leg (10 cm below tibia tuberosity) +1
- Collateral superficial (non-varicose) veins present +1
- Pitting oedema (confined to symptomatic leg) +1
- Swelling of entire leg +1
- Localised tenderness along deep venous system +1
- Alternative diagnosis at least as likely as DVT −2

Assessment

- **Pretest probability:** 2 or higher then 'DVT likely' so don't do D-dimer but get compression ultrasound. If negative, consider repeating USS in 1 week. If score <2 then check D-dimer and if negative DVT excluded. If positive do compression ultrasound: if positive treat, if negative consider repeating in 1 week.
- **Differential diagnosis for DVT:** leg trauma ± haematoma, internal derangement of the knee, muscle tear and damage, ruptured Baker's (popliteal) cyst, cellulitis, obstructive lymphadenopathy, lymphoedema, drug-induced oedema (amlodipine, etc.).

PE probability: two level Wells clinical scoring (see www.mdcalc.com)

- Validated in an outpatient setting. Less valid in inpatient or pregnancy so needs traditional assessment. Assess score from 7 parameters. Only apply test if after history and physical exam suggests that PE is a diagnostic possibility. Not validated for pregnant or postpartum women so use with caution.
- **Calculate scores:** previous PE or DVT +1.5; recent surgery in past 30 days or immobile for 3 days +1.5; malignancy (within <6/12 or palliative) +1; heart rate >100/min +1.5; clinical signs of DVT +3; haemoptysis +1. PE is most/equally likely diagnosis = +3.
- **Outcome:** score 1–4 had PE risk 3% so do D-dimer and if positive CTPA/VQ. If the score is >4 then PE is likely and go straight to CTPA/VQ scan.
- An alternative test is the Geneva score which uses age. VTE experts use the www.mdcalc.com website to get a score and risk estimate. Caution investigating for PE in a patient with an elevated D-dimer if there are no clinical symptoms or signs of PE.

PERC score used to exclude PE (see www.mdcalc.com)

- This is another tool which can rule out PE if all of the following are true (most useful in those <50). Age <50, HR <100, sats >95%, no unilateral leg swelling, no recent trauma or surgery in past 4 weeks with GA, no haemoptysis, no previous DVT/PE, not using hormones HRT/OCP.
- Rules out PE if none of the 8 criteria is present and pre-test probability is less than or equal to 15%.

Investigations

- FBC, U&E, LFTs, CRP, ESR usually normal unless underlying cause.
- **ABG:** medium to large PE: hypoxia and reduced/normal PCO_2 (type 1 RF). Large PE: hypoxic, acidotic and raised lactate.
- D-**dimer assay age adjustment:** a normal D-dimer makes PE/DVT very unlikely in patients with a low or intermediate/moderate pretest, to the extent that no further testing is needed. In those at high risk, skip D-dimer and go straight to diagnostic imaging. A dimer level >500 ng/ml (0.50 µg/ml) is seen in nearly all patients with DVT/PE, and false positives in others. Also elevated in pregnancy, infections, sepsis, anticoagulated, post-op. Degradation product of cross-linked fibrin. Don't test dimer if high probability. *An age-related cut-off can be used now and can exclude VTE in 30% of outpatients with suspected DVT or PE.* Age adjust only if age >50. Age-adjusted upper limit = patient age/50 × usual upper limit; e.g. age 75 is 0.75 mg/L = 750 ng/ml.
- **ECG findings:** sinus tachycardia, new AF. Others include the rare S1Q3T3 pattern. RV strain and right access deviation. New incomplete RBBB. ECG may be normal.
- **CXR: done in all including pregnant.** A normal CXR may be seen with a large PE. Segmental wedge collapse, pleural effusion, area of lung infarction, raised hemidiaphragm, prominent pulmonary artery and a localised absence of vascular markings (Westermark sign), dilated pulmonary arteries. VQ scan not done if abnormal CXR.
- **Markers:** raised troponin, BNP/N-terminal (NT)-proBNP and lactate associated with a worse outcome.
- **Diagnostic imaging for DVT:** contrast venography: largely superseded by compression USS and rarely done. Considered gold standard. **NB:** the superficial femoral vein is a deep vein and thrombosis requires treatment. To avoid confusion, it has been renamed the distal femoral vein. Compression USS of lower or upper limb veins is the preferred diagnostic test. It is non-invasive, relatively inexpensive and readily available. It is particularly useful for pelvic and iliofemoral clots.

Diagnostic imaging for PE

- **SPECT ventilation–perfusion (V/Q) scan** using single-photon emission computed tomography is preferred initial imaging, especially in pregnancy or young with renal failure or allergy to IV contrast. Radiation dose patients receive is roughly half that from a CTPA. Need normal CXR otherwise other lung disease will give abnormalities. Unreliable with bronchospasm and/or infiltrates. Follow local guidance. Look for areas of 'mismatch' with ventilation but low perfusion. Intermediate results seen in 30% and can be unhelpful and will require CTPA or compression USS for DVT to risk assess.
- **CT pulmonary angiography (CTPA):** multislice helical involves giving IV contrast. Identifies PE(s) and/or other pathology – consolidation, aortic syndrome or tamponade. Whole lung scanned with 10 sec breath-hold. Can be done out of hours. Can image sixth-order vessels and visualise thrombi so small that clinical importance is uncertain. Subsegmental PE may not be clinically significant and may not need treatment – take advice. **Right ventricular (RV) dysfunction** caused by acute PE is associated with poor short- and long-term prognosis. RV dilatation as a proxy for RV dysfunction can be assessed by calculating the right-to-left ventricle diameter (RV/LV) ratio on standard CTPA images.
- **Echocardiogram:** consider in those with large PE and haemodynamic impairment unfit for CTPA to make a diagnosis to support lysis or other interventions. RA and RV

dilated, TR, right heart strain, pulmonary hypertension. May see 'clots-in transit' and McConnell's signs with impaired RV contraction. RV hypokinesis has been shown to be associated with double the 30-day mortality.

- **General comments:** CTPA is sensitive and easy to obtain but may lead to overdiagnosis. V/Q scans may be preferable in younger patients (less radiation), patients with normal lungs (a definitive result is more likely), and patients with renal dysfunction (no nephrotoxic contrast). Detection of DVT by ultrasonography of the legs when PE is suspected makes subsequent lung imaging unnecessary because patients need anticoagulation anyway. There is no single pathway. It depends on access to tests and availability of ambulatory testing – this is a complex and challenging area so take advice.

Other tests

- **Cancer testing:** for unprovoked VTE do not offer further investigations for cancer unless they have relevant clinical symptoms or signs.
- **Thrombophilia testing:** if it is planned to stop anticoagulation treatment, consider testing for antiphospholipid antibodies. Test for hereditary thrombophilia (HT) in people who have a first-degree relative who has had DVT or PE. Do not offer testing for HT to those continuing anticoagulation treatment, first-degree relatives of people with a history of DVT or PE and thrombophilia, people who have had provoked PE.
- Several risk scoring systems allow outpatient care for low-risk patients. These are sPESI and MBOVA: MBOVA not discussed here. See online at mdcalc.com.
- **Risks of recurrence:** provoked 5-year recurrence risk 10%. Unprovoked 30%.

VTE and pregnancy

- **Investigations:** options vary. Issue to reduce radiation to fetus or breast tissue (particularly if there is a family history of breast carcinoma). All should have a CXR (screen fetus). Consider USS looking for a DVT which would justify anticoagulation and repeat at day 3 and 7 if scan negative but suspicion high. Consider perfusion component of V/Q scan. Newer CT scanners deliver less radiation so may be best with fetal screening. Follow locally agreed policies. Women with suspected PE should be advised that, compared with CTPA, V/Q scanning may carry a slightly increased risk of childhood cancer but is associated with a lower risk of maternal breast cancer; in both situations, the absolute risk is very small. In women with suspected PE who also have symptoms and signs of DVT, compression duplex USS should be performed. If it confirms the presence of DVT, no further investigation is necessary and treatment for VTE should continue.
- **Management of DVT/PE:** urgent hospital referral if pregnant or have been in past 6 weeks. Commence LMWH. Check peak anti-Xa activity is recommended for women on LMWH weight <50 kg or ≥90 kg or renal impairment or recurrent VTE. High risk of haemorrhage give IV heparin.
- **Massive PE in pregnancy:** collapsed, shocked women who are pregnant or in the puerperium should be assessed by a team of experienced clinicians including the on-call consultant obstetrician. Women should be managed on an individual basis regarding IV UFH, systemic or catheter-directed thrombolytic therapy or thoracotomy and surgical embolectomy.
- **Reference:** RCOG (2015) GTG 37b: *Thromboembolic disease in pregnancy and the puerperium.*

Preventing pulmonary emboli

- **Primary prevention is best:** risk assessment and LMWH, early mobilisation in medical patients. Perioperative LMWH or use of anticoagulants, e.g. DOACs. Early mobilisation post-op. Hydration. Use of LMWH in higher risk pregnancies and those with APLS or thrombophilia up to 6 weeks after. Use of LMWH in oncology patients.

Management of suspected acute pulmonary embolism

- **Assessment ABC:** O_2 if needed, IV fluids if needed. Resuscitation if needed. See below. Risk assess those who can be managed through ambulatory care.
- **Treat if suspicion:** start LMWH or DOAC empirically if no imaging within 4 hours (unless high bleeding risk).

Ambulatory care of suspected PE: consider for those with low sPESI score

- **Simplified pulmonary embolism severity index (sPESI score):** PESI score: age >80 = +1; history of cancer = +1; chronic lung/heart disease = +1; HR >110/min; SBP <100 mmHg = +1; SaO_2 <90% = +1. Combining results of the hsTn T assay with the simplified PESI appears to yield additive prognostic information. Those with a low PESI score can be considered for outpatient management. Score 0: low risk 30 d mortality of 1%; score of 1 or more: 30 d mortality of 10.9% See www.mdcalc.com.
- **Exclusion criteria for ambulatory care:** SpO_2<95% (unless known low baseline saturation), SBP <100 mmHg, Chest pain requiring parenteral analgesia, Active bleeding (even if minor), Severe pulmonary hypertension, High risk of bleeding (stroke <10 days, GI bleed <14 days, plts <50 × 10^9, Severe renal impairment (GFR<30 ml/min), Severe obesity (if using LMWH as dose unpredictable – monitor anti-Xa), Previous intolerance to heparins (HIT or allergy) if using heparin, PE while already on warfarin.

Anticoagulation for VTE prevention

- **Oral therapy:** consider DOAC or treatment dose LMWH if scan delayed and continue if confirmed, e.g. long term: Apixaban 10 mg BD for 1 week post PE then 5 mg BD. Rivaroxaban 15 mg BD for 21 days, then 20 mg OD PO with food. If Dabigatran or Warfarin given, they need 5 days of treatment dose LMWH. Once treated risk assess if can be managed as outpatient.
- **Parenteral therapy: Fondaparinux** 5–10 mg SC OD dose depending on body mass. **Enoxaparin** 1.5 mg/kg OD or 1 mg/kg BD in higher risk patients. Long term switch to DOACs/Warfarin.
- **Duration of anticoagulation:** weigh up bleed risk versus thromboembolism risk. Optimal is 6 weeks to 6 months. Provoked and temporary risk factor, e.g. post-op, then consider 3 months treatment. Recurrence 2–3% per annum. Treatment beyond months does not alter recurrence. If long-term risk factors, e.g. active cancer, then continue anticoagulation long term. Recurrence rate 7–10% per annum which is cumulative and so long-term treatment advocated. Strongest predictors of recurrence are male sex and age <50 and a positive D-dimer assay measured 1 month after stopping anticoagulant therapy. See DASH model. With an unprovoked PE the risks persist and that includes secondary pulmonary hypertension. After 6 months consider **Rivaroxaban** 10 mg OD unless higher risk use 20 mg OD or **Apixaban** 2.5 mg BD.
- **Subsegmental emboli** on CTPA are both small and peripheral and may be asymptomatic or not. Evidence on long-term risks is conflicting with trial saying the opposite. If unsure treat especially where there are ongoing risks, e.g. cancer. Some would treat as standard PE. An active research area.

Treating severely compromised patients

- **Acute massive PE confirmed:** ABC high FiO_2 as per BTS guidelines. ALS algorithm if collapsed and unresponsive, give prolonged CPR. Cardiac monitoring of BP, HR, O_2 sats. Commence 1 L IV crystalloid to ensure adequate RV filling, especially if low BP. Move to CCU/ITU/Resus. Start IV UFH 5000 units bolus. Consider thrombolysis with **Alteplase** if massive PE, persistent SBP <90mmHg and CTPA or echo demonstrates RV dilatation / dysfunction or patient is in peri-arrest. **Alteplase** IV 10 mg over 2 mins followed by 90 mg over 2 hours (max 1.5 mg/kg if <65 kg); if this is not available, consider using local regimen for MI (unlicensed for PE). Continue IV **Heparin** infusion to maintain APTT ratio 1.8–2.8. Major bleeding at 9.24% with thrombolysis vs. 3.4% rate in the anticoagulation cohort. Intracranial haemorrhage: thrombolysed 1.46% vs. 0.19% placebo. Benefits of lower mortality (1.39% vs. 2.92%) with thrombolytic compared to anticoagulation extended to intermediate risk group. Take expert advice in pregnancy. Involve obstetrics/haematology early. Bleeding on/after thrombolysis: (▶Section 8.12).
- **EKOS** was the first interventional device indicated for the treatment of PE and is used for the infusion of physician-specified fluids, including thrombolytics, into the peripheral vasculature. It can accelerate drug dispersion, requiring less lytic agent.
- **Cardiac arrest:** commonly presents as pulseless electrical activity (PEA). Low $ETCO_2$ readings (<1.7 kPa or 13 mmHg) during CPR may support a diagnosis of PE but is non-specific. Consider emergency echocardiography performed by a skilled operator as an additional diagnostic tool. Consider thrombolytic drugs for cardiac arrest when evidence supports PE as cause of cardiac arrest. Take senior advice before thrombolysis as collapse/coma may have other causes such as ICH/SAH. Is it appropriate to continue CPR for 60 minutes? If high index of suspicion of PE then **Alteplase** 50 mg IV bolus. If no ROSC after 15 mins, then a further **Alteplase** 50 mg IV bolus to a max of 100 mg. Continue CPR for 60–90 mins. Use a mechanical chest compression device if prolonged CPR is needed.
- **Catheter-directed thrombolysis:** has been done by cardiology or interventional radiology for submassive PE. Catheters in left/right PA with **Alteplase** eluting 0.5 to 1 mg/h for 8–12 hours. Much lower systemic dose (25 mg vs. 100 mg) and bleed risk but higher dose at thrombus site. Some systemic bleeding risks remain. Consider in PE in pregnancy.
- **Catheter thrombectomy:** mechanically evacuate embolic or thrombotic material within the PA such as a large, proximal pulmonary artery thrombus but techniques, kit and complications vary.
- **Pulmonary surgical embolectomy:** available in some thoracic centres if there is a large central thrombus refractory to lysis. The moribund have little to lose. Discuss with surgeons according to local pathways. Some research has been done on extending use to those with anatomically extensive PE and concomitant moderate to severe RV dysfunction, despite preserved systemic BP; requires cardiac bypass and heparinisation [*Circulation*, 2002;105:1416].

DVT management (see *BNF* for DOAC loading doses)

- **Suspected DVT:** administer LMWH treatment dose or consider **Apixaban** or **Rivaroxaban** and organise dimer/duplex. If DVT present, then commence **Apixaban** or **Rivaroxaban** alone. If **Dabigatran** or **Edoxaban** or **Warfarin** given they need 5 d of treatment dose LMWH. Provoked DVT anticoagulate for at least 3 months (3–6 months if active cancer).

- **Unprovoked DVT consider anticoagulation >6 months (6+ months with active cancer).** See above. If there is a plan to stop anticoagulation treatment, consider testing for hereditary thrombophilia in patients with a 1st-degree relative who has had a DVT or PE, and testing for antiphospholipid antibodies – these tests can be affected by anticoagulants and specialist advice may be needed.
- **Acute massive DVT:** discuss with vascular team or interventional radiologists. Thrombectomy and catheter-directed thrombolytic therapy for patients with symptomatic iliac and proximal femoral DVT who have symptoms <2 weeks, good functional status, a life expectancy of 1 year or more, and a low risk of bleeding. Reduces risk of limb ischaemia and postphlebitic syndrome.
- **Below knee DVT:** repeat USS after 7 d to see if there is extension above the knee. The management of isolated calf DVT is controversial. Those undergoing orthopaedic procedures, malignancy, and the immobile had a higher risk of propagation. Risk of PE and other complications seems low. Most (90%) PEs arise from above the knee thrombus. Mortality rate of proximal DVT > distal DVT. No consensus on whether to treat, observe or not treat. Full dose anticoagulation is not risk-free. Follow local expert guidance. Consider the choice between anticoagulation and serial ultrasound at 1–2 weeks and risk for thrombus extension, bleeding, and patient preference.
- **Upper limb DVT:** treat cause or risks. Anticoagulate for 3 months. SVC filters are available for those where anticoagulation is contraindicated, but efficacy data is limited. Investigate for occult malignancy, lung cancer or lymphoma.
- **IVC filters:** DVT/PE and systemic bleeding contraindicating anticoagulation. May reduce PE but increase DVT risk. No clear mortality benefit or benefit in using them as well as anticoagulation in high-risk patients (*JAMA*, 2015;313:1627). Attractive in concept but robust evidence is lacking. Deaths purely due to IVC filter insertion have occurred. Patients should eventually be anticoagulated when safe to do so. Remove them as early as is possible, e.g. after 2–6 weeks when it is anticipated that anticoagulation can be started in short term or the risk of VTE/PE is short term. Complications include vessel wall erosion, haemorrhage, IVC occlusion because of thrombus, recurrent DVT, and post-thrombotic syndrome with ulcers and leg oedema.
- **References:** NICE (2020) NG158: *Venous thromboembolic diseases: diagnosis, management and thrombophilia testing.* RCOG (2015) GTG 37a: *Reducing the risk of venous thromboembolism during pregnancy and the puerperium.*

4.18 Lung 'white out'

- **About:** get old imaging. Complete opacification usually of one lung field. Position of the mediastinum/trachea is key. Do not insert a chest drain to remove fluid without confirming effusion using ultrasound/CT chest.

Differential using tracheal/mediastinal shift (get CT)

- **Collapse (atelectasis)** of entire lung: volume loss, tracheal shift to affected side. May see signs of obstructed bronchus. Tumour, foreign body, mucus plug.
- **Pleural effusion:** large effusion pushes the trachea away from the affected side.
- **Consolidation:** no shift, air bronchogram, consolidated lung. May have associated effusion even empyema.
- **Mesothelioma:** there is typically no mediastinal shift.

- **Post-pneumonectomy/thoracoplasty:** removed lung/lobe there is volume loss with fluid accumulation and fibrotic opacification of the pleural space. A resected rib may be absent. Thoracoplasty for TB prior to 1944.
- **Congenital absence or hypoplasia of lung:** trachea pulled to affected side.
- **Mixed:** both an effusion and lung collapse. The tracheal position will tell you which of these is greater in terms of volume loss and gain using the above.
- **Clinical:** smoker, cough, weight loss, asbestos exposure, asthma, COPD, old TB. Pyrexia, sputum, haemoptysis, recent pneumonia, previous lung surgery.
- **Investigations:** bloods: FBC, U&E, LFT, CRP/ESR, ABG, calcium. **CXR** (PA ± lateral): position of the trachea is key to see if it is pulled towards the affected side (volume loss) or pushed away (extra volume) or central. Look for other pathology. Absent breast shadow (cancer), hilar mass. **CT chest:** for confirmation and to look for underlying pathology. **Local ultrasound** can distinguish consolidated lung from effusion and can be essential prior to performing a thoracentesis.
- **Management:** ABC, O_2 as per BTS guidelines. Bronchodilators may aid expectoration and help bronchospasm. **Supportive:** manage respiratory failure and infection. Chest physio may help if endobronchial mucus. Determine likely causation and treat. Severe hypoxaemia with RF should lead to intubation and mechanical support. **Old pneumonectomy:** old CXR will show lesion. Signs of old surgery. Optimise ventilation if compromised. **Total lung collapse/atelectasis:** post pneumonia, asthma, COPD. Foreign body inhalation. Consider intrabronchial lesion. If acute may be a sputum plug and chest physio and hydration and mucolytic may help. Bronchial stenosis which may be endobronchial or extrabronchial should be considered. Smoker. Cachexic. Clubbed. May need a fibreoptic bronchoscopy with suction. Consider CT chest. Urgency depending on ABC, O_2 and ABG ± antibiotics if infection. Position involved side uppermost (opposite to haemoptysis) to promote increased drainage of the affected area, vigorous chest physio, and encourage the patient to cough and to breathe deeply. CPAP may help lung expansion. **Consolidation:** needs assessment and appropriate antibiotics. May need HDU/ITU if RF. (See *Pneumonia*, ▶Section 4.14). **Pleural effusion:** consider ultrasound to confirm fluid if unsure and then remove. Urgency depends on the clinical picture. (See *Pleural effusion*, ▶Section 4.13). Heart failure unusual to be unilateral unless patient recumbent on one side. If signs of empyema needs antibiotics and drainage. **Diaphragmatic hernia/pulmonary agenesis:** respiratory support as needed.

4.19 ▶ Lung abscess

- **About:** formation of a pus-filled cavity within the lung parenchyma.
- **Aetiology:** post pneumonia *Staph. aureus*, *Klebsiella*, Gram-negatives, anaerobes. Infected cavity, TB, aspiration pneumonia, bronchiectasis. Trans-diaphragmatic spreads from an amoebic abscess. Distal to endobronchial obstruction, e.g. inhaled foreign body or tumour.
- **Clinical:** fever, malaise, weight loss, breathlessness, pain, foul breath. Clubbing may be seen with chronic untreated suppurative disease.
- **Investigation:** FBC: raised WCC, ESR, CRP. Sputum/blood cultures. CXR and HRCT: infected cavity or tumour, lymph nodes and lung parenchyma.
- **Management:** ABC. Prolonged IV antibiotics and surgical or percutaneous drainage. Bronchoscopy to remove any foreign body or endobronchial biopsy.

4.20 Fat embolism

- **About:** consider if recent fracture with sudden dyspnoea (may not be a PE). A skin rash or new neurology. Consider in sickling crisis chest syndrome.
- **Aetiology:** fat enters the venous circulation and passes into the systemic circulation. Results in vascular occlusion and release of inflammatory mediators. Fat from marrow from long bone (femur usually) or pelvis fractures, lipid infusions, recent steroid administration.
- **Causes:** blunt trauma, bone fractures, acute pancreatitis, sickle cell crisis. Decompression sickness. Parenteral lipid infusion.
- **Clinical:** acute dyspnoea, raised HR, febrile. Type 1 RF, petechiae, confusion, delirium. Coma, retinal haemorrhages with fatty lesions.
- **Investigations:** FBC: low platelets, Hb and fibrinogen. Urinalysis: fat globules in the urine are common after trauma. CXR: infiltrates. ABG: hypoxia and type 1 RF. U&E: AKI. CT chest: ARDS picture, infiltrates. CT head: diffuse white-matter petechial haemorrhages.
- **Management:** ABC and give O_2 as per BTS guidelines. Support, O_2, circulatory support.

4.21 Air embolism

- **About:** air within the circulation results in obstructive shock.
- **Aetiology:** air sucked into negative pressure venous circulation above right atrium. Enters heart and with loss of pumping effectiveness and sudden death. Any operative procedure where the exposed site is >5 cm above right atrium.
- **Causes:** surgical procedures, e.g. neurosurgery or ENT where patients sit upright. Back street abortion – air accidentally injected into pelvic venous plexuses. Penetrating chest injuries with bronchopulmonary venous fistulae. Central venous catheterisation, especially with loss of connections.
- **Clinical:** most episodes are clinically silent or result in mild, transient low BP. Acute dyspnoea, chest pain, agitation or disorientation.
- **Investigations:** ABG: hypoxia, hypo-/hypercarbia, respiratory and/or metabolic acidosis. **ECG:** raised HR, ST/T changes of ischaemia. CXR: oligaemia.
- **Management:** give 100% O_2. Fluid resuscitation. Clamp/remove any central line entry point. Put patient head down and left lateral decubitus (on left side with head down) or Trendelenburg position to trap the air in the RA and not the RV and RVOT. Consider ICU/ECMO. Aspiration of RV possible if there is a catheter already in place in RA/RV. Hyperbaric oxygen.
- **Reference:** McCarthy CJ, et al. (2016) Air embolism: practical tips for prevention and treatment. *J Clin Med*, 5(11): 93.

05 Endocrine and diabetes

Introduction
- Endocrinology testing usually involves a snapshot picture of function. Some hormone secretion is pulsatile, other hormones have diurnal variation and increase with sickness, protein binding can all make results less reliable.
- Dynamic testing provokes suspected underactive glands and suppresses suspected overactive glands and gives a better assessment of true function.

5.1 ▶ Adrenal crisis (addisonian crisis)

- **About:** acutely reduced adrenocortical function (glucocorticoids, mineralocorticoids). Can be progressive and subtle and become life-threatening, provoked by illness, e.g. infection. Iatrogenic due to cessation of medically prescribed steroids. Adrenal cortex produces glucocorticoids, mineralocorticoids and sex hormones. Increased demand during stresses (infection, trauma, illness). Double long-term steroids acutely.
- **Aetiology:** adrenals produce 15–30 mg/d of cortisol and more when under stress. Endogenous production falls with chronic steroid therapy. 8–9 am normal is 110–520 nmol/L (4–19 mcg/dl), but midnight <140 nmol/L (5 mcg/dl). Cortisol – wound healing, BP, immune function, stress response. Adrenal failure causes low glucocorticoids and aldosterone. Failure to retain salt and water causes low BP. Pituitary releases increased ACTH/MSH with pigmentation.
- **High risk patients:** pre-existing Addison's disease, pituitary disease, those on chronic steroids >7.5 mg prednisone or equivalent steroid for >3 weeks in the last 3 months.

Types
- **Primary:** 90% adrenal destruction before detectable. Low cortisol, high ACTH.
- **Secondary:** pituitary disease and ACTH insufficiency. Low ACTH and cortisol.
- **Tertiary:** impaired hypothalamic CRH release. Low CRH and ACTH and cortisol.

Causes of hypoadrenalism
- **Iatrogenic:** exogenous steroid suppresses adrenal production. Abrupt cessation of medically prescribed steroids ± physiological stress (sepsis or surgery). Needs only 3 weeks of steroids to suppress intrinsic production. Taper off steroid doses slowly.
- **Autoimmune adrenalitis:** 70% (lymphocytic infiltration) often with autoimmune disease (Graves' disease, Hashimoto's thyroiditis, pernicious anaemia, hypoparathyroidism or T1DM or vitiligo and primary ovarian failure).
- **Infections:** 5% of those with TB get adrenal destruction (may calcify on AXR), HIV, CMV, adrenalitis. Progressive disseminated histoplasmosis.
- **Haemorrhage/thrombosis:** Waterhouse–Friderichsen syndrome associated with meningococcaemia. Also sepsis, coagulopathy and antiphospholipid syndrome.
- **Malignancy:** bilateral metastases: breast, lung, melanoma, lymphoma.
- **Genetic:** adrenoleukodystrophy, congenital adrenal hyperplasia – 21-hydroxylase (*CYP21A2*) or 11β-hydroxylase (*CYP11B1*) genes.
- **Miscellaneous:** amyloidosis, post-bilateral adrenalectomy, polyglandular autoimmune syndromes.

- **Secondary adrenocortical insufficiency:** pituitary haemorrhage, Sheehan's syndrome.
- **Relative adrenal insufficiency:** suspected in some critical care patients.

Clinical

- Subacute with fatigue, anorexia, weight loss, tiredness, diarrhoea, vomiting. Easily misattributed to virus, chronic fatigue or anorexia or depression.
- Abdominal pain, generalised weakness, precipitated by sepsis, surgery. Postural low BP, raised HR, shocked, confusion, hypoglycaemia.
- Loss of axillary and pubic body hair in females (loss of adrenal androgens). Pigmentation in gums, buccal mucosa, skin, pressure points, skin creases, scars.
- Hypoglycaemia is more common in secondary adrenal insufficiency. May also see type 1 DM, RA, vitiligo, Hashimoto's thyroiditis, coeliac, pernicious anaemia.

Investigations

- **FBC:** raised eosinophils. **U&E:** low Na, high K, low HCO_3, low Cl, low glucose, low or high urea, high Ca. K normal if due to pituitary hypofunction.
- **ABG or venous gas:** low HCO_3 mild metabolic acidosis.
- **Random plasma cortisol:** at 8–9 am value >276 nmol/L is normal and >400 nmol/L makes adrenal insufficiency unlikely. Random cortisol <80–100 nmol/L makes diagnosis very likely unless patient on oral/inhaled steroids. If level between 100 and 400 nmol/L then perform a short synACTHen test.
- **Short synACTHen test:** give synacthen 250 mcg IV or IM (1 vial). Check 30 min cortisol. Diagnosis excluded if cortisol at 30 min >500 nmol/L. Usually a flat response is seen. Treat on clinical evidence if result delayed. Some have relative adrenal insufficiency which manifests with acute illness, infection, bleed, surgery/trauma. A short synACTHen may show a muted response. They may need steroids in their acute phase when unwell and re-evaluate later. In a sick patient testing should never delay steroid replacement. The diagnosis can always be confirmed later post the acute phase.
- **ACTH:** (normal 4.4–22 pmol/L or 20–100 pg/ml) if cortisol low then check ACTH. ACTH >80 ng/L at 9 am with low cortisol confirms adrenal insufficiency.
- **Renin/aldosterone:** low aldosterone and renin is high. Plasma dehydroepiandrosterone (DHEA) and DHEA sulphate are low.
- **Adrenal antibodies to 21-hydroxylase** seen in 80% autoimmune disease.
- **CXR/AXR:** look for active TB and classically small heart. Calcification.
- **CT abdomen:** may show enlarged necrotic glands with calcification. Small adrenals in autoimmune disease. Large with infection or metastases. Haemorrhage may be seen. **Adrenal biopsy** in selected cases.
- **Plasma C26:0 fatty acids** will detect adrenoleukodystrophy.

Differential

- **Hypopituitarism:** see ▶Section 5.9 for pituitary assessment.
- **Anorexia nervosa:** normal/high cortisol, low LH, FSH. Fear of weight gain.

Management

- **ABC and O_2** as per BTS guidelines. 1 L NS over 30–60 min. Check for and manage any hypoglycaemia. Send random cortisol 10 ml in a heparinised tube.
- **Do not** delay glucocorticoids while awaiting laboratory results or attempt endocrine stimulation testing in acutely ill patients. Treat with suspicion alone and confirm later.

- **Immediate: Hydrocortisone** 100 mg IV then 50 mg IM every 6 h. Others **Dexamethasone** 4 mg IV OD. Once stable and able to take oral then start **Hydrocortisone** 8 am 20 mg midday 10 mg evening 10 mg per day in divided doses, usually with a larger morning dose. Then down to long-term doses. Fludrocortisone not needed acutely.
- **Long-term for life: Hydrocortisone** (20–30 mg/d) 10 mg at 8 am, 5 mg at 1 pm, 5 mg at 4 pm (avoid late as may cause insomnia). Later add **Fludrocortisone** 50–200 mcg/d if postural low BP. May not be needed if pituitary insufficiency only. It is only needed in those with primary hypoadrenalism (Addison's). Alternatives are **Prednisolone** 3–5 mg OD. Double dose in times of stress/infection, see below.
- **Relative adrenal insufficiency:** suspected incidence in critical care patients as high as 77%. Management controversial. Trials conflicting. Has been shown that **Hydrocortisone 50 mg IV 6 h** may be beneficial for severe septic shock refractory to fluid resuscitation and vasopressors if given early (<8 h).
- **Determine cause:** investigate and treat for TB or HIV, malignancy, adrenal imaging, etc. Endocrine consult and follow-up for advice and monitoring.
- **Patient advice on sick day rules:** double steroid dose if minor illness or unwell or physiological stress. Family should be aware. Patients should carry a steroid card to alert staff. Ensure know to never stop steroid. Aware that nausea and vomiting may be signs of a crisis and to seek help. Recommended to have an ampoule of **Hydrocortisone** for IM administration in the event of being unable to take oral.
- **Prior to operative procedures** patients should be given **Hydrocortisone** 100 mg IM then 50–100 mg IM 6 h until back on oral therapy.

5.2 Hypoglycaemia

- **About:** prolonged hypoglycaemia causes brain injury and death. Check capillary blood glucose and send lab sample in any confused or comatose patient. Hypoglycaemia is technically <3.0 mmol/L. Treat any symptomatic blood glucose <4.0 mmol/L (72 mg/dl).
- **Note:** starvation in those not on insulin or oral hypoglycaemics or with acute alcohol rarely, if ever, causes significant hypoglycaemia. Be sceptical about diagnosing light-headedness and funny spells as hypoglycaemia unless there is clear evidence, e.g. a laboratory glucose reading.
- **Aetiology:** causes neuroglycopenia and neuronal dysfunction and increased sympathetic drive. Neurons do not need insulin to allow glucose to enter cells. High metabolising brain is dependent on a steady supply of glucose/ketones. Any shortfall in supply quickly leads to neuronal dysfunction.
- **Clinical:** sweating, trembling, palpitations, anxiety, blurred vision, hunger, headache. Lack of coordination, ataxia, stroke mimic – hemiparesis, confusion, aggression. Loss of inhibitions, convulsions, coma, brain damage, death, violence, agitation. Morning headache, night sweats, vivid dreams suggest nocturnal hypoglycaemia or nocturnal seizures.
- **Causes:** drugs: insulin, sulfonylurea, meglitinides (not metformin), pentamidine, quinine, salicylates, acute alcohol, propranolol. Endocrine: Addison's disease, growth hormone (GH) deficiency, hypopituitarism. Liver failure, insulinoma, chronic pancreatitis with a loss of glucagon activity, inborn errors of metabolism. Worsening renal function increases insulin sensitivity.
- **Not usually caused by:** metformin, glitazones, thiazolidinediones, DPP-4 inhibitors, GLP-1 analogues. Starvation: those in fasts or famines or hunger strikes

do not usually succumb to acute hypoglycaemia, due to counter regulatory mechanisms.

- **Impaired awareness of hypoglycaemia** (IAH): acquired syndrome with insulin treatment. Diminished warning symptoms of hypoglycaemia. Increases vulnerability to severe hypoglycaemia. Prevalence increases with duration of diabetes and seen T1DM > T2DM.
- **Investigations:** high morning glucose may suggest overnight hypoglycaemia with stress response. U&E, LFTs, 9am cortisol, sulfonylurea and meglitinide screen, IGF-2 if history of weight loss/malignancy. Insulin / C-peptide (which mirrors endogenous insulin production) should be checked at times of hypoglycaemia. If history suspicious of hypoglycaemia and other causes excluded then a 72-hour fast should be arranged to assess for insulinoma (raised insulin and C-peptide levels). If insulin levels raised/suppressed C-peptide check insulin/insulin receptor antibodies.

Management

- **Hypoglycaemic symptoms:** blood glucose <4 mmol/L (72 mg/dl) treat with 15–20 g glucose as sugary soft drink or sugary tea or juice (not diet drink) or small carbohydrate snack only. Also offer long-acting carbohydrate, e.g. slice of toast. Adults who are conscious but uncooperative but can swallow can give a small snack or 1.5–2 tubes Glucogel/Dextrogel squeezed into the mouth. *If ineffective or oral intake unsafe consider Glucagon 1 mg IM/SC but if no response within minutes then 20–50 ml 50% Glucose IV or 150 ml of 10% dextrose or other equivalent.* Note: there may be a marked disparity between arterial and venous blood glucose which can lead to misdiagnosis of hypoglycaemia based on misleadingly low venous levels when arterial levels are actually normal.
- **Adults with suspected hypoglycaemia (check CBG and send venous blood sample) who are unconscious or fitting** then check ABC + O_2 and give 20–50 ml IV 50% **glucose** through a large vein and place in recovery position and manage as for status epilepticus (▶ Section 11.15). If no venous access or no IV **glucose** then **Glucagon** 1 mg IM/SC. Glucagon may take up to 15 min to take effect because it mobilises glycogen from the liver and so it will be less effective in those who are chronically malnourished (e.g. alcoholics) or in patients who have had a prolonged period of starvation and have depleted liver glycogen stores, or in those with severe liver disease. In this situation, or if prolonged treatment is required, **IV glucose** is better. Once normoglycaemic, assess cause and make changes to diabetic regimen if needed. If there is any suspicion of adrenocortical insufficiency, then **Hydrocortisone** 50–100 mg IV 8 h should be given and later investigated for hypoadrenalism. An insulin and C-peptide assay can be done where hypoglycaemia is unexplained and deliberate or accidental misuse of insulin suspected. Exogenous insulin causes a rise in insulin but not C-peptide. Endogenous insulin release is accompanied by C-peptide release. If hypoglycaemia confirmed with no obvious cause, then one should consider admission for further tests, e.g. a prolonged fast and other assessments of endocrine function.

5.3 Hyperkalaemia

Medical emergency if K >6.5 mmol/L or ECG changes then give 30 ml of 10% calcium gluconate slow IV over 5 min.

- **About:** if the high K is completely unexpected and does not fit clinically quickly send another sample and exclude pseudohyperkalaemia.
- **Clinical:** asymptomatic, arrhythmias, muscle weakness, cramps, paraesthesia. Low BP, low HR, cardiac arrest.
- **Severity: mild** (K 5.5–6.0 mmol/L) or **moderate** (K 6.1–6.4 mmol/L). **Severe** (K ≥ 6.5 mmol/L) or if developing ECG changes.
- **Investigations:** U&E for AKI, VBG. ECG changes. Repeat sample if result unexpected. FBC/LDH: haemolysis. CK: rhabdomyolysis. VBG/ABG: metabolic acidosis.
- **ECG signs:** peaked 'tented' T waves, flat or absent P waves, bradycardia, widened QRS, sine waves, agonal rhythm and VT/VF.
- **Causes** (most commonly drugs – check drug chart) [can get falsely high result: haemolysed sample, laboratory or sampling error]: AKI, CKD, digoxin poisoning (poor prognostic sign). Rhabdomyolysis, tumour lysis syndrome, vigorous exercise, haemolysis, blood transfusion.
- **Drugs:** ACE inhibitors, AT2 blockers, spironolactone, eplerenone, amiloride, NSAIDs, ciclosporin, depolarising muscle relaxants, trimethoprim. Metabolic acidosis, Addison's disease (pigmented, low BP, fatigue), type 4 RTA (diabetes), hyperkalaemic periodic paralysis (AD familial).

Further management

- **ABC. Assess ECG changes.** Stop all potentially offending drugs or infusions immediately. This is easily overlooked. Ensure IV access, repeat any sample if surprise result. Start IV fluids. K >6.0 mmol/L or ECG changes needs telemetry and defibrillator available.
- **Protect the heart: severe** high K ≥6.5 or 6.0 6.4 mmol/L with developing ECG changes. Give 30 ml **10% calcium gluconate** IV or 10 ml of 10% **calcium chloride** into large vein over 5 min.
- **Insulin glucose:** give 10 U Insulin with 25 g of Glucose over 15 mins and then 10% Glucose at 50 ml/h for 5 hours to prevent hypoglycaemia.
- **Salbutamol** 10–20 mg nebulised. Stop K-retaining drugs.
- **Remove K from body: Sodium zirconium cyclosilicate (Lokelma)** 10 g 8 h for 72 h or **Calcium resonium** 15 g 8 h PO OR **Patiromer** 8.4 g/d PO. PR route may be considered for calcium resonium and must be retained for 9 h followed by irrigation to remove resin from the colon to prevent faecal impaction. Bowel perforation is a rare complication. Other methods to remove K include dialysis if AKI and K stays up (talk to renal).
- **Furosemide** 20–40 mg IV may be considered if well hydrated. U&E needs to be repeated every 2 h and blood gas, CBG for 6–12 h. Close ECG monitoring until K normal. These actions only lower K for 4 h.
- **Metabolic acidosis: consider** IV 500 ml NaHCO$_3$ 1.26% in AKI if HCO$_3$ <22 mmol/L and not in fluid overload over 1–2 h, but causes Na overload. These actions work for 4 h. In hyperkalaemic cardiac arrest give 50 ml 8.4% NaHCO$_3$.
- **AKI/CKD:** renal consult. If AKI/CKD and refractory/severe hyperkalaemia despite treatment, then discuss suitability for haemodialysis/haemoperfusion. (AKI: ▶Section 10.4).
- **Diet:** 'low potassium diet', e.g. avoid chocolate, fruit juices.
- **Drugs:** stop amiloride, spironolactone, ACEi, ARB.
- **Reference:** European Resuscitation Council Guidelines (2021) *Emergency treatment of hyperkalaemia.*

5.4 ▶ Hypokalaemia

- **About:** major intracellular cation. In cardiac patients aim for a K of 4.0–5.0 mmol/L. Beware rapid administration of IV potassium can cause lethal arrhythmias. The IV rate of KCl administration should not exceed 20 mmol/h.
- **Aetiology:** the daily intake of potassium is between 80 and 120 mmol. Low K reduces muscle and nerve excitability and enhances digoxin toxicity. Low K and low Mg often coexist. Treatment of low K is unlikely to be successful without reversal of hypomagnesaemia.
- **Causes:** thiazides and loop diuretics, Conn's syndrome, Cushing's syndrome. Severe diarrhoea (villous adenoma, fistulas, laxatives or a VIPoma). Alcohol abuse and magnesium depletion. Renal tubular acidosis 1 and 2, nephrotoxic drugs, severe vomiting with metabolic alkalosis. Insulin therapy in setting of DKA, giving sodium bicarbonate, IV/nebulised salbutamol. Familial (low K) periodic paralysis, amphotericin B, gentamicin, levodopa. Congenital adrenogenital syndromes, Liddle, Bartter (alkalosis, hypocalciuria) and Gitelman syndromes.
- **Clinical:** mild: lethargy, weakness, paralysis, diarrhoea (as a cause). More severe hypokalaemia: muscle pains, rhabdomyolysis, paralytic ileus, palpitations (ectopics). Look for hypertension (Conn's or Cushing's syndrome). Check drugs: loop diuretics, thiazides.
- **Investigations:** U&E: mild K <3.5 mmol/L, moderate <3.0 mmol/L, severe K (<2.5 mmol/L). Normal K 3.5–5.0 mmol/L. Look for/treat low Mg. ECG: atrial/ventricular ectopics, arrhythmias, ST changes, U wave, T wave flattening. TFT: High FT_4 and low TSH if hyperthyroid. **HCO_3 is low in RTA. Endocrine testing** for Cushing's or Conn's syndrome. **Blood gases** may show a metabolic alkalosis.

Management (aim to keep K 4–5 mmol/L on CCU)

- **Mild (2.5–3.4 mmol/L):** give 100 mmol KCl over 24 h PO/NG/IV replacement. Can use multiple routes. Test and treat any hypomagnesaemia. Consider the following Sando-K tablet = 12 mmol KCl; 25 ml Kay-Cee-L = 25 mmol KCl.
- **Severe (<2.5 mmol/L):** replace in total 100–200 mmol KCl over 24 h. Give 40 mmol KCl in 0.5–1 L by an infusion pump over 4 h. Max 10 mmol/h in ward area. May be repeated 2–3 times per day with twice-daily monitoring. Treat any low Mg. Higher rates e.g. 20 mmol/h only given by infusion pump in critical care areas with close ECG/K monitoring.
- **Cardiac arrest:** if hypokalaemia is suspected to be a contributory factor then 10 mmol KCl over 5–10 min and then commence infusion 40 mmol over 1 h. Treat hypomagnesaemia.
- **IV replacement:** solutions with >40 mmol/L can cause phlebitis and pain. Use the largest peripheral vein available. Give only by infusion pump to avoid accidental high flow rates. It is recommended that a second practitioner should check for correct product, dosage dilution, mixing and KCl concentrate and other strong potassium solutions.
- **NB:** if ascites or heart failure consider adding Spironolactone or Eplerenone.
- **References:** Rastergar & Soleimani (2001) Hypokalaemia and hyperkalaemia. *Postgrad Med J*, 77:759. NPSA (2002) Potassium chloride concentrate solution. *Patient Safety Alert*.

5.5 Hypercalcaemia

- **About:** severe high Ca is a corrected calcium >3.5 mmol/L or >3.2 mmol/L and severe symptoms and hypovolaemic. 90% of cases are due to either primary hyperparathyroidism (HPTHM) or malignancy.
- **Severity of corrected calcium** = measured [Ca] + ((40 − [albumin]) × 0.02). If <3.0 mmol/L: often asymptomatic and does not usually require urgent correction; 3.0–3.5 mmol/L: can be well tolerated but if symptomatic then prompt treatment is usually indicated; >3.5 mmol/L: requires urgent correction due to risk of hypovolaemia, dysrhythmia and coma.
- **Aetiology:** body contains 1–2 kg calcium, almost all of which is in bone. Total Ca (2.1–2.6 mmol/L) = free ionised (1.1–1.4 mmol/L) (active) + bound Ca. Calcium is bound to albumin, citrate and phosphate (inactive). A fall in serum albumin leads to a fall in measured total serum calcium.

Causes

- **1° PTHM:** raised PTH and calcium often in an otherwise well patient. Symptoms may be minimal and patients otherwise appear well.
- **Malignancy (low PTH):** if undiagnosed often unwell with weight loss and other malignancy symptoms. Due to bone metastases (lung, breast, renal, thyroid and myeloma) or PTH-related peptide (squamous cell lung). Needs CXR. Symptoms usually marked. Myeloma screen. Note in parathyroid cancer PTH is often markedly raised.
- **Sarcoidosis, TB, lymphoma: raised** ectopic 1,25(OH)$_2$D$_3$.
- **Drugs:** thiazides, calcium, vitamin D and lithium.
- **Endocrine:** Addison's disease, hyperthyroid, phaeo, acromegaly, MEN I / II.
- **Familial hypercalcaemic hypocalciuria (FHH):** autosomal dominant with increased PTH and hypercalcaemia but low urine calcium levels. Usually genetic but autoimmune type found. Genetic tests available.
- **Milk-alkali syndrome:** was seen with milk + excess antacids.
- **Paget's disease:** calcium rises with immobilisation.
- **3° PTHM:** 2° PTHM which becomes autonomous usually with CKD.

Clinical

- Constipation, N&V, confusion, depression, delirium even psychosis and coma. Polyuria and/or polydipsia, hypotonia, hyporeflexia, weakness ± hyperreflexia and tongue fasciculation. Long-standing high Ca may cause band keratopathy. Peptic ulcer disease. Renal stones, pancreatitis.
- Can cause seizures and arrhythmias. Look for malignancy: weight loss, neck, respiratory, abdomen, breasts, lymph nodes, finger clubbing, chest signs.

Investigations

- **FBC and U&E:** raised urea, **ESR** (myeloma/malignancy). **TFT:** hyperthyroid. **Corr calcium:** [Ca] + ((40 − [albumin]) × 0.02). Phosphate: high in 3° PTHM. Urinary calcium low in familial hypercalcaemic hypocalciuria.
- **ECG:** a short QT interval, prolonged PR, risk of arrhythmias.
- **CXR:** squamous cell carcinoma, sarcoidosis, TB.
- **PTH level:** a normal or high PTH in the setting of an increased calcium is suggestive of 1° PHPT. Low PTH / high Ca – malignancy or sarcoid. Check PTH-related peptide in malignancy. A low vitamin D often causes raised PTH and low/normal calcium.

Management (G5W = 5% glucose, NS = 0.9% saline)

- **Emergency:** if corrected calcium level >3.2 mmol/L and/or dehydrated start 3–6 L NS IV (125–250 ml/h) per day titrated to degree of fluid depletion (HR/BP). If CCF consider HDU admission and CVP to avoid fluid overload and the risks of oedema in the elderly.
- **Mild to moderate high Ca** (corrected Ca <3.2 mmol/L) then admission may not be needed and if no cardiac/renal issues. Advise person intake 3–4 L of fluid per day. Encourage mobilisation and return if symptoms worsen. See next day at ambulatory care clinic.
- **Bisphosphonates:** *after rehydration* if the corrected calcium is >3.0 mmol/L and renal function is normal (rehydrate for 12 h and repeat calcium) then IV **Pamidronate** 60–90 mg IV over 4 h. Lower dose in renal failure and GFR <20 ml/min. Alternatives, e.g. **Zoledronate** 4 mg IV infusion in NS over 15 min.
- **Other steps:** drugs: stop any calcium/vitamin D medication (this is often forgotten). **Furosemide** 40–80 mg PO/IV: should not be used until the patient is fully volume-replaced if at all. Consider **Calcitonin** 200 units every 6–12 h until calcium falls. Used rarely nowadays. **Prednisolone:** useful if cause is lymphoma, myeloma, 25(OH)D$_3$ toxicity or sarcoidosis. Steroids inhibit 1,25(OH)D$_3$ production. Start at **Prednisolone** 40 mg daily responding after 2–4 d. Parathyroidectomy: for 1° and 3° HPTHM. Indications in primary disease is for those with stones, renal impairment, bone disease, Ca >3.0 mmol/L and in younger patients. Monitoring may be appropriate for older patients with Ca 2.65–3.00 mmol/L.
- **References:** NICE (2019) *Hypercalcaemia.*

5.6 ▶ Hypocalcaemia

- **About:** normal Ca 2.1–2.6 mmol/L. Total (bound + free) Ca <2.05 mmol/L. Correct a low magnesium first. See *Hypercalcaemia* for pathophysiology.
- **Aetiology:** acidosis reduces protein binding sites and increases the amount of ionised Ca. Alkalosis increases protein binding sites and ionised Ca is lower, causing tetany.

Causes

- **Low PTH:** most common cause is post thyroidectomy with resultant low PTH which can be transient or permanent. Radiation or autoimmune damage.
- **Low albumin:** liver disease or the nephrotic syndrome.
- **Renal failure:** CKD-5 usually (failure of renal hydroxylation).
- **Acute pancreatitis:** seen with moderate–severe pancreatitis.
- **PTH resistance:** pseudohypoparathyroidism. *GNAS1* mutation. Short stature, short metacarpals.
- **High phosphate:** phosphate binds calcium, which precipitates.
- **Malabsorption:** coeliac disease, Crohn's disease, short bowel syndrome, CF or chronic pancreatic insufficiency.
- **DiGeorge syndrome:** hypoparathyroid with thymic aplasia.
- **Miscellaneous:** low Mg (diuretics, alcohol abuse), cinacalcet, tumour lysis syndrome, multiple blood transfusions, rhabdomyolysis, sepsis/toxic shock syndrome, hungry bone syndrome post correction of primary hypoparathyroidism; bisphosphonates, foscarnet.

Clinical

- **Mild:** asymptomatic. **Chronic:** cataracts, basal ganglia calcification, dry skin, pruritus.
- **Moderate:** numbness, paraesthesia, mild muscle weakness, wheezing. Positive Chvostek sign – tapping over facial nerve causes facial muscles to contract. Positive Trousseau sign – inflate BP cuff to 20 mmHg above SBP for 3–5 min – causes muscle spasm, and flexion of the wrist and metacarpal phalangeal joints can be observed with extension of the interphalangeal joints and adduction of the thumb (carpal spasm).
- **Severe:** delirium, seizures, papilloedema, movement disorders, tetany, refractory low BP, or arrhythmias (needs IV calcium + magnesium).

Investigations

- **FBC, U&E, LFTs:** AKI, CKD. Determine estimated glomerular filtration rate (GFR). **Ca, phosphate, PTH, 25(OH)D$_3$, 1,25(OH)$_2$D$_3$: hypoparathyroidism:** low calcium, high phosphate, low PTH. **Pseudohypoparathyroidism:** low calcium, high phosphate and PTH. **Osteomalacia:** calcium/phosphate low, ALP/PTH high, 25(OH)D$_3$ low. **CKD:** high phosphate, ALP, creatinine, PTH high. 25(OH)D$_3$ normal, 1,25(OH)$_2$D$_3$ low. In critically ill patients measure uncuffed sample.
- **Parathyroid antibodies** – autoimmune hypoparathyroidism.
- **Magnesium** <0.5 mmol/L typically results in symptomatic low Ca.
- **Radiographs** for Looser zone and osteomalacia and short 4th metacarpals in pseudohypoparathyroidism. **ECG:** a long QT interval. **Amylase** if pancreatitis considered.

Management

- **Mild/moderate:** start **Adcal-D3** 3 tablets BD or **Calcichew Forte** 2 tablets BD.
- **Severe** (<1.9 mmol/L and/or symptomatic at any level below reference range): give 10–20 ml of 10% **Calcium gluconate** over 15 min in 50–100 ml NS/G5W. Then dilute 100 ml of 10% **Calcium gluconate** (10 vials) in 1 L of NS or G5W and infuse at 50–100 ml/h. Monitor calcium.
- Treat any low Mg: IV **MgSO$_4$** 2 g (8 mmol in 100 ml) over 20 min until symptoms have cleared. Mg avoided in CKD. PPI can cause a low Mg.
- **Vitamin D:** replace as required. Monitor Ca levels. Referral to endocrinology for complex patients, e.g. PTH resistance should be managed by specialists.
- **References:** Hannan & Thakker (2013) Investigating hypocalcaemia. *BMJ*, 346:f2213. Acute Emergency Hypocalcaemia (2013) (www.endocrinology.com).

5.7 Hypothyroid/myxoedema coma

- **About:** may complicate long-standing often undiagnosed/untreated hypothyroidism. May be precipitated by an acute physiological stress event.
- **Tips:** consider hypothyroidism in every older patient with low Na, hypothermia, bradycardia and delirium. Mortality can exceed 20% even with optimal treatment.
- **Risk factors:** mostly older females (mean age = 75) usually during winter. Usually long-standing primary thyroid failure but rarely pituitary failure.
- **Causes:** Hashimoto's disease, post-thyroidectomy, radioactive iodine, antithyroid drugs. Drugs: lithium, amiodarone, iodine deficiency, thalidomide. Congenital, infiltration of thyroid – haemochromatosis, amyloid, Riedel's.
- **Precipitants:** look for infection/sepsis (chest, urine, encephalitis), GI bleed. Drugs (slow metabolism): alcohol, sedatives, tranquilisers, narcotics, amiodarone, lithium,

beta-blockers. Lung disease, stroke, CCF, ACS, upper GI bleed, acute trauma/surgery/ burns. Hypothermia, hypoglycaemia, non-compliance with thyroid replacement.
- **Clinical:** fatigue, increased weight, constipation and cold intolerance. Psychosis with delusions and hallucinations ('myxoedema madness'). Hypothermia, generalised oedema, cool dry rough skin, sparse hair, macroglossia. Seizures, coma, low HR, low BP, hypoventilation. Abdominal distension/pain. Paralytic ileus, megacolon, old thyroidectomy scar. Goitre with Hashimoto's disease, iodine deficiency.

Investigations
- **FBC U&E:** anaemia, high MCV, low WCC, low Na, decreased GFR. **Glucose:** may be low treat hypoglycaemia. Elevated **CK/LDH**, hyperlipidaemia.
- **Short synACTHen test** if hypoadrenalism suspected.
- **TFT:** TSH >10 mU/L (low if pituitary disease), low FT_4. TSH can be unreliable generally in acute illnesses and should at least be accompanied by a FT_4. TFTs should be rechecked when patient is better. Sickness can cause deranged TFTs and this must always be considered.
- **Thyroid autoantibodies** (TPO Ab) in Hashimoto's disease.
- **CSF:** low pressure, high CSF protein.
- **ABG:** type 2 RF may be seen.
- **ECG:** low HR, flat T waves, low QRS. TdP.
- **CXR:** cardiomegaly, pericardial and pleural effusion.
- **Abdominal X-ray:** ileus and distended bowel and faeces.

Management
- **Supportive:** look for precipitant. Admit to ITU to manage hypoventilation, low O_2, low BP, hypoadrenalism and hypothermia. Give O_2 and fluids/inotropes. Gradually rewarm if hypothermic. Overactive warming may vasodilate and drop the BP. Watch for arrhythmias and monitor electrolytes and ABG. Interpretation impaired if hypothermic. Avoid any sedatives or sedating analgesics. Metabolism and drug excretion reduced.
- **Sepsis:** have a low threshold for IV antibiotics as signs of sepsis may be concealed by hypothyroidism, e.g. fever and raised HR.
- **Thyroxine** (T_4) loading dose 50 mcg OD PO or 100–500 mcg IV once followed by 50–100 mcg OD IV/PO. T_4 (a prodrug converted to T_3) may provide a smoother and more gradual though slower onset of action than T_3. Lower doses of T_4, e.g. 25–50 mcg OD in elderly or with cardiac disease.
- **Liothyronine T_3** is available and may be the choice of some. Doses range from 2.5 to 20 mcg 8 hourly. Give T_3 10 mcg bolus IV and then 10 mcg 8–12 hourly for 24–48 h and then start oral T_4. Lower doses in elderly or with cardiac disease. High doses of T_4 >500 mcg IV or T_3 >75 mcg associated with higher mortality.
- **Hydrocortisone 100 mg IV** and then IM 8 h given for first few days and then reduced once no concerns of hypopituitarism and adrenal insufficiency.
- **Hypoglycaemia:** glycogen is often depleted so hypoglycaemia may be seen and so glucose should be monitored. A glucose infusion should be considered.
- **Poor prognosis** associated with hypothermia, advanced age, bradycardia and hypotension, MI/CCF. No indication for prescribing T_4 or any preparation containing thyroid hormones to patients with thyroid blood tests within the reference ranges.
- **Reference:** Wall (2000) Myxoedema coma: diagnosis and treatment. *Am Fam Physician*, 62:2485.

5.8 ▶ Thyroid storm/thyrotoxic crisis

- **About:** rare and life-threatening condition due to excess T_3/T_4. 2% of those with hyperthyroidism. Mortality is quoted as 10–20%.
- **Aetiology of T_4/T_3 excess:** untreated or inadequately treated Graves' disease is the commonest pathology. Toxic adenoma or multinodular goitre, thyroiditis, postpartum thyroiditis. Excessive T_4 ingestion – deliberate or accidental. Recent amiodarone or intravenous iodinated contrast.
- **Precipitant:** recent minor/major illness or post radioactive iodine treatment. Post thyroid surgery or stopping antithyroid treatment.
- **Clinical:** tachycardia, palpitations, AF, heart failure, weight loss, tremor, lethargic. Sweating and agitation, fever, hypo- or hyperactive delirium. Apathetic (more like hypothyroidism) in elderly, abdominal pain. Graves' eye disease: proptosis, lid lag, chemosis, acropachy. Pretibial myxoedema, tender gland suggests thyroiditis. Goitre may be seen with Graves' (bruit) or thyroiditis (tender).
- **Differential:** hyperactive or any form of delirium, septic shock, anticholinergic toxicity. Delirium tremens, acute pulmonary oedema, apathetic cases can be subtle.
- **Investigations:** bloods: FBC, U&E, ESR/CRP: raised Ca. ECG: SR, sinus tachycardia, AF, ST/T wave changes, especially if IHD. TFT: raised FT_3 and FT_4 and TSH <0.05 mU/L. Antibodies: thyroid peroxidase (TPO), thyroglobulin antibodies and TSH receptor antibodies (TRAb) in Graves' disease whose level parallels disease activity. CXR if infection suspected. Blood cultures and CSF if obtunded. Echo: may show a transient rate-induced cardiomyopathy and reduced LV function. Increased ^{123}I uptake in Graves' compared with Hashimoto's thyroiditis.

Management

- **Start ABC.** O_2 as per BTS guidelines. Consider ITU/HDU. Start IV fluids and correct electrolytes. **Antipyretics:** use paracetamol. Avoid Aspirin (displaces protein bound T_4). Look for/treat any sepsis: blood/urine/CSF (if indicated). **Sedation:** if very agitated then **Haloperidol** 1–5 mg or **Lorazepam** 1–2 mg IV/IM or **Diazepam** as needed. **Propranolol** 40–80 mg 12 h PO to rate-control tachycardia/AF.
- **Anticoagulate** any AF as cardioembolic risk using DOACs or warfarin. Cardioversion attempts usually futile until rendered euthyroid.
- **Antithyroid drugs: Carbimazole** 40–60 mg/day or **Propylthiouracil** 400–600 mg daily in divided doses. A high dose may be combined with **Thyroxine** 75–100 mcg as block and replacement therapy. A smaller dose **Carbimazole** 15–30 mg may also be given and titrated against TSH. **Propylthiouracil** 200 mg BD is preferred in pregnancy. PTU reduces T_4 to T_3 conversion.
- **Iodine** is important in reducing the conversion of T_4 to active T_3. **Sodium ipodate**, a radiographic contrast medium (500 mg per day orally), will restore serum T_3 levels to normal in 48–72 hours. Alternatives are **Potassium iodide:** 15 mg 6 h PO or **Lugol's iodine** (8 mg iodine/drop): 10 drops (0.1–0.3 ml) PO/NG every 8 h. Reduces T_4 to T_3 conversion. Give after carbimazole. This is the Wolff–Chaikoff effect.
- **Hydrocortisone** 100 mg 8 h IM/IV to prevent $T_4 \rightarrow T_3$. Immunosuppresses.
- **Plasmapheresis (PLEX):** has been used to treat thyroid storm in adults.
- **Thyroid eye disease** (Graves' orbitopathy) in 15%. Presents with proptosis (Grade 3), redness, pain, diplopia (Grade 4), swelling and oedema. Emergency – those unable to close eyes fully have high risk of corneal ulceration (Grade 5), reduced acuity (Grade 6). Need urgent specialist ophthalmic/thyroid referral. The rest need surveillance, smoking cessation and **Sodium selenite** 100 mcg 12 h.

Manage thyroid disease. Tape eyes closed overnight, artificial tears/lubricants for gritty eyes. High dose steroids: **Prednisolone** 1 mg/kg/d and decompression surgery if sight is at risk. Once controlled refer for radioiodine or subtotal thyroidectomy. Radioiodine avoided if active eye disease as can worsen situation but prophylactic steroids may be given.

- **Heart failure:** chronic tachycardia causes a cardiomyopathy and so an echo may be needed and anti-failure medications.
- **Thyroiditis:** usually self-limiting 1–2 months. Symptom control with **Propranolol** 40 mg TDS. Malaise, fever, pain settles. **Prednisolone** 20–40 mg/d may be given. May be transient hypothyroidism after. A postpartum thyroiditis may be seen in some women <6/12 post-delivery and associated with anti-TPO antibodies in half.
- **References:** Perros *et al.* (2015) Management of patients with Graves' orbitopathy: initial assessment, management outside specialised centres and referral pathways. *Clinical Medicine*, 15:173. Marcocci *et al.* (2011) Selenium and the course of mild Graves' orbitopathy. *N Engl J Med*, 364:1920.

5.9 ▶ Pituitary apoplexy

- **About:** pituitary macroadenoma (>1 cm) undergoes infarction ± haemorrhage. Get urgent CT head. Seen in 1% of pituitary tumours. Apoplexy may be precipitated by anticoagulants or surgery. Rare in pregnancy. The pituitary is shaped like a 6 and releases at least six crucial hormones: ACTH, (MSH), GH, prolactin, TSH, LH, FSH. May need an urgent neurosurgical referral to preserve vision and steroids for any secondary adrenal insufficiency.
- **Aetiology:** rapidly growing tumour outgrows blood supply or compresses its own blood supply. Expanding mass arising from the sella turcica can compress optic nerve and chiasma. Pituitary vascular supply from the inferior hypophyseal branch of the internal carotid artery. Result is hypopituitarism (hypothyroid, hypogonadism) with secondary hypoadrenalism, etc. Secretory pituitary tumour has three effects: hormone excess, space-occupying (headache), hypofunction of other hormones.
- **Clinical:** pre-existing adenoma and severe headache ± eye signs, coma. Low BP with secondary hypoadrenalism. Ophthalmoplegia, bitemporal superior quadrantanopia and loss/reduced visual acuity. Horner's syndrome. Palsy of II, III, IV and VI and V1 (lateral wall cavernous sinuses). Look for signs of prolactinoma, acromegaly and Cushing's syndrome.
- **Differentials:** SAH, bacterial/viral meningitis, brainstem infarction (eye signs/Horner's), cavernous sinus thrombosis.

Investigations
- **Bloods:** FBC, U&E, LFT, clotting screen. **Hormones:** prolactin, GH (pulsatile so check IGF-1), TSH and FT_4, ACTH and cortisol, LH/FSH and testosterone or oestradiol. Commonest tumours secrete prolactin/GH. However, most pituitary tumours that undergo apoplexy are endocrinologically silent. If suspected hypopituitary and ACTH and GH low these can be stimulated with induced hypoglycaemia by an insulin tolerance test. If GH high and acromegaly suspected attempt to suppress with OGTT. These tests and results are assessed in the post-acute phase.
- **CT head:** acutely, haemorrhage in an existing pituitary tumour, subarachnoid bleed or ischaemia and no haemorrhage.

- **MRI/A pituitary:** more sensitive after 24 h showing blood, tumour, pituitary ring sign from central necrosis. MRA shows close vascular anatomy.
- **Formal visual fields** assessment as early as possible (when clinically possible) looking for a bitemporal superior hemianopia suggesting optic chiasmal compression from below. No driving and DVLA referral if visual fields reduced.

Management
- **Hydrocortisone 200 mg IV bolus and then 100 mg IM/IV QDS** to manage acute period. Ensure adequate fluid replacement.
- **Urgent MRI/A (or CT/A if MRI not possible)** and discussion with local neurosurgical and endocrine team. Check visual fields.
- **Cabergoline** or other dopamine agonist *may be sufficient* in non-visually impaired prolactinoma and suffices in 80% and can rapidly reduce tumour size. Need for urgent surgery decided by a neurosurgeon with an endocrinologist. Stop/reverse any coincidental anticoagulation.
- **Neurosurgery:** if vision is at risk or cranial nerve or other pressure effects, then consider urgent trans-sphenoidal surgical decompression to reduce pressure on local structures. Complications include damage to local structures, especially the carotid arteries laterally. GH-secreting tumours are less common than prolactinoma and more likely to need surgery/octreotide/pegvisomant/radiotherapy.
- **Endocrine review:** long-term pituitary hormone replacement may be needed with thyroxine, hydrocortisone, etc. Remember to titrate to the T_4 not the TSH. Posterior pituitary function rarely affected with even a large macroadenoma so if diabetes insipidus is seen, consider inflammatory cause or metastases. Long-term imaging shows an empty sella.
- **Reference:** Rajasekaran *et al.* (2011) UK guidelines for the management of pituitary apoplexy. *Clinical Endocrinology*, 74:9.

5.10 Hyponatraemia

- **About:** low serum Na with low serum osmolality causes movement of water into cells so cerebral oedema, coma and seizures. A rapid uncontrolled normalisation of Na can also lead to permanent neurological deficits.
- **Pathophysiology:** normal Na 135–145 mmol/L. Plasma osmolality is 275–295 mOsm/kg. Any rise in osmolality leads to ADH release and free water retention. ADH causes free water retention and lowers serum osmolality. ADH acts on renal V2 receptors.

Different scenarios
- **Salt level fixed/water excess:** raised ADH release (SIADH) fails to excrete water, excess IV dextrose, potomania, prostate irrigation post TURP, ADH release to pain, opiates, surgery.
- **Excess salt loss/water loss:** diuretics, tubular disorders, surgical drains, Addison's disease.
- **Salt loss/water level constant:** compensated diuresis, Addison's disease.

Assessment
- **Severity:** mild: 125–130 mmol/L: no symptoms or mild lethargy. Not uncommon in elderly. Moderate: 115–125 mmol/L: headache, nausea, cramps, confusion. Severe: <115 mmol/L: confusion, seizure, delirium, coma, cerebral oedema and brain herniation.

Clinical: assess volume status

- **Dehydrated:** oliguria, low BP, tachycardia, thirst, poor skin turgor, weight.
- **Fluid overloaded:** peripheral and/or pulmonary oedema, basal crepitations, S3, raised JVP. Fluid balance shows water taken PO or IV glucose suggests water overload. Salt losses: surgical drains and NG tube may suggest shows excessive salt losses ± water losses.
- **Euvolaemic:** meningitis, brain injury, small cell lung tumour, pneumonia suggests SIADH.

Types

- **Hypovolaemic hyponatraemia:** reduced ECF with low BP, dehydrated, renal or GI or burns or other losses or overdiuresis. **Divide into renal losses** (urine Na >20 mmol/L): diuretics (renal salt loss + ADH stimulation and free water retention), salt-losing nephropathy, RTA, cerebral salt wasting (SAH), Addison's disease, and **non-renal losses** (urine Na <10 mmol/L: gastrointestinal losses, burns, pancreatitis, 3rd space losses. Avoid Na retention and so urine Na <10 mmol/L, and the urine may be low volume and hyperosmolar. **Needs fluid and Na replacement** if normal renal function then salt retention possible so correction should be simpler. Manage underlying cause of losses. Well patient: increase salt intake with slow sodium 80 mmol/d or slow IV NS. If vomiting then simply match losses with IV NS with 20 mmol KCl per litre. If slow to respond or encephalopathic then consider 500 ml of 3% over 6–12 h depending on urgency and response to replacement. Test and treat for any concerns of adrenal insufficiency. Try to limit increases <10–12 mmol/d.
- **Euvolaemic hyponatraemia** (increased ICF and ECF no oedema): causes include thiazide diuretics, SIADH, hypothyroidism, acute porphyria, adrenal insufficiency, Guillain–Barré syndrome. Dilutional hyponatraemia. Avoid excessive hyponatraemic water intake (runners, Ecstasy users, potomania). Correct cause. Increase salt intake with slow sodium 80 mmol/d. Consider IV NS. Give 3% NaCl if urgent correction is needed (e.g. seizures, coma), otherwise bring levels up slowly. IV **Hydrocortisone** 50 mg if hypoadrenalism suspected. Stop thiazides. Limit Na changes < 12 mmol/d. **Demeclocycline** 300 mg BD or **Tolvaptan** 15 mg OD for several days may be used to get rid of free water by inducing a nephrogenic diabetes insipidus.
- **Hypervolaemic hyponatraemia** (increased ICF and ECF, oedema): ascites, raised JVP, CCF, cirrhosis, nephrotic syndrome, renal disease: hyperaldosteronism, diuretic-induced renal salt loss. Dilutional hyponatraemia so the key is fluid restriction to 500–1000 ml per day and diuresis of free water by inducing diabetes insipidus or blocking ADH. In exceptions 3% saline 500 ml over 6–12 h may be given. Saline may be given with **Furosemide** to aid water loss. **Demeclocycline** 300 mg BD or **Tolvaptan** 15 mg OD for several days may be used to get rid of free water by inducing a nephrogenic diabetes insipidus.
- **Spurious hyponatraemia** (normal osmolality) may be due to high triglyceride, protein or glucose.

Investigations

- FBC, U&E, urine Na excretion, glucose, urine and plasma osmolality. In acute correction the U&E should be checked every 2–4 h. TFT: check TSH and cortisol levels. CXR: infection/tumour. Short synACTHen if adrenal failure considered (low BP, low Na, pigmentation).

- **SIADH:** urine inappropriately concentrated when dilute serum and often >100 mOsm/L with hyponatraemic plasma osmolarity. Osmolality = 2 Na + glucose + urea (all in mmol/L).

Management

> **Rises in Na should be managed to not exceed 12 mmol/24 h or 18 mmol/ 48 h. Acute hyponatraemia can be corrected more quickly and more safely than chronic hyponatraemia.**

- **ABC + supportive:** if fitting or low GCS and cerebral oedema then ITU with full support and consider urgent management with hypertonic saline. Manage seizures as per status epilepticus. CT scan if any concern as to cause of coma. General principles depend on likely cause.
- **Principles:** what is the volume status? If severe low Na been present for <48 h then can be reversed more quickly and vice versa. Aim for improvement of 10–12 mmol/d and not immediate normality. Assess fluid balance, osmolality and urinary osmolality, volume and salt loss. Monitor Na closely and frequently and clinical state. Try to break it down into hypo-, eu-, hyper-volaemia, though some have mixed. Chronic hyponatraemia (>48 h) should have the sodium corrected much more slowly. A target of 120 mmol/L attained over 24–48 h depending on baseline should resolve acute symptoms.
- **SIADH:** excessive free water retention. Low serum osmolality and raised urine osmolality (>100 mOsm/kg) and urine Na >30 mmol/L where hypopituitarism, hypoadrenalism, hypothyroidism, renal insufficiency and diuretic use have been excluded. Check and stop any causative drugs and look for other causes (malignancy, Ecstasy (MDMA often combined with excess water), CNS disorders, drugs, lung disease, nausea, postoperative pain, HIV, infections, Guillain–Barré syndrome, acute porphyria). Fluid restriction to 800 ml/d is needed. See above for managing severe hyponatraemia.
- **Drug treatments:** if euvolaemic: **Demeclocycline** 150–300 mg 6 h is given to induce nephrogenic diabetes insipidus and lose free water. Conivaptan or tolvaptan antagonise effects of ADH by different mechanisms to cause free water loss. They may also be used with hypervolaemic/euvolaemic hyponatraemia, e.g. **Tolvaptan** 15 mg (up to 60 mg/d) for short periods. Need to watch for water loss and rapid rises in Na. Specialist use. Fluid status should be monitored closely. Allow patient to drink freely.
- **Adrenal insufficiency** should be treated as per addisonian crisis with IV NS and steroids. (See ▶ Section 5.1).
- **Rapid correction can lead to central pontine demyelination** now called osmotic demyelination syndrome: manifests after 2–3 d as brainstem symptoms of dysarthria, dysphagia, seizures, coma, quadriparesis and can be seen on MRI. Classically seen in malnourished alcoholic with rapid correction. Exact treatment regimens are difficult because multiple factors are involved, but an effort to increase serum osmolality with either NS (or hypertonic saline if volume must be restricted) must be done carefully and cautiously with regular checking of status and bloods; if seizures and coma then more urgency may be applied. Comatose or fitting hyponatraemic patients are best managed in an HDU/ITU setting. It is certainly a time to enlist expert experienced help.

5.11 Hypernatraemia

- **About:** most often free water loss or no access to water. Occasionally excessive salt. Mild hypernatraemia Na >145 mmol/L; severe hypernatraemia >160 mmol/L. Mortality can be up to 50% in elderly patients. Correct slowly at <12 mmol/d. Most often due to an impaired access to water or loss of free water greater than can be replaced by drinking or other routes.
- **Aetiology:** raised serum osmolality causes water to leave cells and cells to shrink. A small rise in osmolality detected by osmoreceptors causes desire to drink. Hypernatraemia occurs where there is limited access to water, e.g. lost in the desert or stuck in a side room and too confused or comatose to drink, or water not to hand.
- **Causes:** water/hypotonic fluid loss or impaired water intake. Polyuria with excess free water loss unmatched by water intake: high Ca, low K, cranial and nephrogenic diabetes insipidus, diabetic ketoacidosis, HONK. Simple dehydration + fever especially older people + impaired access to water. Water losses due to burns, sweat, vomiting, severe diarrhoea. Renal fluid losses: nephropathy, myeloma, obstructive uropathy, adult polycystic kidney disease. Excessive sodium intake: mild hypernatraemia with Conn's or Cushing's syndrome. Salt poisoning, ingestion of seawater, salt tablets, IV $NaHCO_3$, hypertonic saline.
- **Clinical:** dehydration, thirsty, agitation, ataxia, progressively obtunded and comatose. Low BP, thready pulse, sunken eyes, low BP, coma and seizures.
- **Investigations:** FBC, U&E, Ca, K, glucose: exclude AKI, high glucose, high Ca, low K. Raised serum and urine osmolality (>600 mOsmol/kg) unless renal concentrating issue or diabetes insipidus. CT/MRI head if suspect cranial diabetes insipidus. Urine volume and osmolality: diabetes insipidus >3 L/d of a dilute urine despite dehydration.
- **Management:** determine cause: this is fundamental and key. Investigate for free water loss. Assess renal concentrating function and serum and urine osmolality and look for high glucose and calcium or low K which can cause polyuria. May just be failure to match normal losses as listed above in *Causes*.
- **Fluid replacement:** no definite treatment plan. Cautious rehydration if cardiac disease or elderly. Treat and look for a cause if not obvious. Encourage oral fluids. Consider IV G5W slowly with administration guided by plasma Na and urine output. This can be alternated with NS, to avoid too rapid a fall in plasma osmolality which can cause cerebral oedema. Can use a mixture of both. Volume replacement may be up to 4 L/d. Titrate to clinical response. Do not change [Na] by more than 12 mmol/d. Oral fluids may be given as long as losses are replaced and fluid balance maintained.
- **Risk of VTE:** administer VTE prophylaxis with enoxaparin or equivalent.
- **Diabetes insipidus** (>3 L/d of dilute urine despite dehydration) with thirst, headache: nephrogenic: fluid replacement, look for cause, e.g. lithium, correct electrolytes and paradoxically may need to give thiazide diuretics. Cranial: look for cause, replace losses. Consider **Desmopressin** 5–20 mcg nasal spray or tablets. Watch for hyponatraemia and fluid retention. Endocrine review.

5.12 Hypophosphataemia

- **About:** phosphate <0.8 mmol/L. Severe and symptoms <0.35 mmol/L. Reference range is 0.8–1.5 mmol/L. Most phosphate is contained in bone.
- **Causes:** critically ill, DKA, re-feeding syndrome, malabsorption, vomiting, renal loss, antacids, diuretics, insulin, phosphate binders, theophylline.

- **Clinical:** weakness, ileus, cardiorespiratory failure, arrhythmias, rhabdomyolysis. Eventual convulsions and coma.
- **Investigations:** FBC, U&E, phosphate/calcium/magnesium, PTH, vitamin D.
- **NB:** national shortage of Phosphate Polyfusor. Consider (unlicensed) sodium glycerophosphate injection 21.6% has high Na.
- **Management:** correct low Ca. Mild (0.6–0.8) consider Phosphate-Sandoz tablets 1–2 tabs TDS PO with water. Moderate (0.3–0.6): sodium glycerophosphate 20 mmol (2 ×10 ml) in 250 ml G5W/12 h. Severe (<0.3): sodium glycerophosphate 20–40 mmol (4 × 10 ml) in 500 ml G5W/24 h. Low dose in renal failure or weight <40 kg. Treat low vitamin D.

5.13 Hyperphosphataemia

- **Aetiology:** renal reuptake inhibited by PTH. Retained in renal failure.
- **Investigations:** U&E, phosphate >1.4 mmol/L.
- **Causes:** AKI/CKD4/5 ± secondary hyperparathyroid, (pseudo) hypoparathyroidism, tumour lysis syndrome, rhabdomyolysis. Usually causes calcium deposition, acromegaly.
- **Management:** limit phosphate intake. Acutely IV NS if renal function normal. Phosphate binders such as calcium carbonate.

5.14 Hypomagnesaemia

- **About:** normal 0.7–1.0 mmol/L. 1 g = 4 mmol.
- **Causes:** malnourished, (loop) diuretics, alcoholism, diarrhoea, laxative abuse, malabsorption, pancreatitis, Gitelman's syndrome, DKA, severe burns, PPI.
- **Severity:** mild Mg <0.7, mod. Mg <0.5, severe Mg <0.3. Low Mg can cause low Ca/K and will need to be replaced to fix these.
- **Clinical:** weakness, tremor, carpopedal spasm, increased reflexes, adrenal insufficiency, confusion, fits, VT-TdP.
- **Investigations:** U&E: low Ca/Mg, low K. ECG: 1st-degree HB, T wave flattened, widened QRS, VT-TdP. High urine Mg suggests renal problem (Gitelman's syndrome).
- **Management:** mild give magnesium aspartate 10 mmol sachets one BD. It may cause diarrhoea. Correct K/Ca if low. Severe: **Magnesium sulfate** 2 g (8 mmol) IV over 15–30 min. Otherwise 20 mmol (5 g/10 ml ampoule) in 1L NS/G5W over 4 h. Monitor Mg levels.

5.15 Hypermagnesaemia

- **Causes:** Mg >1 mmol/L. Normal 0.7–1.0 mmol/L.
- **Cause:** accidental overdose, e.g. eclampsia or with impaired renal excretion.
- **Clinical:** reduced reflexes, weakness, cardiac arrest.
- **Investigations:** U&E, Mg symptomatic >2 mmol/L. ECG increased PR interval, broadened QRS complex or elevated T waves, AV block.
- **Management:** stop Mg infusion. Suspected high Mg/cardiac arrest give 10–20 ml of 10% **Calcium gluconate.** IV **Furosemide** + IV fluids to aid excretion. Haemodialysis for renal failure. Glucose/insulin as for high K.

5.16 ▶ Lactic acidosis

- **About:** normal <2 mmol/L. Marked increased mortality when >4 mmol/L. A product of anaerobic glycolysis and tissue hypoxia. From skeletal muscle also skin, RBCs, brain, muscle and gut. Increased production and reduced clearance due to tissue hypoperfusion. Other causes are drugs with mitochondrial toxicity e.g. NRTIs/others. The higher the level and the longer the time to normalisation of elevated serum lactate, the greater the risk of death.
- **Aetiology:** pyruvate to lactate in anaerobic conditions and is shuttled to the liver, to undergo gluconeogenesis. Reduces pH. L-lactate is endogenous, D-lactate exogenous, e.g. gut bacteria. High lactate can impair cardiac function.
- **Type A lactic acidosis** (tissue hypoxia): severe sepsis, seizure, diabetes, pancreatitis, malignancy, shock, LVF, renal and liver failure, respiratory failure, carbon monoxide, severe anaemia, local hypoperfusion, e.g. limb ischaemia or bowel ischaemia.
- **Type B lactic acidosis** (no tissue hypoxia): alcohol, iron, salicylates, isoniazid, metformin, zidovudine. Inborn errors of metabolism, thiamine deficiency, pyruvate dehydrogenase dysfunction, cyanide, exercise, seizures, cocaine, paracetamol, propofol, valproate.
- **Clinical:** Kussmaul breathing, low BP, sepsis, shock, hypoxia. Do they take NRTIs (HIV meds), e.g. fatigue, nausea, aches, weight loss?
- **Investigations:** FBC: anaemia, glucose, U&E: AKI, lactate >4 mmol/L with sepsis/metabolic acidosis. **ABG:** hypoxia, hypercarbia may be seen. With mitochondrial dysfunction, e.g. cyanide, O_2 not extracted and so venous O_2 levels maintained. **Metabolic acidosis with raised anion gap:** [Na] – [Cl+HCO$_3$] >12 mmol/L (or >16 mmol/L if K is included).
- **Management:** ABCs, O_2, resuscitate, supportive. Find and treat cause. Stop causative drugs. Low threshold for looking for and treating mesenteric ischaemia, sepsis. IV fluids, antibiotics. Lactate is a useful marker of poor prognosis requiring expert and rapid intervention. Dialysis can be considered in severe cases. Consider inotropes if MAP <65 mmHg. See shock. Get expert help before considering an infusion of 500 ml isotonic 1.26% bicarbonate.
- **References:** Foucher CD, Tubben RE. (2021) Lactic acidosis. In: StatPearls [Internet].

5.17 ▶ Acute porphyria

- **About:** enzyme deficiency in haem pathway. Overproduction of porphyrin precursors.
- **Aetiology:** haem from succinyl-coA + glycine in cytoplasm/mitochondria. Drugs induce some steps in the pathway precipitating acute attacks.
- **Acute:** acute intermittent porphyria, variegate porphyria, hereditary coproporphyria.
- **Clinical:** diagnosis often known. A family history may be available. Severe abdo/back/thigh pain, nausea, vomiting, constipation, tachycardia, hypertension, seizures, weakness less common. Women > men aged 20–40.
- **Non-drug precipitants:** alcohol, fasting, infections, surgery, stress.
- **Drug precipitants:** sulphonamides, rifampicin, OCP, anaesthetic agents, barbiturates, ACEi, carbamazepine, dapsone, furosemide, methyldopa, theophylline, NSAIDs. Check all in *BNF*.
- **Investigations:** FBC, U&E: urea, raised LFTs. Check urine porphobilinogen (PBG) which can be done in local labs. To identify the presence and type of porphyria,

samples of urine, blood and stools (faeces) need to be tested in a laboratory which specialises in porphyria.

- **Management:** supportive: hydration, pain relief, rest, increased carbohydrate intake oral or IV dextrose. Referral to specialist for individual enzyme assays and further tests. If conservative management not effective then consider administering IV **Arginate** 3 mg/kg via large vein (max 250 mg) once daily for four consecutive days which shortens attacks with less risk of complications. Arginate replenishes haem stores and inhibits ALA synthase, thus reducing the production of porphyrins and their precursors, ALA and PBG.
- **Safe drugs: analgesics:** aspirin, diamorphine, dihydrocodeine, ibuprofen, morphine, paracetamol, pethidine. **Anti-emetics:** chlorpromazine, ondansetron, prochlorperazine, promazine. **Hypertension and tachycardia:** atenolol, labetalol, propranolol. **Sedation, seizures:** chlorpromazine, clonazepam, lorazepam, promazine. **Constipation:** bulk-forming (ispaghula), lactulose, senna. **Prevention:** avoid precipitating drugs and alcohol, stopping smoking, stress, fasting or dieting.
- **Reference:** see www.porphyria.org.uk/acute-porphyrias/.

5.18 Diabetic ketoacidosis (DKA)

> **SGLT2 inhibitors, e.g. gliflozins can cause euglycaemic diabetic ketoacidosis with a high anion gap, metabolic acidosis and elevated ketones with normal glucose. Check ketones.**

- **About:** manage with a defined well-documented and communicated plan. 10% of DKA is with new diabetes. Seen in type 1 diabetics with intercurrent illness who reduce/stop insulin. Severe deficit of water, insulin and potassium. Mortality rates have fallen significantly in the past 20 years to <1%. Most DKA is preventable.
- **Goals:** priorities are replacing volume loss, switching off ketone production and removing ketones and normalising blood glucose.
- **Note of caution:** DKA typically most commonly seen with T1DM but can be seen with 'ketosis-prone T2DM' especially in the non-white population. See below.
- **Differential of ketoacidosis:** alcohol ketoacidosis – raised ketones, normal glucose, alcohol misuse. Starvation ketosis – raised ketones, normal glucose.
- **Euglycaemic acidosis:** profound metabolic acidosis, raised ketones, normal glucose. Seen with SGLT2 inhibitors, pregnancy, starvation, liver disease.
- **High risk:** elderly, age 18–25 risk of cerebral oedema, heart, renal failure. Other serious comorbidities. Seek expert help and ITU consult early. **Pregnancy:** ketosis-prone state, high-risk time for DKA in women.
- **Aetiology:** glucose (and K) enters cells by the actions of insulin on the insulin receptor. Insulin deficit leads to cell starvation despite being surrounded by a sea of excess glucose. Switch to beta-oxidation of fats creates acidic products which lower the pH. Ketone bodies include acetone, 3-beta-hydroxybutyrate (main one) and acetoacetate. Dehydration due to profound osmotic diuresis as a result of severe hyperglycaemia. Increased cortisol, adrenaline, glucagon and GH cause hepatic gluconeogenesis and glycogenolysis. Vomiting can compound the fluid losses. All adds to a perfect storm leading to spiralling metabolic derangement.

Capillary blood ketone levels

- <0.6 mmol/L: normal; no action required.
- 0.6–1.5 mmol/L: worsening control. Monitor BG. Seek help if worsens.
- 1.5–3.0 mmol/L: BG >10 mmol/L. High risk of DKA; seek medical advice.
- >3.0 mmol/L: severe ketosis. In the presence of high BG (>10 mmol/L), suggests presence of DKA; seek urgent medical help.

Definition: NB DKA can be seen with T1DM and T2DM

- Diabetes: BG >11 mmol/L or known DM. Normal with euglycaemic DKA.
- Ketonaemia ≥3 mmol/L or significant ketonuria (≥3 on urine sticks).
- Acidosis (raised anion gap): HCO_3 <15 mmol/L and/or venous pH <7.3.

Recent recommendations on managing DKA

- IV NS is the recommended fluid of choice.
- Cautious fluid replacement in young adults to avoid cerebral oedema.
- Measure VBG HCO_3 and pH, blood ketone meters for near-patient testing.
- Continue any long-acting analogue insulin, e.g. Levemir or Lantus.
- DKA, use a fixed rate IV insulin infusion (FRIII) calculated on body weight.
- Avoid priming dose (bolus) of insulin.
- HCO_3 or phosphate administration is not recommended routinely.

Clinical

- Onset over hours/days. Progressive polyuria, polydipsia, tachypnoea.
- Kussmaul's tachypnoea blows off CO_2. Vomiting, tachycardia, low BP.
- Acetone 'nail varnish' smell on the breath (not all can smell it).
- Severe dehydration. Cold peripheries, delayed capillary return, sunken eyes, low BP. Oliguria. Sepsis, chest and urine and other acute illness, e.g. ACS, meningitis, acute abdomen.
- Other precipitants: MI, pancreatitis, alcohol excess, poor control.
- Occasionally self-harm, psychiatric issues, deliberate failure to take insulin.

Markers of severe DKA: needs HDU level 2 bed and CVP/intra-arterial line

- Ketones >6 mmol/L.
- pH <7.0 or HCO_3 <5 mmol/L.
- Initial K <3.5 mmol/L, GCS <12.
- Anion gap >16: (Na + K) minus (Cl + HCO_3).
- Abnormal AVPU score.
- O_2 sats on air <92%.
- SBP <90 mmHg, HR <60 bpm or HR >100 bpm.

Investigations

- **FBC:** raised WCC, raised CRP may suggest infection.
- **U&E:** may have an AKI. Water loss raised Na. Raised K due to acidosis. K levels fall with insulin administration which can lead to severe hypokalaemia.
- **Glucose:** usually >20 mmol/L at presentation. Polyuria, glycosuria. May be normal with euglycaemic DKA – see above. Needs DKA management.
- **Ketones elevated:** ≥3 mmol/L or significant ketonuria (>2+ on urine sticks). Treat to suppress ketonaemia. Monitor ketones to manage treatment. Measures 3-beta-hydroxybutyrate.

- **VBG:** high anion gap metabolic acidosis: [Na] – [Cl + HCO_3] >12 (or 16 if you include K). HCO_3 <15 mmol/L indicates metabolic acidosis with pH <7.30. It can be <7.10 in severe cases.
- **Cardiac troponin** if suspected ACS.
- **CXR** if chest disease, e.g. breathless, fever, coughs.
- **CT head** scan if comatose or neurology to exclude other diagnoses or look for cerebral oedema as a complication.

Assess severity
- Mild: blood pH 7.25–7.30, HCO_3 15–18 mmol/L; the patient is alert.
- Moderate: pH 7.00–7.25, HCO_3 10–15 mmol/L; mild drowsiness.
- Severe: pH <7.00, HCO_3 <10 mmol/L; stupor or coma may occur.

Treatment goals
- Aims are restoration of circulatory volume, clearance of ketones and correction of electrolyte imbalance, particularly potassium, and insulin replacement. Set clear goals and expectations of therapy. Ensure treatment plans are well documented. Ensure good handover between doctors on shifts. Deficits are H_2O 100 ml/kg, Na^+ 7–10 mmol/kg, Cl^- 3–5 mmol/kg, K^+ 3–5 mmol/kg.
- **Treatment goals** are: (1) reduce ketones by 0.5 mmol/L/h and increase venous HCO_3 by 3 mmol/L/h. (2) Reduce capillary blood glucose by 3 mmol/L/h. (3) Maintain K 4.0–5.0 mmol/L. (4) Lower glucose cautiously and start 10% glucose if CBG <14 mmol/L.

Immediate assessment
- Check ABC, good IV access, start IV NS. Assess basic RR, HR, BP, O_2 sats aim for 94–98%, and temperature and GCS. Monitor oximetry. Establish if pregnant.
- Send: blood ketones, CBG, venous plasma glucose, U&E, VBG, FBC, blood cultures. ECG, CXR, urinalysis, culture. Find infection: urine, chest, CNS, skin and soft tissue. Insulin causes a marked drop in K which must be managed. Clinical and biochemical review.

Assess patient: telemetry and pulse oximetry if required
- **ABC:** temp, BP, pulse, O_2 sats, GCS, full clinical exam. Test capillary blood glucose, lab glucose, VBG, U&E, FBC, blood cultures, ECG, CXR, MSU.
- Establish monitoring regimen. Check hourly CBG, capillary ketones.
- Check venous HCO_3/K at 60 min, 2 h and 2-hourly, 4-hourly U&E.

Insulin replacement: given as a fixed rate IV insulin infusion (FRIII)
- **Commence fixed rate IV insulin infusion:** 0.1 unit/kg/h, e.g. 7 unit/h for 70 kg. Give 50 U soluble insulin (Actrapid or Humulin S) in 50 ml NS. Make a FRIII with 50 units of **Actrapid** in 49.5ml 0.9% NS.
- **Continue** any long-acting insulins Lantus/glargine or Levemir/detemir, degludec.

Fluid replacement: initial fluid needs are determined by BP
- Start 0.9% NS infusion. Use large cannula. Give via infusion pump.
- If SBP <90 mmHg give (cautions if heart failure) 500 ml NS over 15 min. If SBP remains <90 mmHg give further 500 ml and get senior/ITU/critical care team input.
- If SBP now >90 mmHg start a 2nd 1 L NS over next 60 min. Give with K as below. If SBP on admission >90 mmHg give 1 L NS over first 60 min.

Potassium replacement (mmol/L)

- Add to second bag of NS or use pre-dosed bags.
- If K >5.5 mmol/L: give none. If K 3.5–5.5 mmol/L: give 40 mmol/L.
- if K <3.5 mmol/L give 40 mmol/L. Senior review if additional K required.

Euglycaemic DKA

- Initiate glucose 10% straight away at 125 ml/h because the glucose is <14 mmol/L. Begin FRIII with 0.1 units/kg/h insulin rate. If glucose falling despite 10% glucose reduce to 0.05 units/kg/h to avoid hypoglycaemia.

Ketosis-prone T2DM

- Afro-Caribbean or Hispanic descent. Treat as DKA. Insulin can be reduced more rapidly. Treat with insulin initially. Needs expert OP follow-up. C-peptide is preserved with T2DM.

1–6 h (see treatment goals above)

- **Reassess patient, monitor vital signs:** hourly blood glucose (lab blood glucose if meter reading 'HI'), hourly blood ketones if meter available. VBG for pH, bicarbonate and potassium at 60 min, 2 h and 2-hourly thereafter.
- **Potassium:** insulin will shift K into the intracellular space causing low K. Add 20 mmol K per litre from the 2nd bag. Check U&E regularly: hourly initially then every 2–4 h when stabilised or more if needed. K >5.5 mmol/L: add none; K 3.5–5.5 mmol/L: give 40 mmol/L; K <3.5 mmol/L: senior review as increased K needed. Use premixed N-saline and potassium bags if possible.
- **Fluid replacement:** *risk of cerebral oedema so recommend more cautious fluid replacement in young people aged 18–25 years, elderly, pregnant, heart or renal failure (consider HDU and/or central line).* 1 L NS + KCl over next 2 h, then another 1 L NS + KCl over next 2 h. 1 L NS + KCl over next 4 h. Add 10% glucose 125 ml/h if blood glucose falls below 14 mmol/L.
- **Insulin infusion rate:** if ketones falling by <0.5 mmol/L/h. Venous HCO_3 not rising by at least 3 mmol/L/h. Plasma glucose not falling by at least 3 mmol/L/h. Continue FRIII until ketones <0.3 mmol/L, venous pH >7.3 and/or venous bicarbonate >18 mmol/L. Reduce rate of FRIII to 0.05 units/kg/h when glucose drops to <14 mmol/L.
- **Treatment not working:** if ketones/glucose not falling as expected always check the insulin infusion pump is working and connected and that the correct insulin residual volume is present (to check for pump malfunction). If equipment working but response to treatment inadequate, increase insulin infusion rate by 1 unit/h increments hourly until targets achieved.
- **Additional measures:** monitor NEWS2. Keep accurate fluid balance chart. Target minimum urine output 0.5 ml/kg/h. Catheter if incontinent or anuric (not passed urine by 60 min).

Other considerations

- **Acidosis:** adequate fluid and insulin therapy will resolve the acidosis in DKA and the use of HCO_3 is not indicated, though some consider treatment with a pH <7.0 and give 500 ml of sodium bicarbonate 1.26% plus 10 mmol KCl – take local expert advice if considered.
- **Urinary catheter:** if concerns about renal function or fluid balance.
- **Consider NG tube** if vomiting. **Give O_2** as per BTS guidance.
- **VTE prophylaxis:** usually LMWH as high risk.
- **Look for precipitants:** acute abdomen to meningitis. Amylase can also go up × 4 in DKA. Give antibiotics if evidence of sepsis/infection.

- **Cerebral oedema** suspected with falling GCS. Consider urgent mannitol or hypertonic saline and CT imaging.

6–12 h management

- At 6 h check venous pH, HCO_3, K, ketones, glucose. Check clinical and biochemical parameters improving. **Start 10% glucose if BG <14 mmol/L.**
- Continue IV fluid at reduced rate of 1 L NS + KCl over 4 h and then 1 L NS + KCl over 6 h. Monitor GCS for cerebral oedema. Review bloods at 6 h.
- Resolution is suggested by pH >7.3 or ketones <0.3 mmol/L.
- If not improving (see treatment goals above) then repeat review and check insulin infusion is working and line is not blocked and that it contains insulin and no errors with making it up.

12–24 h management

- Check venous pH, HCO_3, K, capillary ketones and glucose. Resolution is defined as ketones <0.3 mmol/L, venous pH >7.3. Ensure targets hit and progressive improvement. Ketonaemia and acidosis should have resolved. If not needs urgent senior review. Check lines and FRIII.
- Continue IV fluid replacement if not eating and drinking. If ketonaemia cleared but not eating and drinking move to a variable rate IVII as per local guidelines.
- Look for complications of treatment, e.g. fluid overload, cerebral oedema and continue to treat precipitating factors. Transfer to SC insulin if patient is eating and drinking normally.

After 24 h, discharge planning and follow-up (involve Diabetic team)

- **If DKA not resolved determine why.** Suggests possible failure to get enough insulin or fluids. Check FRIII working. Does the insulin infusion contain insulin? Expert review.
- **Resolving:** transfer to SC insulin when capillary ketones <0.3 mmol/L, pH >7.3 and the patient is ready and able to eat. Give insulin SC and then after 30 min stop IV insulin as there should be some overlap. Conversion to SC insulin should follow local guidelines.
- Some suggest 80% of total 24 hour doses (JBDS recommends 20× the average hourly amount of the last 6 hours) and others a weight-based formula. If the patient is newly diagnosed they need to be seen by the diabetic team prior to discharge or next day. Patients with T1DM should be offered multiple daily injection basal-bolus insulin regimens as the 1st-line choice or twice-daily mixed insulin regimen should be considered if it is preferred.
- **Complications:** cerebral oedema (suspect if fall in GCS – more common in young so go easy on the fluids). Arrhythmias (potassium), circulatory collapse/shock, AKI. Hypoglycaemia with over-treatment, aspiration pneumonia. ARDS, myocardial infarction. Rhinocerebral mucormycosis – destructive lesions affecting face and nose. See ▶Section 9.56
- **Education and prevention: for T1DM, DAFNE** (dose adjustment for normal eating) is recommended and learning how to manage insulin. Ensure patient educated about 'sick day rules': patients need strict advice to never stop their insulin even if ill. If unable to eat/drink then they must come to hospital immediately. Diabetic team should reinforce this message.
- **Reference:** The Joint British Diabetes Societies for Inpatient Care (revised 2021) *The management of diabetic ketoacidosis in adults.*

5.19 Hyperosmolar hyperglycaemic state (HHS)

- **About:** previously called hyperglycaemic hyperosmolar non-ketotic coma (HONK). Mortality 10–20% compared with 3–10% for DKA. Seen more frequently in the elderly. Minimal ketosis or acidosis. Increased risk of VTE so give LMWH. Most do not need insulin if no ketosis.

Definition and diagnosis of HHS: NB minimal ketosis or acidosis

- **Definition:** (1) hyperglycaemia >30 mmol/L (>540 mg/dl); (2) hyperosmolarity >320 mosm/kg (2 × Na + glucose + urea); (3) pH >7.3, bicarbonate >15 mmol/L (mEq/L) (UK), ketones <3 mmol/L; (4) mental state (coma) usually with osmolality >340 mOsm/kg (mmol/kg). NB: one-third of patients with hyperglycaemic crises present with a mixed picture of DKA and HHS. Those with ketones or failing to improve need insulin.
- **Aetiology:** acute stressors increase cortisol/catecholamines, cause hyperglycaemia.
- **Causes:** *new* presentation of T2DM or T2DM + stress, steroids, surgery, thiazides, infection. Pancreatitis, poor/non-compliance with treatment, alcohol, drug abuse, stroke.
- **Clinical:** thirst, polydipsia, polyuria, and mental clouding, seizures, and delirium and coma. Usually known T2 diabetic. Exacerbated by high sugar drinks or water restriction.
- **Investigations:** FBC: raised WCC **U&E:** raised Na often >150 mmol/L, AKI. raised glucose: >30 mmol/L *without significant ketonaemia/acidosis*. Measure and calculate serum osmolarity: >320 mOsm/kg, 2 × [Na] + urea + glucose. **Ketones:** usually <3 mmol/L. **Lactate** >4 mmol/L. **ABG/VBG:** pH >7.3 and HCO_3 >15 mmol unless lactic acidosis.
- **Management:** ABC, good IV access × 2. May need ITU/HDU if in coma/moribund and airway protection needed. Indications for HDU/ITU include serum osmolality >350 mOsm/kg, Na >160 mmol/L, GCS <12, K >6.0 or <3.5, O_2 sats <92%, SBP <90 mmHg, pulse <60 or >100, urine output <0.5 ml/kg/h, hypothermia.
- **Start fluid replacement:** significant fluid losses, e.g. 10 L due to osmotic diuresis due to glycosuria. Fluid replacement alone will lower glucose. Isotonic solutions result in fewer changes in osmolality than hypotonic solutions. Start 1 L NS aiming for 3–6 L over the first 12 h and then replacing rest within 24 h. Losses can be huge: 10–15 L.
- **Potassium:** give added K if serum level <5.0. Suggest 20 mmol/L when K 3.5–5 mmol/L and 40 mmol/L when K <3.5 mmol/L.
- **Hypernatraemia:** a rise in Na is usually seen as water shifts out of the vascular space as glucose levels fall. Consider 0.45% saline if osmolality fails to fall. Rising sodium is only a concern if the osmolality is NOT declining concurrently. Aim to keep falls in Na to <12 mol/L per day. Full normalisation of U&E and osmolality may take 72 h.
- **Insulin:** not needed unless urine ketones >2 or blood ketones >1 mmol/L (some quote 1.5 mmol/L). Target blood glucose 10–15 mmol/L. Lower glucose by <5 mmol/h. Patients need lower doses than in DKA and may be sensitive to large doses. Give insulin if glucose or acidosis fails to improve with hydration. Use a **FRIII (fixed rate insulin infusion) 0.05 units/kg/h**, e.g. 4 units/h in 80 kg person. Discontinue once eating and drinking. IV fluids may be required for longer if intake poor. Most can be transferred to SC insulin if needed. Those with previously undiagnosed diabetes or well controlled on oral agents, can be switched to the appropriate

oral hypoglycaemic agent after a period of stability (weeks or months). Long-term insulin usually not needed and can be discontinued but review diabetes.

- **VTE:** give at least a weight-adjusted prophylactic dose of LMWH as high risk of VTE. Look for and treat cause, e.g. sepsis, MI, pneumonia. Watch for cerebral oedema.
- **Precipitants:** sepsis: treat if any detected – urine, chest, blood cultures, CXR. Remove urinary catheter when possible. Infarction/ischaemia e.g. bowel, cardiac, limb. Antibiotics may be indicated.
- **Hypophosphataemia** (▶ Section 5.12 for replacement details).
- **Education is a key component and NICE recommend DESMOND** (diabetes education and self-management for ongoing and newly diagnosed) **for those with T2DM.**
- **Reference:** Joint British Diabetes Societies Inpatient Care Group (2012) *The management of the hyperosmolar hyperglycaemic state (HHS) in adults with diabetes.*

5.20 ▶ Diabetic foot infections

- **About:** neuropathy and vascular compromise can lead to significant soft tissue damage. Involves bone (osteomyelitis). NB: pain perception impaired.
- **NICE Guidelines:** each hospital should have a care pathway for diabetic foot problems who need inpatient care. Refer. A named specialist consultant should lead the management.
- **Clinical:** may be painless, ulceration, necrosis, loss of pulses, claudication. Inspect foot, toes and soles of feet, peripheral neuropathy (use 10 g monofilament), Charcot's foot: often unilateral swollen erythematous foot with background of neuropathy, which can be mistaken for cellulitis. Neuropathy: painless, high arch, clawed toes, warm good pulses, painless plantar ulcers. Vascular: cold feet, poor pulses, rest pain, hair loss over shin, ulcerated heels and toes. Probe ulcers to see if bone involved.
- **Investigations:** FBC, U&E, glucose **CRP**. Swabs as available. HbA1c, albumin. **Plain X-ray:** may show bony involvement, foreign bodies and fractures. **MRI scan:** show extent of damage and osteomyelitis and marrow oedema early. Vascular studies: **ankle-brachial** pressure index. **Femoral angiography:** if considered for vascular surgery.
- **Management:** multidisciplinary care involving podiatry, diabetic team and nursing, vascular surgery, microbiology, orthopaedics, orthotics. Debridement and removal of dead tissue and appropriate dressings and optimising glycaemic control. Total contact cast if Charcot foot suspected, pending further assessment. Failing to immobilise a Charcot foot immediately can risk permanent deformity (rocker bottom foot). **Ulceration:** uninfected/colonisation: no antibiotics needed. Offloading, Control infection/ischaemia, debridement, dressing. Smoking cessation, nutrition.
- **Infection. Mild:** check MRSA status, if negative **Co-amoxiclav** 625 mg TDS PO. In penicillin-allergic **Clindamycin** 150–450 mg PO QDS. Duration: 7–10d. **Moderate:** check previous MRSA status, if negative **Co-amoxiclav** 1.2 g TDS IV. For penicillin allergy, contact microbiology. **Severe:** blood cultures, swabs from wound. MRSA status. If MRSA negative **Tazocin** 4.5 g 6–8 h IV + **Gentamicin** IV stat (if low BP). If MRSA or penicillin allergy **Teicoplanin** IV (adjust to renal function). **Osteomyelitis:** 6 weeks of antibiotics often with PICC line. Clindamycin is often first line due to its bone penetration.
- **Reference:** NICE (2015, updated 2019) NG19: *Diabetic foot problems: prevention and management.*

5.21 ▶ Managing diabetes during surgery/critical illness

Non-insulin treated diabetics and minor surgery
- **Preoperatively:** random CBG on admission <10 mmol/L – give normal medication until day of op. However, if CBG >10 mmol/L follow as for major surgery (see below).
- **On day of operation:** omit oral hypoglycaemics. Check blood glucose: 1 h pre-op and at least once during op (hourly if op >1 h long) and post-op 2-hourly until eating.
- **Post-operatively:** restart oral hypoglycaemics with first meal.

Insulin-treated diabetics and minor surgery
- This regime only suitable for patients whose random sugar is <10 mmol/L on admission, will only miss one meal pre-op and are first on the list for very minor surgery, e.g. cystoscopy.
- **Pre-op:** normal medication. **Day of operation:** no breakfast, no insulin, place first on list. Blood glucose: 1 h pre-op and at least once during op (hourly if op >1 h long) post-op 2-hourly until eating then 4-hourly. **Post-op:** restart normal SC insulin regime with first meal.

Diabetes and major surgery or critical illness
- Applies to all diabetics who are poorly controlled (blood glucose >10 mmol/L) irrespective of whether on insulin or not at baseline. **Pre-op:** give normal medication until day of operation. **Day of operation:** omit oral hypoglycaemics and normal SC insulin.
- Check capillary blood glucose (and potassium) 1 h pre-op then 2-hourly from start of infusion at least once during operation (hourly if op >1 h long) at least once in recovery area, and 2-hourly post-op.
- One combination is 16 U of soluble insulin + 10 mmol of KCl in 500 ml of 10% glucose. Infusion rate of 100 ml/h with glucose checked every 2 h.
- Alternatively, a variable rate insulin infusion is used, especially in emergency setting and allows insulin to be administered IV and titrated to the CBG.

5.22 ▶ Inpatient diabetes management

Diagnosis of diabetes
- Plasma glucose (PG) in random sample or 2 hours after a 75 g glucose load ≥11.1 mmol/L (200 mg/dl) or fasting PG ≥7.0 mmol/L (126 mg/dl) or HbA1c ≥ 48 mmol/mol.
- In asymptomatic patients, two diagnostic tests are required to confirm diabetes; the second test should be the same as the first test to avoid confusion.

'Pre-diabetes' is classified as:
- Impaired fasting glucose: fasting PG ≥6.1 mmol/L (110 mg/dl) and <7.0 mmol/L (126 mg/dl).
- Impaired glucose tolerance = fasting PG <7.0 mmol/L (126 mg/dl) and 2-h glucose after 75 g oral glucose drink 7.8–11.1 mmol/L (140–200 mg/dl).
- HbA1c range of 42–47 mmol/mol.

New: interstitial continuous glucose monitoring devices
- A new approach to monitoring glucose levels measures interstitial levels continuously. They use a tiny sensor inserted under the skin to check glucose levels

in interstitial fluid. The sensor stays for 2 weeks. It can give real time levels every 1–5 minutes.
- Not perfect so users must still check blood glucose with a glucose meter before driving or changing therapy. It provides useful data on levels especially at night. Alarms can be incorporated into the device to warn individuals about hypoglycaemia.

General principles
- Insulin (from endogenous pancreatic B cells or exogenous IV/SC/IM) allows glucose to enter cells with K for ATP generation. This lowers blood glucose. Excess insulin, sulfonylureas or meglitinides may cause hypoglycaemia. If prolonged or severe, can cause brain injury/death.
- Absence of insulin, e.g. T1DM, leads to hyperglycaemia. Cells starved of glucose which leads them to metabolise fats causing acidosis and ketonaemia/ketonuria. Those with T2DM have enough insulin to stop ketogenesis but not enough insulin to manage their blood glucose. DKA very rarely occurs, but hyperglycaemia and severe fluid loss can, which can cause HHS.
- Physiological stress with cortisol/adrenaline, e.g. illness, surgery, physical trauma, pregnancy can cause hyperglycaemia with polyuria, dehydration and volume loss. This is countered by increased insulin release normally, so the diabetic patient needs to increase insulin dose when unwell or else the result will be a rapid development of DKA.
- In diabetic patients, supply the correct amount of insulin to match the physiological needs, ideally maintaining blood glucose. This can be difficult as physiological demands vary as well as calorific intake and other factors. The primary aim is to avoid severe hypoglycaemia and severe hyperglycaemia (>20 mmol/L). *If the blood glucose is high you must give more insulin. If low you give less.* Insulins come in various formats but the active molecule is the same. The formulation just alters the half-life so that it can be short-acting or long-acting.
- Hospital is the safest place to adjust insulin. Ensure frequent monitoring. Ensure that hyper- and hypoglycaemia can be quickly detected and treated.

Types of commercial insulin
- Insulin concentration usually 100 U/ml. Higher concentrations available for those with high insulin resistance. Insulin is injected SC several times a day into the anterior abdominal wall, upper arms, outer thighs and buttocks. Needle sited at right angle to the skin and given by SC (not IM) route. Two-thirds of the daily insulin is given in the morning. Ratio of short-acting to intermediate-acting is 1:2. Remaining third is given in the evening.
- **Fast-acting short half-life:** Actrapid or Novorapid or Humulin S (soluble/short). These act within a half hour and peak at 2–4 h and last about 6 h in total. They are used to make up sliding scales now called VRIIIs. 1 unit lowers CBG on average by 3 mmol.
- **Intermediate-acting:** Humulin I (isophane), Lente, Insulatard. Normally given in BD doses pre-breakfast and pre-evening meal. Onset 1–3 h and peak 3–8 h. Duration 7–14 h.
- **Long-acting:** glargine (Lantus/Toujeo) or detemir (Levemir) or degludec. Onset 1–2 hours. No peak. Last 18–26 h. Given OD/BD. They mimic the basal level of insulin.
- **Combined insulins:** fast- and intermediate-acting insulins can be combined and so can mimic the basal level and there is a short-acting insulin which can

deal with mealtime hyperglycaemia. BD and TDS insulins are prescribed before meals. In most cases the potential problems can be discussed and control improved pre-operatively and discussed at the pre-operative assessment. There is no such opportunity to optimise diabetic control prior to emergency surgery. Before, during and post-op the aim is to keep the blood glucose level within the range 6–10 mmol/L at all times with a VRIII if needed.

Use of variable rate IV insulin infusion for diabetic patients in hospital

- **About:** in the management of DKA/HHS we use a fixed rate insulin infusion (FRIII) primarily to suppress ketone generation. For unwell hyperglycaemic patients needing glycaemic control we use a variable rate intravenous insulin infusion (VRIII). Use as long as is necessary. Convert to a standard SC insulin regimen as soon as stable. Before stopping a VRIII prescribe appropriate insulin therapy and give 30 min before. In comatose patients, e.g. stroke, very tight control may lead to hypoglycaemia and coma. Set sensible targets to avoid undetected hypoglycaemia.
- **Indications for VRIII:** hyperglycaemia (diabetes) or with hospital-related hyperglycaemia unable to take oral fluid/food and for whom adjustment of their own insulin regime is not possible, e.g. vomiting (exclude DKA), nil by mouth and will miss more than one meal, severe illness with need to achieve good glycaemic control, e.g. sepsis. Other indications are ACS, TPN/enteral feeding, steroid use, pregnancy.
- **NB:** hold usual diabetes treatment during VRIII but continue long-acting insulins.
- **Aims of VRIII are** a CBG in range 6.0–10.0 mmol/L, avoid hypoglycaemia (CBG <4.0 mmol/L) which may increase mortality. Limit use to <24 h where possible, try to avoid using in those patients able to eat and drink.
- **Those on VRIII need:** hourly monitoring of CBG with regular review of insulin infusion rate to achieve target range of glucose, at least daily review of the need for the VRIII, at least daily clinical review of patient including fluid status and daily urea and electrolytes.

Suggested scales for insulin infusion rate

Glucose mmol/L	Insulin rates (ml/hour) Start on standard rate unless otherwise indicated		
	Reduced rate (for use in insulin sensitive patients e.g. ≤24 units per day)	Standard rate (first choice in most patients)	Increased rate (for insulin resistant patients e.g. ≥100 units per day)
NB if a patient is on basal subcutaneous insulin – continue this alongside the VRIII			
<4.0	0*	0*	0*
4.1–8.0	0.5	1	2
8.1–12.0	1	2	4
12.1–16.0	2	4	6
16.1–20.0	3	5	7
20.1–24.0	4	6	8
>24.1	6	8	10

*Treat hypoglycaemia and once CBG >4.0 mmol/L restart IV insulin within 20 minutes. The half life of intravenous insulin is very short (7–8 minutes) and restarting the VRIII promptly minimises the risk of ketosis.
Table reproduced with permission from the Joint British Diabetes Societies.

- CBG check every 1–2 h (mmol/L): **50 U Actrapid in 50 ml 0.9% NS** and run as below (use larger dose if insulin resistance suspected, e.g. obese).
- >20 mmol/L: 8–10 U/h check line (6 U/h insulin sensitive). Ensure insulin was added. Seek medical review.
- VRIII must also be accompanied by IV fluids at 125 ml/h (adjust for patient size, cardiac/fluid status) containing at least 5% glucose, e.g. 1 L 0.45% NaCl with 5% glucose and 40 mmol/L KCl or 5% glucose with 40 mmol/L KCl. If K is >5.5 mmol/L do not add K. If K is <3.5 mmol/L senior review needed as extra K needs to be given.
- **Preparation:** use an insulin syringe/pen to draw up 50 U of a short-acting insulin, e.g. Actrapid. Add to a 50 ml syringe containing 49.5 ml of NS giving 1 U/ml. Always ensure lines and IV access working. Some patients need 100 U/d and others 30 U/d so the VRIII doses need to reflect this. Basal insulin needed will escalate with physiological stress, surgery, sepsis and insulin resistance.
- **Risks:** high/low CBG due to inappropriate insulin infusion rates or inadequate monitoring, rebound hyperglycaemia and possible DKA if IV access Is lost or VRIII is stopped inappropriately, Fluid overload, low K, low Na. Infection related to IV line.
- The insulin is given alongside IV fluid, which must be administered using a **volumetric infusion pump.** This should be 0.45% saline with G5W and 0.15% **or** 0.3% KCl. Omit KCl if K >4.5 mmol/L. The amount of KCl depends on the most recent U&E. For patients with renal impairment and high K, 0.45% saline with 5% glucose **without** KCl should be used. In low Na IV NS may be used.
- Set the fluid replacement rate to deliver the hourly fluid requirements of the individual patient. The rate must not be altered thereafter without senior advice. Insulin must be infused at a variable rate to keep the blood glucose 6–10 mmol/L (acceptable range 4–12 mmol/L).
- Stopping the VRIII: for T2DM **oral hypoglycaemics:** restart when oral intake possible at normal pre-op doses. Reduce or stop sulfonylurea if oral intake likely to be reduced. Metformin avoided if eGFR <50 ml/min. **Restarting insulin:** wait until normal oral intake possible. Restart normal dose but adjust down if oral intake reduced or increase if ongoing sepsis or infection or post-op stress. Aim for a level of 4–12 mmol/L. Involve diabetic specialist team for optimising control. Ensure that the VRIII / IVII overlaps the giving of SC insulin by 30–60 min.

General rules for control in known diabetic

- If blood glucose >12 mmol/L then check capillary ketone levels using an appropriate bedside monitor if available. If capillary blood ketones are >3 mmol/L or urinary ketones greater than +++ then follow DKA guidelines (▶Section 5.18) and contact the on-call medical/diabetes specialist team for advice. For all others with known diabetes see as follows.
- **T1DM: always need insulin.** If blood glucose above target give SC rapid-acting analogue insulin (i.e. Novorapid, Humalog) and assume that 1 U of insulin (Actrapid/Novorapid) will drop blood glucose by 3 mmol/L, BUT wherever possible determine baseline needs. A safe target is 10 mmol/L. Recheck the blood glucose 1 h later to ensure it is falling. If control is still unsatisfactory discuss with medical/diabetic team. Consider VRIII.
- **Insulin pumps and hyperglycaemia:** if hyperglycaemia patient can give insulin 1 unit per 3 mmol drop intended via pump as detailed above. Check ketones to exclude DKA. If there is any question that the pump is not working then give SC insulin. If patient is unwell and control is poor consider removing pump and moving to a VRIII.

- **T2DM:** use SC rapid-acting analogue insulin (i.e. Novorapid, Humalog). Assess using CBG measurement. Always recheck blood glucose 1 h later to ensure it is falling. If worsening or unsatisfactory then contact medical/diabetic team and consider VRIII.
- **New diabetes:** determine if T1DM (young, thin, may be ketotic), will usually need insulin therapy and a VRIII is reasonable initially and an estimate of insulin needed can be made. Involve diabetic team. At earliest reasonable opportunity commence insulin regimen. Older, obese diabetics will usually be T2DM and dietary advice and oral medication can be considered. Use local protocols where available. Ensure enough insulin to render normoglycaemic without any ketones. If this is for DKA, continue insulin at all times (to switch off ketone production, and so reduce acidosis). If for other reasons (e.g. control peri-operatively) <4 mmol/L (72 mg/dl) should stop insulin. Treat hypoglycaemia.
- **Reference:** *Joint British Diabetes Societies (2014) The use of variable rate intravenous insulin infusion (VRIII) in medical inpatients.

Perioperative care guidelines for diabetes: follow local guidance
Diet controlled and non-insulin treated diabetes for minor surgery
- Pre-op: stop SGLT2 inhibitors 3 days pre-operatively. Continue other meds.
- Day of operation: omit oral hypoglycaemia, reduce metformin to BD if given TDS. Check ketones if on SGLT2 inhibitor. Check blood glucose: 1 h pre-op, intraoperatively hourly and post-op in recovery, and 2 hourly until eating. Promote early drinking, eating and mobilisation where appropriate.

Insulin-treated diabetics and minor surgery
- Pre-op: stop SGLT2 inhibitors 3 days before surgery. Otherwise continue usual oral medication. 80% dose of long-acting insulin the evening before the operation.
- Day of operation: stop oral hypoglycaemics. Reduce metformin dose. Blood glucose and ketones (if on SGLT2 inhibitor). Ketones daily if on SGLT2 inhibitor pre-op. 50% dose of mixed insulin morning of surgery. Omit short-acting insulin on the morning of surgery.
- Promote early drinking, eating and mobilisation where appropriate. Restart insulin when eating and drinking. Reduce dose of insulin if reduced meal size, i.e. half normal dose if only able to tolerate half a normal meal size.

Diabetes and major surgery
- Pre-op: stop SGLT2 inhibitors 3 days before surgery. Continue usual oral medication. 80% dose of long-acting insulin the evening before the operation.
- Day of operation: stop oral hypoglycaemics. Reduce metformin dose. Blood glucose and ketones (if on SGLT2 inhibitor). Ketones daily if on SGLT2 inhibitor pre-op. 50% dose of mixed insulin morning of surgery.
- Omit short-acting insulin on the morning of surgery. Promote early drinking, eating and mobilisation where appropriate. Start insulin infusion morning of surgery.

06 Gastroenterology

6.1 Acute diarrhoea

Answering bleep/taking referral

- Diarrhoea: known IBD? Recent antibiotics? Pyrexial, tachycardia, unwell, dehydrated? Frequency and type of stools. Mucus, blood, fatty.
- Bristol stool chart to characterise stools (type 6/7). If suspect infective causes isolation and send stool culture. Wash hands with soap and water. Spores resist alcohol hand washes.
- Why in hospital? When did it start? Frequency? Abdominal pain, guarding, vomiting, recent antibiotics, excessive laxatives.
- Consider AXR – is there faeces ++ is it constipation and overflow? Do PR.

Causes of diarrhoea defined as stool weight >250 g/d

- **Sepsis:** can be a marker of severe sepsis often with rash and low BP.
- **Bacterial infective:** *Salmonella* and *E. coli* usually cause a sudden onset gastroenteritis which can be bloody with a toxic patient. Usually with fever and abdominal pain. *Shigella* – bloody diarrhoea. ▶Section 9.44.
- ***Clostridioides difficile:*** caused by enterotoxins A and B. Associated with antibiotic usage that alters gut flora. Can lead to pseudomembranous colitis, megacolon and perforation and even death. Stop any antibiotic. Needs urgent **Metronidazole** 500 mg 8 h PO or **Vancomycin** 125 mg 6 h PO and surgical consult if abdominal pain. ▶Section 6.11.
- **Viral infective:** norovirus must be isolated quickly. N&V. Spreads quickly. Isolate and infection control and watch for patient/staff in proximity complaining of same.
- **Acute colitis:** known IBD may be on treatment. Bloody stools, fever. Needs stool chart and gastroenterology review and steroids. ▶Section 6.10.
- **Ischaemic colitis:** abdominal pain may exceed clinical signs, older patient, vascular risks, AF, diarrhoea (bloody). ▶Section 6.14.
- **Amoebic:** caused by invasive infection by *Entamoeba histolytica*. Foreign travel. Acute colitis. Check stools. ▶Section 9.49.
- **Laxatives:** overuse and sometimes abuse.
- **Autonomic:** stasis and small bowel bacterial overgrowth. Diabetes.
- **Constipation with overflow:** rectum full of hard stools with liquid stool emerging. PR is helpful and AXR shows faeces. Needs enema and laxatives and medication review.
- **Osmotic diarrhoea:** in hospital commonly seen starting NG or PEG feeding regimens; can cause an osmotic diarrhoea which can be reduced by slowing feed temporarily and stopping laxatives.
- **Neoplastic disease:** colorectal malignancy is certainly a cause of ongoing altered bowel function. However, more altered bowel habit than diarrhoea. Needs colonoscopy.
- **Carcinoid syndrome:** causes flushing, diarrhoea, wheezing. Measure urine 5-hydroxyindoleacetic acid (5-HIAA), plasma chromogranin A. Liver USS for metastases. Octreoscan, Rx: **Octreotide.**
- **Malabsorption:** pancreatic insufficiency, pale bulky stools, diarrhoea, lactose intolerance. Lactose hydrogen breath test. Low B12/folate/Fe.

- **VIPoma:** severe watery diarrhoea, low K.
- **Thyrotoxicosis:** increased frequency rather than diarrhoea. Raised T_4, low TSH and look for signs of Graves' disease. ▶Section 5.8.
- **Toxic shock syndrome:** diarrhoea, rash in patient who may have an infective source, e.g. simple skin wound or tampon. Rapid deterioration with low BP and shock. ▶Section 2.19.

On arrival
- **Review early warning score.** Review notes and drug chart particularly antibiotics and laxatives and stop them if possible. Discuss with microbiology if need for antimicrobials.
- Abdominal examination including PR – may be hard stools with overflow. Check basic bloods if concerned about dehydration. If severe diarrhoea or poor oral intake then IV fluids.
- Caution with loperamide if any suggestion of infective cause. Hand washing. Isolate patient and send stool cultures if infective cause suspected.

Investigations
- **Bloods:** FBC, U&E, LFT, TFT, CRP.
- **Request stool culture:** cysts, ova, parasites and *C. difficile* toxins A and B.
- **AXR:** features of IBD, toxic megacolon if pseudomembranous colitis.
- **Sigmoidoscopy:** inflamed mucosa, rectal biopsy if diarrhoea persists.
- **Colonoscopy:** if colitis or polyps/tumour suspected. Colonoscopy is best investigation to diagnose colonic cancer in those without significant comorbidities. If there are such issues then CT colonography may be considered or flexible sigmoidoscopy and barium enema.
- **CT/MRI:** rarely needed. Get if suspected intra-abdominal pathology. MRI best for pelvic Crohn's disease or other inflammatory bowel disease.
- **Rare:** look for carcinoid syndrome, VIPoma, etc.

General management
- Isolation if an infective cause suspected. Gown up and wear gloves, which should be placed in bin in patient's room. Ensure hands washed with soap and water to remove any *C. difficile* spores.
- See individual cases above, but all patients need to maintain adequate hydration either orally or IV depending on losses. Monitor fluid balance and U&E and general observations.
- Use codeine/loperamide sparingly in lowest dose for short period if severe symptomatic diarrhoea if infective causes suspected. Use with caution, concern is that they may delay resolution. Avoid if suspected *C. difficile* and pseudomembranous colitis. Surgical review if acute abdomen.

6.2 ▶ Constipation

- Has there been dietary intake? When did bowels last open? Is patient in pain or discomfort? Patient taking opiates or dehydrated or bed-bound or Parkinson's disease or hypothyroid?
- Rarely an acute issue unless nil PR is a sign of obstruction with pain and abdominal distension and abnormal bowel sounds.

On arrival

- Review notes, observations and drug chart. Assess patient and usual bowel frequency. Once a week may be normal for some. Is it physical/psychological, e.g. having to use bed pan or commode?
- Pain, e.g. anal fissure or haemorrhoids will make patient avoid defecation. Needs stool softeners. If there are signs of bowel obstruction then nil by mouth, bloods and AXR and surgical consult. If not obstructed and mild may simply require improved hydration, high fibre diet and oral laxatives. If constipated (AXR may show stool ++) with watery diarrhoea and an enema, e.g. Microlax enema or a Picolax (sodium picosulphate) enema, can be very effective in emptying the rectum.
- **Examination:** tenderness, bowel sounds, peritonism, masses. PR examination: anal pain or discomfort, rectal tumour or impacted faeces. Spinal cord disease or multiple sclerosis usually already known. Hirschsprung's disease usually from childhood. Myxoedema: look for clinical signs, raised TSH.

Causes of constipation

- **General:** multiple factors, poor dietary intake or lack of dietary fibre, immobility or dehydration.
- **Drugs:** opiates, anticholinergic, diuretics, CCBs, e.g. verapamil, iron, ondansetron.
- **Metabolic:** low K or Mg. High Ca, hyperglycaemia, dehydration, hypothyroid.
- **Physical:** volvulus, stricture, ileus, colorectal tumour, anal pain, difficulty toileting.
- **Others:** acute porphyria, spinal cord disease, Hirschsprung's disease, Parkinson's disease, depression, dementia.

Management

- Hydrate orally if possible and high fibre diet and early mobility and provide time and access to optimal toileting conditions with as much privacy as can be provided. Make use of gastrocolic reflex – toileting patient after eating.
- Ongoing or new constipation for several weeks warrants consideration to exclude a colorectal malignancy. Try stool softeners (e.g. **Sodium docusate** 200 mg TDS), bulking agents (e.g. **Fybogel** one sachet BD), stimulants (e.g. senna 1 tab BD is useful especially if stools are large, soft and bulky).
- **Osmotic laxatives** (e.g. **Lactulose** 10–20 ml BD) really are to be avoided if possible, except to improve stool output with hepatic encephalopathy. **Movicol** (contains polyethylene glycol or codanthramer). Enemas, e.g. glycerin suppository or **Picolax** enema are useful for distal stool.
- Occasionally all fails and you may be asked to perform a manual evacuation, which is digital removal of rectal faeces. Be sure to wear two pairs of gloves and have lots of pads. Constipation is common but significant complications are very rare, but include faecal impaction where the rectum fills with 'rocks' of hard stool with soft stool leaking around sides and overflow diarrhoea.
- Can even cause intestinal obstruction and perforation and megacolon leading to sigmoid volvulus. Rectal prolapse can be seen. It may provoke urinary retention and UTI.

Laxatives and bowel preparation

- **Stimulant laxative: senna** 15 mg (2 tabs) BD. SE: cramps, diarrhoea and low K. Avoid if bowel obstruction. **Bisacodyl** 5–10 mg nocte.
- **Osmotic laxative: lactulose** 10–30 ml 12 h, higher doses in hepatic encephalopathy (30–50 ml TDS) to have 2+ soft stools/d.
- **Bulk-forming laxative: ispaghula husk** 3.5 g BD or one sachet BD.

- **Bowel cleansing for severe cases:** sodium picosulfate 10 mg and review.
- **Enema:** Microlax one PR and the more potent phosphate enema.

6.3 ▶ Dyspepsia

- **Definitions:** recurrent epigastric pain, burning, fullness, early satiety or discomfort. Symptoms often poorly localising and several tests may be needed. Symptoms are defined to be present for at least 4 or 12 weeks depending on definitions.
- **Red flags needing endoscopy:** age >55, bleeding, anaemia, vomiting, dysphagia, abdominal mass, early satiety. Finding gallstones does not mean that this is the cause and often find those with continuing symptoms post-cholecystectomy.

Causes of dyspepsia

- **Peptic ulcer disease:** epigastric pain with food and weight loss suggests GU, better with food suggests DU. OGD – gastritis or erosions; mucosal breaks <5mm are erosions, otherwise ulcers. Gastric and duodenal. Presents: iron-deficiency anaemia. Outflow obstruction. Haematemesis. GU epigastric pain. DU pain to back – patient points to epigastrium. Risks: NSAIDs, steroids, aspirin and combinations of same. *Helicobacter pylori*. Prevention: **misoprostol** reduces NSAID ulcers or PPI for those on long-term aspirin/steroids/NSAIDs aged >60 or with symptoms. Stop smoking. Needs OGD. FBC, haematinics, test for *H. pylori* and treat.
- **Oesophageal cancer:** weight loss, progressive dysphagia to solids then fluids, regurgitation. Needs endoscopy ± stenting, biopsy and staging.
- **Gastric cancer:** weight loss, bleeding, anaemia, early satiety, vomiting. Needs endoscopy ± stenting, biopsy and staging.
- **GORD:** reflux causes heartburn and waterbrash. Worse on lying or bending. OGD may show oesophagitis or erosions.
- **Gastroparesis:** impaired gastric motility. Type 1/2 DM. OGD shows food still present.
- **Biliary colic/gallstones:** RUQ pain. Stone in gallbladder or cystic duct. Needs USS and LFTs. May need ERCP.
- **Irritable bowel:** abdominal pain and bloating and intermittent diarrhoea or constipation or mucus. Feeling of incomplete evacuation. Bloods should be normal. No red flags – bleeding, anaemia, no weight loss or family history and age <60, no abdominal mass or rectal mass and negative CA125 where ovarian cancer is possible. Normal faecal calprotectin can help distinguish from inflammatory disease and avoid colonoscopy when cancer is not suspected.
- **Non ulcer dyspepsia:** OGD normal. Functional. Reassurance.
- **Pancreatic cancer:** weight loss, pain, anaemia, early satiety, vomiting. Needs ERCP ± stenting, biopsy and staging.
- **Pancreatitis:** elevated lipase/amylase. Epigastric pain. Gallstones and alcohol. See below.
- **Coeliac disease:** check FBC, duodenal biopsies, antibody testing for coeliac disease (endomysial antibodies (EMA) or tissue transglutaminase (TTG)).
- **Medication:** most drugs in *BNF* cause dyspepsia. Ask about all medication given. Steroids, aspirin, NSAIDs, L-dopa-containing meds, macrolides, bisphosphonates, nitrates, calcium channel blockers, codeine, theophylline, etc.
- **Chronic alcohol abuse:** dyspepsia is common.
- **Metabolic:** uraemia and renal failure, hypercalcaemia.
- **Cardiac:** ACS as inferior MI can classically cause epigastric discomfort. Needs ECG and troponin. Myocarditis and pericarditis.
- **Aortic disease:** dissection or aneurysm. Chest pain to back. CT aortogram.
- **Ischaemic bowel:** uncommon but should be considered.
- **Pulmonary:** PE, pneumonia, malignancy. Get CXR and other tests as needed.
- **Lactose intolerance:** ingestion of lactose (milk) increases symptoms. Try without. Need lactose hydrogen breath test.

- **Investigations:** diagnostics can help where cause not evident. Send FBC. U&E, LFT, Ca, amylase/lipase, CRP, troponin (if needed), ECG, USS biliary tracts and pancreas, endoscopy, urea breath test for HP. HP serology identifies only prior exposure.
- **Management:** treatment can be with **Sucralfate** 2 g BD PO, **ranitidine** or **PPI.** *H. pylori* eradication – see *BNF* for latest regimen. Transfuse if anaemia Hb <80 g/L or bleeding. Iron replacement. See below for acute upper GI bleed and for gallstones. Always ask if this could be an ACS.

6.4 ▶ Acute upper gastrointestinal bleeding

- **About:** bleeding from above the ligament of Treitz. Nasopharynx, oesophagus, stomach, duodenum. Multiple causes may coexist – varices and gastritis and a duodenal ulcer. Epistaxis and swallowed blood can mimic GI bleed. If physicians can't stop life-threatening bleeding it's a surgical problem. 90% of non-variceal bleeds (VBs) and 50% of VBs stop spontaneously. Mortality is 10%, rising to 26% in patients who bleed when in hospital for other reasons. Use the Blatchford and Rockall score to assess patients.
- **NB:** With a suspect GI bleed first make sure there are at least two good wide-bore IV lines before all peripheral venous access disappears.
- Check Glasgow-Blatchford Score (GBS) is at presentation with AUGIB.

Causes of acute upper GI bleeding

- **Peptic ulcer disease (38%):** usually lesser curve of stomach or duodenal bulb where an ulcer can erode into a large vessel. *H. pylori* positive, NSAIDs. Multiple ulcers with Zollinger–Ellison syndrome. Needs OGD and endoscopic therapy and **PPI** and *H. pylori* eradication. Rarely surgery.
- **Oesophageal ulcer/severe oesophagitis (13%):** pain on swallowing, dysphagia, GORD symptoms. In HIV, infections with candida, CMV, HSV. Local ulceration with bisphosphonates and NSAIDs. Consider PPI. Treat GORD.
- **Oesophageal/gastric cancer (7%):** progressive dysphagia to solids then liquids. Weight loss, bleeding, adenocarcinoma. **Gastric cancer:** chronic blood loss more usual. Early satiation and weight loss.
- **Coagulopathy:** warfarin or liver disease or antithrombotics or DOACs or heparin or severe thrombocytopenia with any other gastric pathology.
- **Oesophageal varices (16%):** OGD + **Terlipressin** 2 mg IV QDS + **Tazocin** 4.5 g TDS IV + endoscopic management, Sengstaken tube and TIPSS. Bleed due to portal HTN due to: cirrhosis (alcohol, NAFLD, viral hepatitis, haem, PBC, PSC, idiopathic, etc.), schistosomiasis (commonest worldwide), extrahepatic portal vein thrombosis, idiopathic portal hypertension, cardiac fibrosis. Assess cirrhosis mortality with Child–Pugh score (▶ Section 7.12). Useful prognostic marker of cirrhosis and varices. Has been used to aid selection of those for further interventions. Cirrhosis causes portal pressure >12 mmHg and so blood rediverted to lower oesophagus and small vessels become distended and thinner walled. Alcohol history, signs of chronic liver failure and caput medusae. Splenomegaly suggests portal hypertension. Look for causes of cirrhosis and portal hypertension.
- **Aorto-enteric fistula:** previous AAA surgery with fistula with 3rd part of duodenum causing severe GI bleeding. Left untreated they are universally fatal. Surgical repair carries a very high mortality.
- **Mallory–Weiss tear (4%):** history of retching and often alcohol misuse. Linear mucosal tear found near the oesophagogastric junction. Mucosal tear can be injected with adrenaline. If this fails haemoclips or band ligation.
- **Gastric vascular ectasias (6%):** may be found and also seen with hereditary haemorrhagic telangiectasia, arteriovenous malformation and other vascular lesions. Angiodysplasia with CKD.
- **Dieulafoy's lesion (2%):** a large-calibre arteriole, which lies just below the mucosa and causes an arterial bleed through a pinpoint mucosal lesion. Most commonly on the lesser curve.
- **Spurious:** swallowed epistaxis blood or from nasopharynx can cause haematemesis and melaena. Ask about these. Epistaxis can be severe with swallowed blood but the history should be clear if asked.
- **Right colonic bleed:** may cause melaena-type stools but this is rare.

- **Clinical history/risk factors:** most of the time the story is difficult with dark material passed orally or rectally and the usual 'coffee grounds', which may be bile. Ask about liver disease, peptic ulcer disease, alcohol intake, aspirin usage, NSAIDs, warfarin, steroids. Ask about a history of bleeding problems – dental extractions, etc. Bright red haematemesis implies active bleeding from the oesophagus, stomach or duodenum. This can lead to circulatory collapse and constitutes a medical emergency. Coffee ground vomitus refers to the vomiting of black material assumed to be blood. Its presence implies that bleeding has stopped or has been relatively modest. It may simply be bile. Often over-reported. Melaena is the passage of tarry black stool usually due to acute upper GI bleeding but occasionally from bleeding within the small bowel or right colon. Iron preparations will cause some black faeces. Haematochezia is the passage of fresh blood per rectum usually due to colonic bleeding but occasionally due to profuse upper GI bleeding.
- **Examination:** look for signs of liver disease and portal hypertension suggests varices but bleeding may be other pathology. Liver disease – ascites, jaundice, gynaecomastia, Dupuytren's contracture, clubbing, spider naevi, caput medusae, palmar erythema, etc. Liver decompensation, e.g. jaundice, encephalopathy, asterixis. Liver flap. Evidence of significant blood loss: postural fall in SBP >20 mmHg, postural HR Increase >30 bpm (lying/sitting when too ill to stand). Signs of shock and haemodynamic compromise. Thready pulse, thirst, poor skin turgor, cold nose. Increased capillary refill time. Oliguria – measure urine output. Rectal exam for melaena. Facial telangiectasias (HHT).
- **Warnings:** elderly patients decompensate early; healthy younger patients (<50) decompensate late and quickly so take care and don't be lulled into a false sense of security. Be careful with those on beta-blockers where normal raised HR response may be muted. Steroids can mask perforation and acute abdominal pathology.

Investigations
- **FBC:** Hb acutely is of no value as haemodilution yet to take place. Check platelets. Target Hb 80 g/dl. Recent evidence suggests that higher Hb targets associated with increased mortality.
- **U&E:** raised urea suggests UGIB and protein load in gut. May see AKI.
- **LFT** and **coagulation screen:** at baseline and repeat as needed.
- **Blood group** and **cross-match** 2–4 units depending on estimated losses.

Management of GI bleed irrespective of cause
- Also see also Haemorrhagic shock (▶Section 2.22).
- **ABC, give O$_2$ if shocked. Get good IV access and protect it especially** if low BP and raised HR or melaena or witnessed haematemesis. Prefer a grey venous cannula in each antecubital fossa. If difficult IV access get immediate help from registrar or anaesthetist. A central line is too long and fine for giving volume quickly. Once access gained send bloods FBC, U&E, LFT, clotting, and group and cross-match 4 units or more if needed. Upper GI endoscopy: usually within 24 h or sooner. They want patients as haemodynamically stable as possible and anticoagulation reversed first if possible.
- **Observations:** repeat frequent assessments of BP, HR and JVP and titrate volume and blood replacement with these. Take care not to volume overload the frail and elderly and those with poor cardiac function. A urinary catheter can be the poor man's central line because it can give some measure as a surrogate marker of renal and general perfusion. If you can get the patient to an HDU/ITU bed then that is ideal for the shocked bleeder.

- **Reverse anticoagulants or coagulopathy:** see ▶Sections 8.8–8.12.
- **Fluids:** start 500 ml NS over 15 min.
- **Transfuse:** acutely checked Hb/Hct of little value. Red blood cell transfusion should follow a restrictive protocol (trigger: Hb <70 g/L; target: 70–100 g/L). A higher trigger should be considered in patients with ischaemic heart disease or haemodynamic instability. Give blood O negative if exsanguinating.
- **Keep nil by mouth:** so they can go for urgent endoscopy if needed. Unless actively bleeding, patients should be NBM for 4 h before endoscopy. Otherwise stable non-bleeding patients should be allowed to eat.
- **Starting PPI: IV Pantoprazole** 40 mg BD is used only in patients with severe active bleeding from ulcers after endoscopy. Otherwise give **Omeprazole** 20 mg PO after endoscopy, unless endoscopy is likely to be delayed. NICE recommends that PPI treatment is not started before endoscopy. Although it is logical to begin treating bleeding peptic ulcers with PPIs as soon as possible, there is no evidence that treatment before endoscopy alters outcome. Treatment with PPIs makes testing for *H. pylori* less reliable. Follow local guidance.
- **Risk assess:** Glasgow-Blatchford Score (GBS) or modified GBS to assess on admission and full Rockall post-endoscopy to guide management. Escalate high score or unstable patients. Resuscitate those who are actively bleeding and discuss need for urgent endoscopy. In suspected GI bleeding, consider the patient for non-admission or early discharge if before endoscopy the Blatchford score is 0, i.e. no melaena and no haemodynamic disturbance, no significant comorbidity and normal FBC and normal urea. Low score patients may be managed as outpatients on a next day list.
- **Transfuse** if bleeding or Hb <70 g/L. Treat INR >1.3 with FFP. Fibrinogen <2 with cryoprecipitate. Keep platelet count >50,000/µL.
- **Prolonged PT: IV Vitamin K** 5–10 mg slow IV. See below if on warfarin.
- **Fibrinogen level** <1.5 g/L. Raised INR/PT >1.3. Consider FFP at 15 ml/kg (each unit is about 150–200 ml) or cryoprecipitate (2 units) as per transfusion policy.
- **UGIB and anticoagulation:** ▶Section 8.8. **Warfarin:** vitamin K and 4 factor PCC ▶Section 8.9. **DOAC:** ▶Section 8.11. **Heparin/Fondaparinux:** ▶Section 8.10. **Low platelets:** ▶Section 8.4.
- **UGIB and stent or metal valves:** risk of bleeding usually is the more pressing and anticoagulation/antiplatelets should be stopped and reversed acutely. Stent thrombosis is a concern if bleeding occurs soon after PCI and stenting; however, so is anaemia-induced cardiac ischaemia and exsanguination. Liaise closely with cardiologists and gastroenterologists to manage risk. You can give/continue aspirin.
- **Cardiac/stroke patients:** patients with critical CAD or new or drug-eluting stents should be discussed with cardiology prior to next dose. **Aspirin can be continued but stop Clopidogrel/Prasugrel** until discussed. Uncontrolled bleeding and anaemia exacerbates IHD.
- **ITU/HDU:** patients may be best on HDU/ITU, especially if need for intubation or ventilation or inotropic support or multi-organ failure. Speak to ITU team and involve them early in a deteriorating patient. **Vasopressin** may be used where available if bleeding persists.

Pre-endoscopy GBS score at admission (some use modified version)
- **Blood urea:** 6.5–7.9 (**+2**), 8.0–9.9 (**+3**), 10–25 (**+4**), >25 (**+6**)
- **Hb** (men g/L): 120–129 (**+1**), 100–119 (**+3**), <100 (**+6**)
- **Hb** (women g/L): 100–119 (**+1**), <100 (**+6**)

- **Systolic BP:** 100–109 (**+1**), 90–99 (**+2**), <90 (**+3**)
- **Pulse:** >100 (**+1**), **melaena (+1)**, **syncope (+2)**, **hepatic disease (+2)**, **cardiac failure (+2).** Score >6 suggests need for intervention. GBS ≤1 at presentation are considered for outpatient management.

Calculate pre-endoscopy score used to risk assess
- Helps gastroenterologists to select those for urgent endoscopy. Those with an additional low score may not require urgent endoscopy and some may be managed as outpatient.
- Score: <u>very low risk</u>: 1–2 can be considered for instant discharge and OP OGD and PPI and follow-up. <u>Low risk</u> <3: 0% expected mortality and 5% rebleed – good prognosis; consider discharge, outpatient endoscopy on PPI. <u>Intermediate</u> 3–8: monitor as inpatient. <u>High risk</u> >8: high (41%) mortality and (42%) rebleed – consider urgent endoscopy.

Endoscopy can determine bleeding source(s)
- Should be done in high-risk patients using GBS to assess. First attempt resuscitation and reversal of any coagulopathy. Needs sedation and airways management and close monitoring.
- In practice most bleeding vessels go into spasm and stop bleeding after the initial rupture. In patients who continue to bleed or re-bleed following admission, endoscopic therapy or surgery may be necessary. The decision on the timing of endoscopy is individualised for patients depending on the severity of the bleed and their comorbidities. If endoscopy is required out of hours contact the on-call consultant endoscopist. All other patients with upper GI bleeding should have endoscopy within 24 h of admission.
- The endoscopist can use a heater probe as well as injecting dilute adrenaline to get haemostasis. TC-325 (Hemospray, Cook Medical) is a powder agent for endoscopic haemostasis in patients with upper gastrointestinal bleeding (UGIB) not amenable to standard endoscopic treatment (e.g. diffuse bleeding) or as salvage therapy after failure of conventional methods. There were high immediate haemostasis rates with Hemospray in oesophageal and peptic ulcer bleeds.
- **Interpretation of endoscopic findings:** risks of rebleeding – active bleeding 90%, non-bleeding visible vessel 25%, adherent clot 25–30%, oozing without visible vessel 10–20%, flat spot 7–10%, clean ulcer base 3–5%.

Failed endoscopic haemostasis and role for surgery for ulcer disease
- **Rebleeding** is from large GU >2 cm and lesser curve and posterior wall DU. Visible clot and visible bleeding increase bleed risk. The risk of rebleeding from a peptic ulcer decreases significantly 72 h after the initial episode of bleeding.
- Start IV PPI if signs of risk of rebleeding. If there is evidence of high-risk ulcers with active bleeding, adherent clot, visible vessel start **Omeprazole** 80 mg IV bolus and 8 mg/h for 72 h. PPI raises gastric pH and aids clot stability and haemostasis. Continue for 3 d when rebleeding most common. Reduces bleeding and need for transfusion. For the remainder start an oral PPI, post-endoscopy, which should be used for at least 4 weeks to heal ulcers, e.g. **Omeprazole** 20–40 mg OD. *H. pylori* should be eradicated if present (biopsy result or CLO test). Some consider this to be unnecessary if the patient is going to be on long-term PPI treatment.

Surgical care for peptic ulcer disease

- It is useful for the surgeon to be present at the time of endoscopy, as important anatomic information will be gained during the endoscopic procedure. Failure of initial endoscopic haemostasis attempts is one of the indications for surgery in bleeding peptic ulcers. Early elective surgery for bleeding peptic ulcer does not reduce the mortality risk, but it does reduce the risk of re-bleeding. It seems reasonable to consider early elective operative intervention in those patients who are at high risk of recurrent bleeding such as those with ulcers >2 cm, hypotension on presentation, with posterior duodenal or lesser curvature gastric ulcers. This recommendation must be balanced against significant risk of complications and death in this elderly frail patient population and requires the exercise of careful surgical judgment.
- Excision or biopsy of the gastric ulcer is important with ulcer type surgey. For a bleeding DU a duodenotomy is performed and the gastroduodenal artery is ligated in the ulcer crater. A pyloroplasty is performed.
- Perforation is rare (rigid abdomen, toxic, masked in those on steroids) but commoner with DU than GU. Needs surgical closure and abdominal drainage.

Interventional radiology

- Angiography with embolisation is used in refractory cases and is generally preferred over surgery. 85% of upper GI haemorrhage is from the left gastric artery territory. Extravascular contrast extravasation indicates the site of active bleeding.
- Upper GI embolisation is well tolerated due to the rich collateral blood supply. Even with no identifiable active bleeding but active GU haemorrhage on endoscopy, embolisation of the left gastric artery is sometimes performed. With a bleeding DU embolisation of gastroduodenal artery territory is recommended as a life-saving procedure.

Post-endoscopy Rockall score (*Gut*, 1999;44:331)

- **Age:** <60 (+0), 60–79 (+1), >80 (+2).
- **Shock:** HR <100 SBP >100 mmHg (+0), HR >100 SBP >100 mmHg (+1), SBP <100 mmHg (+2).
- **Comorbidities:** none significant (+0), IHD/CCF or other major comorbidity (+2), liver failure/kidney failure/metastatic cancer (+3).
- **Post-endoscopy findings**
- **Endoscopic diagnosis:** Mallory–Weiss tear (+0), all other diagnoses (+1), gastrointestinal malignancy (+2).
- **Bleeding at endoscopy:** none/dark spots only (+0), blood, spurting vessel, adherent clot (+2).
- **Severe oesophagitis: Omeprazole** 40 mg OD PO. Manage blood loss. Consider also **Sucralfate** 2 g BD PO.
- **Surgery:** see above.
- ***H. pylori* eradication:** all should have CLO test and *H. pylori* eradication if positive. Early pre-endoscopy PPI can reduce sensitivity of *H. pylori* detection at endoscopy. Eradication is **Omeprazole** 20 mg + (**Metronidazole** 400 mg OR **Amoxicillin** 1 g) + **Clarithromycin** 500 mg ALL given BD for 7 d. **Follow-up: all** *H. pylori* positive need testing for successful eradication. All gastric ulcers need to be rescoped at 4–6 weeks to ensure healed and no gastric malignancy.

- **Aspirin** discontinuation is associated with a threefold increased risk of cardiovascular or cerebrovascular events, the majority of which occurred within 7–10 d. It may be continued if felt necessary for IHD/stroke prevention at a small risk of further bleeding.
- **P2Y12 inhibitors** should be stopped (e.g. clopidogrel) until haemostasis is achieved unless the patient has coronary artery stents, in which case, a decision should be taken after discussion with a cardiologist.
- **Additional:** SSRIs should be used with caution in those at risk of upper GI bleed particularly if on NSAID, clopidogrel or aspirin. Consider switching to non-SSRI.
- **Repeat OGD for a GU at 6–8 weeks.** This is because occasionally gastric ulcers are malignant even though at first presentation they appear benign.

Oesophageal variceal bleed

- **Resuscitate.** ABC, ITU, intubation: failure to control severe bleeding, encephalopathy, hypoxia, aspiration. Terlipressin and antibiotics may be started pre-endoscopy if portal hypertension and varices likely. Target pulse <100 bpm, SBP >90 mmHg, CVP 8–10 cm and urine output >30 ml/h. Once stable consider urgent endoscopy.
- **Antibiotics:** give a broad-spectrum antibiotic when acutely unwell, e.g. **Tazocin** 4.5 g TDS IV (unless penicillin allergy when suggest **Gentamicin or Metronidazole**) to any patient with cirrhosis who presents with an upper GI bleed. Another option is **Co-amoxiclav** IV 1.2 g every 8 h or **Ciprofloxacin** 400mg 12-hourly IV. If ascites is present perform an ascitic tap looking for infection.
- **Active management:** 40% will not settle conservatively and need active treatment to control bleed. Admit HDU.
- **Transfusion target Hb 80 g/L.** Over-transfusion may increase bleeding. Endoscopic bleeding risk factors: severity of cirrhosis, raised hepatic vein pressure, variceal size, tense ascites, endoscopic appearance, e.g. haematocystic spots, diffuse erythema, bluish colour, cherry red spots, or white-nipple spots. Large varices >5 mm diameter. Prophylactic treatment to prevent variceal bleeding is recommended with large oesophageal varices irrespective of the presence or absence of red colour signs.
- **Terlipressin** 2 mg IV followed by 2 mg 4-hourly for 3 d (C/I if severe IHD or stroke or peripheral vascular disease); mesenteric/splanchnic vasoconstrictor decreases portal venous inflow. 34% reduction in mortality for VB. Give immediately prior to endoscopy if varices likely.
- **Octreotide** 50 mcg/h infusion for 3–5 d is the alternative to Terlipressin (can be used in those with IHD) but evidence base poorer and it is unlicensed. Take senior specialist advice.
- **Laxatives:** reduce risk of encephalopathy: **Lactulose** 30–50 ml TDS and **Phosphate enemas** to get >2 soft bowel motions per day.
- **Endoscopic management: variceal band ligation** is first choice option for oesophageal varices where a rubber band placed around varix. **Sclerotherapy:** first choice for gastric varices and may also be used for bleeding from oesophageal varices.
- **Balloon tamponade:** Sengstaken tube with gastric and oesophageal balloons. Placed in intubated patient in Level 3 care by experienced operator. Gastric balloon placed in stomach via mouth and filled with 200–300 ml of water as per instructions. AXR to check position. Gentle retraction pressure on balloon can stop bleeding – usually the weight of a 500 ml or 1 L bag of fluids. Oesophageal balloon rarely needs filling. Sedation, intubation and ventilation will aid airway protection and tolerance of the procedure.

- **Transjugular intrahepatic porto-systemic shunt (TIPSS):** drops portal pressures. Use if persistent bleeding. Radiological guidance. Guide wire inserted into internal jugular to IVC to hepatic vein into liver. Stent passed over wire to create communication, allows high-pressure portal veins to shunt into systemic veins. This drops portal pressure, reducing bleeding and shunts portal venous blood bypassing liver to IVC, but can worsen encephalopathy. Local gastroenterologists will suggest when appropriate. Usually done at tertiary centre for uncontrolled VB.
- **Long term: Carvedilol** 6.25 mg OD PO up-titrate to 12.5 mg OD if tolerated. Otherwise **Propranolol** 40 mg BD and up-titrate to 160 mg OD sustained release. Beta-blockers for varices decrease rebleed by 40%. Re-banding for varices until obliterated. Liver transplantation.

Other causes

- **Gastritis/duodenitis:** oral PPI therapy and *H. pylori* eradication if CLO test positive.
- **Gastric/oesophageal cancer:** treat much the same as peptic ulcer disease. Argon laser or other comparable interventions may be tried. Some need surgery.
- **Dieulafoy's lesion:** cautery or angiographic embolisation. Surgical over-sewing if other management fails.
- **Reference:** Siau *et al.* (2020) British Society of Gastroenterology (BSG)-led multisociety consensus care bundle for the early clinical management of acute upper gastrointestinal bleeding. *Frontline Gastroenterology.*

6.5 ▶ Lower gastrointestinal bleeding

- **About:** bleeding from beyond the ligament of Treitz. May be from small bowel or colorectal. If source unclear do OGD. A torrential upper GI bleed can cause fresh PR bleeding. Always exclude a colorectal cancer.
- **Causes:** diverticular disease (blood, mucus), haemorrhoids (fresh bright blood on toilet paper), colorectal cancer (anaemia, bowel habit, weight loss), ulcerative/Crohn's colitis (known IBD), ischaemic colitis (AF, atherosclerosis, smoker), pseudomembranous colitis (recent antibiotics + *C. difficile*). Angiodysplasia, colorectal polyps, Meckel's diverticulum. Radiation enteropathy, e.g. for gynaecological malignancies. Use of NSAIDs, anticoagulants, antiplatelets. Localised trauma – foreign bodies, sexual assault with anal fissure (severe pain on defecation, tear can be seen).
- **Clinical:** look for signs of shock and volume loss/anaemia. A history of pain and weight loss and altered bowel habit suggests cancer. Check if patient on warfarin, antiplatelet or a DOAC. Evidence of coagulopathy – liver failure. Gynaecological malignancies and bowel irradiation (radiation proctitis). Perform digital rectal examination and proctoscopy. Any local trauma.

Investigations

- **FBC, U&E, coagulation** if coagulopathy suspected or warfarin. **Group and cross-match** 2–4 units or more as needed.
- **Colonoscopy:** usually with good bowel can visualise entire colon. Often difficult to see source when bleeding acutely and often deferred to allow bleeding to settle.
- **OGD:** if source unclear. A torrential upper GI bleed can cause fresh PR bleeding. May be multiple sources.
- **Flexible sigmoidoscopy:** for the rectum and left side of the colon. Can be done without full bowel preparation. Proctoscopy to examine anal canal and useful to identify haemorrhoids.

- **Mesenteric angiography:** for angiodysplasia and occult bleeding lesion. The yield is low and therefore usefulness in question. Needs an arterial bleeding rate of at least 0.5 ml/min. It may allow for embolisation to take place.
- **Technetium-labelled red cell scan:** for occult and active bleeding.
- **CT and CT angiography** may localise pathology. CT colonography being used increasingly to look for colonic polyps and cancer.

Markers of poor prognosis
- **Age:** acute lower GI bleeding occurs most often in the elderly.
- **Acute haemodynamic disturbance:** raised HR, low BP, shock.
- **Gross rectal bleeding** on initial examination ($\times$ 2.3–3).
- **Comorbidity:** 2+ conditions double the chance of a severe bleed.
- **Aspirin or NSAIDs:** increased risk of severe lower GI bleeding $\times$ 1.8–2.7.
- **Inpatients:** (any cause) who bleed after admission have a mortality rate of 23% compared with 3.6% in those admitted to hospital because of rectal bleeding.

Management
- **Supportive:** ABC, high flow O_2 if shocked and resuscitate. See Haemorrhagic shock, ▶ Section 2.22. Correct any coagulopathy and transfuse and replace fluids as required. Most cases settle conservatively. In the acute stage, colonoscopy can be difficult and the usual first lower GI investigation will be a flexible sigmoidoscopy following an enema bowel preparation. If no bleeding cause then consider colonoscopy which may help haemostasis as an effective means of controlling haemorrhage from active diverticular bleeding or post-polypectomy bleeding, when appropriately skilled expertise is available. Other options include CT abdomen, technetium-labelled red cell scanning, angiography and emergency surgery.
- **Surgery:** rarely needed as most bleeding self-limiting and can be managed medically/endoscopically. The exceptions would be massive ongoing bleeding (>5 units in 24 h). Involve surgeons early if bleeding does not settle, especially if there is a suspected underlying malignancy, failed medical therapy for ulcerative colitis or ischaemic colitis or ongoing recurrent bleeding from a diverticulum. Localised segmental intestinal resection or subtotal colectomy is recommended.
- **Catheter mesenteric angiography** and embolisation may be attempted (evidence on which this practice is based is limited).
- **Reference:** SIGN (2008) 105: *Management of acute upper and lower gastrointestinal bleeding: a national clinical guideline.*

6.6 Acute abdomen

- **About:** rapid onset of abdominal pain, vomiting, pyrexia and possibly low BP. This is a surgical emergency potentially requiring operative management. However, may be admitted mistakenly under medical teams or *de novo* presentation in medical patients.
- **Atypical 'understated' presentations** seen in: elderly, immunocompromised, high-dose steroids which mask symptoms and signs when gravely ill and septic. Get urgent help if high NEWS, peritonism, bleeding, pregnant or high lactate.
- **Frequency of causes:** acute appendicitis 30%, acute cholecystitis 10%, small bowel obstruction (SBO) 5%, perforated peptic ulcer 3%, pancreatitis 3%, diverticular disease 2%.

- **Urgent senior review needing resuscitation and possible surgery: (1) severe haemorrhage** (low BP, raised HR, low Hb appears late with bleeding due to AAA or ectopic pregnancy or splenic rupture). **(2) Perforation or rupture of a viscus** (toxic appearance, rigid abdomen, absent bowel sounds, *in extremis*, air under diaphragm), ascending cholangitis (jaundice, rigors, RUQ pain). **(3) Viscus necrosis,** e.g. ischaemic bowel from atherosclerosis, embolism or strangulated hernia, pancreatitis, intussusception, volvulus. **(4) Missed ectopic pregnancy** can lead to death; is she pregnant?
- **Historical clues:** previous surgery – adhesions suggest causes of obstruction. Known IBD. Peptic ulcer disease and perforation: use of NSAIDs, steroids. Previous appendectomy excludes appendicitis. Warfarin – psoas/retroperitoneal haematoma. Known AAA. Immunosuppression.
- **Volume status:** look for raised HR, low BP on sitting or standing suggests significant hypovolaemia, e.g. acute haemorrhage and blood loss (GI bleed, leaking AAA) or volume loss into obstructed bowel.
- **Abdominal pain:** examine abdomen carefully looking for area of maximum tenderness. Pain tends to come on suddenly or sub-acutely. Mechanism is either peritonitis with well-localised pain that is painful on coughing and movement and patient lies still with guarding and a rigid abdomen. Pain may also be colicky in nature and patient moves about and suggests a more obstructive luminal mechanism, e.g. intestinal obstruction. Associated N&V.
- **Position:** sitting bending forward – chronic pancreatitis; lying still – perforation; restless – renal colic.
- **Visible peristalsis and distension:** suggests obstruction.
- **Radiation of pain:** to shoulder – diaphragmatic irritation; to the back – consider AAA or acute pancreatitis or posterior perforation; to umbilicus – acute appendicitis.
- **Guarding:** reflex contraction of abdominal muscles due to light abdominal palpation suggests perforation and peritonism.
- **Rebound tenderness:** increase in severe pain and discomfort when the examining hand abruptly stops pressing on a localised region of the abdomen or on percussion suggests peritonitis (25% don't have it).
- **Rigid abdomen:** contraction of abdominal muscles. Abdomen feels hard like a wooden board. Suggests perforation and peritonism.
- **Fever:** >38°C suggests infective or inflammatory process.
- **Jaundice:** common bile duct obstruction, liver failure, gallstones, haemolysis.
- **Dehydration:** peritonitis, small bowel obstruction, DKA, high Ca.
- **Ascites:** bulging flanks, abdominal distension with shifting dullness. Bowel floats and ascites gravitates to lowest point. Consider spontaneous bacterial peritonitis and diagnostic paracentesis in liver disease.
- **Murphy's sign:** palpation over RUQ causes acute severe pain stopping inspiration. Acute cholecystitis.
- **Don't forget:** check groin hernial orifices as well as scrotal sac and contents.
- **Per rectum examination** – tenderness, induration, mass, frank blood.
- **Per vaginum examination** where indicated – bleeding, discharge, cervical motion tenderness, adnexal masses, and tenderness, uterine size.
- **Bowel sounds:** listen for 2 min at least. May be high-pitched and tinkling.
- **Check hernial orifices**, e.g. strangulated femoral hernia, and the testes of men for a testicular torsion or hernia. Can identify cause of bowel obstruction.

6.7 Acute abdomen – surgical causes

- **Cholecystitis:** gallstones, RIF pain, Murphy's sign, fever, jaundice if stone in CBD risk of cholangitis with fever, jaundice, rigors.
- **Acute appendicitis:** pain begins peri-umbilical and moves to RIF as becomes more peritonitis.
- **Leaking abdominal aortic aneurysm (AAA):** midline pulsatile expansile mass, low BP, may have lost a femoral pulse.
- **Acute pancreatitis:** history of gallstones or alcohol and raised amylase.
- **Bowel ischaemia:** older, raised lactate, abdominal pain often much worse than clinical signs suggest, melaena, AF. May need resection of necrotic bowel.
- **Adhesions causing bowel obstruction:** previous surgery, abdominal scars and old incisional wounds.
- **Incarcerated or strangulated hernia:** SBO/LBO check hernial orifices.
- **Pelvic inflammatory pain:** vaginal discharge, history of STIs.
- **Acute diverticulitis:** left iliac fossa pain, older patient.
- **Abdominal wall:** haematoma, anticoagulants/antithrombotics. Coughing. Localised tender.
- **Gastrointestinal malignancy:** stomach, pancreas, small bowel, colonic.
- **Budd–Chiari:** prothrombotic, RIF pain, jaundice.
- **Inflammatory bowel disease:** Crohn's disease predominantly a small bowel obstruction picture. Ulcerative colitis. Watch for toxic megacolon.
- **Testicular torsion:** acute severe testicular pain.
- **Ureteric colic/renal stones:** renal angle to loin pain, restless, paroxysmal. Stone on CT KUB. Don't be caught out as a AAA can mimic renal colic in an older patient.
- **Meckel's diverticulum:** pain in RIF. May perforate. Seen in adolescents and young adults. Can mimic appendicitis.
- **Gynaecological: endometriosis:** recurrent pain. Ectopic pregnancy: positive pregnancy test and abdominal pain. Acute salpingitis: on right can mimic appendicitis. Ovarian torsion: on right can mimic appendicitis. Mittelschmerz: ovulation mid-cycle pain. May need urgent gynaecological consult and urgent surgery.

6.8 Acute abdomen – medical causes

- **Gastroenteritis:** vomit, diarrhoea, vague pain, tenderness; gradually settles.
- **Myocardial infarction** (inferior): ECG – ST/T changes and troponin.
- **Lower lobe pneumonia:** fever, breathless, chest signs, late CXR signs.
- **Pyelonephritis:** positive urinalysis, tender renal angle, female.
- **Addisonian crisis:** pale, pigmented creases and scars, low BP.
- **Diabetic ketoacidosis:** hyperglycaemic, polyuric, dehydrated, ketotic.
- **Sickle cell crisis:** Afro-Caribbean, known sickle, anaemia. Hyposplenism.
- **Herpes zoster:** rash may be late, rash/pain fits dermatome and one-sided.
- **Acute porphyria:** variegate, AIP, hereditary coproporphyria.
- **Familial Mediterranean fever:** Turkish/Middle Eastern. Mesenteric adenitis: viral-type illness – younger patients. Mimics appendicitis.
- **Tabes dorsalis:** as part of tertiary syphilis.

Pain and localisation: variability seen, e.g. late pregnancy, appendicitis

- **RUQ:** cholecystitis, gallbladder empyema, hepatitis, liver abscess, duodenal ulcer, pneumonia, subphrenic abscess, hepatic flexure of colon.

- **LUQ:** gastroenteritis, splenic disease (infarction/rupture), splenic flexure of colon, subphrenic abscess, perinephritis, acute pancreatitis.
- **Epigastrium:** oesophageal/gastric disease (perforation, gastric/duodenal ulcer), ruptured AAA, acute pancreatitis, myocardial infarction, PE, pancreatic cancer.
- **Right flank:** ureteric colic (loin to groin), pyelonephritis (renal angle), retrocaecal appendix, muscle strain, perinephric abscess.
- **Periumbilical:** early appendicitis, small bowel obstruction, IBD, gastroenteritis, pancreatitis, ruptured AAA, ischaemic bowel.
- **Left flank:** ureteric colic (loin to groin), pyelonephritis (renal angle), muscle strain, perinephric abscess.
- **RIF:** appendicitis, mesenteric lymphadenitis, perforated duodenal ulcer, caecal obstruction, Meckel's diverticulum, ectopic pregnancy, ovarian pathology, terminal ileal disease (Crohn's/*Yersinia* pseudotuberculosis) or very rarely RLQ diverticulitis, biliary colic with low-lying gallbladder, acute salpingitis.
- **LIF:** sigmoidal diverticulitis, constipation, ectopic pregnancy, ovarian pathology, ischaemic colitis, rectal cancer, IBS, ulcerative colitis.
- **Suprapubic:** cystitis, UTI, acute urinary retention, testicular torsion, pelvic inflammatory disease, ectopic pregnancy, uterine disease, diverticulitis.

Investigations

- **Bloods:** FBC, CRP, U&E, pancreatic amylase/lipase. LFT and INR if any suggestion of liver disease or gallstones. Group and cross-match if suspected AAA, ectopic pregnancy or laparotomy or frank bleeding. Get VBG, lactate.
- **Erect CXR** and **erect AXR** can help exclude pathology. Perforation of viscus with free air visible under the diaphragm or between viscera and subcutaneous tissue on lateral decubitus. Distended central small bowel proximal to small bowel obstruction with air–fluid levels. Thickened oedematous valvulae conniventes span entire wall of small bowel unlike colonic haustra. Large bowel obstruction loops more peripheral. ▶ Section 6.12. Renal stones may be seen best with AXR or CT. Normal AXR does not exclude ileus or many other pathologies. Toxic megacolon if diameter >7 cm in midtransverse colon. Pancreatic calcification may suggest acute or chronic pancreatitis. 'Thumb printing' with ischaemic bowel.
- **CT abdomen:** imaging important but does not substitute for good clinical assessment – appendicitis shows inflamed appendix fluid-filled with fat stranding and a hyper-attenuated wall with IV contrast. Uncomplicated sigmoid diverticulitis can show fat stranding and focal thickening of the colonic wall in an area with diverticula. Abscess formation or fistulas may or may not be seen. Colonic cancers may be seen. Renal stones. Obstruction with transition zone showing level of blockage.
- **USS:** imaging of choice for cholecystitis with gallstones and thickened wall hydropic gallbladder. A stone may be seen blocking cystic duct. Sludge or stone material may be seen in the gallbladder. Gallstones may also suggest pancreatitis. Collections in the pelvis or subdiaphragmatic. Abscesses.
- **Urinalysis:** blood, protein, stones. **Pregnancy test** in all fertile women.

General management

- **Supportive:** ABC, O_2 as per BTS guidance. Get good IV access and protect it. Start IV crystalloid fluids with good IV access and monitor physiology. Give 1 L Hartmann's or IV NS over 1–2 h as needed. Most patients are dry.
- **Analgesia: Morphine** 5–10 mg IV + **Cyclizine** 50 mg IV. If tachycardic, low BP or bleeding then get senior help urgently. Fertile female consider ectopic pregnancy

for all acute abdominal pain and/or low BP. Full monitoring BP, HR, temperature and urinary output. Catheterise. FBC, U&E, clotting if liver disease, amylase, group and hold/cross-match if haemorrhage or laparotomy.

- **Severe haemorrhage:** IV access, cross-match, give O-negative blood.
- **Sepsis suspected:** then **Tazocin** 4.5 g 6–8 h IV and fluid resuscitation (see Sepsis, ▶Section 2.21). Maintain NBM until senior review decides otherwise. Normal important meds can sometimes be given with sip of water. Diabetic patients need to be started on a VRIII and keep CBG 4–12 mmol/L. AXR is helpful and depending on findings may need abdominal CT. Laparoscopy may reduce rate of unnecessary laparotomy and improve diagnostic accuracy.

6.9 ▶ Gastric outlet obstruction/pyloric stenosis

- **About:** weight loss, food regurgitation.
- **Causes:** pancreatic cancer (10–20%) or gastric malignancy. Peptic ulcer disease with scarring and oedema of pylorus. Gastric polyps, duodenal malignancy, cholangiocarcinoma.
- **Clinical:** fullness and vomiting (HCl loss) postprandial which is non-bilious. Weight loss, succussion splash if NBM for 2–3 h. Palpable abdominal mass and gastric dilation. Malnutrition is seen late. Aspiration pneumonia. Supraclavicular lymph nodes. Hepatomegaly and jaundice if liver metastases.
- **Investigations: FBC, U&E,** raised urea and creatinine, low K develops later after 2–3 weeks. **LFT:** raised ALP or bilirubin may suggest malignancy. **VBG:** vomits HCl loss, increased HCO_3 and low Cl. Alkalosis increases serum K (K excreted to preserve Na). Results in hypochloraemic (hypokalaemic) metabolic alkalosis. **Plain AXR:** calcification, masses, perforation. **Barium upper GI studies:** can be helpful to identify the gastric silhouette and site of obstruction. **USS abdomen:** liver metastases, obstructive jaundice. CT abdomen with oral contrast: will define and stage any masses or mets. **Upper GI endoscopy:** may still be food residue in stomach and difficulty passing probe. A lesion may be seen and biopsies taken. A stent may be passable.
- **Management:** ABC, IV rehydration and fluid and electrolyte replacement and nutrition. Prolonged vomiting causes loss of hydrochloric (HCl) acid and produces an increase of bicarbonate in the plasma to compensate for the lost chloride and sodium. The result is a hypokalaemic hypochloraemic metabolic alkalosis. Alkalosis shifts the intracellular potassium to the extracellular compartment, and the serum potassium is increased factitiously. With continued vomiting, the renal excretion of potassium increases in order to preserve sodium. The adrenocortical response to hypovolaemia intensifies the exchange of potassium for sodium at the distal tubule, with subsequent aggravation of the hypokalaemia. Manage electrolytes and acid–base disturbances. Specific management depends on cause. Stenting may be possible depending on circumstances. Surgical referral in appropriate cases. (Hypovolaemia, ▶Section 2.20).

6.10 ▶ Acute severe colitis

- **About:** combined medical/surgical approach is best. Always exclude *Clostridioides difficile* even in those with known ulcerative colitis.
- **NB:** stools >8/d or CRP >45 on day 3 of admission predicts an 85% likelihood of requiring a colectomy during that admission.

- **Causes:** IBD: ulcerative colitis, Crohn's disease, colitis of undetermined type and aetiology (CUTE) infection, e.g. *Shigella* and certain *E. coli* (risk of HUS). *C. difficile*: recent antibiotics. Amoebiasis or CMV colitis can mimic ulcerative colitis. Others: radiation colitis, ischaemic colitis (older, AF, vascular disease).
- **Clinical:** diarrhoea, mucus, tenesmus, bloody often 10–20/d and urgency. IBD flare-up can be provoked by infection, stress, NSAIDs, antibiotics. Crampy abdominal pain, weight loss, fevers, raised HR. Silent rigid abdomen suggests perforation but steroids mask signs and perforation may not be dramatic. Rebound suggests peritonism. Distension, vomiting suggests obstruction. Look for signs of sepsis and volume depletion. Enquire if infective source – chicken, contact with livestock, salads.
- **Findings suggesting IBD** (most will have a known diagnosis): mouth ulcers, eye disease – conjunctivitis, iritis, episcleritis. Erythema nodosum – painful red lesions usually over the lower legs. Joint pain – large joints, migratory, asymmetrical. Ankylosing spondylitis seen with Crohn's disease, sacroiliitis – low back pain. Pyoderma gangrenosum pustule, expands as a large ulcer with violaceous margins. Pleuritis, primary sclerosing cholangitis.

Different presentations of IBD
- **Distal ulcerative colitis:** starts distally and confined to sigmoid colon and rectum (proctitis). Contact bleeding. Left-sided cramps, diarrhoea, mucus and bleeding, tenesmus and pain. Ulcerative colitis affecting only the rectum tends to have a better prognosis than other forms.
- **Ulcerative colitis:** pancolitis: where the whole colon is affected from caecum to rectum. Risk of megacolon. Severe diarrhoea fluid loss, bleeding. Abdominal distension, fever.
- **Crohn's disease:** anywhere mouth to anus, skip lesions, often affects terminal ileum, can be perianal involvement, colitis/proctitis, transmural and often penetrating and fistula with abscess forming inflammation.

Differentials
- *Clostridioides difficile* infection (CDI): see ▶Section 6.11.
- *Campylobacter* infecton: see ▶Section 9.41.
- **CMV colitis** usually in immunocompromised patients mimics ulcerative colitis but biopsies show inclusion bodies and PCR CMV DNA is positive and needs IV Ganciclovir. ▶Section 9.26.
- **Ischaemic colitis** causes bloody diarrhoea with abdominal pain in older patients, with AXR appearance and low BP and AF and raised lactate and atherosclerosis. Surgical consult is needed. ▶Section 6.14.

Severity (modified Truelove and Witt's criteria)
- **Mild:** bloody stool <4/d and at least one of temp <37.5°C, HR <90/min, ESR <20 mm/h, CRP <5 mg/dl, Hb >115 g/L.
- **Moderate:** bloody stool 4–6/d and at least one of temp ≤37.8°C, HR ≤90/min, ESR ≤30 mm/h, CRP <30 mg/dl, Hb >105 g/L.
- **Severe:** bloody stool >6/d and at least one of temp >37.8°C, HR >90/min, ESR >30 mm/h, CRP >30 mg/dl, Hb <105 g/L.
- **Fulminant:** 10 stools/d, continuous bleeding, toxicity, abdomen tender or distension, transfusion requirement, colonic dilation on AXR.

Investigations

- **FBC:** low Hb, low MCV if low Fe, raised MCV if low B12/folate. CRP, raised ESR raised ferritin: acute phase response. **U&E:** AKI. **LFTs:** low albumin. Raised ALP and AST with liver disease. **Serology:** antineutrophil cytoplasmic antibodies **pANCA** positive in ulcerative colitis, anti-*Saccharomyces cerevisiae* antibodies (ASCA).
- **Stool:** culture and sensitivity × 3, ova cysts and parasites and *C. difficile* **toxin testing** if suspected. Exclude an infective cause.
- **Plain AXR:** look for megacolon with colonic diameter >6 cm, perforation, no faeces, mucosal oedema, mucosal islands, thumb printing. Extent of disease can be assessed with reasonable accuracy by the distal extent of faecal residue visible on a plain abdominal radiograph. Should be repeated daily whilst the patient fulfils the criteria for severe colitis and with any evidence of worsening such as an increase in pulse rate, temperature or stool frequency.
- **Small bowel imaging:** suspected Crohn's disease and abdominal symptoms.
- **Flexible unprepared sigmoidoscopy with air insufflation:** can be considered in the absence of colonic dilation. It confirms diagnosis and shows erythematous inflamed, even haemorrhagic, mucosa with contact bleeding and allows biopsies. Ulcerative colitis shows continuous areas of inflamed mucosa.
- **Colonoscopy:** can also be done but not in the acute phase. It can show extent of disease and used to exclude malignancy in long-standing colitis.
- **Barium enema:** may show loss of haustral pattern and featureless colon. Avoided during acute flare-up. Biopsies – goblet cell depletion, inflammatory, mucosal ulcers, crypt abscesses.
- **Abdominal CT or MRI:** if intra-abdominal infection, e.g. abscess suspected or an acute abdomen or perforation suspected. MRI preferred for pelvic Crohn's disease.

Management of severe disease: ensure senior gastroenterology/ colorectal surgical review

- **General:** severe cases admitted with daily senior review at least. AXR to exclude toxic megacolon (>6 cm), stool for culture and *C. difficile* toxin, frequent CRP. Fluid and electrolyte (K) balance. Stool chart. Often dehydrated then ensure IV access and volume replacement. Transfusion as required to match losses to maintain Hb >100 g/L. Potassium replacement at up to 60–100 mmol/d. Stop any antidiarrhoeals, anticholinergics, NSAIDs, opiates which could precipitate megacolon.
- **Aminosalicylates:** mild–moderate: acute attack **Mesalazine** up to 4.8 g PO OD in divided doses until remission (or 12 weeks) then 2.4 g OD or **Balsalazide** 2.25 g TDS until remission. Distal disease: **Mesalazine** foam enemas 1–2 g OD for 4–6 weeks or **Mesalazine** suppository 1 g OD or **Sulfasalazine** 1–2 g QDS PO ± steroids until remission.
- **Steroids severe: Hydrocortisone** 100 mg IV QDS × 5 d – convert to oral when improves. **Prednisolone** 0.5 mg/kg/d PO for 4 weeks then reduce by 5 mg/week. **Distal disease: Prednisolone** foam 20 mg PR or suppository 5 mg or **retention enema** 20 mg/100 ml. Oral and local applied steroids may be combined in moderate–severe disease. If ongoing steroid needs, consider **Omeprazole** 40 mg OD and calcium and cholecalciferol (current formulary preparation is **Calceos** 1 tablet BD). A failure to respond, perforation or toxic megacolon all demand urgent surgical review. Typical clinical signs of perforation may be minimal, because patients are being treated with steroids. Response rate to IV steroids in acute severe colitis is 40%. Oral steroids, e.g. prednisolone, can be used and continued as an outpatient.

- **Treatment failure** after 4 d may lead to a decision to treat with **Ciclosporin** 2 mg/kg/d or **Infliximab** the antibody to TNF administered as a single dose IV infusion of 5 mg/kg under specialist care or colectomy. Side-effects of infliximab are a risk of infection and disseminated TB. This is for specialist use only.
- **Surgery:** a colorectal surgeon should review those with acute severe ulcerative colitis early in their stay. IBD may be complicated by either toxic megacolon, uncontrolled colonic bleeding or failure to settle with optimal medical therapy. Surgery can be life-saving. Early review can help prepare the patient for possible colectomy and introduce them to a stoma therapist. Surgery is either total colectomy with ileo-anal anastomosis and pouch or panproctocolectomy with ileostomy.
- **Enteral feeding:** should be continued as long as tolerated, often in conjunction with other agents including biologicals. Nutrition is fundamental to a good outcome.
- **VTE prophylaxis: LMWH** should be given because this is a prothrombotic period even with mild–moderate bloody stool but watch Hb.

Crohn's disease
- Can develop a severe colitis but in 'unwell patients' exclude any coexisting complex transmural penetrating disease with localised abscess/fistula formation which needs to be treated first where steroids alone could be harmful. Get early expert review. Collections may be seen on USS/CT/MRI.
- Management is with antibiotics, abscess drainage (surgical or USS guidance) and liquid formula diet. Complications of Crohn's include stricture and abscess, fistula formation, perianal disease, infection, colorectal cancer with long-term Crohn's colitis. MRI is best imaging modality for perianal disease. Antibiotics, e.g. **metronidazole** or **ciprofloxacin.** Smoking cessation helps.

Management of mild–moderate disease
- **Mild–moderate colitis:** treated with oral steroids (**Prednisolone** 30 mg reducing dose for 8–10 weeks) and/or an aminosalicylate with telephone or direct advice from IBD specialist nurses, and regular consultant review as needed.
- **Distal disease affecting rectosigmoid:** steroid and mesalazine enemas and suppositories. Mild and moderate cases may go home on steroids if sensible, coping and knowing to return if worsens. Direct telephone access to IBD nurse specialists. Senior assessment if unwell.
- **Reference:** Jakobovits & Travis (2006) Management of acute severe colitis. *Br Med Bull,* 131:75.

6.11 ▶ *Clostridioides difficile* infection

- **About:** diagnosis needs diarrhoea plus a positive toxin test or diarrhoea and clinical suspicion and pending toxin result.
- **Aetiology:** large Gram-positive anaerobic spore-forming bacteria. Found in the soil, bowel or environment as spores. Found in 5–15% of healthy adults. Ribotype 027 causes a virulent form of infection with higher toxin production and quinolone resistance.
- **Risks:** exposure to organism + broad-spectrum antibiotics, elderly, PPI usage, antidepressants. Comorbidities, IBD.
- **Pathophysiology:** toxin A: enterotoxin inactivates Rho-GTPase; toxin B: cytotoxin. Toxins cause hypersecretion, disruption of tight junctions and death of colonic luminal cells. Together these cause ulceration and diarrhoea.

- **Clinical:** diarrhoea 4 d to 6 weeks after antibiotic treatment. Mild diarrhoea to severe colitis with bloody diarrhoea. Copious liquid stool with fever, malaise, abdominal pain, distension, toxic megacolon. Acute abdomen, peritonitis and perforation and death.

Investigations
- **Bloods: FBC:** raised WCC, CRP. **U&E:** prerenal AKI failure.
- **Stool culture:** only test stools for toxin from patients with Type 6–7 diarrhoea for *C. difficile*. Nucleic acid amplification tests (NAAT) such as PCR for *C. difficile* toxin genes are superior to toxins A + B EIA testing. Anaerobic culture on cycloserine, cefoxitin and fructose (CCFA) media. EIA for detecting toxins A and B has sensitivity of 80% and specificity of 98%.
- **AXR/CXR:** look for perforation, ileus, megacolon.
- **CT abdomen and pelvis:** severe disease.

Severity
- **Mild infection:** normal WCC. <3 episodes of loose stools per day.
- **Moderate infection:** raised WCC (<15 × 10^9/L). 3–5 loose stools per day.
- **Severe infection:** WCC >15 × 10^9/L, creatinine >50% increase above baseline), or temp >38.5°C or severe colitis (CT/AXR or clinical).
- **Life-threatening infection:** hypotension, partial or complete ileus, toxic megacolon or CT evidence of severe disease.

Management
- ABC. Supportive. Side room with toilet. IV fluids, VTE prophylaxis. Prevent spore transmission by hand washing with soap and water. Gloves and gowns. Assess severity. Stop Loperamide or drugs which slow GI motility. Stop PPIs and laxatives. Stop NSAIDs, ACEi, ARBs and diuretics.
- **Mild–moderate:** oral **Vancomycin** 125 mg 6 h 14 days.
- **Severe life-threatening:** oral **Vancomycin** 250–500 mg 6 h along with **Metronidazole** 500 mg IV TDS for 10–14 days. Consider adding intracolonic **Vancomycin** 500 mg in 100–500 ml saline 4–12-hourly. Keep oral antibiotics going even if NBM. Take expert help early.
- **Indications for surgery:** low BP needing vasopressors, age >65, WCC >20 × 10^9/L, lactate >5 mmol/L, peritonism, severe ileus, perforation or toxic megacolon, failure to improve after 5 d of medical therapy. Prognosis poor in elderly patients. About 25% can have a relapse.
- **Surgery:** if necessary for severely ill patients, perform subtotal colectomy with preservation of the rectum. Diverting loop ileostomy with colonic lavage followed by antegrade vancomycin flushes is an alternative approach that may lead to improved outcomes.
- **Recurrent or subsequent episodes:** discuss with microbiology fidaxomicin, intracolonic vancomycin or faecal transplantation. **Fidaxomicin** 200 mg BD PO for 10 d, which is non-inferior to vancomycin in curing patients with mild–severe *C. difficile* infection.
- **Reference:** McDonald *et al.* (2018) Clinical practice guidelines for *Clostridium difficile* infection in adults and children: 2017 Update. *Clin Infect Dis.* 66(7):e1.

6.12 Small and large bowel obstruction

- **About:** bowel obstruction can cause bowel ischaemia, infarction, and perforation, peritonitis, sepsis and death. How severe is the obstruction, what level is it at – large bowel obstruction (LBO) or small bowel obstruction (SBO)? What is likely aetiology? Is strangulation present?
- **Aetiology:** ileus, functional **SBO:** adhesions, scars, strictures, hernias, malignancy, Crohn's. **LBO:** colorectal tumours, volvulus, diverticulitis.
- **Complications:** bowel perforation, sepsis, death.
- **Functional obstruction/paralytic ileus:** no mechanical block but does not work. Cause is inflammation, electrolytes, or recent surgery.

Clinical

- **SBO:** crampy abdominal pain, high-pitched tinkling, nausea and early vomiting and central distension and look for an inguinal, femoral hernia.
- **LBO:** colic and abdominal pain. Constipation, ribbon stools and no flatus PR. High-pitched bowel sounds, silent abdomen. PR for a mass or LIF mass. Vomiting uncommon with LBO.

Investigations

- **Bloods:** FBC: raised WCC. U&E: AKI, Ca, LFTs, raised CRP, raised INR if on warfarin, ECG – AF? VBG. SBO – metabolic alkalosis.
- **AXR: SBO:** plain AXR shows many multiple central air–fluid levels. Central small bowel loops dilated >3 cm.Valvulae conniventae across lumen. No gas in large bowel. **LBO:** dilated right and left side of abdomen, large bowel <8 cm and haustra, and the absence of small bowel dilatation on a AXR is worrying as they indicate a competent ileocaecal valve and closed loop large bowel obstruction. A patent ileocaecal valve prevents the pressure in LBO being released into the small bowel. If the obstruction is not relieved, perforation of the caecum and generalised peritonitis eventually occur.
- **CT abdomen scan with IV contrast:** SBO shows dilated small bowel loops (diameter >3 cm from outer wall to outer wall) proximally to normal calibre or collapsed loops distally. LBO dilated bowel and a transition point and cause.

Management

- ABC, NG suction. NBM. IV fluids often several litres deficient, anti-emetics. Analgesia. IV antibiotics if sepsis or perforation. Monitor U&E, CRP, WCC, lactate. Surgical involvement if mechanical obstruction.
- **Small bowel obstruction:** usually adhesions treated conservatively initially as may result in the formation of further adhesions. A strangulated obstruction of the small bowel is a surgical emergency because of the possibility of ischaemic necrosis of the intestinal segment that is distal to the point of strangulation. Surgery. If bowel resection is required, the re-joining of obstructed bowel is often not possible, and a stoma may be necessary.
- **Large bowel obstruction: Ileus** correct fluid and electrolytes and treatment of the underlying disorder. NG decompression may be helpful. Stop medications that slow colonic motility. **Pseudo-obstruction:** neostigmine or colonoscopic decompression. **Volvulus:** endoscopic reduction and decompression of a sigmoid volvulus. Flexible sigmoidoscopy can be both diagnostic and therapeutic – passage of the scope beyond the obstruction often results in a dramatic release of flatus and liquid stool. Caecal or transverse colon volvulus may need surgical resection

and anastomosis. **Intussusception:** a contrast enema (barium or air) may help. Surgery if there are signs of peritonitis or bowel perforation. **Colonic obstruction:** endoscopic dilation and stenting of colonic obstruction or surgery. May help palliative disease.

6.13 Acute colonic pseudo-obstruction

- **About:** colonic obstruction and severe dilation usually in elderly without an obstructive lesion. Consider surgical review to ensure no physical cause.
- **Complications:** colonic dilation, perforation (caecal), peritonitis, death. Risks of perforation if caecal diameter >14 cm, delayed decompression, elderly.
- **Clinical:** abdominal distension (measure abdominal circumference at umbilicus), pain, vomiting, constipation, acute abdomen if perforation.
- **Causes/precipitants:** comorbidities, e.g. CCF, sepsis, renal and respiratory failure, spinal injury. Recent trauma, surgery, burns. Diabetes. Opiates, antimuscarinics, calcium channel blockers, TCA, electrolyte abnormalities.
- **Investigations: FBC:** low Hb, raised WCC. U&E: AKI/dry. Ca, Mg, TSH? hypothyroid. **AXR:** massive colonic dilation most pronounced at caecum so repeat and measure diameter daily if needed. Look for free gas and evidence of perforation. **Abdominal CT scan:** contrast enema or colonoscopy to exclude a physical cause of colonic obstruction. **Water-soluble contrast enema:** can exclude lesion and break up hard faeces. **Colonoscopy:** can exclude obstructive lesion and aid decompression.
- **Management:** supportive: daily review. Exclude a physical obstructive cause. Treat/remove any identifiable cause. Review medications. Correct electrolytes and hydration. **Treat infection.** If vomiting NBM and NG tube to decompress from above. Encourage mobilisation as tolerated, e.g. sit out. **Nutrition:** if prolonged may even need total parenteral nutrition (TPN). Consider **Prucalopride** 1–2 mg PO OD (unlicensed). Anticholinesterase **Neostigmine** 1–2 mg IV over 5 min (treats 85–90% of cases; may be repeated after 3 h). May cause low HR (give **atropine** if significant). **Decompression:** flexible sigmoidoscopy/colonoscopy and/or insertion of a rectal tube considered if caecal diameter >8–9 cm. Repeated until condition settles. **Surgical caecostomy** if not settling conservatively.

6.14 Acute bowel/mesenteric ischaemia

- **About:** seen in older population at risk of atherosclerosis and thromboembolism particularly with AF. Can be small or large bowel, be segmental or diffuse, acute or chronic.
- **Aetiology:** occlusion of vascular supply to gut or low BP causes ischaemia and sepsis. AF, IHD, HTN, smoker, cholesterol, AAA, shock, dissecting aorta, embolism to superior mesenteric artery (SMA). Mechanical – twisting of the blood supply, rarely venous or vasculitis. Very rare – antiphospholipid syndrome, PAN, etc.
- **Anatomy:** coeliac axis supplies distal oesophagus to the descending duodenum. SMA: the transverse and ascending duodenum, the jejunum and ileum, and the large bowel to the splenic flexure. Inferior mesenteric artery (IMA): left colon from the splenic flexure to the rectum.
- **Clinical:** crampy diffuse abdominal pain, vomiting, diarrhoea (bloody), lower GI bleeding, atrial fibrillation, murmurs, chest pain if ACS, low BP and septic or cardiogenic shock, pyrexia, absent or altered bowel sounds, incarcerated hernias.
- **Investigation:** FBC: raised WCC, CRP. Elevated lactate, glucose. Metabolic acidosis. U&Es: AKI. Amylase: exclude pancreatitis. **Erect CXR:** exclude perforation.

AXR: thumb printing due to mucosal oedema, sentinel loop, distended bowel due to ileus, gas due to dilatation caused by ileus, intramural gas from necrotic bowel. **CT abdomen:** thickened bowel loop, oedema, embolism in SMA. ECG: AF, ACS, troponin, TFT, exclude MI. May need echocardiogram.

- **Differential:** AAA, pancreatitis, renal colic, biliary disease, dissection.
- **Management:** ABC, NBM, IV fluids. Analgesia. Manage nutrition – may need TPN post-op. Suspicion of ischaemic bowel warrants laparotomy and resection of compromised section. Percutaneous interventional vascular radiology in acute mesenteric artery occlusion may be considered to aspirate thrombus, thrombolyse or stent. Manage any AKI – good volume support, treat infection. Ongoing AF – assess for later anticoagulation.

6.15 Acute diverticulitis

- **About:** protrusions of mucosa/submucosa through muscular wall of colon.
- **Aetiology:** pouches of mucosa and submucosa herniate through the muscular wall of the bowel at points of weakness. Mainly sigmoid colon. Possibly high intraluminal pressures. Low fibre western diets may play a role.
- **Clinical:** diverticulae are clinically silent in 90% and very common. Diverticulitis classically causes left-sided iliac fossa pain. Fever, N&V, constipation or diarrhoea. Frank bleeding PR which can be significant. Fistula to bladder or vagina with subsequent UTI and foul discharge.
- **Investigations: FBC:** raised WCC. U&E: AKI. raised ESR, raised CRP. **Abdominal USS:** show mucosal thickness, excludes an abscess and pericolic fluid. **Barium enema:** presence of diverticulae. **Flexible sigmoidoscopy and colonoscopy** can show diverticulae but acutely risk of perforation. **Spiral CT of abdomen or CT colonography:** can show diseased sections, narrowing of lumen and thickening of bowel wall and lack of clarity of pericolic fat.
- **Management:** supportive: ABC. If unwell start IV fluids, e.g. 1 L NS. Associated haemorrhage usually managed conservatively. Surgical involvement especially if any signs of bowel perforation or peritonitis. Perforation can lead to fistula formation. If markers of infection consider **Tazocin** 4.5 g TDS IV. Mild attacks may be managed with oral antibiotics as an outpatient. Laparoscopic surgery may be considered. An open Hartmann's procedure may be needed.
- **Complications:** diverticulitis, pericolic abscess. Perforation and peritonitis and/or fistula formation to bladder, uterus, small intestine. Local narrowing and stricture formation and intestinal obstruction.

6.16 Re-feeding syndrome

- **About:** restarting nutrition after a period of starvation. Need to manage low potassium, phosphate, magnesium and give thiamine. Re-feeding (whether it's oral, enteral or parenteral nutrition) triggers a switch from fat to carbohydrate metabolism, with consequent insulin release, and uptake of potassium, phosphate, magnesium and water into cells.
- **Screening for those at risk – any 2 of:** (1) BMI <18.5 kg/m^2, (2) unintentional weight loss >10% in past 3–6 months, (3) little or no nutritional intake for over 5 d, (4) history of alcohol excess or chemotherapy.
- **Clinical:** Wernicke's encephalopathy – encephalopathy, ataxic gait, oculomotor dysfunction, ophthalmoplegia. Look for cardiac or respiratory failure, arrhythmias, rhabdomyolysis, seizures, coma, death.

- **Investigations:** FBC: low Hb. U&E: low K, low Mg, low phosphate. Check lactate and VBG.
- **Management:** prevent by monitoring phosphate and starting re-feeding slowly at 25% normal requirement to minimise rise in insulin. Close involvement of dietitian. Watch potassium, phosphate, magnesium prior to and for the first few days of feeding. Give IV fluids as required. **Potassium:** K 3.0–3.5 mmol/L give **Sando K** (12 mmol each) – 2 TDS, K 2.5–2.9 mmol/L IV KCl 40 mmol in 1 L NS or G5W over 8 h (at 125 ml/h). Concentration must not exceed 40 mmol/L peripherally. Maximum infusion rate is 20 mmol/h unless via a central line with ECG monitoring. **Phosphate:** level 0.5–0.8 mmol/L give **Phosphate Sandoz** (16 mmol each) 2 TDS, level 0.3–0.49 mmol/L give 25 mmol **Phosphate Polyfusor** (250 ml) over 12 h peripherally, level <0.3 mmol/L give 50 mmol PO_4 Polyfusor (500 ml) over 24 h peripherally, measuring PO_4 at 12 h. **Pabrinex** IV paired vials (vitamin B and C) TDS for 1–2 d before giving any carbohydrate. **Magnesium:** level: 0.5–0.7 mmol/L give **Magnaspartate** 1 sachet BD (10 mmol/sachet), level: <0.5 mmol/L give IV **Magnesium sulfate** 35–50 mmol in 1 L NS or G5W over 12–24 h peripherally.

6.17 Ingested foreign bodies and food impactions

- **About:** foreign body and food impactions are seen mainly in children but do occur in adults with learning difficulties and in those who are self-harming. In most cases the risk of harm is minimal and objects pass harmlessly but there are exceptions, which must be noted for early escalation as needed. The need and urgency of intervention depend on patient age and clinical condition. Also depends on size, shape, content, anatomic location and orientation of the ingested object, and the time since ingestion.
- **Clinical:** there may be no symptoms, ranging up to severe chest discomfort and difficulty swallowing or breathing and inability to swallow even saliva. With distal perforation, abdominal pain and symptoms of bowel obstruction or perforation or GI bleeding.
- **Investigations:** lateral and AP radiographs of neck, chest and abdomen can help locate object as well as exclude any mediastinal or peritoneal air. CT scan is possibly more useful. Some materials – small chicken and fish bones or plastics may be difficult to see radiologically.
- **Management:** ABCs. Initially keep NBM and avoid emetics. Avoid oral contrast as this may make endoscopic removal more difficult.

Urgency of endoscopy
- **Emergency:** complete oesophageal obstruction (i.e. unable to manage secretions), disc batteries in the oesophagus, sharp-pointed objects in the oesophagus.
- **Urgent:** oesophageal foreign objects that are not sharp-pointed, oesophageal food impaction in patients without complete obstruction, sharp-pointed objects in the stomach or duodenum, objects >6 cm in length at or above the proximal duodenum, magnets within endoscopic reach.
- **Non-urgent:** coins in the oesophagus may be observed for 12–24 h before endoscopic removal in an asymptomatic patient. Objects in the stomach with diameter <2.5 cm. Disc batteries and cylindrical batteries that are in the stomach of patients without signs of GI injury may be observed for as long as 48 h. Batteries remaining in the stomach longer than 48 h should be removed.

Management of ingested substances

Urgency	Indications for endoscopy
Disc batteries	The current generates NaOH causing localised alkali burns and perforation even within 2 h of ingestion, particularly in the oesophagus. Symptoms can, however, be late up to 28 d. Batteries >2 cm diameter are particularly dangerous. The negative smaller side is more harmful if opposed against mucosa. Batteries only retrieved if signs of injury to the GI tract. A large-diameter battery (>2 cm) in the stomach longer than 48 h, shown by AXR, should be removed. Once past the duodenum, 85% pass out of the body within 72 h. AXR every 3–4 d is adequate to assess progress through the GI tract.
Food bolus impaction	Meat or other materials can become stuck in the oesophagus and endoscopy is needed to either extract piecemeal/advance the bolus. Stricture dilation can be attempted if present. Caution with advancing food if distal oesophagus may be ulcerated particularly with a bolus present for a period of time or a history of eosinophilic oesophagitis.
Miscellaneous	Objects longer than 6 cm are likely to have difficulty passing the duodenum and should be removed.
Magnets	More than one magnet or combined with any metallic object needs to be removed as the adhesion between bowel can cause obstruction and perforation. Consider urgent removal of all magnets within endoscopic reach and for the rest close observation and surgical consultation for non-progression through the GI tract.
Body packers	See ▶ Chapter 14: Toxicology for management.

07 Liver disease

7.1 Jaundice

Pathophysiology

- Jaundice is due to excess circulating bilirubin in the tissues. It is a breakdown product of haem with blood levels >50 μmol/L when it becomes detectable clinically (normal <17 μmol/L). Seen most easily in pale skin in good light or in the scleral part of the eye. It may be seen in 3% of population as Gilbert's syndrome. It must be viewed in clinical context. It is included here as a sign of liver function. Is the patient toxic and unwell, is there pale stool and dark urine, wasting, cachexia and likely cancer? Bilirubin is conjugated with glucuronate within the liver so pre-hepatic is excess unconjugated form. Excreted in urine and faeces and gives them their distinctive yellow and brown colours, respectively. Look for IV drug use, alcohol, toxins, all drugs, history of gallstones, pregnancy. Most commonly the question is whether it is hepatic or post-hepatic and the most critical test is abdominal USS. Severe liver damage causes loss of synthetic function making procoagulant: fibrinogen, prothrombin, factors V, VII, IX, X and XIII. Anticoagulant proteins C and S. NOT gammaglobulins. Antithrombin, transferrin and caeruloplasmin. Albumin $t_{1/2}$ about 20 d. Glucose homeostasis – controlling blood sugar.

Causes of jaundice

- **Pre-hepatic haemolysis** with increased (unconjugated = indirect) bilirubin formation, raised reticulocytes, anaemia, high LDH. Gilbert's syndrome. LFTs are normal.
- **Hepatic:** alcoholic/non-alcoholic and other causes of cirrhosis, hepatitis A/B/C, toxins, drugs, anaesthetic agents, paracetamol, ALF, ischaemia, malignancy, severe right heart failure. Needs liver USS and usual work-up. Viral studies, cirrhosis work-up. Defined by aetiology. Raised ALT/AST, bilirubin. ALP may be elevated.
- **Post-hepatic:** pale stool, dark urine, abdominal pain, fever. Gallstones, worms, strictures, tumour, pancreatic cancer occluding CBD. Cholangitis. Elevated GGT and ALP. AST/ALT may also be raised. Obstruction seen on USS or MRCP. Needs mechanical release – ERCP/surgery.

7.2 Acute liver failure

- **About:** fulminant hepatic failure is where encephalopathy develops in under 2 weeks with a previously normal liver. Prothrombin time is a marker of synthetic function. Get good drug history and ask about over-the-counter and herbal and other natural remedies obtained from shops or internet.
- **Classification based on time from appearance of jaundice to developing encephalopathy.** Hyperacute <1 week: (paracetamol or viral). Massive necrosis. Acute <4 weeks: viral, drugs, others. Subacute 12 weeks: viral, drugs, others.

Causes	Details and notes
Infectious	**Viral hepatitis:** see below. **Bacterial:** leptospirosis, severe bacterial infections. **Protozoal:** amoebic infection.
Paracetamol overdose (1/2 of UK cases)	Within 4 h of presentation give activated charcoal just prior to starting *N*-acetylcysteine. NAC should be used promptly in all patients where paracetamol-induced liver injury is anticipated or there is concern of such and may be given acutely even if cause is unclear. ▶ Section 14.28 for paracetamol overdose protocol.
Other drugs and toxins	MAOIs, halothane, isoniazid, phenytoin, sulphonamides, amiodarone, propylthiouracil, Ecstasy, herbal remedies. *Amanita phylloides* mushroom, carbon tetrachloride. Enquire about all drugs taken, environmental toxins, herbal and natural remedies. Tetracycline, valproate and nucleoside reverse-transcriptase inhibitors can cause fatal liver disease. Many others so check all.
Inherited	**Wilson's disease:** autosomal recessive. Low serum Cu, low caeruloplasmin. Haemolysis. Raised urinary Cu. Treat with penicillamine. **Haemochromatosis:** AR. Iron overload, high ferritin. Transferrin saturation >50%. HFE gene mutation positive >95%. MRI ferriscan or liver biopsy. **Alpha-1 antitrypsin deficiency,** low alpha-1 antitrypsin.
Ischaemic	Circulatory failure and shock. Raised AST. Manage underlying cause.
Venous	**Venous thrombosis: Budd–Chiari syndrome:** acute ascites, USS diagnostic with thrombosed hepatic vein. Consider thrombolysis and TIPS. Hepatic failure is an indication for liver transplantation, provided underlying malignancy is excluded.
Pregnancy	Acute fatty liver of pregnancy, HELLP syndrome with haemolysis, raised AST/ALT and low platelet count. Expeditious delivery needed.
Reye's syndrome	Inhibition of beta-oxidation and uncoupling of oxidative phosphorylation in mitochondria. Acute encephalopathy with fatty infiltration of the liver. Precipitated by aspirin ingestion and viral infections.
Mushroom poisoning	ALF patients with known or suspected mushroom poisoning. Consider administration of **penicillin** G and **silymarin** (III) and should be considered for urgent orthoptic transplantation, the only life-saving option.
Autoimmune hepatitis	Patients with ALF (usually a biopsy is done) due to autoimmune hepatitis should be treated with corticosteroids (**prednisolone** 40–60 mg/d). In ALF patients with evidence of ischaemic injury, cardiovascular support is the treatment of choice.
Malignancy	Hepatoma: check USS and alpha-fetoprotein.
Miscellaneous	**Others:** idiopathic: viral, ischaemia: severe RHF, non-alcoholic steatohepatitis.

- **Clinical:** history of drug/toxin exposure key. Encephalopathy: flapping tremor, poor concentration. Reversal of day/night cycle, jaundice usually but not always – date when first appeared, bleeding and coagulopathy. Hypoglycaemia, fetor hepaticus, look for Kayser–Fleischer rings. RUQ tenderness, NO splenomegaly or ascites, exception is Budd–Chiari syndrome.

- **Identify likely precipitants of acute on chronic decompensation:** sepsis, spontaneous bacterial peritonitis, fluid overload, albumin. Transjugular intrahepatic porto-systemic shunt, renal failure, CNS suppressants. Electrolyte abnormalities, diuretic overuse, GI bleeding.
- **Clinical:** reversal of day/night sleeping, psychomotor dysfunction, impaired memory. Sensory abnormalities, poor concentration, disorientation, tremor, shuffling gait. Melaena, haematemesis. Fetor hepaticus, flapping tremor, asterixis. See Encephalopathy, ▶Section 7.11.
- **Investigations:** FBC: raised WCC, ESR and CRP, low platelets (alcohol, HELLP). Haemolysis in Wilson's disease: low Hb, raised reticulocytes, raised LDH. **Raised** prothrombin time. Raised bilirubin: elevated unconjugated. LFT: raised AST, raised ALT often >1000 (transaminases fall eventually). U&E: raised creatinine. Check paracetamol levels and salicylates. **VBG:** metabolic acidosis and raised arterial lactate and arterial ammonia. **Viral serology:** anti-HAV IgM, HBsAg, anti-HBc IgM, anti-HEV, EBV, CMV, HSV, HIV, anti-HCV (rare cause). **Others:** paracetamol level, caeruloplasmin and 24 h urine copper, ammonia levels. Autoimmune: ANA, anti-smooth muscle actin, anti-liver/kidney microsomal antibodies and immunoglobulins. **USS Doppler:** liver size and pathology, and hepatic veins for Budd–Chiari syndrome. **Miscellaneous:** pregnancy test. ANA, anti-smooth muscle, immunoglobulin, HIV status. **NB:** focal neurology not typical and suggests need for CT brain.
- **Management:** stop all potentially implicated drugs. Regard all as potentially hepatotoxic if no other evident cause. Consider *N*-acetylcysteine (NAC) infusion – possibly useful in both paracetamol and non-paracetamol ALF. **Supportive:** ABCs and O_2 to get and maintain sats >92% and admit to an HDU/ITU environment.
- **Hypovolaemia/low BP:** cross-match blood and transfuse if bleeding or anaemia. 4.5% human albumin solution is the colloid of choice to elevate CVP to 10 cmH_2O or until clinically euvolaemic. G5W if fluids needed (but can worsen hyponatraemia). Give 100 ml 20% human albumin solution per 2.5 L of ascites during paracentesis, or if SBP. Avoid NS (worsens fluid overload).
- **Hypoglycaemia:** stat dose 20 ml 50% IV **Glucose** and then 10% **Glucose** infusion as needed. **Glucagon** 1 mg IM/SC has limited effectiveness if no liver glycogen. ▶Section 5.2.
- **Low K, phosphate, magnesium:** replace as needed (▶Sections 5.4, 5.12, 5.14).
- **Hyponatraemia:** may need hypertonic 3% saline. ▶Section 5.10.
- **Pabrinex IV ×2** TDS for 1–2 d. Provide **thiamine** if alcoholic or malnourished. If suspected Wernicke's syndrome give for 7 d to prevent Korsakoff psychosis. Give before any nutrition/IV glucose. Long-term **Thiamine** 100 mg OD PO.
- **Cerebral oedema:** nurse at 20° head elevation. Consider mechanical hyperventilation to reduce PCO_2. **Mannitol** 200 ml of 20% (20 g/100 ml) IV over 20–30 min may repeat.
- **Stress ulcer prevention:** start IV PPI or **Ranitidine** 150 mg BD PO. PPI is a risk for *C. difficile* and SBP.
- **Antivirals:** Aciclovir for HSV or VZV and ganciclovir for CMV.
- **Antibiotics:** low threshold to treat any infection. Bacterial and fungal. Impaired immunity. Treat if encephalopathy. **Tazocin** 4.5 g 6–8 h IV is often 1st-line.
- **Coagulopathy: Vitamin K** 2–5 mg slow IV, 2–4 units FFP, platelets if <50 × 10^9/L and bleeding. Vitamin K replaces any deficit, so any resulting coagulopathy is entirely due to reduced liver function. However, PT is not always a good indicator of bleed risk in ALF and giving FFP can lead to portal vein thrombosis so assess risk and benefits.

- **Hepatic encephalopathy:** avoid the use of FFP unless actively bleeding. FFP renders the PTT (a vital prognostic marker) less useful. Give **Lactulose** 20 ml BD ± enemas to ensure three bowel movements per day. Use phosphate enemas if unsuccessful. ▶Section 7.11.
- **Ascites and spontaneous bacterial peritonitis,** ▶Section 7.9.
- **Acidosis:** take expert advice and consider IV **NaHCO₃**. A pH <7.3 at >24 h after paracetamol overdose is a poor prognostic indicator.
- **Renal failure** and AKI common with ALF and may require haemofiltration or haemodialysis. ▶Section 10.4.

King's College criteria for liver transplant (discuss early)	
Discuss when	INR >3.0, hepatic encephalopathy, low BP despite resuscitation. Metabolic acidosis. Prothrombin time (seconds) > time from overdose (hours).
Transplant ALF due to paracetamol	pH <7.30 OR (INR >6.5 (PT >100 s) and serum creatinine >300 μmol/L (>3.4 mg/dl) in patients with grade 3 or 4 hepatic encephalopathy).
Transplant ALF due to other cause	INR >6.5 (PT >100 s), OR any 3 of the following: age <10 or >40 y; aetiology non-A, non-B hepatitis, or idiosyncratic drug reaction; duration of jaundice before hepatic encephalopathy >7 d; INR >3.5 (PT >50 s); serum bilirubin >300 μmol/L (>17.6 mg/dl).

7.3 ▶ Viral hepatitis

Causes	Details and management
A	Faeco-oral spread. Incubation 2–6 weeks. Malaise, jaundice. Usually self-limiting. 10% hospitalised. Prevent with vaccination. No chronicity. Check anti-HAV IgM.
B	Commonest viral cause of fulminant hepatitis. Sexual and maternal transmission (90% chronic). Blood, HBsAg, anti-HBcIgM. Incubation 6 weeks to 6 months. Currently no antiviral improves clinical outcome, some may advocate lamivudine. Infants born to HBsAg-positive mothers must receive hepatitis B immunoglobulin and be vaccinated within 12 h of birth. Fulminant hepatitis 1 in 1000.
C	Mild to severe illness. Sharing needles or from maternal route (6 out of 100), sexually rare. Malaise, fever, jaundice. Elevated ALT. Anti-HCV antibodies, HCV RNA. Nearly 10% prevalence in Egypt. Fulminant hepatic failure rare but is seen in HIV-positive men who have sex with men and has been reported sporadically in Asia. Acute infection treated with pegylated interferon.
D	Seen in those with hepatitis B. Prevent by hepatitis B vaccination.
E	Hepatitis E is generally mild unless pre-existing liver disease or pregnant. Causes acute and chronic disease. 4 genotypes. Faeco-oral transfer so need good hand hygiene. Flu-like illness, malaise, jaundice. Send anti-HEV IgM antibodies. Usually self-limiting. 1 in 20 may develop GBS.
Non- A/E	Acute hepatitis of presumed viral cause with negative serology. Due to unknown viruses or variants of hepatitis B.

Others	CMV, EBV, VZV, yellow fever, adenovirus, parvovirus. Patients with known or suspected HSV or VZV as the cause of ALF should be treated with **Aciclovir. Ganciclovir** for CMV.
General	Consider virus-specific therapy for HCV, all with acute viral hepatitis should avoid alcohol consumption and paracetamol. Sexual contact should be avoided if the partner is not immune. Those with sub-fulminant or fulminant hepatitis should be referred early for possible liver transplantation and supported in an ITU setting. The ALT level is not prognostic, but PT and bilirubin and lactate are prognostic.

7.4 Alcoholic hepatitis

- **About:** the aim of the liver clinician is to keep the patient alive long enough to allow them to benefit from alcohol cessation (Hazeldine *et al.*, 2015).
- **Acute liver dysfunction** with jaundice in known alcoholic. Poor prognosis. Discriminant function >32 implies >50% mortality at 1 month. Reversible if patients are non-cirrhotic. The term hepatitis is a misnomer as transaminases (AST and ALT) are marginally elevated.
- **Causes:** acute exacerbation in known alcohol abuser. Look out for SBP. Quantity of alcohol ingested is not always directly proportional to risk of liver disease. Steatohepatitis (fat + hepatocellular injury + inflammation ± fibrosis). Loss of liver function.
- **Clinical:** pyrexia, raised HR, jaundice, encephalopathy, anorexia. Hepatomegaly (tender), abdominal discomfort, nausea, worsening ascites. Alcoholic neuropathy, cerebellar degeneration, cardiomyopathy, AF. Evidence of hepatitis B/C/HIV infection.
- **Aetiology:** polymorphs + necrosis in zone 3. Mallory bodies seen
- **Investigations: FBC, U&E, LFT: raised** WCC, raised reticulocytes (haemolysis suggests Zieve's syndrome), raised CRP, raised bilirubin, AST, ALT (usually <200 rarely >400 U so not a severe biochemical 'hepatitis').
- **Abdominal USS:** hepatomegaly, coarse edge, increased echogenicity, free fluid.
- **Ascitic tap:** if spontaneous bacterial peritonitis suspected – neutrophil count >250 cells/mm^3. Infection seen in 10%. Transudate total protein <30 g/L, e.g. cirrhosis, CCF/RHF, nephrotic syndrome. Exudate has a total protein >30 g/L, e.g. cancer, infection, TB.
- **Specialist tests:** 'hepatic screen': immunoglobulins, anti-mitochondrial antibody, anti-smooth muscle antibody; ANA/dsDNA; ferritin (high in acute illness, check iron studies and transferrin saturation), caeruloplasmin (if <45 y); αFP; anti-HA IgM, HBsAg, anti-HCV ± EBV, CMV ± tumour markers (CA125, CA15-3, CA19-9, CEA, AFP) ± haptoglobin/LDH (haemolysis).
- **Liver biopsy:** histological confirmation is required where there is uncertainty about the diagnosis. 25% of presumed alcoholic hepatitis not confirmed on histology. Trans-jugular biopsy is required if coagulopathy.

Severity scorings to determine prognosis and need for abstention

- Several prognostic scores are available but the most practical one to assess severity is the Glasgow alcoholic hepatitis score (GAHS, see table below). This predicts 28-d and 3-month mortality and can be used as a guide for treatment with corticosteroids or pentoxifylline. It has an overall accuracy of 81% in predicting 28-d mortality.
- **Management:** supportive. Long-term abstinence from alcohol – refer to appropriate support on discharge. Management is supportive care to allow liver

regeneration without additional 'toxin' exposure. Nutrition must be maintained with enteral feeding if required.

- Manage alcohol withdrawal, complications of portal hypertension, ascites, encephalopathy, variceal haemorrhage. **Pabrinex** IV paired vials TDS for 1–2 d + IV **vitamin K.** Commence and continue **Thiamine** 200 mg PO OD. Signs of agitation of alcohol withdrawal consider **Chlordiazepoxide** PO or **Diazepam** PO.

- **Active treatment:** the role of steroids has been questioned by the STOPAH trial. However, some may consider in those with GAHS ≥9 (severe alcoholic hepatitis) either **Prednisolone** 40 mg OD for 28 days (reassess at Day 7) or **Pentoxifylline** 400 mg PO TDS for 28 days. Take local expert advice as some continue to use. If advice to give steroids, ensure all infection is excluded/treated. NAC has also failed to improve 6-month survival. Reassess at Day 7 to decide on continuing steroid/pentoxifylline therapy.

- **Severe liver dysfunction: liver failure (INR >2, albumin <30, encephalopathy)** discuss with local or regional liver centre. In those with decompensated cirrhosis or alcoholic hepatitis then any rise in creatinine by 50% must be met with stopping diuretics and nephrotoxins with plasma expansion with albumin (▶Section 7.11) and renal advice. If signs of encephalopathy give **Lactulose** 20 ml 12 h ± enemas to ensure two bowel movements per day. ▶Section 7.11.

- **Best supportive care** involves access to 24 h endoscopy, expert fluid management, variceal banding and **Terlipressin** 2 mg 4 h for bleeding and early active management of sepsis – the commonest cause of death.

- **Antibiotics:** broad-spectrum antibiotics indicated for variceal bleeding. Prophylactic antibiotics after spontaneous bacterial peritonitis (SBP) such as **norfloxacin** or **ciprofloxacin** should be considered.

- **Early transplantation:** consider with severe alcoholic hepatitis because it reduces mortality, though some will go back to alcohol.

- **References:** European Association for the Study of the Liver (2010) EASL clinical practice guidelines. *J Hepatol*, 533:97. Hazeldine *et al.* (2015) Alcoholic liver disease – the extent of the problem and what you can do about it. *Clinical Medicine,* 15:179. O'Shea *et al.* (2010) Alcoholic liver disease. *Am J Gastroenterol*, 105:14.

Glasgow alcoholic hepatitis score (poor prognosis if score >9)			
Score	1	2	3
Age (y)	<50	≥50	
WCC (× 10^9/L)	<15	≥15	
Urea (mmol/L)	<5	≥5	
Prothrombin ratio	<1.5	1.5–2.0	≥2
Bilirubin (µmol/L)	<125	125–250	>250

7.5 Alcoholic ketoacidosis

- **About:** seen with severe alcoholic liver dysfunction + alcohol and/or starvation. Exclude spontaneous bacterial peritonitis.

- **Clinical:** signs of advanced alcoholic liver disease, raised HR, dehydration. Jaundice, alcoholic hepatitis, ascites, coagulopathy, encephalopathy. Anorexia, N&V may be prominent. May follow 2–3 days after a binge. Ketones detectable in breath, Kussmaul's respiration.

- **Investigations:** FBC, U&E, LFT: low urea or AKI. Raised LFTs. Anaemia. Measure Mg, Ca, phosphate. **Glucose:** hypoglycaemia. Urine: ketones. **Venous blood gas:** raised AG **metabolic acidosis** with raised ketones (beta-hydroxybutyrate). Metabolic alkalosis if vomiting. **Ascites:** test as may have SBP – always aspirate.
- **Management:** supportive as for advanced alcoholic liver disease: IV fluids and IV **Glucose** and IV **Pabrinex** paired vials TDS for 1–2 d. Replace electrolytes and phosphate and magnesium as needed. Long-term abstinence from alcohol and refer to appropriate support on discharge. Alcoholic hepatitis, ▶Section 7.4.

7.6 Alcohol abuse

- **About:** alcohol is a colourless odourless liquid and liver toxin freely available for adults to consume in harmful amounts. Additives give the associated smell. It is a CNS depressant and sudden withdrawal can cause hyperexcitability, delirium and seizures. Alcohol misuse is common.
- **Alcohol history** from all patients. In those suspected of alcohol abuse start by suggesting one bottle of spirits a day and see what they say. Patients will often under report. Ask about the alcoholic life – what time they have their first and last drink, who gets the drink, falls, head injuries, violence, if children at risk involve social services, the central role alcohol takes, do they drink with someone, are they suicidal. What is their view, do they want to stop or simply cut back. Drinking is legal and a competent patient can self-discharge and go and do very little.
- **Recommended** limit of 14 units/week (males and females). 1 unit = 8 g alcohol = small glass of wine or half pint of beer. The liver effect of alcoholism is one facet compared to its effects on relationships, children, violence, unemployment, drink driving, hypertension, mental health issues.
- **Alcohol cessation:** sudden acute alcohol withdrawal can lead to DTs 1–3 days later and is potentially lethal. Patients should be encouraged to gradually reduce their alcohol intake over time.

CAGE questionnaire is recommended
Alcohol problem very likely if 2 or more positive answers to the following:
- Have you felt you should **C**UT down on drinking?
- Have you been **A**NGERED by suggestions you cut down?
- Have you felt **G**UILTY about drinking?
- Have you used alcohol as an **E**YE-opener in the morning?

Clinical presentations of alcohol abuse
- **Alcoholic hepatitis:** jaundiced, toxic, unwell, elevated ALT. ▶Section 7.4.
- **Liver failure:** jaundice, coagulopathy, encephalopathy, ascites. ▶Section 7.2.
- **Delirium tremens (DTs):** hyperactive delirium. Agitated, fever, sweating, picking at bedclothes (now is the time to treat), hallucinations, e.g. rats, terrified – can progress to acute seizure. ▶Section 7.8.
- **Suicide:** always ask about suicidal thoughts. Needs mental health review.
- **Trauma:** assaults, brain injury from falls and assaults, RTC.
- **Alcoholic cerebellar ataxia:** chronic cerebellar disease with ataxia.
- **Social:** spending one's life focused on obtaining and consuming alcohol leads to unemployment, divorce, homelessness, malnutrition, violence.
- **Cancer risk:** hepatoma, pancreatic cancer, oesophagus, head and neck.
- **Medical and social costs of alcoholism:** head injury, falls, assaults, road traffic accidents, seizures, overdoses, suicidal attempts, self-harm. Cerebral haemorrhage,

hypothermia, meningitis and chest infections, cardiomyopathy. Ketoacidosis, pneumococcal infections, low potassium, magnesium and calcium. Renal failure, Wernicke's and Korsakoff's psychosis and B_1 deficiency. Variceal haemorrhage and liver disease, peptic ulcer disease. Peripheral neuropathy, cerebellar degeneration, atrial fibrillation. Social and family break-up, abuse, divorce, poverty, violence.

- **Management:** alcohol-induced liver damage is silent often until a late stage when it presents in 80% as decompensated cirrhosis or alcoholic hepatitis. Long-term abstinence from alcohol is needed to allow liver regeneration. All attempts should be made to identify and change harmful behaviour early with information and coping strategies. A coordinated approach from primary and secondary care is needed as well as governmental and societal changes and attitudes to alcohol. Screening tools involve questionnaires in those at risk, GGT has a high predictive value in terms of liver disease and death. **Liver elastography** can assess fibrosis and is helpful. Various blood markers of fibrosis are being examined. See ▶ Section 7.4 on alcoholic hepatitis for further information on acute presentation.

7.7 Zieve's syndrome

- **About:** rare, differential of bleeding in alcoholic liver disease.
- **Clinical:** jaundice, RUQ pain (alcoholic hepatitis), alcohol-related issues.
- **Investigations:** FBC: low Hb, raised reticulocytes, raised LDH, low haptoglobins. U&E/LFTs: raised bilirubin.
- **Blood film:** anaemia, spherocytosis due to haemolysis. Raised triglycerides.
- **Management:** supportive. Alcohol avoidance. Haematinics as needed.

7.8 Delirium tremens/alcohol withdrawal

- **About:** a cause of seizures and coma. Exclude SDH, pneumococcal bacterial meningitis, drugs. Best predictor is a past history of alcohol-related DTs.
- **Aetiology:** related to alcohol withdrawal. 1–4 days after last drink. Mortality is 15%. It is a central depressant. Withdrawal causes a hyperadrenergic state.
- **Clinical:** delirium, agitation, autonomic instability tachycardia, hypertension, low-grade fever, and diaphoresis. Develop seizures, aspiration, respiratory failure, arrhythmias. Fever, visual hallucinations and seizures occur after 24 h, peaking at 50 h. Signs of advanced alcoholic liver disease, dehydration. Jaundice, alcoholic hepatitis, ascites, coagulopathy, encephalopathy.
- **Differential:** opiate or cocaine use, hypoglycaemia, head injury (SDH/stroke/skull fracture). Sepsis, hepatic encephalopathy, psychotic illness. Encephalitis, non-convulsive status.
- **Investigations:** FBC, U&E and LFT. CRP: exclude infection and liver failure. **CXR:** exclude tumour, infection, TB, aspiration, perforation. **Sepsis screen:** chest, urine, aspirate ascites to exclude spontaneous bacterial peritonitis. ECG: exclude MI, AF. **Coagulation screen** if possible liver failure. **CT head:** if concerned about head injury or stroke or subdural haematoma, or some other pathology. Have a low threshold to scan if concerned. **LP:** if suspected meningitis (pneumococcal seen in alcoholics).
- **Management:** supportive: ABC, O_2 as per BTS guidelines. Manage in a well-lit area; involve family or known trusted carers to reduce anxiety. If significant sedation is needed then consider HDU/ITU environment for ABC. Monitor glucose, Mg and K and dehydration and treat accordingly. Agitated confused patient: start a

reducing dose regimen of **Chlordiazepoxide** or **Diazepam.** Determine when was last drink. Fits tend to classically occur about 48–96 h later. Titrate the dose to the level of agitation. Fixed dose schedule: (consider higher doses in very agitated and those with high body weight; watch for over-sedation): <u>days 1–2</u>: **Chlordiazepoxide** 10–30 mg 6 h. <u>Days 3–4</u>: **Chlordiazepoxide** 10 mg 8 h. <u>Days 5–6</u>: **Chlordiazepoxide** 10 mg 12 h and stop. Early discharge (>48 h) possible if asymptomatic and 24/7 supervision until days 5–6.

* **Seizures:** manage as status epilepticus (▶Section 11.15). Monitor GCS and ABCs. May need nasopharyngeal airway, recovery position and HDU bed or even ITU. Take advice if GCS <9. Low threshold to CT head if any concerns about head injury, SDH, meningitis, delirium, stroke. In the case that you are unable to convince the patient to take medications then **Lorazepam** 1–2 mg IV/IM or **Diazepam** IV/PO could be considered. **Avoid Haloperidol.** Identify early and sedate patients likely to 'go off' when they are compliant. Start as soon as any hyperactive features appear or high risk, e.g. a patient with previous delirium tremens and now off alcohol. Watch for over-sedation and precipitating encephalopathy. Consider HDU/ITU. Prophylactic anticonvulsants not usually recommended.

* **Wernicke–Korsakoff syndrome:** ataxia, ophthalmoplegia, nystagmus, low BP, memory disturbance, comatose, confusion, hypothermia. Give IV **Pabrinex** two sets of paired ampoules TDS for 3–5 d and then **Thiamine** 200 mg PO OD. ▶Section 15.16.

7.9   Cirrhosis, ascites and bacterial peritonitis

* **About:** decompensated cirrhosis is a medical emergency with a high mortality. Effective early interventions can save lives and reduce hospital stay. Complete checklist in all with decompensated cirrhosis within the first 6 h of admission.

* **Clinical:** jaundice, increasing ascites, hepatic encephalopathy, renal impairment, GI bleeding, signs of sepsis/hypovolaemia, occasionally signs may be minimal. May be mild to severe abdominal pain, ascites and generalised tenderness and signs of liver disease. Document current alcohol intake and other drugs.

* **Ascites grading:** grade 1 (mild) – detectable only by USS. Grade 2 (moderate) – moderate symmetrical distension of the abdomen. Grade 3 (large) – marked abdominal distension.

* **Precipitants:** GI bleeding (variceal and non-variceal), infection/sepsis (SBP, urine, chest, cholangitis, etc.), alcoholic hepatitis, acute portal vein thrombosis, development of hepatocellular carcinoma, drugs (alcohol, opiates, NSAIDs, etc.), ischaemic liver injury (sepsis or low BP), dehydration, constipation.

Investigations

* FBC, U&E, LFT, coag. screen, glucose, Ca/Mg/phosphate, blood cultures, urine dip/ MSU and CXR for infection, CRP.

* **Liver USS:** liver size, coarse edge, increased echogenicity, free fluid throughout abdomen, hepatocellular carcinoma, portal vein or hepatic vein thrombosis, renal tract abnormalities.

* **Aspirate of ascites:** in all within 24 h (SBP can be clinically silent): a 10 ml aspirate with a blue/green needle in all unwell patients with ascites to exclude SBP: raised WCC and CRP. Neutrophil count >250 cells/mm^3 and low pH of ascitic fluid. Gram stain and aerobic and anaerobic culture. Measure ascitic protein because SBP more common with ascitic albumin <15 g/L and may need antibiotic prophylaxis.

Secondary peritonitis is likely if ascitic fluid shows >1200 cells/mm^3. Serum/ascites albumin gradient: >11 g/L suggests portal hypertension. Cirrhotic patients with low ascitic fluid protein concentration (<10–15 g/L) and/or high serum bilirubin levels are at high risk of SBP so consider prophylactic antibiotics.

- **Management: ABC, HDU** if worsening NEWS and liver failure. **Sodium restriction:** moderate restriction of salt intake to sodium of 80–120 mmol/d, which corresponds to 4.6–6.9 g of salt/d. No added salt diet. Avoid pre-prepared meals. Avoid IV NS. Alcohol ingestion then give IV **Pabrinex** 2 pairs of vials TDS for 1–2 d.

Managing ascites

- **Spontaneous bacterial peritonitis:** diagnostic paracentesis >250 polymorphs/ mm^3 (0.25 × 10^9)/L. Treat with antibiotics, e.g. **Tazocin** 4.5 g TDS IV or **Ceftriaxone** 1–2 g IV OD for at least 5 d or as per local policy. EASL guidelines recommend **human albumin** (HAS) (day 1 give 1.5 g/kg and day 3 give 1 g/kg); reduced the incidence of hepatorenal syndrome from 30% to 10% and mortality from 29% to 10%. Following an episode of SBP patients should be considered for **Norfloxacin** 400 mg OD as prophylaxis. **Quinolones** have been used but increase risk of *C. difficile.* ▶Section 6.11.
- **Fluid/salt balance:** restrict dietary Na <90 mmol/d (5.2 g). Lowers diuretic requirement and increases resolution of ascites and shorter hospital stay.
- **Diuretics:** start **Spironolactone** 100 mg OD. There is a 3–5 day lag before natriuresis (urine Na > K) then add a loop diuretic, e.g. **Furosemide** 40–160 mg/d. Use spironolactone and furosemide in a ratio 50 mg to 20 mg, respectively. Spironolactone max dose 400 mg. Review diuretics and take advice if Na <125 mmol/L or serum creatinine rising >0% from baseline.
- **Steroids:** have been advocated for severe alcohol hepatitis but evidence is contentious. They increase risk of serious infections. Exclude/treat infection first. Use under expert guidance. Pentoxifylline has also been recommended but evidence again is not clear.
- **Therapeutic paracentesis:** recommended with large ascites. If renal function normal then administer **1 unit (100 ml) HAS 20%** following every 3 L drained or for every 2 L if there is impaired renal function. Failure to volume expand risks circulatory dysfunction + renal failure. Albumin better than artificial plasma expanders. Ascites recurs in 90% of patients if diuretics not begun and in 20% despite diuretics. **Do NOT leave drain *in situ* overnight or more than 6 h.** ▶Section 21.6.
- **Hyponatraemia:** ratio of Na >126 mmol/L, no need for H$_2$O restriction and continue diuretics if renal function stable. If Na <125 mmol/L consider stopping diuretics, especially if Na <121 mmol/L if creatinine rising (>150 μmol/L), volume expansion maintaining renal function is crucial. The maximum recommended weight loss during diuretic therapy should be 0.5 kg/d in patients without oedema and 1 kg/d in patients with oedema. ▶Section 5.10.
- **Prevent AKI:** increase in serum creatinine ≥26 μmol/L within 48 h, or ≥50% rise in serum creatinine over the last 7 d, or urine output <0.5 ml/kg/h for more than 6 h based on dry weight, or clinically dehydrated then suspend all diuretics and nephrotoxic drugs. Fluid resuscitates with 5% HAS or 0.9% NS (250 ml boluses with regular reassessment: 1–2 L will correct most losses). Monitor daily weights and aim for MAP >80 mmHg to achieve urine output >0.5 ml/kg/h based on dry weight. At 6 h, if target not achieved or EWS worsening then consider escalation to higher level of care. ▶Section 10.4.

- **GI bleed:** fluid resuscitate according to BP, pulse and venous pressure (aim for MAP >65 mmHg), suspected variceal bleed **Terlipressin** IV (caution if IHD or PVD; perform ECG in >65 y). If PT prolonged give IV **Vitamin K** 10 mg stat. If PT >20 s (or INR >2.0) – give FFP (2–4 units). If platelets <50 give IV platelets. Transfuse blood if Hb <7.0 g/L or massive bleeding (aim for Hb >8 g/L). Early endoscopy after resuscitation (ideally within 12 h). ▶Section 6.4.
- **Encephalopathy: lactulose** 30 ml QDS or phosphate enema (aiming for 2 soft stools/d). CT if SDH in differential. ▶Section 7.11.
- **Antibiotics:** sepsis start **Tazocin** 4.5 g TDS IV or **Ceftazidime** 1–2 g 8 h IV. Alternatives include **Ciprofloxacin** 500 mg BD PO/400 mg BD IV. Resolution is seen in 90%. Prophylaxis should also be considered.
- **Liver transplant:** those who survive an episode of SBP should be considered for liver transplantation.
- **Transjugular intrahepatic portosystemic shunt** (TIPS) for refractory ascites. 25% risk encephalopathy. Can cause heart failure.
- **VTE prophylaxis:** prescribe prophylactic LMWH (patients with liver disease are at a high risk of thromboembolism even with a prolonged PT; withhold if patient is actively bleeding or platelets <50).
- **References:** European Association for the Study of the Liver (2010) EASL clinical practice guidelines. *J Hepatol*, 533:97. Wiest *et al.* (2012) Spontaneous bacterial peritonitis: recent guidelines and beyond. *Gut*, 61:297.

7.10 Hepatorenal syndrome

- **About:** AKI with acute liver failure and cirrhosis – presents with oliguria. Exclude other causes of AKI first especially prerenal.
- **Aetiology:** splanchnic vasodilation with renal vasoconstriction, afferent renal vasoconstriction. Exclude prerenal failure by a trial of volume expansion.
- **Causes:** 40% of those with cirrhosis and ascites develop AKI. Causes are shock, diarrhoea, diuretics, sepsis, ATN, prerenal disease, drugs, paracentesis, obstruction or parenchymal renal disease. Exclude SBP as a cause.
- **Risk factors:** MAP <80 mmHg, dilutional hyponatraemia, urinary Na <5 mmol/L.
- **Differentials: prerenal failure, ATN,** nephrotoxic drugs, parenchymal renal disease (proteinuria/haematuria, abnormal renal USS), obstructive nephropathy, glomerulonephritis.
- **Classification. Type 1:** rapid AKI with oliguria. Creatinine quickly >350 µmol/L. Precipitated by spontaneous bacterial peritonitis (25% of patients), bleed or infection. Characterised by diuretic-resistant ascites, encephalopathy. Most die within 10 weeks. May respond to **terlipressin** which reduces splanchnic vasodilation (see below). **Type 2:** moderate and stable reduction in the GFR, median survival of 3–6 months. Slower. Creatinine rarely >180 µmol/L.
- **Criteria for diagnosis of hepatorenal syndrome in cirrhosis:** (1) cirrhosis with ascites + serum creatinine >133 µmol/L (1.5 mg/dl). (2) No sustained improvement of serum creatinine (to <133 µmol/L) despite 2 d of diuretic withdrawal and volume expansion with albumin (1 g/kg of body weight per day up to a maximum of 100 g/d). (3) Absence of shock. No current or recent nephrotoxic drugs, e.g. NSAIDs, etc. No parenchymal disease (no proteinuria >500 mg/d or microhaematuria (>50 RBC/high powered field)) and normal renal USS.
- **Clinical:** fatigue, malaise, progressive uraemia with oliguria without significant proteinuria. Chronic liver disease, ascites, jaundice, encephalopathy. Abdominal pain/ascites, e.g. SBP, ▶Section 7.9.

- **Investigations:** FBC, U&E, creatinine >130 µmol/L, creatinine clearance <40 ml/min. Check LFTs, PT. Urine culture and urinalysis: urine volume <500 ml/d. Proteinuria <500 mg/d. Urine Na <10 mmol/d. Urine osmolarity > plasma osmolarity. Urine RBC count <50 cells/high powered field.
- **Abdominal USS:** no renal parenchymal disease or obstruction to explain AKI, cirrhosis, ascites.
- **Sepsis screen:** diagnostic paracentesis for SBP, CXR, urinalysis, blood cultures.
- **Management:** specialist supportive care and nephrology review. Exclude other causes of AKI such as shock, ongoing infection or recent treatment with nephrotoxic drugs. Treat hypovolaemia with fluid challenge. Failure to respond suggests hepatorenal. Withdraw diuretics and other nephrotoxic drugs. Look for SBP and treat usually with **cefotaxime. In alcoholic hepatitis: pentoxifylline** 400 mg PO TDS may be used. **Vasopressin** and **noradrenaline** may be used but get specialist help. **Terlipressin,** a vasoconstrictor predominantly in the splanchnic circulation, is given as a dose of 0.5–2.0 mg IV QDS especially in type 1 in addition to day 1: 1 g HAS/kg; days 2–16: 20–40 g HAS/d. Diuretics are usually avoided. Continue until serum creatinine falls below 130 µmol/l. Where creatinine is rising despite treatment, 60 g HAS/d may be clinically indicated. As ever take expert guidance. **Octreotide** 100–200 mcg SC TDS may be used instead of **terlipressin.** Liver transplantation is usually indicated in types 1 and 2 and is the main definitive therapy. Transjugular intrahepatic porto-systemic shunting may be considered. Also see AKI, ▶Section 10.4.
- **References:** European Association for the Study of the Liver (2010) EASL clinical practice guidelines. *J Hepatol*, 533:97. Ginès & Schrier (2009) Renal failure in cirrhosis. *N Engl J Med*, 361:1279.

7.11 Hepatic encephalopathy

- **About:** potentially reversible neuropsychiatric disorder in those with liver failure. Exclude unrelated neurologic and/or metabolic abnormalities.
- **Aetiology:** associated with arterial NH_4 levels and other protein breakdown products crossing blood–brain barrier.
- **Identify likely precipitants: sepsis:** chest, urine, biliary, spontaneous bacterial peritonitis. **Metabolic:** fluid overload or electrolyte, e.g. low Na, low K, diuretic overuse. Transjugular intrahepatic porto-systemic shunt, renal failure. **Drugs:** sedatives, NSAIDs, CNS suppressants. **GI bleeding:** which may be variceal or non-variceal. Ischaemic liver injury: low BP, sepsis. **Acute portal vein thrombosis:** needs USS. Development of hepatocellular carcinoma continued alcohol intake.
- **Clinical:** reversal of day/night sleeping, psychomotor dysfunction, impaired memory. Sensory abnormalities, poor concentration, disorientation, tremor, shuffling gait. Melaena, haematemesis. Fetor hepaticus, flapping tremor, asterixis.

Grades of encephalopathy
- I: anxiety, mild confusion, reversed sleep/wake cycles, apathy, asterixis.
- II: + moderate confusion, disorientation, rigidity.
- III: + severe confusion, somnolence, incontinent, Babinski's sign.
- IV: + coma, decerebrate posturing.

Investigations
- **FBC, U&E and LFT:** raised WCC, AST/ALT, PT, alpha-fetoprotein.
- **Abdominal USS:** cholangitis, hepatocellular cancer, ascites, liver size.

- **Blood ammonia level:** raised due to GI bleeding, renal failure, hypovolaemia, urea cycle disorder, TPN, urosepsis, valproic acid.
- **CT head:** rules out acute bleeding.
- **Lumbar puncture:** if encephalitis suspected (check coag and plt first).
- **Diagnostic ascitic tap:** for spontaneous bacterial peritonitis.
- **EEG:** symmetrical slowing with (non-specific) triphasic waves.
- **Others:** exclude hypoxia, hypercarbia, uraemia, hypoglycaemia.
- **Ascitic tap always:** exclude spontaneous bacterial peritonitis.

Management

- **Supportive:** manage dietary input including adequate protein (1.5 g/kg/d) and calories (30 kcal/kg/d). Watch for re-feeding issues. Assessment by a dietitian with experience in liver disease is useful. Grade III or more encephalopathy consider intubation to protect airways and other supportive treatment often needed.
- **Drugs:** avoid opiates, NSAIDs, benzodiazepines. Check drugs for safety.
- **Precipitants:** look for and treat any cause, e.g. antibiotics for infection, paracetamol overdose, dehydration, manage bleeding, volume replace cautiously, avoid alcohol, diagnostic paracentesis for SBP and review all drugs.
- **Lactulose 20–50 ml BD** to give 3 loose stools per day. **Phosphate enema** BD may be needed. Lactulose is metabolised by bacteria in the colon to acetic and lactic acid, which reduces colonic pH, decreases survival of urease-producing bacteria in the gut, and aids conversion of ammonia (NH_3) to ammonium (NH_4), which is less readily absorbed by the gut.
- **Antibiotics: Ceftriaxone** 1–2 g/d. Consider **Rifaximin** 600 mg BD for 6 months, maintained remission from hepatic encephalopathy compared with placebo and significantly reduced hospitalisation (91% of the patients were using concomitant lactulose). **Metronidazole** 250 mg BD is also useful. Avoid neomycin.
- **L-ornithine L-aspartate** has a possible beneficial effect on mortality, hepatic encephalopathy, and serious adverse events in comparisons with placebo or no-intervention, but the quality of the evidence is very low.
- **References:** Bass *et al.* (2010) Rifaximin treatment in hepatic encephalopathy. *N Engl J Med*, 362:1071. Ginès & Schrier (2009) Renal failure in cirrhosis. *N Engl J Med*, 361:1279.

7.12 ▶ Chronic liver disease

- **About:** chronic liver disease (CLD) contrasts with ALF as management of declining liver function. Complications such as SBP, varices, acute decompensation need management. The aim is to preserve function long enough for transplant if possible.

Initial investigation for CLD of unknown aetiology

- FBC, LFTs, clotting screen, immunoglobulins – increased IgG in autoimmune, IgA in alcohol, IgM in PBC.
- Anti-mitochondrial (PBC), anti-smooth muscle, ANA in autoimmune hepatitis and renal failure in the presence of cryoglobulins (seen in viral disease specifically).
- Hepatitis viral/bacterial serology, alpha-1-antitrypsin, alpha-fetoprotein.
- Ferritin, copper, caeruloplasmin and urinary copper ± penicillamine challenge test (in patients <40 with unexplained CLD or seronegative hepatitis).
- Urinalysis and 24 h urine for creatinine clearance and protein, ECG, CXR, ultrasound and Doppler studies of abdomen, CT, MRI/MRCP studies may be needed.

Complications/associations of CLD

- Ascites in liver disease and spontaneous bacterial peritonitis (▶Section 7.9).
- Hepatic encephalopathy (▶Section 7.11).
- Coagulopathy: upper GI bleed and varices (▶Section 6.4).
- Renal impairment or hepatorenal syndrome (▶Section 7.10).

Assess mortality risk in cirrhosis: use Child–Pugh score	
Encephalopathy	None = +1, controlled/minimal = +2, advanced = +3.
Ascites	None = +1, mild = +2, moderate/severe = +3.
Bilirubin	(µmol/L): <34 = +1, 34–51 = +2, >51 = +3; in PSC/PBC the score levels are set higher: 68 = +1, and 170 = +2.
Albumin	(g/L): >35 = +1, 28–35 = +2, <28 = +3.
Prothrombin time (INR)	<4 s (INR 1.7) = +1, 4–6 s (INR 1.7–2.2) = +2, >6 s (INR >2.2) = +3.
Add scores	5–6: Class A has 100% 1 y survival 7–9: Class B has 81% 1 y survival 10–15: Class C has 45% 1 y survival

7.13 ▶ Liver abscess

- **Three types:** local bacteria, amoebic (*Entamoeba histolytica*), echinococcus (*E. granulosus*).
- **Clinical:** fever, abdominal pain, hepatomegaly, jaundice. Right pleural effusion, pleural rub. Occasionally abscesses are well tolerated and may present as PUO. Anaphylaxis (*E. granulosus*).
- **Investigations:** FBC: low Hb, raised neutrophil, raised CRP, raised ALP, raised B12. Serology can be useful – see below. CXR: raised right hemidiaphragm. Abdominal USS and CT diagnostic for liver abscess.
- **Differential:** liver cyst, hepatoma, metastases.
- **Management:** antibiotics are the 1st-line in therapy and then some require open or radiologically guided percutaneous drainage depending on the response (see below).

Causes

- **Pyogenic:** from appendicitis, cholecystitis, diverticulitis. Older patients. Multiple lesions, possible bowel malignancy. Diagnosis: USS, raised LFTs. Management: IV antibiotics and drainage. Foul smelling pus. Treat **Co-amoxiclav** 1.2 g 8 h or **Tazocin** 4.5 g TDS IV. Alternatives are **cefotaxime.** Consider adding **metronidazole** if causative organism unclear.
- **Amoebic:** see Amoebiasis, ▶Section 9.49.
- **Hydatid disease:** tapeworm infection. *E. granulosus* cysts in liver, lungs and bones usually asymptomatic and patients are well unless secondarily infected. Hydatid cyst rupture can lead to anaphylaxis. Hydatid serology 90% positive. Mortality is related to anaphylaxis and sudden death reported. Management: surgery remains the primary treatment and the only hope for complete cure. The puncture, aspiration, injection, and reaspiration (PAIR) technique is suggested with open surgery as a further option along with appropriate agents such as **albendazole** and **mebendazole** combination. Risk of anaphylaxis is, however, significant.

7.14 ▶ Gallstone disease and local complications

- **About:** commoner in women. Gallstones 10% of the population. Most are silent.
- **Risks:** mainly in females, middle age and beyond, obesity, those on octreotide. Liver disease, e.g. cirrhosis, rapid weight loss and fasting. Rare in black people other than sickle cell disease with haemolysis.
- **Aetiology:** lithogenic bile, raised insoluble cholesterol and insufficient bile acids. Obstruction of the gallbladder neck or cystic duct by a gallstone. Inflammation is more likely chemical rather than infective as bile is usually sterile.
- **Bacterial infection:** *E. coli*, *Klebsiella*, *Strep. faecalis*, and anaerobic organisms.

Pathophysiology and clinical presentations of gallstones	
Biliary colic	Gallstone stuck at cystic duct. Waves of RUQ or epigastric pain, N&V. Lasts 20 min then may return.
Acute cholecystitis	Inflamed gallbladder. Blocked cystic duct. May be bacterial infection and infected bile. Severe RUQ pain, fever. Murphy's positive pressure on RUQ catches patient on inspiration.
Emphysematous cholecystitis	Gas-producing bacteria in gallbladder. Blocked cystic duct. Classically male diabetics. Similar to cholecystitis. Toxic. Gas seen on AXR/CT.
Acalculous cholecystitis	Seen in critical care. Trauma or burns, those on TPN, etc. High mortality (see below). Possibly due to poor GB emptying.
Chronic cholecystitis	Ongoing inflamed gallbladder. Colic. May be asymptomatic. Develops 'porcelain gallbladder'.
Gallbladder perforation	Gallbladder perforates due to erosion and ischaemia. Stones pass into peritoneal cavity. Peritonitis. Fever, RUQ mass. High mortality.
Acute cholangitis	Fever, jaundice, rigors, sepsis (▶ Section 7.15).
Acute pancreatitis	With stones in common bile duct (▶ Section 7.16).

Investigations

- **Bloods:** FBC and U&E: raised WCC, CRP, creatinine, urea. LFT: bilirubin, ALP, GGT (esp. if common bile duct blocked), raised mild ALT and AST.
- **Abdominal USS:** gallstones, enlarged hydropic gallbladder with a thickened wall in the region of maximum tenderness. Gallstones in gallbladder and/or cystic duct or common bile duct. USS is more sensitive than CT for acute gallstone disease. USS can pick up stones as small as 2 mm. Identifies thickened wall gallbladder and gallbladder distension (>4 cm short axis) and pericholecystic fluid. Operator can also look for a positive Murphy's sign. Stones in common bile duct suggested if duct diameter >7 mm.
- **ERCP with cholangiogram** and sphincterotomy be needed for ductal stones.
- **Complications:** biliary sepsis, cholangitis, empyema (pus) of the gallbladder. Perforation and peritonitis, death occasionally.

Management

- ABC, O_2 as per BTS guidelines + IV access + NBM. NG tube if vomiting. **Fluids:** 1 L crystalloids (NS or Hartmann's) over 2–4 h and assess volume needs and replace.

- **Pain relief:** IM NSAIDs or **Morphine** 5 mg IV. Anti-emetics: **Cyclizine** 50 mg slow IV or **Ondansetron** 8 mg PO/IV BD. **Antibiotics: Tazocin** 4.5 g TDS IV for 10 d. Penicillin allergy **Cefuroxime** 1.5 g TDS IV + **Metronidazole** 500 mg TDS IV.
- **Surgical management:** a lap cholecystectomy is standard of care and should be carried out urgently within days of onset of symptoms unless frailty precludes it otherwise the patient is prone to further episodes. Early surgery has shorter stay, less pain and less mortality than open surgery. Those unfit for surgery may have temporary drainage. Commonest complication is bile leak which can be managed by ERCP and stenting. Conversion to open surgery is commoner in older, males, obesity, previous abdominal surgery. A fistula between GB and small bowel may result in a stone causing small bowel obstruction.
- **Biliary colic alone which settles within 6 h and no cholecystitis can go home with adequate pain control and have surgical review later.** Ask to return if worsens especially fever or worsening pain or severe vomiting. Murphy's negative.
- **Acalculous cholecystitis** can occur with no stones seen but a typical acute cholecystitis picture. Prognosis is worse. Seen with diabetes, fasting, TPN, sepsis, trauma, burns, opiates, IHD. Treat with antibiotics and supportive management. Gangrene and perforation are more common. Urgent cholecystectomy may be indicated. Other methods to treat chronic stones are oral bile acids (**Ursodeoxycholic acid**) or extracorporeal shock wave lithotripsy (ESWL).

7.15 Acute cholangitis

- **Aetiology:** bacterial infection of the biliary tree usually due to stones or impaired drainage within the common bile duct. Mortality 5–10%. Early ERCP and early antibiotic therapy.
- **Causes:** gallstones predominantly, strictures, sclerosing cholangitis, chronic pancreatitis, HIV-related cholangiopathy. **Rare:** clonorchis, ascarisis.
- **Clinical:** Charcot's triad of non-colicky RUQ pain to right shoulder, jaundice and fever. Biliary obstruction – dark urine and pale stool.
- **Investigations:** FBC, U&E, LFT: raised WCC, raised bilirubin, raised ALP, raised GGT, raised ALT. Blood cultures positive in half.
- **Abdominal USS:** enlarged hydropic gallbladder with a thickened wall and stones. Stones in common bile duct suggested if duct diameter >5–7 mm.
- **Abdominal CT:** can be useful to see obstruction and measure common bile duct. Can also exclude pancreatic carcinoma/other pathologies.
- **Magnetic resonance cholangiopancreatography (MRCP):** can visualise biliary tree anatomy and stones. Not possible if patient has non-compatible pacemaker, etc.
- **ERCP:** see stones in CBD and exclude tumour. Sphincterotomy can release impacted stones. Stenting if needed.

Management

- **Supportive:** IV fluids, crystalloids and basic ABC, O_2 as per BTS guidelines. NBM, NG if vomiting. Get abdominal USS as soon as possible.
- **Antibiotics: Tazocin** 4.5 g TDS IV for 7–10 d. Alternative consider **Cefuroxime** 1.5 g TDS IV + **Metronidazole** 500 mg TDS IV.
- **ERCP ± sphincterotomy:** allows bile drainage and passage of a stone ± spontaneously or pulled out with a basket device. If malignant lesion or stricture a stent can be placed.
- **Laparoscopic cholecystectomy** at 6–12 weeks for gallbladder stones.
- **Complications:** sepsis, ARDS, multi-organ failure.

7.16 ▶ Acute pancreatitis

- **About:** significant morbidity/mortality. Calculate Modified Glasgow Score.
- **Diagnosis:** needs 2/3 of typical abdominal pain, high amylase, high lipase and imaging. Admit under surgeons or gastroenterology.
- **Aetiology:** activation of trypsin, lipase and amylase and autodigestion leads to an inflamed oedematous/haemorrhagic pancreas. Ongoing tissue damage activates complement with a progressive systemic inflammatory response syndrome.

Causes

- **Gallstones (45%):** in ampulla of Vater allows bile reflux into pancreatic duct activating enzymes causing inflammation.
- **Alcohol (45%):** chronic alcohol for several years or occasional binge.
- **Hypertriglyceridaemia:** look at fundi for lipaemia retinalis.
- **Primary hyperparathyroidism,** hypercalcaemia: check Ca and PTH.
- **Cancer:** pancreatic cancer, biliary cancer.
- **Miscellaneous:** trauma, snakebite, HIV, CMV, EBV, sphincter of Oddi dysfunction.
- **Iatrogenic:** post ERCP reduce with IV hydration before.
- **Drugs:** steroids, thiazides, azathioprine, sulphonamide, octreotide, valproate.
- **Congenital:** pancreas divisum, familial non-X-linked dominant.

Clinical

- Raised HR, low BP, shock from sepsis, haemorrhagic pancreatitis. Severe epigastric pain to back eased with sitting up and forwards. Peritonitis with guarding, signs of causes, e.g. gallstones, alcoholism. Shocked, sepsis – generalised, pneumonia, low Hb.
- Bruising in flanks – Grey Turner's sign (associated 40% mortality). Peri-umbilical bruising – Cullen's sign (haemorrhagic pancreatitis). Coagulopathy from DIC. Cyanosed, dyspnoea from ARDS. Oliguria from AKI and/or hypovolaemia.

Diagnostic criteria for acute pancreatitis

- Requires two of the following three features: (1) abdominal pain consistent with acute pancreatitis (acute onset of a persistent, severe, epigastric pain often radiating to the back), (2) raised serum lipase activity (or amylase activity) >3× upper limit of normal (ULN), (3) characteristic findings on contrast-enhanced CT or MRI or USS.
- If clinical picture suggests acute pancreatitis, the serum amylase/lipase activity is <3× ULN (e.g. delayed presentation); imaging is needed to confirm the diagnosis otherwise the clinical picture + raised serum pancreatic enzyme activities suffices and a CT is not usually required for diagnosis acutely.

Investigations

- **FBC:** low Hb with haemorrhagic pancreatitis; raised MCV with alcohol. **U&E:** AKI, low Ca, raised triglycerides (familial hypertriglyceridaemia). **CRP:** >200 within first 4 days suggests acute severe attack – risk of complications, e.g. infection, pseudocyst, abscess formation.
- **Pancreatic lipase** raised (>3× ULN): more sensitive and specific than amylase. Elevated longer than amylase after disease presentation.
- **Amylase** (>3× ULN is diagnostic): usually >1000 IU/ml (levels up to 10,000 may be seen). Mild elevations >200 IU/ml not unique to pancreatitis but may also be seen in abdominal pain due to perforation of a viscus, small bowel obstruction, leaking AAA, ectopic pregnancy. A level of >1000 is more diagnostic, *but there is not a close*

correlation between amylase level and clinical severity. Very rarely a normal amylase suggests little remaining amylase-producing pancreatic tissue left. Amylase may be normal if alcohol-induced or high triglycerides. False positive serum amylase with macroamylasaemia – the level is constant.

- **Urinary trypsinogen-2** is now considered as a new test in development.
- **IL-6 and IL-8** may predict severity.
- **ABG:** low pH, low HCO_3, low PO_2 in severe cases, raised lactate.
- **Imaging: erect CXR/AXR:** exclude perforation, small bowel obstruction. Left pleural effusion may be seen. Look for calcification and sentinel loop. Bowel gas is seen in small bowel in centre of abdomen.
- **Contrast-enhanced CT/MRI abdomen:** reserved for patients in whom the diagnosis is unclear or who fail to improve clinically within the first 48–72 h after hospital admission or to evaluate complications. Best done at or after 3 days to support diagnosis and determine full extent of pancreatic necrosis and the presence of any fluid. CT may show fat-stranding surrounding the inflamed pancreas. Fluid may be aspirated to detect infection. Necrotic pancreas is identified by failure to opacify when CT with contrast is carried out. Gas bubbles may suggest infection. In a patient >40 y, look for a pancreatic tumour.
- **USS abdomen:** pancreatic mass, gallstones, pseudocyst, liver disease.
- **ERCP:** when aetiology unclear. May show a cause, e.g. ampullary tumour, stricture, gallstones, pancreas divisum and allow sphincterotomy. In those at high risk of pancreatitis post ERCP advise guidewire cannulation, pancreatic duct stents, rectal NSAIDs.

Severity scoring

- **Balthazar CT Severity Index: calculated on the basis of CT findings:** (A) normal pancreas +0, (B) focal or diffuse enlargement of the pancreas, contour irregularities, heterogeneous attenuation, no peripancreatic inflammation +1, (C) grade B plus peripancreatic inflammation +2, (D) grade C plus a single fluid collection +3, (E) grade C plus multiple fluid collections or gas +4. Percentage necrosis present on CT score: none +0, <33% +2, 33–50% +4, >50% +6. **Severe = score >6.**
- **Modified Glasgow Score:** PaO_2 <60 mmHg; **A**ge >55 years; **N**eutrophils (WCC) >15 × 10^9/L; **C**alcium <2 mmol/L; **R**aised urea >16 mmol/L; **E**nzyme LDH >600 units/L; **A**lbumin <32 g/L; **S**ugar (glucose) >10 mmol/L. Note spells out PANCREAS. A score >3 suggests severe and ITU/HDU care should be considered (Moore (2000) A useful mnemonic for severity stratification in acute pancreatitis. *Ann R Coll Surg Engl* (2000); 82:16–17).

Local and systemic complications

- **Acute kidney injury:** multiple factors. Optimise fluid status, treat infection, stop nephrotoxins. AKI, ▶Section 10.4.
- **Pancreatic pseudocyst and fluid collections:** can form around the pancreatic mass and may need laparoscopic drainage.
- **Necrotising pancreatitis:** >50% of gland necrosed on imaging. Can lead to infection and abscess formation. Needs antibiotics ± surgery. May get walled-off necrosis. Can erode into retroperitoneal vessels, e.g. splenic artery with acute haemorrhage.
- **Pancreatic abscess:** CT shows a ring-enhancing fluid collection with gas. Surgical or percutaneous drainage. IV antibiotics.
- **Others:** exocrine: fat malabsorption (low faecal elastase), endocrine: secondary diabetes.

- **Systemic:** recurrent acute pancreatitis, ARDS, AKI, DIC, multi-organ failure, sepsis.
- **Chronic pancreatitis:** repeated episodes of pancreatic injury, often alcohol-related, and frequent admissions. Alcohol cessation is the key in those who drink. Symptoms mimic acute pancreatitis. Develops exocrine and later endocrine dysfunction with steatorrhoea and weight loss. **Diagnosis with CT/USS/ERCP.** Exclude gallstones. **Differential** is autoimmune pancreatitis, inherited causes that start in early adult life and pancreatic cancer. Treatment is alcohol avoidance, nutritional support, manage exocrine and endocrine needs. Acutely these patients may be seen for mainly pain relief and managing acute flares. Pancreatic duct stenting if local stenosis.
- **Portal vein/splenic thrombosis:** localised inflammation. Develop portal hypertension with splenomegaly and variceal bleeds.

Management

- **ABC** and O_2 as per BTS guidance. Give early aggressive hydration (250–500 ml/h depending on cardiac/renal status) with 0.9% NS or Hartmann's solution to give urine output >30 ml/h. Baseline volume loss is 4–6 L but assess case by case. Consider CVP monitoring, monitor urine output, and clinical assessments of hydration, oxygenation, etc. There may be significant '3rd space' losses, which will need to be accounted for. ITU/HDU admission with any signs of organ failure. Look for and correct any significant hypocalcaemia. Severe cases need CT at 3–7 d and assess severity with CT severity score.
- **Nutrition:** in mild/mod disease normal oral feeding can be considered if no significant gastroparesis and there are normal bowel sounds and no signs of ileus. Early feeding by naso/gastric/jejunal (NG/NJ) tube is advised if there is ongoing vomiting. Enteral feeding is preferred to TPN. However, those with severe disease may be initially NBM. Calcium and magnesium should be checked and replaced if needed and adequate hydration given.
- **Analgesia: tramadol** IV is preferred. **Morphine** 1–5 mg IV every 4 h is widely used. **Pethidine** 25–50 mg IV/SC/IM historically advocated as concerns that **morphine** increased sphincter of Oddi tone or caused spasm. Combine with anti-emetic **Ondansetron** 2–4 mg IV every 4–6 h when required.
- **Diabetes: may be new,** consider **variable rate insulin infusion** to control any hyperglycaemia.
- **Alcohol withdrawal:** consider **Chlordiazepoxide** or **Lorazepam** 1–2 mg PO/IV/IM 8 hourly and **Pabrinex** IV paired vials TDS for 1–2 d.
- **Antibiotics:** are given if evidence of specific infections. Advice now against prophylaxis. Fever often due to inflammatory nature of the disease. If infected necrosis suspected then either **Cefuroxime** 750 mg – 1.5 g TDS IV or **Tazocin** 4.5 g TDS IV or **Meropenem** 1 g TDS IV if penicillin allergic (choice of carbapenems, quinolones, metronidazole).
- **Nutrition:** can feed normally if mild, no N&V, and abdominal pain resolved. In moderate–severe disease try to continue enteral nutrition which may be by NG/NJ tube. Try to avoid parenteral nutrition unless the enteral route is not available, not tolerated, or insufficient for caloric requirements.
- **ERCP ± sphincterotomy** should be considered, usually within 24 h where there is a cholangitis or jaundice and a common duct stone, which requires removal. A sphincterotomy may be performed and/or stone removed. ERCP is not needed in most patients with gallstone pancreatitis without evidence of biliary obstruction. Manage gallstones with either cholecystectomy or ERCP; or ursodeoxycholic acid can be considered.

- **MRCP or endoscopic ultrasound** (EUS) rather than diagnostic ERCP should be used to screen for choledocholithiasis if highly suspected.
- **CT-guided FNA:** consider infected necrosis in those with pancreatic or extrapancreatic necrosis who deteriorate or fail to improve after 7–10 d; consider either CT-guided FNA for Gram stain and culture to guide antibiotic prescribing, or empiric use of antibiotics without CT FNA.
- **Respiratory support:** patient with severe upper abdominal pain can experience basal atelectasis and hypoventilation and develop respiratory failure and may need a mixture of analgesia with a trial of high FiO_2 with humidification, chest physiotherapy to help expectorate secretions, CPAP or even invasive ventilation on ITU.
- **Surgery** may be required where there is a **severe necrotising pancreatitis** or if there is an **abscess or pseudocyst.** Usually delayed about 4 weeks. A pancreatic necrosectomy involves removing dead pancreatic tissue, which may be done by laparoscopy. Minimally invasive methods are preferred to open necrosectomy. Consider cholecystectomy prior to discharge if gallstone pancreatitis. Asymptomatic pseudocysts may be observed and often resolve but some may need to be managed endoscopically.
- **Behaviour:** offer advice and help with good nutrition and in cessation of alcohol and smoking.
- **References:** Tenner *et al.* (2013) Management of acute pancreatitis. *Am J Gastroenterol*, 108:1400. UK Working Party on Acute Pancreatitis (2005) UK guidelines for the management of acute pancreatitis. *Gut*, 54(Suppl III):iii1. Banks *et al.* (2013) Classification of acute pancreatitis. *Gut*, 62:102.

7.17 Budd–Chiari syndrome

- **Introduction:** uncommon (1 in 100,000) condition characterised by obstruction of the hepatic venous outflow tract. Requires accurate, prompt diagnosis and aggressive therapy.
- **Causes:** hepatic vein thrombosis and post-sinusoidal portal hypertension. There may be hepatic vein thrombosis due to prothrombosis, stenosis or webs. Portal hypertension, liver congestion and centrilobular cell necrosis. Idiopathic. Prothrombosis, malignancy.
- **Clinical:** RUQ pain, asymptomatic to fulminant liver failure in days. Often with jaundice, renal failure and coagulopathy and encephalopathy.
- **Investigations:** FBC, U&E, LFTs, CRP. High AST/ALT/bilirubin and PT. Liver USS shows enlarged caudate lobe and hepatomegaly and regional echogenicity and ascites. CT/VT venography is also useful and MRI shows absence of blood flow in the occluded veins. If no local cause then needs a full thrombophilia screen. *JAK2* mutation. Catheter venography is considered the standard for the diagnosis of this condition.
- **Management:** medical, surgical and endovascular. Treat any cause. Best treated in tertiary care centres where liver transplantation is available. Endovascular interventions include angioplasty, stenting, catheter-directed mechanical thrombolysis, and creation of transjugular intrahepatic portosystemic shunts (TIPSS).

08 Haematology

8.1 Anaemia

- **About:** normal Hb depends on sex and age. Look at Hb, MCV and MCH. Anaemia may be acute or chronic but is better tolerated in young. Anaemia Hb <130 g/L in men, 120 g/L in women, 110 g/L pregnant women.
- **Pathophysiology:** we require bone marrow, B12, folate, iron, erythropoietin to produce RBCs with Hb. Haem: Fe^{2+} + protoporphyrin IX. Globins are haem-containing O_2-binding proteins. B12 and folate and bone marrow needed to make white cells and platelets.
- **Aetiology of anaemia:** deficiency of B12/folate causes megaloblasts in bone marrow and increased MCV. Deficiency of iron causes microcytosis with insufficient Hb (low MCV and MCH concentration). Lack of both causes a dimorphic anaemia with a mixture of small and large RBCs. Reduced bone marrow function: congenital, chemotherapy, infiltration, drugs, parvovirus B19, CKD. Excess blood loss/ destruction of red cells, acute or chronic bleeding, chronic or acute haemolysis.

Causes/notes on anaemia	
Acute haemorrhage	Acute blood loss. Baseline Hb then haemodilution later to lower Hb. Usually obvious: external wound or GI with melaena/urinary/pelvic fracture/retroperitoneal. Hb/Hct are of little use in an acute bleed. See also Haemorrhagic shock, ▶Section 2.22; Bleeding disorders, ▶Section 8.8.
Iron deficiency	Menstrual blood loss, GI blood loss. Low Hb, low MCV, low MCHC, low ferritin (falsely elevated if CRP high), low serum iron, high TIBC, high soluble transferrin receptor. Iron/TIBC <19%. Upper and lower GI endoscopy, coeliac screen (duodenal biopsy, IgA TTG, anti-endomysial antibody). Capsule endoscopy. CT abdomen. Bone marrow – lack of iron and erythroid hyperplasia. Look for and treat cause. Give iron.
B12 deficiency	Megaloblastic marrow. Low Hb, high MCV. Low B12 <50 ng/L and folate low too. Raised bilirubin, LDH. Low WCC, low platelets. Neuropathy, SACD, optic atrophy. Usually pernicious anaemia, malabsorption, gastric surgery. Check intrinsic factor/parietal antibody. Give IM or oral B12 2 mg/d.
Folate deficiency	Diet/malabsorption, drugs. Megaloblastic marrow. Raised MCV >100. Low red cell folate. Folic acid 5 mg OD.
Anaemia chronic disease	CKD, malignancy, connective tissue disease, RA, hypothyroid (macrocytic). Usually small or normal-sized red cells.
Haemoglobinopathy	Abnormal Hb reduces red cell half-life with chronic anaemia, e.g. thalassaemia (very low MCV), sickle cell. ▶Section 8.2.
Pregnancy	Dilutional anaemia is normal. Give folate and iron.
Haemolytic anaemia	Short-lived RBC. Low Hb, low haptoglobin, elevated bilirubin, high LDH. Structural issues (spherocytosis/elliptocytosis), abnormal Hb (sickle/ thalassaemia), faulty RBC metabolism (phenylketonuria/G6PD), immune (warm IgG/cold IgM), physical, e.g. metal valves, malaria, microangiopathic haemolytic anaemia, PNH.

Causes/notes on anaemia	
Sideroblastic anaemia	Rare. Dysfunctional synthesis. Marrow ringed sideroblasts. Alcohol, lead, isoniazid. Treat cause. Give vitamin B6.
Aplastic anaemia	Congenital, acquired, bone marrow infiltration, radiation, cytotoxic drugs, HIV, TB, PNH, drugs. Low RCC/WCC/platelets. Aplastic bone marrow. May be pancytopenia or more selective. Low/no reticulocytes. Identify cause and support. May need bone marrow transplant so caution with blood products. Urgent haem review. If neutropenic, see Neutropenic sepsis, ▶ Section 17.5.
Pancytopenia	Aplastic anaemia, B12/folate loss, TB, sepsis, leukaemia, myeloma, malignancy, PNH, SLE, drugs.

Clinical signs of abnormal FBC

- **Low Hb:** pale sclerae, hand creases. Fatigue, headache, breathlessness. Symptoms depend on rapidity of onset, cardiorespiratory status, age.
- **Low WCC** if affected: fever, sore throat, sepsis.
- **Low platelets:** petechiae, menorrhagia, epistaxis, haematuria.
- Broad assessment of any coexisting illness which can be very varied. Look for fever, large spleen/liver/lymph glands. Look at congenital, racial (thalassaemia/sickle), contacts, travel.
- **Examine drug chart/recent drugs:** phenytoin, cytotoxics, alcohol, quinine.
- **Investigation: FBC:** low Hb, WCC, platelets. **Haematinics:** B12, red cell folate, ferritin/serum iron/TIBC, reticulocytes. **U&E:** AKI/CKD and CRP. TSH and T_4. Bilirubin (red cell breakdown). CXR: infection, malignancy, TB. **Blood film:** schistocytes, fragmented, deformed, irregular, or helmet-shaped RBCs suggests DIC. **Reticulocytes:** usually increased except in aplastic anaemia. **Bone marrow:** hypocellular with aplasia, ringed sideroblasts, megaloblastic. Lack of iron. **Infiltration** – cancer, infection. **Intravascular haemolysis:** raised LDH, reticulocytes, bilirubin, low haptoglobin, Coombs test negative. AKI (HUS/TTP or uraemic platelet dysfunction). **Upper GI endoscopy** with D2 biopsies for coeliac, **lower GI endoscopy, capsule endoscopy and CT** abdomen for iron-deficiency anaemia.

Management (see Blood products ▶ Section 8.14)

- **ABC, resuscitation.** Establish cause. Treat and replace. Supportive measures – blood components. Caution with giving Hb in pernicious anaemia with circulatory overload, if future need for bone marrow transplant, check if need irradiated blood (▶ Section 8.17). Those with severe iron deficiency may receive IV iron. Those with B12 deficiency should get oral/IM B12. Folate may then also be given.
- **Blood transfusions** needed to increase oxygen carriage when Hb <7 g/dl or 8–9 g/dl in ACS or when bleeding. Each unit is 350 ml of packed red cells and has a Hct of 60%. Contains red cells, some white cells and plasma. Cross-matched takes about 40 min if no antibodies. One unit raises the Hb by about 1 g/dl.
- **Take haematology advice if unsure.** Bone marrow transplant recipients and patients with cellular immunodeficiency should be considered for CMV-negative blood. Focused management on determining cause and replacing components or treating disorder.

8.2 Sickle cell crisis

- **About:** chronic haemolytic anaemia. Abnormal Hb first described by Linus Pauling in 1946. Commoner in black patients but may also affect other groups. Homozygous inheritance of HbSS or HbSC. Most painful crises are managed at home. **NB:** early diagnosis of acute chest syndrome/stroke enables red cell transfusion and exchange transfusion.
- **Aetiology:** HbSS contains 2 defective β-globin chains due to a valine to glutamate substitution on the β6 position. Structural change and HbS polymerisation and sickling at low O_2 tensions. HbAS: symptoms with extreme hypoxia (sickle cell trait).
- **Acute crises seen with HbSS:** (sickle cell anaemia) HbSS who only have HbS. HbSC: HbS and HbC from either parent. HbS–βO: sickle cell + β-thalassaemia.
- **Clinical:** crises triggered by infections and other illness or hypoxia. Usually severe chest/bone/back/limb/abdominal pain and anaemia. Anaemia from shortened RBC half-life needs transfusion but cost is iron overload.

Complications

- Haemolytic anaemia, aplastic crises, lung fibrosis, stroke, hepatosplenomegaly.
- *Salmonella* osteomyelitis, sickling crisis, avascular necrosis of the hips, Hib infection.
- Renal failure, renal concentrating defects, renal papillary necrosis.
- Priapism – sequestration of red cells in corpus cavernosum.
- Acute chest syndrome due to pneumococcal pneumonia, lung infarction or fat embolism, bleeding in anterior chamber of eye (hyphaema).
- Osteoporosis: vertebral collapse, avascular necrosis of femoral head or dactylitis or swollen joints, skin ulcers, pigment gallstones, splenic infarction – autosplenectomy.
- Stroke – seen mainly in children (see below).

Investigations

- **FBC:** low Hb 60–90 g/L, raised retics.
- **Blood film:** sickled RBC, target cells, polychromasia.
- **U&E, LFT, LDH, CRP, CXR, ABG.**
- **ECG, troponin** and D-**dimer** if SOB/chest pain.
- **Exclude infection:** blood/urine cultures and CXR. USS abdomen.
- **Sickle solubility test:** positive in disease and trait.
- **Hb electrophoresis** 80–95% HbSS and no HbA.
- **Cross-match** if symptoms severe and transfusion needed. Close matching of blood is needed to reduce antibody formation.

Acute general management (consult with haematology early)

- **Supportive:** most painful crises are self-managed in the community with NSAIDs/paracetamol. Admission for uncontrolled pain or suspicion of complications. ABC, O_2 as per BTS guidelines. Eat and drink freely as able. If not able to take oral fluids then IV fluids to maintain good hydration.
- **Analgesia:** pain is often the dominating symptom and reason for admission. Offer analgesia within 30 min of presentation if needed. Avoid pethidine. Mild pains try **Paracetamol** 1 g TDS and **Ibuprofen** 400–600 mg TDS or **Diclofenac** 50 mg TDS PO. If severe pains then in addition to NSAID give IV **morphine** repeated until pain-free, usually with an anti-emetic e.g. **Cyclizine** 50 mg PO/IM/IV. Consider continuous infusion pump or patient-controlled anaesthesia. Add a laxative, e.g. **Senna** 15 mg

PO and/or **Lactulose** 10–20 ml. **Hydroxyzine** 25 mg 12 h may be given for itch. **Haloperidol** 1–3 mg PO/IM for anxiety.

- **Exchange blood transfusion used for severe chest syndrome and stroke:** basically venesect and transfuse (e.g. 6 units in and 6 units out). Used for acute ischaemic stroke, multiple organ failure, acute chest syndrome, hepatic sequestration. Outcome for acute chest syndrome improved. Replacement of sickle cells by normal cells can help prevent further vaso-occlusion, although pre-existing vaso-occlusion may not be reversed. The goal for acute stroke and acute chest syndrome is a HbS under 30% (for patients with SCD-SS) while keeping the Hb at 10 g/dl. Get urgent senior haematology advice.
- **LMWH:** VTE prophylaxis reduces the length of stay of patients with an acute painful sickle cell episode.
- **Crizanlizumab:** a monoclonal antibody medication that binds to P-selectin. Used to prevent sickle cell crises in sickle cell disease and available on NHS since early 2022 under managed care agreement.
- **Hydroxycarbamide (hydroxyurea):** raises HbF, reduces crisis by 50% so consider in all with severe disease.
- **Folate:** ensure supplementation given.
- **Prophylaxis:** hyposplenism consider **Penicillin** 500 mg OD PO prophylaxis and pneumococcal/Hib vaccination.
- **Allogeneic bone marrow transplantation:** cure success in 90–95%. Usually from matched siblings. Requires myeloablative therapy. Outcome excellent.
- **Pregnancy:** screen pregnant patients. Acute care is the same. Transfuse to reduce proportion of HbS and so sickling crises. Liaise with obstetric team.

Specific syndromes

- **Acute chest syndrome:** chest pain, cough, fever, CXR infiltrates (may appear late), hypoxia. Precipitated by excess opiates/PE/fat embolism/microvascular infarction/infection or fluid overload. Give O_2 as per BTS guidance. Bronchodilators for wheeze. Consider CPAP with escalation to ITU admission and ventilation if unable to keep PO_2 >8 kPa despite an FiO_2 of 0.6. May need a CTPA and anticoagulation if PE suspected. Take haematology advice and ITU help early. Antibiotics and antivirals if H1N1 suspected. May be prevented using incentive spirometry. Consider blood/exchange transfusion. Need antibiotic coverage which also covers atypical, e.g. **co-amoxiclav** and **clarithromycin.** Penicillin-allergic – **Ceftriaxone** 1–2 g 12 h and **clarithromycin.** May develop pulmonary arterial hypertension. Screen with transthoracic echo. PAH associated with increased mortality. Treat with hydroxyurea, chronic transfusions, O_2. Consider prostacyclin and bosentan, and sildenafil. Incentive spirometry can prevent the development of complications associated with acute chest syndrome in patients with sickle cell disease.
- **(Splenic) sequestration crisis:** painful rapidly enlarging liver/spleen due to occluded organ venous outflow. In children the spleen is involved. Severe anaemia, low BP and fatal. In adults the liver more affected with severe RUQ pain and liver enlargement. Treat with good IV hydration, O_2, analgesia and blood transfusion. Exchange transfusion may be warranted. Treat infection. Rare in adults except with haemoglobin SC disease or SB + thalassaemia.
- **Aplastic crisis:** temporary red cell aplasia due to infection by parvovirus B19. Low Hb and low reticulocyte count. Supportive management.

- **Priapism:** penile venous outflow obstructed with a sustained painful erection. Can result in impotence. Treatment is ice, IV hydration, analgesia, transfusion if needed and urology referral. Injected α-blocker. May settle with conservative therapy.
- **Renal:** tubular necrosis and haematuria and potential urinary obstruction. Damage to collecting ducts can lead to impaired concentrating ability and dehydration. Nephritic syndrome and chronic kidney disease can develop.
- **Sickle cell stroke:** children/young adults. Transfuse to reduce the sickle fraction to <30%. Screen children with transcranial Doppler. If high velocity flow should receive a preventative transfusion regimen. This has a 90% absolute risk reduction of first stroke.
- **Avascular necrosis of the femoral and humeral heads.** Adults. Plain films show advanced changes. MRI gold standard diagnostic tool. Needs analgesia and steroid joint injections, and some may need joint replacement.
- **References:** Howard *et al*. (2015) Guideline on the management of acute chest syndrome in sickle cell disease. *Br J Haematol*, 169:492. NICE (2012) CG143: Sickle cell acute painful episode: Management of an acute painful sickle cell episode in hospital.

8.3 ▶ Disseminated intravascular coagulation

- **About:** DIC is seen in 1% of inpatients. Uncontrolled microvascular clotting causes a consumptive coagulopathy and thrombocytopenia leads to massive haemorrhage, organ failure. Very poor prognosis. The cornerstone of supportive treatment of this coagulopathy is management of the underlying condition. See Blood products ▶Section 8.14.
- **Aetiology:** endothelial disruption and other initiators lead to a procoagulant state. Formation of microvascular thrombi consumes clotting factors, fibrinogen and platelets. Microthrombi can cause organ dysfunction. Bleeding due to coagulopathy. In malignancy, DIC can be a more chronic process over weeks and months.
- **Clinical:** severe spontaneous bleeding and bruising in an unwell patient. Haemorrhagic shock due to bleeding from lines, GI tract, genitourinary tract, epistaxis. Spontaneous intracerebral haemorrhage, post-operative wound bleed. Bleeding may be hidden, e.g. retroperitoneal, psoas. See also Haemorrhagic shock, ▶Section 2.22. DIC with purpura fulminans may rarely be a presentation of acute promyelocytic leukaemia.
- **Causes:** trauma and tissue damage, sepsis and septicaemic shock (Gram –ve). Malignancy, acute promyelocytic leukaemia/M3, massive transfusions. Obstetric emergencies (placental abruption, amniotic fluid embolism, eclampsia). Pancreatitis, vascular abnormalities, snake bites, recreational drugs. ABO transfusion incompatibility, transplant rejection, severe liver failure. Severe Covid-19 infection.

Investigations
- **FBC, blood film:** anaemia, low platelets, fragmented red cells.
- **U&E:** AKI, raised LDH and evidence of haemolysis.
- There is no one test but progressive coagulopathy and low platelets suggestive. Use the scoring algorithm when clinical context supports DIC **Scoring Algorithm: platelets** >100 = 0, <100 = 1, <50 = 2. **FDP/dimers:** no increase = 0, <5× upper limit

of normal = 2, strong increase (≥5× upper limit of normal) = 3. **Prothrombin time** <3 s = 0, ≥3 s but <6 s = 1, ≥6 s = 2. **Fibrinogen level** (often late to fall) >1.0 g/L = 0 ≤1.0 g/L = 1. A score of ≥5 points is compatible with DIC. Note that if the score is <5, consider repeating after 1 to 2 days. The severity of DIC according to this scoring system is a strong predictor for mortality in sepsis.

Differentials
- **TTP and HUS** (low plts no coagulopathy minimally raised dimers).
- **MAHA** microangiopathic haemolytic anaemia: (low plts no coagulopathy dimers minimal elevated). Severe HTN, pregnancy: pre-eclampsia, HELLP syndrome.
- **Heparin-induced thrombocytopenia**; arterial and venous thrombosis: dimer may be elevated but no coagulopathy.
- **Coagulopathy of liver disease:** coagulopathy but ascites splenomegaly and stable platelets suggest liver disease rather than DIC.

Management: manage underlying condition/cause
- **ABC, supportive care:** admit ITU. ABC, O_2. Care with central lines, coagulopathy. Find and treat the underlying cause. Involve haematology.
- **No major bleeding or thrombosis:** prophylactic LMWH.
- **Active bleeding or need for a procedure:** give platelets, target 30–50 × 10^9/L, Give FFP or prothrombin complex concentrates to keep PT <3 sec prolonged and keep fibrinogen >1.5 g/L. Give **Vitamin K** 10 mg slow IV if deficiency suspected. Tranexamic acid IV if hyperfibrinolysis (high FDPs).
- **Clinically overt thromboembolism:** thrombosis and organ failure, purpura fulminans or acral ischaemia: consider IV Heparin.
- **Acute promyelocytic leukaemia** needs urgent haematology review for **all-*trans* retinoic acid** (ATRA) and chemotherapeutic agents.
- **References:** Levi M. & Scully M. (2018) How I treat disseminated intravascular coagulation. *Blood*, 131: 845. British Committee for Standards in Haematology (2009) Guidelines for the diagnosis and management of DIC. *Br J Haematol*, 145:24.

8.4   Severe thrombocytopenia

- **About:** platelet count <150 × 10^9/L. Spontaneous bleeding if count <10 × 10^9/L. If bleeding then target platelet count >50 × 10^9/L or higher for CNS procedures or bleeding. See Blood products ▶ Section 8.14.
- **Bleeding risk:** at its simplest platelet count, platelet function and structural issues and presence of any coagulopathy.
- **Pathophysiology:** platelets survive 7–10 d. 35% of all platelets are found in the spleen. Reaction to vessel wall injury is rapid adhesion of platelets to the subendothelium and formation of a haemostatic plug, composed primarily of platelets. This is further stabilised by a fibrin mesh generated in secondary haemostasis. Significant quantitative or qualitative platelet dysfunction results in mucocutaneous bleeding.
- **Aetiology:** platelets formed from developing megakaryocytes in the bone marrow. Low platelets can be due to a fall in production or increased consumption or sequestration. Platelet dysfunction with antiplatelets, drugs and diseases, e.g. uraemia.

Causes of low platelets

- **Sampling error:** platelet clumping can spuriously lower count. Repeat. It is evident on a peripheral smear by the presence of platelet clumps.
- **Acute idiopathic thrombocytopenic purpura (ITP):** all ages. Immune- destruction of platelets/ megakaryocytes due to the platelet GP IIb/IIIa complex. May be post-viral or drug-induced. Rarely SLE or HIV. Treat with steroids (**prednisolone** 1 mg/kg) or other immunosuppression and IVIg and splenectomy if severe and persisting. Avoid platelets if possible. ITP in pregnancy can lead to low plts in fetus with neonatal intracranial haemorrhage. **Other agents:** danazol, eltrombopag, rituximab, romiplostim.
- **Chronic ITP:** adults with low plts. Slow onset. Smear shows giant platelets.
- **Heparin-induced thrombocytopenic purpura (HIT/T):** on UFH/LMWH. Develops low platelets + thrombosis. Stop all heparins even flushes. Test for **heparin-dependent platelet antibodies.** ▶Section 8.5.
- **HUS/TTP: CNS** involvement, renal failure, diarrhoea. ▶Sections 8.6 and 8.7.
- **Pregnancy-related thrombocytopenia:** mild thrombocytopenia in an otherwise healthy pregnancy. May resemble a mild ITP. Infant unaffected. ▶Section 8.4.
- **Pre-eclampsia/eclampsia syndrome:** increased platelet turnover. Controlling BP. Delivering the fetus leads to restoration of the platelet count. ▶Section 16.6.
- **HELLP syndrome:** thrombocytopenia with haemolysis and raised liver enzymes and low platelet (HELLP) syndrome. Treat BP and deliver fetus.
- **Post-transfusion purpura:** typically occurs 10 d following a transfusion.
- **Disseminated intravascular coagulation:** pathological thrombin generation. There is consumption of platelets with thrombosis and bleeding. Seen in those with other overwhelming pathology. ▶Section 8.3.
- **Drug-induced thrombocytopenia:** drugs such as gold, ibuprofen, quinine, quinidine, methotrexate, amiodarone, valproate, cimetidine, captopril, carbamazepine, sulfonamides, glibenclamide, tamoxifen, ranitidine, phenytoin, vancomycin, piperacillin, cocaine.
- **Bone marrow failure:** malignancy, myelodysplasia, marrow failure.
- **Severe fever with thrombocytopenia syndrome:** infectious disease with a 12% case-fatality rate in China due to a novel bunyavirus.
- **Dengue fever, HIV:** HIV test, CD4 count, viral load. ▶Sections 9.8 and 9.34.
- **SLE:** check ANA dsDNA. Look for classical signs and laboratory results.
- **Hypersplenism:** thrombocytopenia rarely below $40 \times 10^9/L$.
- **Platelet dysfunction:** platelet numbers normal. Aspirin, clopidogrel, prasugrel, ticagrelor, uraemia, etc. all prolong bleeding time.
- **SARS-CoV-2** reduces the number of platelets.

- **Clinical:** spontaneous petechiae, purpura, bleeding. Mouth may show evidence of bleeding. Check drug chart. Look for splenomegaly and lymph nodes, which may suggest a cause. Menorrhagia, epistaxis, haematuria.

Investigations

- **FBC:** low Hb, low platelets. **Blood film:** schistocytes, fragmented, deformed helmet-shaped RBCs suggests DIC. **U&E:** AKI, check B12, folate, ferritin.
- **Intravascular haemolysis:** raised LDH, reticulocytes, bilirubin, low haptoglobin, Coombs test negative. (HUS/TTP/uraemic platelet dysfunction).
- **Coagulation:** normal PT, APTT, D-dimer and fibrinogen levels. Increased bleeding time. Renal biopsy if HUS may be indicated to see degree and nature of kidney damage. ADAMTS13 levels of limited use.
- **Management:** treat cause: look for underlying sepsis, drugs, other causes, and treat. Use local physical methods/surgery to stem bleeding. Avoid NSAIDs,

antiplatelets e.g. aspirin, clopidogrel, ticagrelor, prasugrel, warfarin, heparins and DOACs. Pre-eclampsia/eclampsia/HELLP: **BP control and delivery.**

When to transfuse platelets

- **General advice:** spontaneous bleeding uncommon if platelets >30 × 10^9/L. Post trauma/surgery/bleeding target is platelets >50 × 10^9/L. CNS trauma or ICH then target is 70–100 × 10^9/L. If bleeding and platelets >30 × 10^9/L look for additional cause. Preventive levels in non-bleeding patient is keep the count above 10 × 10^9/L. May replace to higher levels if patient has taken antiplatelets or has platelet dysfunction. Take haematological advice. Must determine cause before transfusion and exclude TTP by examining blood film. Platelets not usually indicated for ITP/TTP/HUS/HIT syndromes. In acute ITP only used for real risk of or actual bleeding. The decision to transfuse should be supported by the need to prevent or treat bleeding. There may be a role for desmopressin in patients taking aspirin or uraemia.
- **Platelets (× 10^9/L) and advice when to transfuse platelets: 0–10:** prophylactic transfusion. **10–20:** bleeding, fever, infection, platelet dysfunction, coagulopathy. **20–50:** prior to minor procedures or in actively anticoagulated patients or in the presence of active bleeding. **50–100:** sufficient for most invasive procedures, including gastroscopy and biopsy, insertion of indwelling lines, transbronchial biopsy, liver biopsy, laparotomy or similar procedures. **50–75:** prior to general surgery/childbirth. **100:** prior to ophthalmic surgery or neurosurgery.
- **Reference:** Lin & Foltz (2005) Proposed guidelines for platelet transfusion. *Br Columbia Med J*, 47:245.

8.5 Heparin-induced thrombocytopenia

- **About:** heparin-induced thrombocytopenia (HIT) + thrombosis (HITT). Heparin induces formation of antibodies with thrombosis and a fall in platelets. Consider HIT in any patient with low platelets on heparin started within past 5–10 d.
- **Type I HIT:** common, non-immune, clinically innocuous, benign reaction.
- **Type II HIT:** rare, immune-mediated, can be serious; causes thrombosis.
- **Aetiology:** formation of platelet-rich thrombosis 5–10 d after starting heparin therapy. It can also occur with exposure within 100 d and one single re-exposure. Target antigen is a complex between heparin and platelet factor 4 (PF4). Common with UFH, rare with LMWH. IgG activates platelets via their FcIIa receptors.
- **Clinical:** venous thrombosis: DVT/PE. Arterial thrombosis: limb, stroke, MI, PE, renal artery, mesenteric arteries. Skin necrosis at injection sites. Adrenal failure due to vein thrombosis and haemorrhagic necrosis. Severe DVT with venous limb gangrene is seen.
- **The 4Ts pre-test probability score:** This can assist in determining if HIT is present. Generally, scores of <3 suggest the absence of HIT. Higher scores send ELISA for heparin/PF4 antibodies. Not included here for brevity but scoring can be found on www.mdcalc.com. Strong features in 4Ts are >50% plt fall, onset days 5–10, new thrombosis/skin necrosis, no other causes of platelet count drop.
- **Investigations: FBC:** platelets <150 × 10^9/L or fall by 30–50% after starting heparin therapy (the platelet count may still be normal). **U&E:** look for AKI. **Blood film:** fragmented RBCs. **Specific test:** ELISA test for heparin/PF4 antibodies.
- **Management:** Check plts every 2–3 d from days 4 to 14 or until heparin is stopped. If detected **stop all heparins** (UFH/LMWH/heparin line flushes/catheters with

heparin) in suspected HIT. Urgent haematology consult. Rivaroxaban may be considered for acute HIT. Apixaban and dabigatran have also been used. Other drugs used are Argatroban, danaparoid, fondaparinux or bivalirudin – see local licensing. Long-term warfarin may be used.

- **Reference:** Nilius H *et al.* (2021) Comparative effectiveness and safety of anticoagulants for the treatment of heparin-induced thrombocytopenia. *Am J Hematol.* 96(7):805–15.

8.6 ▶ Haemolytic uraemic syndrome

- **About:** children with diarrhoea and AKI. Adults no diarrhoeal illness.
- **Triad:** thrombotic microangiopathy, thrombocytopenia and AKI.

Aetiology

- **Children:** AKI due to shiga-like toxin-producing *E. coli* strain 0157:H7.60.
- **Adults:** drugs that damage endothelial cells. Familial (congenital) HUS – deficiency of factor H, a plasma protein synthesised by the liver, which regulates the complement pathway. MAHA = microangiopathic haemolytic anaemia.
- **ADAMTS13** is a protease which breaks down clumps of vWF and deficiency can stimulate thrombosis and cause atypical TTP/HUS. Toxin-producing *E. coli* cause endothelial cell damage and renal microvascular thrombosis. Platelet aggregation causes consumptive thrombocytopenia. MAHA as RBCs circulate through partially occluded microcirculation.

Classification of haemolytic uraemic syndrome

- **Typical HUS: shiga toxin/verotoxin producing *E. coli* (STEC/VTEC-HUS) or *Shigella dysenteriae* type 1 infection.** Usually in children/infants but can be in adults causing haemodialysis-dependent AKI in 50%. Single episode. Normal ADAMTS13 levels. *E. coli* strain 0157:H7 from cattle or sheep. Verocytotoxin (shiga toxin 1/2). New strain *E. coli* O104:H4 with high rate of complications. Toxins damage endothelium. *Shigella* and *Streptococcus pneumoniae*.
- **Atypical HUS:** low ADAMTS13 levels due to a defect in complement levels. Familial recurrent character and familial history. Other drugs – mitomycin C, ticlopidine, ciclosporin, tacrolimus, quinine, chemotherapy. Congenital, malignancies – prostate, gastric, pancreatic, scleroderma, SLE/APLS. Often severe, with respiratory, neurology, coma; the mortality rate is 12%. Genetic – several genes detected. Treat with eculizumab, which blocks complement C5 activation.

Clinical

- **Shiga toxin EC HUS:** haematuria, AKI, oliguria, diarrhoea, children.
- **Atypical HUS:** AKI, illness (HIV, *Strep.*), genetics, drugs.
- **Both:** red/brown urine, petechial rash (low platelets), malaise, hypertension, uraemia. Jaundice, easy bruising and pallor from anaemia.

Investigations

- **FBC:** Hb <8 g/dl (haemolysis), low platelets. Increased retics, high LDH.
- **U&E:** AKI. **LFTs:** raised bilirubin. Raised LDH. **Coombs test** negative.
- **Blood film:** schistocytes, fragmented, deformed, irregular, helmet-shaped RBCs.
- **Intravascular haemolysis:** raised LDH, raised reticulocytes, low haptoglobin.
- **Coagulation:** normal PT, APTT, D-dimer, fibrinogen.
- **Stool samples:** will be cultured for *E. coli* 0157:H7 and *E. coli* O104:H4.

- **Renal biopsy** may be indicated to see degree and nature of kidney damage.
- **ADAMTS13** levels normal in VTEC/ETEC disease. Low in atypical HUS.
- **Others:** ANA, dsDNA, HIV test.
- **Complement** functional assays: CH50, AP50 (factor H function). Serum levels: C3, C4, factor H, factor I, factor B.

Management of HUS (urgent renal/haematology consult)
- **Typical HUS: ETEC/VTEC HUS:** children. Avoid antibiotics possibly release more toxin, antimotility agents, NSAIDs. Can precipitate HUS and worsen severity. Avoid platelet transfusions unless life-threatening bleeding with low platelets. Renal replacement therapy in 50%. Most go on to make a full recovery. Manage hypertension, input/output, anaemia, K. Daily plasma exchange (plasmapheresis + FFP replacement) is treatment of choice. No role for steroids. Children often recover completely. Irreversible renal damage and death in more severe cases. AKI, ▶ Section 10.4. **Avoid plasmapheresis** with HUS post *Strep. pneumoniae*. **Unresponsive cases** consider **Vincristine** or **Ciclosporin** A.
- **Atypical HUS:** prognosis worse. Initial mortality 10–15% and 70% go on to end-stage renal failure. Consider PLEX. Consider **Eculizumab** (Soliris) which binds terminal complement C5. NICE and the FDA approved use but very expensive. Improves platelet count, reduces thrombotic episodes and maintains or improves kidney function. Main side-effects are headache and leukopenia. Congenital disease may need liver transplant.
- **References:** *ASH Education Book*, 15. NICE (2015) *HST1: Eculizumab for treating atypical haemolytic uraemic syndrome*.

Comparing causes of microangiopathic anaemia

Disease	Schistocytes	Platelets	PT APTT	Fibrinogen	Dimer
HELLP	Yes	Low	Normal	Normal	Normal
TTP/HUS	Yes	Low	Normal	Normal	Normal
DIC	Yes	Low	Prolonged	Low	Raised

8.7   Thrombotic thrombocytopenic purpura

- **About:** activation and consumption of platelets, vessel occlusion, microangiopathic anaemia. Neurological events. Early diagnosis to enable therapeutic plasma exchange (TPE) improves outcome.
- **Aetiology:** inhibition or congenital/acquired lack of ADAMTS13 increases platelet adhesion to endothelium by vWF. Causes thrombosis, platelet consumption. Schistocytes normal clotting and fibrinogen. Platelets consumed.
- **Causes:** low ADAMTS13, acquired due to antibodies to ADAMTS13. Ticlopidine, clopidogrel, ciclosporin, OCP, pregnancy, SLE, HIV, hepatitis.
- **Pathophysiology:** platelet activation causes cerebral renal/gut microvascular thrombosis. Platelet aggregation and a consumptive thrombocytopenia. RBCs damaged passing through partially occluded microcirculation.
- **Differential:** DIC (coagulopathy), drugs, e.g. quinine, simvastatin, interferon and calcineurin inhibitors, malignant hypertension, viral infections, CMV, autoimmune disease (lupus nephritis, acute scleroderma), vasculitis, HUS (diarrhoea positive/negative), malignancy, catastrophic APLS.

- **Clinical:** anaemia, fever. Thrombosis: phlebitis with superficial vein thrombosis. Thrombotic stroke, delirium, coma, cardiac/gut/renal ischaemia/infarction. Bleeding, e.g. mucosal, petechiae, purpura, bruising.

Investigations

- **FBC:** Hb <8 g/dl, low platelets. **Clotting:** normal PT, APTT, D-dimer, fibrinogen. **Blood film:** microangiopathic haemolytic anaemia (MAHA) with schistocytes. Fragmented, deformed, irregular or helmet-shaped RBCs.
- **Intravascular haemolysis:** raised LDH, reticulocytes, bilirubin, low haptoglobin. **U&E:** AKI. **Kidney biopsy** may be indicated.
- **ADAMTS13 levels** ADAMTS13 activity of <10%.
- **Renal CT/MRI** may show areas of infarction.
- **Serology:** HIV (+CD4 count), HAV, HBV, HCV. CT brain (if CNS signs).
- **CT chest/abdomen/pelvis** to check for underlying malignancy (if indicated).
- **Pregnancy test** where appropriate.

Management (urgent haem consult and transfer to tertiary centre)

- **Medical emergency.** High risk of preventable, early deaths in TTP. Needs plasma exchange as soon as possible, preferably within 4–8 h. May need immediate transfer to specialist haematology centre that offers PLEX.
- **Therapeutic plasma exchange (TPE)** reduces 3-month mortality from 90% to almost 15%. Removes circulating antibody and ADAMTS13. Replace total plasma volume daily (1.5 × plasma volume). Low BP with ACE inhibitors.
- **Steroids:** after TPE consider steroids; either IV **Methylprednisolone** 1 g/d for 3 d or oral **prednisolone** 1 mg/kg/d with PPI especially for first event.
- **Rituximab:** a chimeric monoclonal ab to CD20 found on B cells.
- **Caplacizumab** blocks platelet vWF interactions. Prevents formation of microvascular thrombosis in small arterioles and capillaries.
- **HIV-positive**, then consider starting HAART.
- **Platelets** avoided generally as can cause thrombosis. Take specialist advice if active bleeding and low platelets. Watch daily bloods for response. Relapses may require steroids. Others may need a splenectomy.
- Give **packed red cells** as needed for anaemia. Give **Folate** 5 mg OD. Low dose **Aspirin** 75 mg OD started once platelets >50 × 10⁹/L. Long-term avoid quinine and oestrogen-containing medications which can cause relapse.
- **Reference:** Long Zheng X *et al.* (2020) ISTH guidelines for treatment of thrombotic thrombocytopenic purpura. *J Thromb Haemost.* 18(10): 2496–502.

8.8 ▶ Bleeding and reversal of anticoagulation

- **About:** the body tries to maintain a constant balance of clot formation and breakdown. We produce prothrombotic as well as antithrombotic factors. Effective haemostasis requires vessel endothelial integrity, platelets, clotting factors as part of the coagulation cascade, vWF and fibrinogen.
- **Coagulation cascade:** two systems which function together to ultimately produce nets of fibrin. Extrinsic is initiated by tissue factor, a molecule found on smooth muscle, fibroblasts. Exposure-activated factor VIIa forms factors IXa and Xa. Alternative contact pathway involves formation of XIIa by high molecular weight kininogens and calcium. This activates XI to XIa, which forms Xa and then IX to IXa. This forms VIIIa which activates X to Xa which is the common focal point. Factor Xa

converts prothrombin to thrombin and thrombin cleaves fibrinogen to fibrin which forms on the surface of platelets.

- **Platelets:** damage to vascular endothelium causes localised vasoconstriction and platelet activation. Platelet adhesion to damaged endothelium requires vWF.
- **Presentation:** bleeding may be obvious or occult with evidence of shock. It may be more chronic with progressive anaemia. Inherited conditions. There may be a long-standing history of excess bleeding, e.g. with challenges such as dental extraction, circumcision and other surgery, menstruation, etc. Current bleeding – bruising, petechiae. GI – melaena, PR bleeding, retroperitoneal. Renal – haematuria. Mucosal – epistaxis or from gums, bleeding into joints or intracerebral haemorrhage.
- **Investigations:** FBC: MCV may show anaemia, thrombocytopenia and low ferritin. PT (tissue factor and VII to VIIa) and APTT (XIIa/XIa, IXa), raised D-dimers in DIC, raised APTT with haemophilia A/B. Raised PT in vitamin K deficiency/warfarin and liver disease. Individual factors can be assayed as needed.

Clinical actions (see Blood products ▶ Section 8.14)

- **Drug-induced bleeding:** warfarin, heparin and DOACs covered below.
- **Consumptive coagulopathy:** inappropriate activation of coagulation system with low platelets, low fibrinogen (see DIC, ▶ Section 8.3).
- **von Willebrand disease:** seen in 1–2% population on testing but fewer clinically ever have problems. vWF binds platelets and endothelium and it also carries factor VIII. Different forms mean that vWF can be reduced or simply faulty. Mucosal bleeding is main issue. Nose bleeds, menorrhagia. Can treat with tranexamic acid 25 mg/kg TDS or desmopressin. Severe bleeding factor VIII and vWF concentrates may be given. Most are autosomal dominant, potentially mild to moderately severe. Test: low vWF antigen, low ristocetin cofactor activity, and in some low factor XIII.
- **Haemophilia A/B:** haem A is commonest form. Lack of factor VIII or IX, respectively. Clinically identical. Half of haem A have *de novo* mutations with unaffected parents. Affects males – X-linked recessive. Can be mild/moderate/severe. Treat with recombinant factors. Suffer from bleeding into joints or related to minor traumas or post-surgery.

Bleeding while anticoagulated

- A careful balance must be struck if anticoagulation is important. The risk of death from active haemorrhage usually outweighs risk of lack of anticoagulation acutely and achieving haemostasis should be the priority in the first 24 h.
- Take cardiology advice with metal valves (mitral INR 2.5–3.5 and aortic 2–2.5 lower in some newer valves) and recent stents. Direct pressure and surgical ligation and even radiological embolisation can assist in controlling bleeding. 'Bleeding comes first'. Risk of further PE may be reduced with an IVC filter.

Bleeding with thrombocytopenia

- **Platelet disorders:** qualitative and quantitative defects. Thrombocytopenia is covered elsewhere. Antiplatelet agents, e.g. aspirin, clopidogrel. NSAIDs. Impaired function – uraemia, liver disease, acquired von Willebrand disease, cancer. New drugs – prasugrel, ticagrelor. Thrombocytopenia ▶ Section 8.4.

8.9 ▶ Bleeding on warfarin/vitamin K antagonists

- **NB:** take expert advice in patients with metal valves who will need restarted on warfarin once bleeding stops. In non-valve patients consider if a DOAC will improve safety. In guidance treat VKA as Warfarin. Acenocoumarol and phenindione are used in patients who cannot tolerate warfarin.

Clinical	Escalation actions (see Blood products ▶ Section 8.14)
Limb or life-threatening bleeding, or active bleeding with haemodynamic compromise; intraocular bleed	High risk patients: age >70; hypertension; diabetes; renal failure; previous MI, stroke or GI bleed. ABC, STOP warfarin, get IV access and resuscitate depending on bleeding source. Check INR, FBC, LFTs. **Four-factor Prothrombin complex concentrate** (PCC) 25–50 U/kg. Round to nearest 500 units, maximum 5000 units, plus 5 mg IV vitamin K. Recheck coagulation 15 min after **4 factor PCC**. If inadequate correction, consider other factors such as DIC, liver disease or inadequate **4 factor PCC** dose. If adequate correction repeat testing at 4–6 h.
Possible CNS bleed	Patients with rapid onset neurological signs on Warfarin. Perform an urgent INR and CT scan (<1 h). Consider urgent reversal with **4 factor PCC** if CT is delayed while these results are awaited if high suspicion of intracranial bleeding.
Non-major bleeding	IV **Vitamin K** 1–3 mg. Recheck INR daily until stable, or at 6 h if bleeding continues. IV vit K produces a more rapid correction of the INR than oral and is preferred in the bleeding patient.
INR >8.0 (no bleeding)	**Vitamin K** 1–5 mg PO. Recheck INR daily until stable.
INR 5.0–8.0 (no bleeding)	Omit warfarin until INR <5 and reduce maintenance dose. Consider vitamin K 1 mg PO if high bleeding risk, e.g. 70 y, uncontrolled hypertension, liver disease, renal impairment, previous bleeding, recent surgery, anti-platelet drugs or thrombocytopenia. Recheck INR daily until stable. Give extra consideration before administering high doses of vitamin K with metallic heart valves as will delay restarting oral anticoagulation.
Warfarin and needs surgery	For surgery that requires reversal of warfarin and that can be delayed by 6–12 h, the INR can be corrected by giving IV vitamin K 5 mg. For immediate surgery that cannot be delayed, the INR can be corrected by giving **4 factor PCC** and IV **Vitamin K** 5 mg. 4 factor PCC may induce a prothrombotic state. Use with caution in patients with DIC or decompensated liver disease.

8.10 Bleeding on heparins and fondaparinux

Unfractionated heparin (UFH) reversal with Protamine
- It may not be necessary to routinely reverse prophylactic subcutaneous heparin unless the aPTT is significantly prolonged (take Haem advice).
- Significant bleeding on treatment dose heparin. Consider reversal with **Protamine sulphate** over 5–10 min. Dose 1 mg/100 units of LMWH given over the past 2–3 h. Max 50 mg.
- If the aPTT remains elevated, consider further **Protamine** 0.5 mg/100 units of UFH (conditional recommendation, low quality of evidence).

Low molecular weight heparin (LMWH) partial reversal with Protamine
- It may not be necessary to routinely reverse prophylactic subcutaneous LMWH unless the aPTT is significantly prolonged (take Haem advice).

- **Enoxaparin:** give **Protamine** slow IV over 10 min. If given <8 h give 1 mg **Protamine** sulfate per 1 mg drug up to max dose 50 mg. If enoxaparin given 8–12 h ago, then dose 0.5 mg/1 mg.
- **Dalteparin: Protamine** 1 mg/100 U given or 100 anti-Xa units of LMWH in the past 3–5 half-lives of the drug, up to a maximum single dose of 50 mg.
- **Tinzaparin: Protamine** 1 mg/100 anti-Xa units of LMWH administered in the past 3–5 half-lives of the drug, up to a maximum single dose of 50 mg.
- If life-threatening bleeding persists/renal insufficiency, consider redosing protamine at half the dose already given. Consider **Recombinant factor VIIa** (90 mcg/kg IV) if protamine is contraindicated.
- **Bleeding on fondaparinux:** a synthetic inhibitor of factor Xa. No antidote to fondaparinux. Levels can be assessed by anti-factor Xa activity. Manage through cessation of drug and haemostatic measures. Consider **rFVIIa** if continued life-threatening bleeding.
- **Reference:** Frontera A *et al.* (2015) Guideline for reversal of antithrombotics in intracranial hemorrhage. *Neurocrit Care*, 24(1):6–46.

8.11 ▶ Bleeding on direct oral anticoagulants

- **About:** some of the new anticoagulants have specific antidotes which should be reserved for severe/life-threatening bleeding. Take expert advice early.
- **Direct Xa** inhibitors: **Apixaban, Edoxaban, Rivaroxaban**.
- **Direct IIa (thrombin)** inhibitors – Dabigatran.
- **Assessment:** determine bleed severity. Clotting tests and factors can be measured. If life-threatening and medication taken then treat.
- **Investigations:** get IV access, use local haemostatic measures to control bleeding – mechanical compression. Check FBC, U&E and clotting screen for PT, APTT, TT. Send group and save sample.

Management: consult with haematology (see Blood products ▶ Section 8.14)

- **Basics:** If minor bleed, then omit next dose and observe. Otherwise, ABC, IV access, CT head if ICH/SDH/EDH suspected.
- **Moderate bleeding** consider omitting next dose, observe, **Activated charcoal** (50 g) can be considered if DOAC ingested within 8 h of **rivaroxaban**, 6 h of **apixaban** and 2 h of **dabigatran** ingestion. Consider **Tranexamic acid** IV.
- **Severe bleeding/life-threatening: ABC**, bleed management. No antidote. Consider Activated Charcoal, IV **Tranexamic acid** and **4 factor PCC (II, VII, IX, X). FFP** has been used but evidence lacking in efficacy.
- **Dabigatran (thrombin inhibitor):** can be assessed with APTT. Antidote is **Idarucizumab (Praxbind)** IV infusion as one split dose of 5 g (2 × vials of 2.5 g). Not available, consider **4 factor PCC/Tranexamic acid.** It is dialysable. Do not give **Idarucizumab** and **4 factor PCC together** as risk of prothrombotic state.
- **Rivaroxaban, Edoxaban and Apixaban:** if life-threatening/severe consider **Andexanet-alfa** (recombinant form of human factor Xa protein). It is very expensive so may need senior approval. It is not yet licensed for Edoxaban. If not available **4 factor PCC/Tranexamic acid.** Do not give **Andexanet-alfa** and **4 factor PCC together** as risk of prothrombotic state.

8.12 ▶ Bleeding post thrombolysis

- **About:** alteplase used for stroke, PE, ischaemic stroke, STEMI. Monitor for bleeding. Reteplase, streptokinase, etc. Work by breaking down fibrinogen.
- **Intracranial/systemic:** CNS: low GCS, headache, new seizure, acute BP rise, N&V, dilated pupil. Systemic: melaena, haematemesis, low BP, high HR, flank bruising. Epistaxis. Shock.
- **Investigations:** check fibrinogen, PT, APTT, FBC.
- **Management:** ABC, IV access. Stop alteplase or other agent. CNS bleed get urgent CT scan. Systemic bleed. Resuscitate. Quickest way to replace fibrinogen is with **Cryoprecipitate** 10 units or 4 units FFP which is much more dilute fibrinogen. Target fibrinogen level of 1 g/L. **Tranexamic acid** may be considered. For ICH Neurosurgical consult once coagulation normalised. ENT for persisting epistaxis, Gastroenterology for melaena, haematemesis. Direct pressure if possible to control bleeding from arterial or venous puncture sites. See Blood products ▶ Section 8.14.

8.13 ▶ Blood transfusion

- **About:** risk of death is 3 in 1 million transfusions. Infection transmission is rare. Most deaths occur from transfusion-associated circulatory overload (TACO). In general, red cell needs are falling but platelets and plasma rises. Helped by using **tranexamic acid** in major traumatic haemorrhage and evidence is that a restrictive policy in red cell transfusion in critical care/surgical patients is safe. There is increasing recognition of the lack of a precise trigger point but that this should reflect the patient's clinical needs and quality of life and symptomatology. Important issues are to ensure that transfusion is necessary, the right blood, right patient, right time and right place and the right amount. Use only if benefits outweigh risks. Ensure informed consent of risks of blood and alternatives considered. Indications must always be recorded. Transfusion must never happen if there is any uncertainty about identity. Monitoring is vital.
- **NB:** never give Rh- or Kell-negative girls or fertile females Rh/Kell-positive blood as they develop IgG anti-D antibodies which may cause haemolytic anaemia of the newborn.
- Whole blood is rarely used and instead individual products are used so 'blood' transfusion is a misnomer. It's a 'blood product' transfusion.

8.14 ▶ Blood products

- **About:** Blood products are red cells, platelets, FFP and cryoprecipitate. See below. Plasma comes only from males to reduce TRALI and derivatives include albumin, IVIg, coagulation factors. ABO compatibility is desirable for FFP and cryoprecipitate but not for plasma. No need to worry about rhesus or irradiation. Determine which product best fits the clinical need. Blood stocks come from unpaid altruistic donors and are tested for HBsAg, anti-HIV1/HIV2, anti-HCV, anti HTLV-1 and -2, syphilis antibodies. CMV may be tested to deliver stocks of CMV-negative blood. May also be tested for serology to malaria, West Nile virus and *Trypanosoma cruzi*. Those at risk of CJD are excluded from donor pool.
- <u>**Packed red cell concentrates.**</u> Volume 350 ml. Hct 60%. Each unit raises Hb by 1 g/dl. Contains white cells. For bleeding/anaemia. Find and treat underlying cause. Red cells needed for O_2 carrying and delivering capacity but due to low

levels of DPG this can take several days to optimise. It is thought that transfusion in non-haemorrhagic anaemia may not be needed until Hb <70–80 g/L. Severe sepsis, traumatic brain injury or brain ischaemia, consider if <90 g/L. Consider for chronic anaemia (sickle cell, marrow disease, etc.) if Hb <70–80 g/L, though the exact threshold for transfusion depends on symptoms and context. In the setting of acute bleeding the Hb may be an unreliable indicator of need for transfusion. <30% loss (1500 ml adult) then replace with crystalloid, 30–40% crystalloid + red cell concentrates, >40% (2000 ml) rapid replacement with red cells. Blood with plasma and as many leucocytes removed as possible (reduces risk of vCJD) and an additive solution added. Stored at 4°C. Laboratory need to ensure ABO and rhesus compatibility. A bag of packed cells lasts 35 d and is kept refrigerated at 4°C. Risks of infection, TACO, transfusion reactions, etc.

- **Platelets.** Platelet function is reduced by drugs such as aspirin, ticlopidine, clopidogrel, abciximab, tirofiban, prasugrel and ticagrelor, and systemic disease, e.g. renal failure. Platelet count can be a poor estimate of platelet functional activity. Each bag contains 300×10^9/L platelets in 300 ml and raises count by $20–30 \times 10^9$/L. **Indications:** any severe thrombocytopenia with significant bleeding or very high risk of bleeding. Try to avoid in HITT and TTP / ITP if possible. Use to prevent bleeding when platelet count $<10 \times 10^9$/L or when $<20 \times 10^9$/L and use in those with active bleeding with level $<50 \times 10^9$/L or higher if CNS bleed. Use pre-procedure (LP, biopsy/central line) to give count $>50 \times 10^9$/L. Target $>80–100 \times 10^9$/L before spinal epidural, brain or eye surgery. Massive surgery then maintains levels $>75–100 \times 10^9$/L. ABO-compatible platelets are more effective. Side-effects: as for blood transfusion. One therapeutic dose for adults.
- **Fresh frozen plasma (15 ml/kg typical dose).** For acquired coagulation deficiencies. Stored at −25°C. Plasma derivative. Contains stable components of the coagulation, fibrinolytic and complement systems, proteins that maintain oncotic pressure and modulate immunity and others. **Indications:** used for single/ multiple clotting factor deficiencies, acute DIC with bleeding, TTP with plasma exchange, or for inherited coagulation deficiencies undergoing major surgery, major haemorrhage in a ratio of 0.5–1 unit FFP per unit of red cells, aiming for a PT and APTT ratio of <1.5 and a fibrinogen level of >1 5 g/L. Dose: **FFP 15 ml/kg body weight (equivalent to 4 units for an adult).** For warfarin reversal (use only if PCC unavailable). **SE:** reactions can include all those seen with a blood transfusion.
- **Cryoprecipitate.** Used for DIC and low fibrinogen and bleeding, is a plasma derivative from FFP and contains 100 IU of factor VIII (missing with haemophilia A) and 250 mg of fibrinogen, vWF, factor XIII and fibronectin. Used originally for haemophilia. Used with FFP unless isolated deficiency of fibrinogen. **Indications:** DIC with bleeding and a fibrinogen level <1.5 g/L, advanced liver disease, to correct bleeding or as prophylaxis before surgery, when the fibrinogen level <1.5g/L, bleeding associated with thrombolytic therapy causing low fibrinogen, renal failure or liver failure associated with abnormal bleeding where DDAVP is contraindicated or ineffective. Inherited hypofibrinogenaemia, where fibrinogen concentrate is not available. **SE:** reactions can include all those seen with a blood transfusion. Dose: 2 pooled units, equivalent to 10 donor units, for an adult (contains 3 g of fibrinogen).
- **IV immunoglobulins** for treatment of ITP and GBS.
- **Severe low albumin:** human albumin solution (HAS) is a plasma derivative. No cross-matching needed. Isotonic forms 50–500 ml of 4.5–5% used in burns,

pancreatitis, trauma or plasma exchange. Concentrated amount of 20% 50–100 ml in nephrotic syndrome, liver cirrhosis, removal of ascites.

- **4 factor prothrombin complex concentrates (PCC):** use for immediate reversal of warfarin (or equivalent) and DOAC-induced bleeding. It is a combination of blood clotting factors II, VII, IX and X, as well as proteins C and S. It is used to reverse the effect of warfarin, rapidly reducing INR to 1.0.
- **Reference:** Norfolk (ed.) and the UK Blood Services (2013) Indication codes for transfusion. In: *Handbook of Transfusion Medicine* 5e.

8.15 ▶ Cross-matching

- **About:** blood transfusion has significant risks as well as benefits. The report *Serious Hazards of Transfusion* (SHOT) highlights potentially fatal mistakes in the administration of blood. Follow hospital policy on pre-transfusion sample collection, which should detail who can collect samples. Do not use addressograph labels to label blood samples for cross-matching.
- **Vital steps:** identify patient in whom a cross-match sample is indicated. Prepare kit and bring to bedside – do not pre-label bottle yet. Identify patient by asking **name** and **DOB** and check with **wristband**; take blood at bedside and label and date and sign the sample. Only cross-match and bleed one patient at a time to minimise the risk of error. Label the sample immediately at the bedside after taking the blood, before leaving the patient.
- **Never prelabel sample tubes.** Labelling of request: last name, first name(s) in full, DOB (not age or year of birth), NHS number or address or other unique patient identifier, reason for the request. Labelling of sample tubes: patient last and first name in full, NHS number or other unique patient identification number, DOB (not age or year of birth), date and time of collection, signature or initials of the collector. As the sample collector you must sign the request form and the sample label to verify patient identification.
- **Check identity** by asking the patient to state and spell their name, and check the wristband and check that the request form and sample match the patient and wristband. If not possible, e.g. coma or confused then check identity with spouse or carer at the bedside and then check wristband.
- **Transfusion monitoring:** pulse, BP, temp and RR every 15 min and most transfusions can be given over 90–120 min. Observation continued for additional 60 min.
- **References:** British Committee for Standards in Haematology (1999) The administration of blood and blood components and the management of transfused patients. *Transfusion Med*, 9:227. Norfolk (ed.) and the UK Blood Services (2013) *Handbook of Transfusion Medicine* 5e.

8.16 ▶ Acute transfusion reactions

- **Febrile non-haemolytic** (temp >38°C, can be seen with blood, FFP, platelets): febrile non-haemolytic reactions are usually clinically mild. If unsure, slow blood and observe patient over minutes. If worsening or any haemodynamic compromise, then stop transfusion and start crystalloid and take senior advice. Minor symptoms are not uncommon. Check the name and the bag and ensure no identification errors. Seen in 1% of transfusions. Check correct patient/transfusion. Restart about 30 min of observations. Slow transfusion, paracetamol, continue if settles. Due to pyrogens and leucocyte antibodies.

- **Allergic transfusion reactions** (with blood, FFP, platelets): can range from urticaria to anaphylaxis. Urticarial: check correct patient/transfusion. Consider **Chlorphenamine** 10 mg IV/IM. Continue if settles. Mucosal swelling: consider checking IgA levels. Anaphylaxis: stop transfusion, treat as for anaphylaxis with 1 L NS IV and **Hydrocortisone** 200 mg IV. Consider **Adrenaline** 0.5 ml of 1 in 1000 IM. May occur with IgA deficiency being exposed to IgA. Consider checking IgA levels. Check mast cell tryptase immediately and at 3 and 24 h. Get a CXR if dyspnoea. Anaphylaxis, ▶Section 2.18.

- **ABO incompatibility (with blood, rarely with platelets and FFP):** even 30 ml of type A to group O can be fatal. Keep the implicated blood unit. Transfused red cell antigen meeting recipient's anti-A and/or -B antibodies rapidly leads to complement-mediated haemolysis to DIC, AKI and haemoglobinuria/-aemia. Acutely unwell, tachycardic and low BP and progressively worse. Fever, chills, pain, flushed face, vomiting, diarrhoea all due to complement fragments. If transfusion reaction, stop blood. Take full bloods from patient and repeat cross-match. Direct antiglobulin test (DAT), LDH, haptoglobin. Coagulation screen. Start IV NS. Give **Adrenaline** IM if anaphylaxis. Consider **furosemide** IV to initiate diuresis. Discuss with ITU. Discuss with haematologist. Keep opened unit and any unused units and return to lab for checking. If low BP, oliguria and anuria may cause AKI and need **furosemide** IV. ABO incompatibility has 10% mortality. Extravascular lysis is milder with fever and chills and is usually delayed with anaemia and jaundice and usually due to anti-D. Check all bloods and coagulation screen. Commonest cause is mislabelling pre-transfusion samples and failures in identity checking. There is only a 30% risk of ABO incompatibility reactions so errors may go undetected.

- **Bacterial contamination:** commoner with platelets as stored at 20–24°C. Fever usually >39°C, low BP, rigors, septic shock, oliguria, DIC. Usually immediate and often lethal. Stop transfusion. Take blood cultures. Consider antibiotic.

- **Viral contamination:** HBV, HTLV, HIV, HCV. Testing is done for these. Use CMV-negative donors for those receiving bone marrow transplants or solid organ transplants on immunosuppression.

- **Other infections:** include syphilis and malaria and toxoplasmosis. Syphilis is screened for.

- **Transfusion-associated circulatory overload (TACO):** usually elderly medical; TACO any age but more in age >70. Leads to breathlessness and cardiogenic pulmonary oedema within 6 h, CXR changes. Treat as cardiogenic pulmonary oedema. It is one of the more common causes of transfusion-related death. Patients should be monitored and reassessed between transfusions. JVP raised, BP high, O_2 sats low. Worsens with fluid challenge. Improves with diuretics. Abnormal echo.

- **Transfusion-related lung injury (TRALI):** haematology and surgical patients. Plasma antibodies react to host white cell antigens and pulmonary endothelium. Comes on acutely usually <2–6 h with breathlessness, rigors, non-cardiogenic pulmonary oedema, cough, CXR changes. Due to donor antibodies to white cells. Treat as ARDS. Seen with plasma or platelets. JVP low, BP low. CXR bihilar shadowing. Low O_2 sats. Low WCC. Improves with fluid challenge. Worsens with diuretics.

- **Transfusion-associated graft-versus-host disease (TA-GvHD):** immunocompromised host. TA-GvHD occurs when donor lymphocytes from transfused blood engraft in the recipient and cause disease and destroy recipient's bone marrow. Occurs 10–14 d post-transfusion with clinical features of fever, skin

rash, hepatitis, diarrhoea and pancytopenia. It is fatal in >90% of cases. Prevent by giving irradiated blood to groups at risk. See table below.
- **Post-transfusion purpura:** later fall in platelets after 10–14 d. Recipient develops antibodies to human platelet antigen 1a. Treat with IVIg or plasma exchange.
- **Reference:** Serious Hazards of Transfusion website: www.shotuk.org.

8.17   Indications for irradiated blood

Indications for irradiated blood products in adults to prevent TA-GvHD

- Blood from a 1st/2nd-degree relative. Receiving a granulocyte transfusion.
- Patients receiving HLA – selected components even if immunocompetent.
- Purine analogues (fludarabine, cladrabine, deoxycoformicin, etc).
- Hodgkin's lymphoma, at any stage of the disease (for life).
- Patients receiving allogeneic haemopoietic stem cell (HSC) grafts, from the start of conditioning therapy and while the patient remains on GvHD prophylaxis (usually 6 months post-transplant). If chronic GvHD is present or the patient is taking immunosuppressants, continue irradiated blood components indefinitely.
- Allogeneic HSC donors being transfused 7 d before harvest of their HSC.
- Patients who will have autologous HSC graft: any transfusion 7 d prior to/during the bone marrow/stem cell harvest.
- Transfusion from start of conditioning chemo-radiotherapy until 3 months post-transplant (6 months if total body irradiation was used).
- Patients receiving anti-thymocyte globulin (ATG) and/or alemtuzumab (anti-CD52).
- Patients with known/suspected T-cell immunodeficiency, e.g. DiGeorge syndrome irradiation.
- There is also no indication for routine irradiation of cellular blood components for adults who are HIV antibody positive or who have AIDS.

8.18   Immunocompromised patients

Introduction
- Those with HIV or acquired/congenital immune deficiency.
- Those on steroid therapy – depends on dose and duration.
- Those on drugs for organ rejection post-transplant.
- Immunosuppression for RA, SLE and autoimmune disease.
- Use of ciclosporin, tacrolimus, azathioprine, mycophenolate, steroids.
- Myeloma, lymphoma, hypersplenism, asplenia.
- Diabetes, hypophosphataemia (on TPN).
- Infections – influenza, rubella, measles, AIDS. Malnourished, malignancy.

Problems
- Meningitis. Severe overwhelming sepsis. Fewer typical signs and symptoms.
- Pneumonias, meningoencephalitis, PCP pneumonias.
- Mucocutaneous and systemic fungal infections.
- Severe gastroenteritis, diarrhoea.
- Viral infections – isolate and need prophylactic and treatment antivirals.
- Avoid live vaccines. Culture, LP, treat with lower threshold.
- Stop immunosuppressive agents if significant infection detected.
- Increased malignancy risk – skin, renal, cervical.
- Take expert infectious diseases or transplant team help early.

8.19 ▶ Plasmapheresis/plasma exchange (PLEX)

- **About:** plasmapheresis means removal of plasma 'take away', which either involves some form of filtering by centrifugation or membrane separation that can remove products from plasma at a rate greater than the body can make and distribute the toxic immunoglobulins. With centrifuge devices, citrate is the anticoagulant of choice and this can cause hypocalcaemia. Plasmapheresis is used when a substance in the plasma, such as immunoglobulin, is acutely toxic and can be efficiently removed. It may be combined with other treatments such as rituximab which destroys both normal and malignant B cells that have CD20 on their surfaces. These make immunoglobulins.
- **Indications:** GBS, myasthenia gravis, CIDP, hyperviscosity in monoclonal gammopathies, TTP, Goodpasture syndrome (anti-GBM disease), atypical HUS (autoantibody to factor H), neuromyelitis optica.
- **Method:** patients require central line placement. Dose 40–50 ml/kg of plasma is removed and the plasma replaced with albumin or saline. Up to 3–6 exchanges on a daily or alternate day regimen.
- **Side-effects:** include a flu-like illness, haemodynamic instability with arrhythmias and low BP, and autonomic dysfunction. There may be problems from the access with thrombophlebitis, bleeding, line infections and PTX.

8.20 ▶ Vaccine-induced immune thrombocytopenia and thrombosis (VITT)

- **About:** venous thrombosis <30 days of Covid-19 vaccination.
- **Aetiology:** anti-platelet factor 4 antibodies arise after Covid-19 vaccination.
- **Clinical:** new onset of severe headache, which is getting worse and does not respond to simple painkillers. Unusual headache worse when lying down or bending over, or may be accompanied by blurred vision, nausea and vomiting, difficulty with speech, weakness, drowsiness or seizures. New unexplained pinprick bruising or bleeding. Dyspnoea, chest pain, leg swelling or persistent abdominal pain.
- **Investigations:** FBC for low platelets. If low check coagulation screen, including fibrinogen (Clauss) assay, D-dimer, blood film to confirm true thrombocytopenia and exclude alternative diagnoses. VITT unlikely if D-dimer low and platelets normal. If diagnosis suspected and symptoms suggest CVST then CT/CTV or MRV, CTPA if PE, duplex if DVT, USS/CT abdomen if portal or splanchnic vein thrombosis. If confirms do ELISA for platelet factor 4.
- **Differential:** TTP, cancer, APLS, HIT, PNH.
- **Management:** start anticoagulation (avoid heparin), consider DOAC, fondaparinux, danaparoid sodium, argatroban.
- **Reference:** NICE (2021, updated 2022) NG200: *COVID-19 rapid guideline: vaccine-induced immune thrombocytopenia and thrombosis (VITT)*.

09 Infectious diseases

Introduction
- This chapter covers infections which are easily grouped here rather than under specific organs. Infections are those most commonly seen in a UK population but occasionally we pick up less common illnesses from abroad where early suspicion is key. 'Influenza' could easily be cerebral malaria if recent travel to an endemic area is discovered.
- Delayed diagnosis and treatment could be deadly. Also see ▶ Section 23.2 on antibiotic prescribing. Finally, ID and microbiology staff are usually accessible and helpful and will provide excellent advice and should certainly be spoken with for any severe infection.
- Many tropical diseases are here briefly and very rarely, but basic knowledge to cause clinical suspicion and to aid discussions with ID are included.
- The UK has designated certain infections as HCIDs to be aware of.

High consequence infectious diseases (HCIDs) defined
- Acute infectious disease.
- Typically has a high case-fatality rate.
- May not have effective prophylaxis or treatment.
- Often difficult to recognise and detect rapidly.
- Ability to spread in the community and within healthcare settings.
- Requires an enhanced individual, population and system response to ensure it is managed effectively, efficiently and safely.

Two main categories (Covid-19 not now included)
- **Contact HCID:** Argentine haemorrhagic fever (Junin virus), Bolivian haemorrhagic fever (Machupo virus), Ebola virus disease (EVD), Crimean Congo haemorrhagic fever (CCHF), Lujo virus disease, Marburg virus disease (MVD), Lassa fever.
- **Airborne HCID:** Andes virus infection (hantavirus), Avian influenza A H7N9 and H5N1, Avian influenza A H5N6 and H7N7, Middle East respiratory syndrome (MERS), Monkeypox (Clades I and IIa only), Nipah virus infection, Pneumonic plague (*Yersinia pestis*), severe fever with thrombocytopenia syndrome (SFTS), severe acute respiratory syndrome (SARS).

Imported fever service (IFS) in the UK
- Clinical advisory and specialist diagnostic service for medical professionals managing travellers who've returned to the UK with fever.
- 24-hour, 7-days a week telephone access to expert clinical and microbiological advice.
- 24-hour on-call molecular diagnostic service for viral haemorrhagic fevers.
- Next working day diagnostic service for a range of other acute imported fevers, panels of diagnostic tools designed for 10 world regions, with the aim of delivering a positive diagnosis, rather than ruling out single infections.

Referrals (www.gov.uk/guidance/imported-fever-service-ifs)
- Hospital doctors can contact the IFS after discussion with the local microbiology, virology or infectious disease consultant.

- Call 0844 778 8990 for direct access to one of the on-call experts.
- See the enquiries process and list of patient details you need before you access the IFS.

Links to important topics
- Sepsis ▶Section 2.21.
- CNS infections ▶Sections 11.8–11.13.
- Urinary tract infections ▶Section 10.6.
- Febrile neutropenia ▶Section 17.5.
- Cellulitis ▶Section 19.3.
- Necrotising fasciitis ▶Section 19.6.
- Animal and human bites ▶Section 19.5.
- Infective endocarditis ▶Section 3.22.
- Respiratory infections ▶Sections 4.14–4.16.

9.1 Pyrexia of unknown origin

- **About:** fever persisting for >2 weeks, with no clear diagnosis despite intelligent and intensive investigation. Temp >38.3°C. Specialist PUO scenarios – HIV-positive and neutropenic PUO. Most are infection, malignancy or inflammatory, autoimmune diseases.
- **Causes and strategy:** comprehensive history and repeated examination.
- **Common:** TB, endocarditis, gallbladder disease and HIV infection.
- **Rare:** tropical unless clear travel history or exotic diseases. Always consider exposure to an infection, travel to a high-risk area, environmental exposure, contact with an infected individual, occupation and leisure activity history, e.g. canoeing (leptospirosis), animal exposure, sexual contacts, IV drug use/needles, blood transfusion, vaccinations. HIV test should be done in all.
- **Factitious:** seems well, temp >41°C, self-harm or self-injection, bizarre, normal CRP/ESR, secondary gain.

Clinical clues: check frequently and observe fever
- **Lymphadenopathy/hepatosplenomegaly** give foci for tissue diagnosis.
- **Top to toe exam including orifices:** mouth, throat, perineum, axillae, skin.
- **Tenderness:** skin abscess, spinal tenderness, bone pain, dental pain.
- **Abscesses:** skin, subphrenic, perineum, pelvic, brain. Pain, pneumonia.
- **Tuberculosis:** weight loss, cough, confusion, immigrant.
- **Perinephric abscess:** complicated UTI, renal TB.
- **Endocarditis:** look for signs. Get TTE/TOE. Blood cultures, HACEK group.
- **Cholangitis:** LFTs may be minimally deranged, USS, look for stones.
- **Drugs can cause a fever.** Consider stopping any likely ones.
- **PAN/RA/SLE:** autoantibodies, U&E, urine, juvenile idiopathic arthritis.
- **Others:** sarcoidosis, Crohn's disease, ulcerative colitis.
- **Rare:** familial Mediterranean fever, thyrotoxicosis.
- **Kikuchi's disease:** histiocytic necrotising lymphadenitis, young women, rare, benign condition, cervical lymphadenopathy and fever.
- **Malignancy:** lymphomas, leukaemia, solid tumours, renal, liver.
- **Brucellosis:** travel to affected areas, work with animals, food preparation and ingestion of unpasteurised dairy or raw meats.
- **Dental abscesses:** check the mouth and dentition and tap the teeth for pain and discharge and get dental review. Arrange orthopantomogram (OPG) X-ray.

- **Bioterrorism:** anthrax, plague, smallpox (was eradicated, fever, aches, vomiting, centrifugal pustular rash use vaccination, cidofovir/ST-246), tularaemia.
- **Dog/cat saliva:** *Capnocytophaga canimorsus* and *Pasteurella multocida*.

Investigations

- **FBC and DWCC:** neutrophils suggest bacterial infection. Lymphocytes: a viral infection. Lymphopenia: HIV, Covid infection. Neutropenia: viral infection. Eosinophilia: parasitic infection, low platelets, malaria (parasites on film indicative).
- **ESR/CRP:** elevated confirms disease but poor specificity for aetiology.
- **Serology:** HIV1 and HIV2, HBV, HCV, monospot, CMV/EBV.
- **Blood cultures:** preferably before antibiotics started. Aerobic and anaerobic bottle using strict asepsis. Contaminants jeopardise diagnosis and care.
- **LFTs:** hepatitis, cholangitis, alcoholic liver disease. Imaging/liver biopsy.
- **Imaging:** CXR in all. Consider USS abdomen and pelvis or CT chest/abdomen/pelvis for pus collection, malignancy.
- **Biopsy:** nodes or liver biopsy or bone marrow can help with diagnosis.
- **Labelled white cell scanning:** can help isolate any white cell collection.
- **Echocardiogram:** transthoracic initially and then transoesophageal if endocarditis suspected and need to see vegetation and valve damage.
- **Lumbar puncture:** if suggestion of CNS infection – headache, delirium.
- **TB suspected:** culture urine, sputum, CSF, Mantoux test. CXR/CT chest. Interferon-gamma assay (IGRA), fewer false positives from BCG vaccination.
- **Therapeutic trials** can be considered as a test if a diagnosis is strongly suspected, e.g. tuberculosis, brucellosis.
- **Autoimmune screen:** ANA, dsDNA, ANCA, RF, anti-CCP.
- **Syphilis:** TPHA/FTA/FTI. **Leptospirosis:** IgM, cultures. **Lyme disease** serology. **Dengue:** non-structural protein 1 (NS1). **Malaria films** on three consecutive days or a malaria rapid diagnostic test (RDT).
- **Procalcitonin:** increased levels in patients with bacterial sepsis, especially severe sepsis and septic shock. May aid decisions relating to antibiotic requirements. PCT <0.50 ng/ml represents a low risk of severe sepsis and/or septic shock. PCT >2.00 ng/ml represents a high risk of severe sepsis and/or septic shock. It is not a substitute for good clinical judgement and cannot be used in isolation. May be falsely elevated in SCLC or medullary C-cell carcinoma of the thyroid.

Management

- **Resuscitate:** ABC. Severe sepsis ▶Section 2.21; Hypovolaemia, ▶Section 2.20. If possible try to avoid starting antimicrobials without first getting CSF and multiple blood cultures off and discussing with infectious diseases or microbiology.
- Logically work through common diagnoses first. Consider second opinion as these can be challenging and arrange rheumatology review.

9.2 ▶ Assessment of the febrile traveller

- **About:** 1 in 12 travellers acquire an infection needing medical attention. Differential is all the home-grown local infective and perhaps non-infective causes plus exotic ones. In any infective presentation a travel history should always be obtained. Anyone with fever and flu-like illness who has travelled to an endemic area has falciparum malaria until proven otherwise.

- **Main killers:** meningococcaemia, cerebral malaria and viral haemorrhagic fevers. They are uncommon but rapidly fatal. If malaria considered determine what prophylaxis taken, areas visited and likely dates of infection.
- **Clinical:** business, leisure. Where stayed, town vs. countryside, medications taken, night nets, unprotected sex with new person(s). Game parks, farms, caves, health facilities, exotic foods, activities involving fresh or salt-water exposure. Any bites/saliva, e.g. bats (rabies), dogs (*Capnocytophaga canimorsus* and *Pasteurella multocida*).
- **Symptoms:** malaise, photophobia, rash, dysuria, cough, phlegm, rash, eschar on legs/inguinal/axilla (typhus), rose spots on torso (typhoid), hepatosplenomegaly, lymphadenopathy or jaundice.
- **Consider usual causes first:** always consider the usual familiar causes – influenza, UTI, chest infection, meningitis, endocarditis, TB or a lymphoma, Lyme disease.

Clues to infective causes where unclear
- **Raised lymphocytes:** viral infection, TB, pertussis, brucellosis, syphilis.
- **Low lymphocytes:** HIV, *Legionella*, steroids.
- **Raised neutrophils:** bacterial infection.
- **Low neutrophils:** sepsis, viral, brucella, typhoid (WCC normal), kala-azar, TB.
- **Raised eosinophils:** parasites, drugs, polyarteritis nodosa, COPD.

Sources of infection endemic locations
- **Anywhere:** HIV, bacterial sepsis, UTI, meningitis, HSV encephalitis, influenza, leptospirosis, rabies.
- **Africa:** malaria, dengue fever, rickettsial disease, enteric fever, viral haemorrhagic fevers, Ebola, amoebic liver abscess, Katayama syndrome.
- **African safari:** rickettsial disease, African trypanosomiasis.
- **West Africa** (Nigeria, Niger, Mali, Senegal, etc.): viral haemorrhagic fever.
- **Horn of Africa:** visceral leishmaniasis.
- **Southeast Asia:** malaria, dengue fever, enteric fever, chikungunya disease, rickettsial disease.
- **Africa, Asia, Caribbean, South America:** malaria, typhoid 'enteric' fever, viral hepatitis, dengue fever, poliomyelitis.
- **USA:** coccidioidomycosis in **southwestern** (desert areas): **Rocky Mountain spotted fever:** USA commonest in North Carolina and Oklahoma and so beyond the Rocky Mountains.

Mode acquired
- **Foodborne:** typhoid, paratyphoid, bacillary dysentery and amoebic dysentery are persisting causes of symptoms >48 h.
- **Sexual contact:** HIV, gonorrhoea, syphilis, Chlamydophila, chancroid, hepatitis.
- **Blood-borne:** hepatitis B/C, HIV, Ebola, VHF, Lassa fever.
- **IV drug users:** *Staph. aureus*, hepatitis B/C, HIV, anthrax, botulism.
- **Mosquito bite:** malaria, dengue fever, chikungunya disease, tularaemia, filariasis, Zika virus, yellow fever, West Nile virus, Japanese encephalitis.
- **Tsetse fly:** African trypanosomiasis.
- **Animals:** brucellosis, rabies, Q fever, plague, tularaemia.
- **Dog, fox, skunk, bat contact (bite):** rabies.
- **Bats:** rabies, histoplasmosis, Marburg haemorrhagic fever, Nipah virus encephalitis, Hendra virus disease.
- **Faeco–oral:** hepatitis A and E, enteric fever, gastroenteritis.

- **Water-borne:** cryptosporidiosis, giardiasis, amoebiasis, hepatitis A but concentrated dose from oysters and shellfish in contaminated waters.
- **Airborne:** meningococcal meningitis, MERS, TB, coronavirus, influenza.
- **Fresh water:** leptospirosis (canoes, windsurfers), schistosomiasis (Katayama fever).
- **Tick bites:** often painless. Rickettsia, Lyme disease, Rocky Mountain spotted fever, ehrlichiosis. Scrub typhus.
- **Hotels and air conditioning and shower heads:** *Legionella.*

Incubation period infection to symptoms/signs
- The time between acquiring pathogen and disease symptoms/signs.
- **Early before 21 days:** typhoid fever, malaria, dengue, rickettsia, leptospirosis. May begin whilst away.
- **Late after 21 days:** TB, viral hepatitis, malaria, Katayama fever. Occurs when returns home.
- **Malaria:** can be early and late.

Clinical signs
- **Eschar:** 'patch of black necrotic tissue'. Tick bites. Scrub and other Typhus/rickettsia infection, anthrax, *Pasteurella multocida.*
- **Buboes:** bubonic plague, gonorrhoea, tuberculosis, chancroid or syphilis.
- **Cold sores:** *Herpes simplex* encephalitis, pneumococcal pneumonia.
- **Sore throat:** teenager, adult <30, infectious mononucleosis (EBV or CMV), epiglottitis, tonsillitis, quinsy, Lemierre's syndrome.
- **Fever without tachycardia** (ignore if on beta-blockers): typhoid fever, legionnaire disease, malaria, dengue, yellow fever, VHF, chlamydial pneumonia.

Other considerations
- **Preventative measures:** vaccines against hepatitis A/B, and yellow fever usually rules out these infections. *Anti-malarial chemoprophylaxis does not exclude malaria.* Protective clothing, use of netting, avoiding being outdoors in peak times for feeding, etc.
- **Historical clues:** travel itinerary: the risk of acquiring a travel-related infection depends on the precise geographic location and the length of stay at each destination. Modern hotel or with locals or family. Infections can be acquired en route, so layovers and intermediate stops should be recorded. Mode of transport should be recorded.
- **Sexual history:** with whom, male/female, frequency, protected, prostitution, condom use, what type of sex. Risk of infection. Other STIs.

Management of pyrexia in a traveller
- Consider local and visited areas for infective causes, inflammatory, malignancy and drugs.
- **Cerebral/falciparum malaria:** if in endemic malarial area then assume falciparum malaria until you have a total of 3 negative smears which should be obtained 8–12 h apart over the course of 2 d. Discuss with infectious diseases specialist. If any signs of complications, then consider starting treatment immediately (▶ Section 9.3).
- **Bloods:** get FBC, blood film, U&E, LFT, HIV test, acute viral serology, blood cultures and CXR and CT head if any neurology. Lumbar puncture if CNS symptoms (check coagulation first). Serology and liver USS if liver abscess suspected. If bacterial meningitis or HSV encephalitis are a possibility, then treat appropriately.

- **Echocardiogram, cultures, CRP** if any cardiac signs. TFTs as thyrotoxic crisis could resemble infection. Repeat history and examination to make sure all information extracted. Take expert advice. Work through differential.
- **Others:** is there another cause – medications, malignancy, vasculitis, rheumatological, factitious?

9.3 ▶ Falciparum malaria

- **About:** incubation period (IP) <4 weeks but cases seen up to 6 months.
- **Biology:** systemic protozoal infection due to *Plasmodium falciparum, P. vivax, P. ovale* (subspecies *curtisi* and *wallikeri*). Falciparum most severe as it invades red cells of all ages but especially young cells and trophozoites adhere to vascular endothelium. Take expert advice early if Falciparum suspected, from local ID team or contact numbers for Liverpool School of Tropical Medicine and Birmingham in *BNF*. Follow UK malaria treatment guidelines 2016.
- **High risk groups:** children, pregnant, HIV/immunocompromised, travellers.
- **Protective:** sickle cell trait, G6PD deficiency.
- **Assume malaria** until proven otherwise if patient has been in endemic area within the incubation period. Fatal disease may present like 'flu' and moribund before post take ward round. Asking about travel is the golden question with urgent serial thick and thin films which can be falsely negative. Rapid stick tests. Treat quickly on clinical acumen as it can kill within hours. Appropriate prophylaxis with full adherence does not exclude fatal falciparum malaria. Take expert advice.
- **Endemic areas:** Africa, Asia, Papua New Guinea, South America, Western Pacific. Milder disease in older children and adults from endemic areas.
- **Aetiology:** a bite from an infected female *Anopheles* mosquito injects sporozoites which infect hepatocytes. Hepatocytes release merozoites which infect erythrocytes. Bite to RBC infection takes 7–30 d. Infected RBCs release more merozoites which infect more RBCs and cause pyrexia. Lethality due to cytoadherence of infected red cells to the walls which block post-capillary venules. Mechanism is formation of *P. falciparum* erythrocyte membrane protein (PfEMP)-1. Rosetting where infected cells adhere to uninfected RBCs.
- **Clinical:** flu-like malaise, fever >39°C (may be absent), headache, vomiting, myalgia. Coma, fits, hemiparesis, blindness, brisk reflexes, extensor plantars, decorticate or decerebrate posturing, diarrhoea, rigors, backache, drenching fevers, hepatosplenomegaly. AKI needing dialysis in 10%, intravascular haemolysis, jaundice, haemoglobinuria. Malaria does not cause lymphadenopathy or rash (consider other or additional diseases, e.g. HIV, malignancy).
- **Complications:** low GCS, seizures, oliguria <20 ml/h, ARDS/pulmonary oedema. Spontaneous bleeding/DIC, shock (algid malaria BP <90/60 mmHg). Haemoglobinuria (without G6PD deficiency). DIC, ▶Section 8.3.
- **Markers of severity:** Hb <8 g/dl, glucose <2.2 mmol/L, HCO_3 <15 mmol/L, pH <7.3, lactate >5 mmol/L, parasites >2%. Creatinine >265 µmol/L, raised bilirubin and jaundice.
- **Differential:** malaria must first be excluded in any pyrexial illness from, or in, an endemic area. Typhoid, hepatitis, dengue, avian influenza, SARS, HIV. Meningitis/encephalitis and viral haemorrhagic fevers.

Investigations

- **FBC and U&E:** low Hb, haemolysis, raised reticulocytes, raised urea and raised creatinine, raised LDH.

- **Thick and thin peripheral blood films:** (EDTA sample) to identify parasite infection. Thick films identify parasite. Thin films show the number of red cells infected and type. Need serial 3× thick/thin negative slides over 48–72 h to fully exclude malaria. Consider stopping antimalarial prophylaxis, as these may reduce parasitaemia and so reduce test sensitivity. Examination should identify the degree of parasitaemia.
- **Antigen tests:** send malaria antigens (e.g. HRP-2 for *Plasmodium falciparum* or parasite-specific LDH for *P. falciparum* and *P. vivax*).
- **Coagulation screen:** DIC seen: CXR: non-cardiogenic pulmonary oedema, exclude pneumonia and other causes of fever.

Management supportive plus antimalarials (watch CBG)

- **ABC, oral/IV** rehydration may be needed with fever, polyuria, poor intake. Give O_2 to achieve 94% saturation. Treat hypoglycaemia with IV **glucose**. Admit complicated malaria to the ITU. See antimalarial management below. Do not delay antimalarial if patient has signs of complicated falciparum malaria.
- **Pregnancy** (take expert advice. Higher risk of complications). Falciparum malaria in pregnancy may be more severe than suggested by the peripheral blood film due to marked placental sequestration. Most dangerous in 3rd trimester. Use **quinine** and **clindamycin** (as per *BNF*). Avoid **doxycycline** in pregnancy or breastfeeding. Fetus usually unaffected. Quinine is safe and effective in all stages of pregnancy and is used in standard doses. IV **artesunate** may be used in severe cases under expert guidance.

Antimalarial treatment (follow expert guidance)

- Record what anti-malarial prophylaxis. May Influence treatment.

Complicated falciparum malaria: artesunate or quinine

- Consider for seriously ill or unable to take tablets, or if >2% of red blood cell are parasitised. **Artesunate:** drug of first choice (34% reduced mortality) used on named patient basis under specialist advice. Rapid effect on parasite clearance. Most effective with parasitaemias >10%. If not available, then quinine. Artesunate 2.4 mg/kg as an IV injection at 0, 12, 24 h, then daily for 7 d. **Doxycycline** 200 mg OD for 7 days should also be given as above.
- **Quinine** 20 mg/kg in G5W over 4 h. Followed by quinine 10 mg/kg every 8 h for first 48 h (or until patient can swallow). Reduce dosing frequency to 12 h if IV quinine continues >48 h. Once able to take oral therapy then quinine sulphate 600 mg TDS for 5–7 d. Must be accompanied by a second drug: **Doxycycline** 100 mg BD PO for 7 d (or **Clindamycin** 450 mg TDS for pregnant women) from when the patient can swallow. Note there are quinine-resistant areas of SE Asia and artesunate may need to be considered. Quinine IV/PO is safe in pregnancy for treatment of falciparum malaria.

Complications

- **ABC for coma** (cerebral malaria): exclude other causes (e.g. hypoglycaemia, bacterial meningitis). Avoid steroids, heparin and adrenaline; intubate and ventilate if necessary. Paracetamol.
- **Hyperpyrexia:** tepid sponging, fanning, cooling blanket and antipyretics.
- **Convulsions:** ABC; treat promptly. IV/PR **diazepam** if ongoing.
- **Hypoglycaemia:** monitor glucose and treat hypoglycaemia. Treat acutely and consider IV 10% dextrose infusion.

- **Severe anaemia:** (Hb <5 g/100 ml, PCV <15%) transfuse with screened fresh whole blood.
- **Acute pulmonary oedema:** over-enthusiastic rehydration should be avoided. Prop patient up at an angle of 45°, give O_2, give a diuretic, stop IV fluids, intubate and add PEEP/CPAP in life-threatening hypoxaemia.
- **Acute kidney injury:** exclude pre-renal causes, check fluid balance and urinary sodium; if severe AKI consider haemofiltration or haemodialysis, or if unavailable, peritoneal dialysis. The benefits of diuretics/dopamine in acute renal failure are not proven (▶Section 10.4).
- **Spontaneous bleeding and coagulopathy:** transfuse with screened fresh whole blood (cryoprecipitate, FFP, platelets if low); vitamin K injection.
- **Metabolic acidosis:** exclude or treat hypoglycaemia, hypovolaemia and septicaemia. If severe, add haemofiltration or haemodialysis.
- **Shock:** suspect septicaemia, take blood for cultures; give parenteral antimicrobials, correct haemodynamic disturbances.
- **Hyperparasitaemia:** treat as below.

Non-falciparum malaria in adults
- **Chloroquine** 600 mg PO stat then 300 mg at 6, 24 and 48 h. If vivax/ovale then **Primaquine** 30 mg (15 mg if ovale) base/d for hypnozoites for 14 d, but check for G6PD deficiency first as can cause haemolysis.

Uncomplicated falciparum malaria
(1) **Quinine** 600 mg PO 8 h + (**Doxycycline** 200 mg OD or **Clindamycin** 450 mg 8 h) all for 7 d. **Quinine** is treatment of choice; if pregnant avoid **doxycycline** and use **clindamycin.**
(2) **Malarone** 4 'standard' tablets daily for 3 d.
(3) **Riamet** (artemether and lumefantrine) 8 tablets 12 h for 3 d.

9.4 ▶ African trypanosomiasis

- **About:** African trypanosomiasis, 'sleeping sickness', is caused by microscopic parasites of the species *Trypanosoma brucei.*
- **Transmission:** tsetse fly (*Glossina* species) from sub-Saharan Africa. Two very similar parasites cause very different disease patterns in humans.
- **Types:** *T. b. gambiense*: slowly progressive disease in western and central Africa. *T. b. rhodesiense* is more acute African trypanosomiasis in eastern and southern Africa.
- **Clinical:** two stages: blood then CNS. Chancre at inoculation site. Develops headache, malaise, weakness, fatigue, pruritus, and arthralgia. Hepato-splenomegaly, weight loss and intermittent fevers lasting 1 day to 1 week. Lymphadenopathy, mainly posterior cervical but in some cases axillary, inguinal or epitrochlear, may also occur. Posterior triangle nodes are commonly seen in *T. b. gambiense* infections. Later somnolescence, sleepiness. Awake all night, sleeps in day. Psychiatric manifestations. Myocarditis. Progressive neurology.
- **Investigations:** light microscopy of lymph node aspirate. CSF: observing trypomastigotes.
- **Management:** sleeping sickness is curable with medication but is fatal if left untreated. Pentamidine and others – take expert advice.

9.5 ▶ Tick typhus

- **About:** tick bite. Rickettsia. Obligate intracellular, Gram-neg bacteria. African tick typhus. Walking with uncovered arms/legs.
- **Clinical:** IP <10 d, high fever, headache, myalgia, maculopapular rash, eschar at site of tick bite, lymphadenitis and reactive arthritis.
- **Complications:** pneumonitis, meningo-encephalitis. DIC, AKI. Death 20%.
- **Diagnosis:** exclude malaria. Confirm diagnosis retrospectively on paired initial and convalescent-phase serum sample.
- **Management: Doxycycline** 100 mg BD PO/IV for 7 d very effective. Prevention 0.5% permethrin to treat clothing. Avoid wooded and brushy areas with high grass and leaf litter. Walk in the centre of trails.

9.6 ▶ Rocky Mountain spotted fever

- **About:** tick bite is source of rickettsia. *Rickettsia rickettsia*. USA: Oklahoma and South Carolina (far from the Rockies). Treat early if suspicious.
- **Aetiology:** Gram-neg intracellular coccobacillus. Endothelial vascular injury.
- **Clinical:** fever, headache, myalgia, maculopapular rash, no eschars. Reduced GCS, gangrene, focal neurology, organ failure, fatality 5%.
- **Diagnosis:** low Hb, raised WCC, raised LFT, AKI. Send serology.
- **Management: Doxycycline** 100 mg BD PO/IV can prevent death/severe illness.

9.7 ▶ Schistosomiasis (Katayama fever)

- **Source:** endemic in parts of Africa. From freshwater lakes/rivers allows cercariae from snails to penetrate intact skin. *Schistosoma mansoni, S. haematobium* and *S. japonicum*. Also called bilharzia.
- **Clinical:** (1) Swimmer's itch following skin penetration with papular rash. (2) Katayama fever 4–10 weeks (longer than other traveller-acquired febrile illnesses, e.g. dengue, leptospirosis). Systemic schistosomal infection, fever, lethargy, myalgia, arthralgia, cough, headache. Urticarial rash, diarrhoea ± blood, hepatosplenomegaly and wheeze. (3) Chronic infection liver, GI tract/bladder. Urinary obstruction, spontaneous abortion, bladder cancer.
- **Diagnosis:** stool or urine samples can show eggs (stool: *S. mansoni* or *S. japonicum*, urine: *S. haematobium*). Eggs passed intermittently and may not be detected. It may be necessary to perform a blood (serologic) test.
- **Management: Praziquantel** 40 mg/kg may be given for 1–2 d.

9.8 ▶ Dengue

- **Source:** flavivirus with 4 serotypes endemic in Asia, S America, Caribbean; transmitted by day-biting mosquito *Aedes aegypti*. Incubation period 7 d (3–14 d; mean 7 d) of mosquito bite. No effective vaccine.
- **Aetiology:** primary infection usually benign. Secondary infection with a different serotype or multiple infections with different serotypes may lead to severe disease with dengue haemorrhagic fever (DHF) or dengue shock syndrome (DSS).
- **Clinical: initial infection:** mild febrile, headache, retro-orbital pain, myalgia, arthralgia (back pain) and erythrodermic rash which may become petechial. Positive tourniquet test **2nd exposure** (local or staying >2 weeks): initial fever often abrupt spiking at 40°C for 5–7 d then signs of DHF with petechiae, melaena,

drop in Hb ± DSS with capillary leak, postural low BP, narrow pulse pressure, ascites, effusion, SBP <90 mmHg. Secondary infection rare in travellers. Critical phase of DSS/DHF lasts 24–48 h. **Pregnancy:** neonatal dengue possible if mother has infection <5 weeks prior to delivery.

- **Investigations:** FBC: low WCC, low platelets and raised PCV due to plasma leak, low protein. AST/ALT >1000 IU/L. DIC. Test for non-structural protein 1 (NS1) in dengue (antigen detection). PCR or positive IgM-capture ELISA. Needs daily FBC and haematocrit and platelet count.
- **Management:** ABC. ITU and supportive care of organ failure. Transfuse if required. IV crystalloids/colloids given rapidly in severe disease. Avoid aspirin as antipyretic. Mortality 1–2%. Steroids/antivirals have no evidence base. See Hypovolaemia, ▶Section 2.20; Sepsis, ▶Section 2.21; DIC, ▶Section 8.3.

9.9 Viral haemorrhagic fever

- **About:** strict isolation of infected individuals and barrier practices for healthcare workers are key to preventing transmission.
- **RNA viruses:** arenaviruses, filoviruses, bunya viruses and flaviviruses. Urgent isolation and senior advice if contact with Ebola or from affected area. Do not do bloods without discussing with infectious disease specialist.
- **Source:** Africa, S. America and Asia. Very rare with a handful of cases per decade in the UK. Delayed diagnosis leads to further cases. Zoonosis. Usually from monkeys. As viruses depend on a host they are usually restricted to the geographical area inhabited by those animals. Humans are not the natural host for these viruses, which normally live in wild animals.
- **Types:** Lassa fever: visitors to Nigeria, Liberia, Sierra Leone. Crimean–Congo haemorrhagic fever, Marburg/Ebola. Contact with dead. Sick animals.
- **Pathogenesis:** haemorrhage, severe capillary leak and shock.
- **Clinical:** incubation <3 weeks. Some cause mild illnesses, others cause severe, life-threatening disease. Fever, fatigue, dizziness, muscle aches, loss of strength and exhaustion. Petechiae, bruising, haemorrhage, mucosal bleeding, PR bleeding. Hypovolaemic shock, coma, delirium and seizures. AKI.
- **Investigations:** (take advice if safe to do bloods as high risk) send serology, **FBC:** fall in Hb raised Hct, **U&E:** AKI, coagulation screen, sickle test, ABG, raised LFT. Blood films for malaria.
- **Management:** isolate. Personal protective equipment. Exclude/treat for malaria if suspected. Contact local infectious disease specialist and follow local policy. Immediately isolate patient, protective clothing, waste disposal. Largely supportive. *Person-to-person spread possible so strict precautions must be taken.* IV **Ribavirin** has been effective in treating some individuals with Lassa fever or HRS. Convalescent-phase plasma has been used in some patients with Argentine haemorrhagic fever. Transfer to specialist unit. See Hypovolaemia, ▶Section 2.20; Sepsis, ▶Section 2.21; DIC, ▶Section 8.3.

9.10 Chikungunya

- **Source:** alphavirus transmitted by day-biting *Aedes* mosquitos. Africa/SE Asia.
- **Clinical:** flu-like, malaise, headache, rash, severe joint pain.
- **Rare sequelae:** encephalitis, GBS, seizures.
- **Management:** check serology. Supportive care.

9.11 ▶ Plague/tularaemia

- **Source:** *Yersinia pestis*. Sub-Saharan Africa. Gram-neg coccobacillus. Reservoir in rodents. Passed by bites containing blood-stained vomit from fleas who bit infected rodent. Untreated mortality >70%. Potential bioterrorism. Tularaemia can present similarly. Same treatment.
- **Clinical:** bubonic plague – swellings (buboes) in groin, axilla, neck lymph nodes, septicaemia, pneumonia (haemoptysis), meningitis.
- **Investigations:** diagnosis by blood culture or from aspirate from bubo.
- **Management:** isolate, protection. **Gentamicin** 5 mg/kg OD IV, **Ciprofloxacin** 400 mg IV BD, **Doxycycline** 100 mg IV BD.

9.12 ▶ Brucellosis

- **About:** *Brucella abortus, B. melitensis, B. suis, B. canis.*
- **Biology:** Gram-neg intracellular infection.
- **Source:** animal contact (goats, sheep, cattle, camels, pigs, dogs), unpasteurised milk, cheeses. S. Europe, India. Incubation period 2–4 weeks.
- **Clinical:** undulant fever. Enlarged nodes, liver, spleen, foul-swelling sweat, arthritis, osteomyelitis, meningoencephalitis. Scrotal pain.
- **Investigations:** WCC and CRP may not be increased. Diagnosis serology. Culture is prolonged – blood, CSF, lymph nodes.
- **Management: Doxycycline** 200 mg OD 6 weeks. **Rifampicin** + streptomycin for 2 weeks.

9.13 ▶ *Pseudomonas* infection

- **Source:** *Pseudomonas aeruginosa*, Gram-neg, rod-shaped bacterium.
- **Aetiology:** produces PEEP: phospholipase C (degrades cell membranes); endotoxin (fever, shock); exotoxin A (inactivates EF-2).
- **Clinical:** HAP, UTI, soft tissue, wounds, chronic lung disease, cystic fibrosis with chronic pneumonia due to biofilm formation, skin infections (e.g. hot tub folliculitis, wound infection in burn victims).
- **Investigations:** WCC and CRP may or may not be raised. Culture.
- **Management: Ciprofloxacin** 500–750 mg BD PO or 400 mg IV BD/TDS, **Tazocin** 4.5 g 6–8 h IV, **Meropenem** 0.5–2 g 8h, Gentamicin.

9.14 ▶ *Coxiella burnetii* (Q fever)

- **About:** *Coxiella burnetii*. Animals. Zoonosis.
- **Source:** dust, aerolised media, spores, unpasteurised milk. IP 2–4 weeks.
- **Clinical:** fever, headaches, myalgia, pneumonia, hepatitis, endocarditis.
- **Investigations:** diagnosis by serology. FBC, U&E, CRP, LFT, CXR, echo.
- **Management: Doxycycline** 100 mg BD ×14 d. See Endocarditis, ▶ Section 3.22.

9.15 ▶ *Bacillus anthracis* (anthrax)

- **Source:** Gram-positive rods. Endemic zoonosis. Found naturally in soil as spores. May be used in bioterrorism (*anthrax* – Greek for coal).
- **Aetiology:** releases a 3-protein exotoxin with oedema factor and lethal factor causing oedema and tissue necrosis.

- **Clinical:** (1) **Cutaneous:** handling infected material – painless blisters, itching, black eschar. Lymphadenopathy. (2) **Pulmonary:** inhaled spores – breathless, haemoptysis, chest pain, cough, sweats, haemorrhagic mediastinitis.
  (3) **Gastrointestinal:** eating raw infected meat – fever, chills, neck lymphadenopathy, bloody diarrhoea. (4) **Injection:** a few cases of a heroin batch contaminated with spores – fever, skin abscess.
- **Investigations:** FBC, U&E, CRP. Cultures blood/sputum/CSF/skin swab for *B. anthracis* before antibiotics. Serology for *B. anthracis*.
- **CXR/chest CT:** enlarged mediastinum, nodes, bloody pleural effusion.
- **Management:** person-to-person only with cutaneous form. Full protection should be used. Isolate. Those at risk without symptoms: anthrax vaccination can be considered. **Ciprofloxacin** 500 mg BD. **Benzylpenicillin** 2.4 g IV 4 hrly. Gentamicin may be added if severe. **Doxycycline** can be given to exposed individuals before symptoms. **Cutaneous disease: doxycycline** PO for 7–14 d as outpatient. **Systemic/inhalational anthrax:** ABC, ITU, antibiotics (**ciprofloxacin** IV and/or **doxycycline** IV) and antitoxin. **Raxibacumab** (a monoclonal antibody) may be useful against an anthrax bacterial antigen, or **obiltoxaximab.** Prognosis poor for those with pulmonary/mediastinal, gastrointestinal or meningeal anthrax. Death is toxin-mediated and results in haemorrhagic/septicaemic shock. Sepsis, ▶ Section 2.21.

9.16 Leptospirosis

- **Source:** *Leptospira interrogans*. Zoonotic. Worldwide infections. Worse in warm climates. SE Asia peaks with monsoons.
- **Risks:** water sports, canoes, windsurfers, river/lake swimming. Enters via cuts or mucous membranes. Exposure to infected urine of rats (*L. ictero-haemorrhagiae*), dogs (*L. canicola*), cattle and other animals.
- **Clinical:** IP 1–2 weeks. 2 peaks. (1) Intense headache, congested conjunctiva, fever, muscle pain, tender calf ± diarrhoea/vomiting. (2) 10% develop fever, myalgia, jaundice, erythematous rash, haemorrhage. May develop aseptic meningitis, AKI, liver failure, myocarditis, pancreatitis, purpura, ecchymosis, pulmonary and gastrointestinal haemorrhage. Most are self-limiting but occasionally severe and even fatal. Jaundice, hepatomegaly and bleeding, respiratory failure, pulmonary syndrome with ARDS, DIC.
- **Differential in tropics:** malaria, dengue, typhoid, scrub typhus, hantavirus.
- **Investigations: FBC:** raised neutrophils, low platelets, low Hb if haemorrhage. U&E: AKI, raised bilirubin and ALT. High CK. **Coagulation screen:** may have raised PT. Bleeding due to capillary fragility. **Urinalysis:** may show proteinuria and haematuria. Urine is not a suitable sample for the isolation of leptospira seen in 2nd week. **Serology:** cultures slow. Serology positive early. Diagnosis IgM titre >1 in 320 and convalescent serology >10 d for IgM ELISA and microscopic agglutination test (MAT). CSF and aerobic blood cultures: (if done early, before antibiotics) Refer to UK Leptospira Reference Unit. Keep blood cultures at room temperature prior to sending. Detection of leptospiral DNA by PCR.
- **Management:** ABC, symptomatic and supportive. Severe AKI may need renal replacement. Blood transfusion as needed. **Doxycycline** 100 mg BD ×7 d or **Ceftriaxone** 1 g OD IV if more severe. Evidence for antibiotic effectiveness is unproven. Note penicillin can cause Jarisch–Herxheimer reaction with fever, low BP, myalgia, raised HR. Those with jaundice can become very unwell despite therapy and may need liver support. Severe disease is probably immunologically mediated. No role for steroids.

9.17 *Listeria monocytogenes* (listeriosis)

- **About:** *Listeria monocytogenes*. Small Gram-positive rod.
- **Source:** sewage, salads, soft cheese, undercooked meat, chicken, patés.
- **Risk:** HIV, transplant, elderly, pregnant, renal/liver disease, malignancy.
- **Clinical:** (1) Self-limiting mild gastroenteritis. (2) Listeriosis: severe, invasive illness with mortality rate 20%. Brainstem meningitis, septicaemia, rare bone/joint infections. (3) Fetal infection and loss in pregnancy.
- **Investigations:** high WCC/CRP/ESR. MRI sign of encephalitis. CSF culture and PCR. Raised WCC and normal glucose.
- **Management:** IV **Amoxicillin** 2 g 4 hourly or **Co-trimoxazole** 120 mg/kg/day (not if pregnant/breastfeeding) in 2–4 divided doses if pen allergic. Treat for 21 days. Always take specialist advice. Bacterial meningitis, ▶Section 11.10.

9.18 *Clostridium botulinum* (botulism)

- **About:** *Clostridium botulinum* produces a potent neurotoxin. Causes a neuroparalytic disease. Botulism (latin *botulus* for sausage). Most powerful neurotoxin known. Used cosmetically/medically to paralyse muscles.
- **Source:** large rod-shaped anaerobic Gram-positive spore-forming bacillus. Found in soil, canned food, injection drug abuse, honey, trauma. Bacilli grow best when warm O_2 free low pH. Destroyed by boiling 10 min.
- **Pathology:** bacillus releases neurotoxin. It blocks presynaptic Ach transmission causing smooth/skeletal muscle paralysis. Also blocks autonomic conduction.
- **Clinical:** IP 18–36 h. Food-borne, intestinal, wound infection. Progressive blurred vision, bulbar and facial weakness, dysphagia, unable to speak. Progressive (descending) symmetrical flaccid paralysis, respiratory failure. Death in 10%. Diarrhoea, vomiting, dry mouth, constipation.
- **Clues:** no fever or meningism or headache, symmetrical neurology. Cognition intact, normal/slow HR, normal BP. No sensory deficits except blurred vision.
- **Differential:** GBS, myasthenia gravis, tick paralysis – look for and remove.
- **Investigations:** FBC, U&E, ABG: hypoxia and hypercarbia, FVC measurements TDS. NCS show defect is at neuromuscular junction. Tensilon test false positive seen. Identification of toxin in serum, stool, vomitus or food sources several days. Anaerobic cultures take up to 6 d.
- **Management:** diagnosis is clinical. ABC, ITU, severe cases (FVC <1 L) may need mechanical ventilation to avoid respiratory failure. Respiratory therapy. Recovery may take 4–6 weeks. **Antibiotics and debridement** if wound-based infection (IV **benzylpenicillin** or **clindamycin or metronidazole**). NG/PEG feeding if no swallow. PPI or ranitidine to prevent stress ulcer. Urinary catheterisation if needed, DVT prophylaxis. Wound infection: debridement and antitoxin and antibiotics. **Equine Botulinum anti toxin** halts but does not reverse neurology. Recovery takes months.

9.19 *Clostridium perfringens*

- **About:** *Clostridium perfringens* forms gas. Gram-positive anaerobic spore-forming rods. Forms exotoxins. Spores found in guts of large animals and soil, dust. From meat and poultry.
- **Clinical:** (1) Self-limiting nausea, watery diarrhoea and vomiting. (2) Clostridial necrotising enteritis (CNE) or pigbel. Can be fatal. Pork meat. Ischaemic necrosis of

jejunum. Caused by a β-toxin of *C. perfringens*, type C. (3) Clostridial myonecrosis (gas gangrene) muscle necrosis due to exotoxins, alpha/theta. Severe pain, oedema, tenderness, pallor, haemorrhagic bullae, and gas at the site of wound. Shock AKI, coma and death. (4) Anaerobic cellulitis or infection of ischaemic limb. (5) Meningitis or encephalitis.

- **Investigations:** culture and characterisation of the bacteria. Gram stain. PCR for enterotoxin (cpe) gene responsible for toxin production, detection of cpe in faeces through toxin assay, cell culture assay, ELISA or other tests.
- **Management:** ABC. Hydration for self-limiting GI symptoms. Bowel resection if very severe. Systemic infection high dose **Benzylpenicillin** 1.2–2.4 g QDS IV + **Clindamycin** 0.6–1.2 g QDS IV. Soft tissue surgical debridement. Also see Necrotising fasciitis, ▶Section 19.6.

9.20 ▶ Acute bacterial sepsis

- **About:** source, renal, bladder, skin, chest, cardiac, GI, cholecystitis, bone and joint, consider CNS and intrabdominal sources. See Sepsis, ▶Section 2.21.
- **Investigations:** screen if pyrexia, hypothermia, raised WCC, malaise, confusion. FBC, U&E, LFT raised CRP. Screen urine, aerobic and anaerobic blood cultures, CXR, lumbar puncture, ascitic aspirate, echocardiogram, joint aspirate, serology where useful. CT head, USS abdomen/pelvis. CT abdomen/pelvis. MRI spine.
- **Management:** if unwell send samples. See Sepsis, ▶Section 2.21.

9.21 ▶ Measles

- **Note:** prevent with vaccine (MMR). Severe in the immunocompromised patient (take urgent advice). Paramyxovirus. Notifiable. Highly infectious.
- **Source:** IP 12 d. In unvaccinated non-immune. Respiratory droplets. Severe infection in older children/adults. Lifelong immunity. Infectious for 1–2 weeks.
- **Clinical:** prodrome of URTI, Koplik spots in buccal mucosa, macular papular rash. Lymphadenopathy, diarrhoea, otitis media, bacterial pneumonia. Viral encephalitis, seizures acutely. Malnourished/immunocompromised get pneumonitis, encephalitis. Secondary bacterial pneumonia or severe diarrhoea or cancrum oris. Can be lethal particularly in developing countries.
- **Diagnosis:** clinical, serology or PCR. **Complications:** viral, later bacterial pneumonia, encephalitis; very late: subacute sclerosing panencephalitis.
- **Management:** IVIg may help immunocompromised if given early. Vitamin A can help. Antibiotics for bacterial superinfections.

9.22 ▶ Chickenpox/varicella-zoster virus

- **About:** more severe in adults, immunosuppressed, pregnant. Varicella pneumonia has a 10% mortality. Lives in dorsal root ganglion and can reactivate. Increased risk with pregnant, smokers, immunosuppressed.
- **Virology:** human alphaherpesvirus 3 (HHV-3) is the varicella-zoster virus (VZV). Causes chickenpox (varicella) and shingles (herpes zoster).
- **Clinical:** crops of vesicles to pustules, crust and dry on face, scalp and trunk. Feverish. IP from contact to symptoms 2–3 weeks. Hypoxia, breathlessness and respiratory failure. Can recur in later life as shingles with a dermatomal or trigeminal (ophthalmic usually) spread of vesicles with redness, pain and inflammation.
- **Investigations:** ABG: hypoxia, serology if immunity unclear. Long-term calcification on CXR. Viral DNA on PCR or electron microscopy.

- **Management:** stop any immunosuppression. Take expert guidance. HDU/ITU care for respiratory support in severe varicella pneumonia. Broad-spectrum antibiotics for secondary bacterial infection (*Staph. aureus*, pneumococcus, haemophilus). Normal: **Aciclovir** 800 mg PO QDS for 5 days. Immunocompromised: consider **Aciclovir** 10 mg/kg IV TDS for 7 days.
- **Prevention of zoster/shingles.** Vaccination in those >50 seems to dramatically lower the risk of post-herpetic neuralgia.
- **Post-herpetic neuralgia: Amitriptyline** 25–100 mg ON, **Gabapentin** 300–600 mg OD or **Pregabalin** 75 mg BD to 200 mg TDS if needed.
- **Adolescents/adults:** childhood uncomplicated infection needs only supportive care. Age >16 presenting <3 d of onset needs to be treated. Shingles/adult chickenpox: oral **Aciclovir**. Severe complicated infection: IV **Aciclovir**. Get Ophthalmic consult if eye affected as affects ophthalmic branch of trigeminal.
- **Pregnant women:** need Zoster immune globulin (ZIG). They need **aciclovir** if they develop signs. Take advice.

9.23 ▶ Mumps infection

- **About:** paramyxovirus. Sterility is uncommon with orchitis. IP is 2 weeks.
- **Clinical:** parotitis, orchitis, meningitis, pancreatitis, encephalitis is rare.
- **Investigations:** CSF: lymphocytic. (Salivary) amylase may be high due to parotitis and confuse pancreatitis diagnosis. Serology/PCR for confirmation.
- **Management:** isolate if admitted. Analgesia. Supportive management. No evidence for steroids for orchitis. Prevent with MMR.

9.24 ▶ Herpes simplex 1 and 2

- **About:** usually benign but watch for Herpes simplex encephalitis.
- **Clinical:** severe mucocutaneous lesions – mouth, genital, anorectal, vaginal, oesophagus, systemic. HSV2 more genital. Often reactivation rather than new infection. Visceral involvement can be fatal, e.g. encephalitis.
- **Investigations:** LP for CSF if HSE suspected. Stop immunosuppression. Expert consult. HSV DNA PCR on lesions.
- **Management** (see *BNF* for dosing): topical, **Aciclovir** 200 mg 5/day for 1 week. Non-genital, **Aciclovir** 200 mg 5/day PO for 5 days. Severe non-genital immunocompromised, **Aciclovir** 400 mg 5/day PO for 5 days or 5–10 mg/kg IV 8 h. Encephalitis, IV **Aciclovir** 10 mg/kg TDS for 14–21 days, also consider **Valaciclovir** and **Famciclovir.** Look for and treat any bacterial superinfection. Viral encephalitis, ▶Section 11.8.

9.25 ▶ Infectious mononucleosis

- **About:** seen with EBV (HHV4), HHV6, CMV, HIV and toxoplasmosis.
- **Clinical:** syndromic presentation with severe sore throat and fever and malaise. Teenagers or young adults. Pharyngeal oedema/respiratory obstruction, rash with ampicillin, post-viral fatigue. Hepatitis 80%, jaundice, myelitis, encephalitis. GBS, low platelets, splenomegaly, nephritis, myopericarditis, splenic rupture.
- **Investigations:** positive monospot with EBV. Viral serology for usual causes. Elevated LFTs. Atypical lymphocytes (activated CD8-positive T lymphocytes) may be seen. USS abdomen if splenomegaly.

- **Management:** largely supportive. Avoid sports and trauma with splenomegaly. Manage complications as they arise. Steroids may be given for encephalitis, thrombocytopenia and other complications. Avoid amoxicillin/ampicillin.

9.26 Cytomegalovirus

- **About:** close contact human to human, saliva. Screen blood to ensure CMV non-immune not exposed if immunocompromised.
- **Clinical:** immunocompetent: get hepatitis and infectious mononucleosis, rarely GBS. Immunocompromised: (solid organ and stem cell transplant) get a CMV pneumonitis usually 1–4 months post-transplant. Mortality of 50%. AIDS patients CD4 <50: retinitis, CMV colitis, polyradiculopathy. Pregnancy: primary infections can affect fetus. Rash, hepatosplenomegaly and CNS complications.
- **Investigations:** swab, microscopy, serology (high incidence in population) and biopsy. PCR samples. Biopsy: owl eye inclusion bodies and giant cells.
- **Management:** CMV retinitis **Valganciclovir** 900 mg PO BD 21 days, then maintenance 900 mg daily (solid organ transplant patients), otherwise IV **Ganciclovir** 5 mg/kg BD for 14–21 days then maintenance. Needs expert help, particularly if pregnancy or immunosuppressed. Others **Foscarnet, Cidofovir.** Consider HAART if AIDS.

9.27 Influenza

- **About:** influenza A/B. Orthomyxoviruses. Outbreaks due to influenza A.
- **Virology:** surface haemagglutinin (H) and neuraminidase (N) antigens. Haemagglutinin binds erythrocytes and initiates infection. Neuraminidase cleaves haemagglutinin and releases virus from cells.
- **Variants:** avian influenza: influenza A infection (H5N1) caused a more severe pneumonia. Seen mainly in SE Asia. Treat as for influenza with neuraminidase inhibitors. Swine influenza: Mexico 2009. Influenza A infection (H1N1).
- **Clinical:** comes on within days of contact. Fever, headache, severe myalgia and malaise. Cough, sputum, dyspnoea. Diarrhoea. Secondary infection with *Staph. aureus,* pneumococcal or *H. influenzae* pneumonia.
- **Complications:** secondary bacterial pneumonia, myositis, GBS, myocarditis, transverse myelitis, encephalitis, pericarditis.
- **Investigations:** FBC, U&E, LFT, CRP, PCR of nose swab. CXR cavitating secondary pneumonia.
- **Management:** supportive, hydration, analgesia, isolation, hand washing. Pandemic flu: needs special isolation and barrier nursing with staff wearing appropriate masks, goggles, gloves, and protective gear. Patient wears a surgical mask. Neuraminidase inhibitors: **Oseltamivir** (Tamiflu) treatment dose 75 mg BD for 5 days (10 days if immunocompromised). PO or inhaled **Zanamivir** 10 mg BD for 5 days inhibit neuraminidase and work against influenza A and B, but must be given within 48 h to reduce duration of illness. Can also be given IV. Susceptible to bacterial pneumonia. Sepsis, ▶Section 2.21; Pneumonia, ▶Section 4.14.

9.28 Severe acute respiratory syndrome (SARS)

- **About:** isolate suspected SARS immediately. SARS is a coronavirus respiratory illness (SARS-CoV). Since 2004, no known cases of SARS anywhere in the world. Prior to 2004, patients had had close contact with infected person.

- **Clinical:** sore throat, rhinorrhoea, chills, rigors, myalgia, headache, D&V.
- **Investigations:** FBC. Raised WCC, CRP, ALT, CK and LDH. CXR. Blood cultures, test for viral respiratory pathogens, influenza A and B and respiratory syncytial virus. Legionella and pneumococcal urinary antigen testing if CXR/CT evidence of pneumonia (adults only).
- **Management:** supportive. Isolate, analgesia, O_2. See advice for MERS below regarding PPE. Take local expert advice. Sepsis, ▶ Section 2.21; Pneumonia, ▶ Section 4.14.

9.29   Middle Eastern respiratory syndrome (MERS)

- **About:** isolate immediately. Coronavirus new to humans. Travel from Saudi Arabia and environs should raise suspicion.
- **Clinical:** severe respiratory illness, fever, cough, dyspnoea, fatality 52%.
- **Management:** supportive. Isolate, analgesia, O_2. Deadlier than SARS. Ensure respiratory isolation. Ask patient to wear a surgical mask. Wear personal protective equipment (PPE) – this should be a correctly fitted FFP3 respirator, gown, gloves and eye protection. If not available, wear a surgical mask, plastic apron and gloves. Take local expert advice. Sepsis, ▶ Section 2.21.

9.30   Acute Covid-19

- **About:** infection with novel coronavirus (SARS-CoV-2). Origin China end of 2019. Mutations – Delta and Omicron so far. Appears more infectious.
- **Aetiology:** enveloped virus. Binds to ACE-2 receptor. Respiratory spread.
- **Clinical:** IP 5–6 d. Fever >37.8°C, dyspnoea, sore throat, anosmia, fatigue, malaise, sputum, headache, delirium, falls, respiratory failure (hypoxia but not breathless), RR >30, sats <93%. Severe disease 7–10 d after onset.
- **Investigation:** lung infiltrates on CXR/CT. CXR can be normal. Most mild to moderate. A positive viral PCR 'rules in' the diagnosis but is not 100%. CT scan: ground glass opacities, crazy paving, peripheral consolidation, air bronchograms, reverse halo/perilobular pattern. Low lymphocytes, high dimer, high CRP, high AST, raised troponin and BNP.

Management (take latest advice as guidance changes rapidly)

- Isolate, protect staff, VTE prophylaxis. IV fluids, low flow O_2 15 L/min. Target >92%. Avoid aerosol generating where staff not protected: sputum induction (avoid). CPR needs full protection.
- **CPAP/BIPAP:** consider if hypoxaemia despite FiO_2 of 0.4 and when mechanical ventilation not yet needed or where CPAP is ceiling.
- **High-flow nasal O_2 (HFNO):** consider for those on CPAP when they need a break from CPAP, such as at mealtimes, humidified O_2, weaning from CPAP.
- **Nebulisers** are NOT a risk as the mist seen is from the nebuliser and not the patient. Pressurised humidified O_2 is also NOT a risk.
- **VTE prophylaxis:** double the standard prophylactic dose of LMWH for medical patients. Alternatives are fondaparinux sodium or unfractionated heparin (UFH).

Therapeutics constantly changing – discuss with ID team

- **Steroids:** those with an O_2 requirement give **Dexamethasone** PO/IV 6 mg OD or **Prednisolone** 40 mg PO OD or **Hydrocortisone** 50 mg IV 8 h for 10 d or until discharge with PPI. Monitor CBG. Hyperglycaemia is seen.

Non-hospitalised high risk with mild to moderate Covid

- Neutralising monoclonal antibodies bind to the spike protein of SARS-CoV-2. Evidence suggests significantly improve clinical outcomes in unvaccinated non-hospitalised patients with Covid-19 who are at high risk of progression to severe disease and/or death.
- **Casirivimab** and **Imdevimab** (Ronapreve): an nMAB combination that binds specifically to two different sites on the spike protein of the SARS-CoV-2 virus particle. Use in aged ≥12 hospitalised because of PCR positive with no detectable antibodies (seronegative). Hospitalised with acute Covid give 2.4 g. Hospital onset Covid-19 then 1.2 g is given.
- **Sotrovimab (Xevudy):** an nMAB that both blocks viral entry into healthy cells and clears cells infected with SARS-CoV-2 Give 500 mg as single infusion.
- **Molnupiravir:** oral antiviral for those with mild–moderate Covid-19 and at least one risk factor for developing severe illness. Such risk factors include obesity, older age (>60 y), diabetes mellitus, heart disease.

Others

- **Remdesivir:** for Covid-19 pneumonia in adults and children age ≥12 in hospital needing low-flow supplemental O_2 (≤15 L/min). Not for those on high-flow nasal O_2, CPAP/NIV or mechanical ventilation.
- **Tocilizumab:** in hospital with Covid-19 in addition to steroids unless steroids contraindicated. No other IL-6 inhibitor during this admission. No evidence of bacterial or viral infection (other than SARS-CoV-2) that might be worsened by tocilizumab. Needs supplemental O_2 and CRP ≥75 mg/L, or are within 48 h of starting HFNO, CPAP, NIV or mechanical ventilation.
- **Sarilumab:** affected adults in hospital if tocilizumab is unavailable for this condition or cannot be used. Use same eligibility criteria as with tocilizumab.
- **Antibiotics:** bacterial infection unusual (<5%). If uncertain treat as CAP.
- **New agents:** discuss with ID. Cancer patients: withhold all oral anti-cancer medicines, chemotherapy and biological modifiers, in hospitalised patients. Notify their specialist team. Do not administer granulocyte colony stimulating factor (GCSF) without specialist input.
- **Convalescent plasma:** administer only as part of a clinical trial.

9.31 Zika virus infection

- **About:** flavivirus. Brazil 2015. Birth defects (microcephaly). Affects pregnancy and can harm fetus.
- **Clinical:** fever, rash, joint pain and conjunctivitis (red eyes). Usually mild. Symptoms several days to a week. GBS seen. Severe disease uncommon.
- **Investigations:** pregnant women with symptoms get RT-PCR or serology.
- **Management:** avoid mosquito bites. Found in semen. Avoid unprotected sex with infected person. Mosquitoes that spread Zika virus also spread dengue and chikungunya viruses.

9.32 Needlestick injury

- **About:** concern is potential infection with HBV, HIV, HCV. Needle used to take blood or give IM/IV/SC injection pierces the skin of another. Infected fluids in eyes or ingested or on contact with mucocutaneous surfaces. Hepatitis C risk 3%, HIV risk 0.3%. All NHS staff need immunised against hepatitis B.

- **Aetiology:** passage of blood-borne viruses. HBV risk in HBV patient much higher but clinical staff should have been immunised. If there is a reasonable risk that the patient is HIV positive, then treat as a medical emergency and seek urgent help – see below.
- **Management:** encourage wound to bleed freely and then wash with soap and water. Don't scrub such that further tissue damage occurs. Cover with waterproof dressing. If oral or eye contamination, then wash and irrigate thoroughly with IV NS via giving set or tap water. Mouth contamination should rinse but don't swallow. Report incident promptly to line manager and complete incident form when appropriate. In working hours contact occupational health, out of hours go to local emergency department (A&E). Do not try to manage this on the ward yourself or with your team.
- **Inform the patient and explore any particular risks** for HIV/HBV/HCV, e.g. IV drug use, sexual history. Patient may allow a clotted sample for HBV/HCV/HIV. Patient should be aware that results will be divulged to the injured person. The consent should be recorded in their notes. All NHS clinical staff should be immunised against hepatitis B. Hepatitis B immunoglobulin may be given if required following expert assessment with emergency department or occupational health who may liaise with microbiology. The risk of hepatitis C is 3% and there is no post-exposure prophylaxis (PEP) but follow-up should be carried out. For HIV the risk is 0.3% and depends on depth of wound, visible blood on device, needle from artery or vein and terminal HIV disease. Risk of HIV transmission = risk that source is HIV positive × risk of exposure. As part of risk assessment record size and volume of the inoculum, i.e. whether the needle was hollow, etc. Depth of injury. Visible blood on the device that caused the injury. Injury with a needle that had been placed in an artery or vein. If HIV possible, AZT reduces infection 5-fold.
- PEP is given which involves three antiretrovirals for 1 month and is started immediately. Should begin within 24 h but can be taken up to 72 h. Check baseline HIV. PEP should be taken following local expert risk assessment and guidance and policies; an exact protocol is not included here because local practice should be followed.
- **Reference:** Kuhar *et al.* (2013) US Public Health Service Guidelines for the management of occupational exposures to HIV and recommendations for post-exposure prophylaxis. *Infection Control and Hospital Epidemiology*, 34:875.

9.33 Tuberculosis

- **About:** *Mycobacterium tuberculosis* is the most common form in humans. *M. bovis* seen in developing countries from infected milk products (non-pasteurised). Pulmonary cavitation is synonymous with infectivity but may be absent in those with AIDS. Isolate patient.
- **Risks:** HIV/AIDS, homelessness, alcohol dependency. Immigrants from sub-Saharan Africa, Bangladesh, India, Pakistan. Drug and multidrug-resistant TB is a problem. Age, malignancy, alcohol, immunodeficiency, malnutrition. Use of immunosuppression, anti-TNF-alpha drugs.
- **Multidrug-resistant TB:** TB resistant to two first line anti-TB drugs (usually Rifampicin and Isoniazid two best drugs). Typical risks HIV-positive male, London,

born in a country that has a high TB incidence, previously treated for TB, poor compliance, contact with a known case of MDR-TB.
- **Extensively drug-resistant tuberculosis:** resistant to isoniazid, rifampicin, a fluoroquinolone, and an injectable agent. Patient from South Africa.
- **Pathology:** classed as one of the granulomatous inflammatory conditions. Th1 reaction with epithelioid macrophages, Langhans giant cells, lymphocytes. Central caseous necrosis and production of interferon-gamma by T helper cells. The Ghon focus + local hilar lymphadenopathy is called a Ghon complex.
- **Clinical:** night sweats, fevers, weight loss, cervical or generalised lymphadenopathy, hepatosplenomegaly. Pyrexia of unknown origin, cervical lymph node (scrofula). **Gastro:** TB of terminal ileum with a RIF mass, peritonitis, ascites, psoas abscess. **Resp:** breathless, cough, sputum and consolidation and upper lobe scarring on CXR, pleural effusion. **Renal TB:** sterile pyuria with WCC in urine and normal cultures negative. **Skin:** lupus vulgaris and erythema induratum. **CNS TB:** TB meningitis – headache, cranial nerve palsies, etc. **Vertebral disease:** back pain – spinal infection, discitis, disc collapse, spinal cord compression. **Cardiac:** TB pericardial effusion and constrictive pericarditis. **Endocrine:** Addison's disease with adrenal TB.

Investigations
- **FBC:** low Hb, raised WCC, ESR, CRP, raised AST and ALT.
- **CXR:** pleural effusion, hilar lymphadenopathy, consolidation, fibrosis, upper and middle lobe infection, millet seed-like opacities on chest film <5 mm with miliary TB. Cavitatory disease suggests infectivity, right mid-zone collapse. Pneumothorax.
- **Sputum smear:** direct staining and microscopy of a smear from recently expectorated sputum. If bacilli seen it is classed as 'smear positive' and is infectious. Inducing sputum is said to be as effective as broncho-alveolar lavage. Auramine O is an alternative to Ziehl–Neelsen especially as the dye fluoresces under UV light and so the bacilli are easier to see.
- **Sputum cultures/analysis** are the gold standard but take 3–6 weeks to grow and then identify species. DNA PCR identifying serotype/drug sensitivity.
- **Serology:** HIV test and CD4 count.
- **Tuberculin test:** uses purified protein derivative (PPD) to elicit a delayed-type hypersensitivity response which is mediated by T lymphocytes. The reaction is maximal at 2–3 d after inoculation. Positive tuberculin testing does not always suggest active disease, it suggests a prior immune response, previous infection or BCG. So only a grade 3/4 (10 mm induration) or a negative test are useful in those with history of BCG. It is important to elicit a weal to demonstrate that it is intradermal and not subcutaneous. Most with active TB will have a positive skin test (=10 mm). Must measure the induration, not erythema. Tuberculin skin tests are not contraindicated in BCG-vaccinated people and skin test reactivity should be interpreted and treated as for unvaccinated people. False negatives occur in immunosuppressed, steroids, malnourished, HIV, severe TB (e.g. miliary disease), early primary disease – becomes positive 2–12 weeks post primary infection.
- **Lumbar puncture:** CSF raised lymphocytes and protein low glucose. Smears rarely positive in TB meningitis. Check CT exclude any space-occupying lesion.
- **Early morning urines** to culture for TB in suspected renal disease.
- **Renal imaging:** image with CT or intravenous urogram.
- **Bronchoscopy and lavage:** may be useful to get samples in difficult cases when there is an unproductive cough and high clinical suspicion. It may help to exclude other causes such as tumours with a potential for biopsy of abnormal tissue.

Microbiological culture from sputum analysis, gastric aspirate (used in children), urine for renal TB, bone marrow biopsy, CSF, liver biopsy, bronchoalveolar lavage.
Interferon gamma release assays: raised level does not differentiate active and latent disease. Main use is alongside Mantoux testing to detect latent disease.

Management
- Needs to be a high level of suspicion in the high-risk groups identified and TB with widespread manifestations should always be considered. Those with smear-positive disease need to be isolated. It is a notifiable disease. Smear-negative patients are rarely infectious. Smear-positive patients can be considered not infectious after 2 weeks of treatment. Should be referred to specialist. Adequate tissue samples for diagnosis should be taken before treatment started. Patients should be treated with 4-drug regimen (RIPE) for 2 months and 2-drug regimen for 4 months. In those with a low chance of resistance then **Rifampicin, Isoniazid** and **Pyrazinamide** only without **Ethambutol** may be used (RIP): RIPE 2 months and RI 4 months; RIP 2 months and RI 4 months – low chance of resistance. Exceptions: TB of CNS – treatment is for 12 months. Resistance to any of the drugs (isoniazid or rifampicin) means a 9-month course.

9.34 ▸ HIV infection

- WHO guidelines now agree that all HIV-positive patients should receive antiretroviral therapy (ART) after diagnosis regardless of CD4 count. When to start depends on a person's unique needs and circumstances.
- Evidence strongest with CD4 count <350 cells/mm^3 (WHO Guideline HIV, September 2015).

Seroconversion illness/acute retroviral syndrome
- **About:** HIV testing should be routine if sexually active or who use IV drugs.
- **Source:** 2–6 weeks post contact. HIV1 Euroasia/America, HIV2 Africa.
- **Risk groups:** men having sex with men. IV drug use and needle sharing. Casual unprotected sex with sex worker. Their sexual partners. Children of HIV-positive mothers.
- **Clinical** (seroconversion 2 weeks after contact): fever, rash, joint pains, malaise, lymphadenopathy, headache, myalgia, pharyngitis. Lasts for days to 3 weeks. Medical attention often sought as severe. Highly infectious period. Differential diagnosis of acute seroconversion: exclude malaria in endemic area, glandular fever, influenza and dengue.
- **Investigations:** HIV1/HIV2 antibody not detected but there is HIV RNA or HIV p24 antigen in plasma. HIV test. Repeat after 6 weeks. Check CD4 count and viral titres. CXR and ABG if suspected *Pneumocystis carinii* pneumonia (PCP). High viral loads >100,000 copies/ml.
- **CD4 count** varies daily ± 20%. Normal >500/mm^3. CD4 <200/mm^3 that severe immune suppression seen. If the CD4 <50 then high risk of CMV and atypical mycobacterial infections, e.g. disseminated *Mycobacterium avium* intracellulare. Untreated over time the CD4 count falls.
- **Management:** patient highly infectious. Test also for syphilis and other sexually transmitted infections. Take expert advice as to need for post-exposure prophylaxis. Refer to GUM for contact tracing and treatment with ART.

Acquired immunodeficiency syndrome (AIDS)

- It is later with the clinical occurrence of infections and malignancies in the setting of a low CD4 count that AIDS is defined. All those with symptomatic disease should be offered ART, usually as the count is <350 cells/mm^3.
- Those who are pregnant, need treatment for hepatitis B infection or have HIV nephropathy are treated regardless of CD4 count. Aim is to reduce the plasma viral load (PVL) and improve CD4 count and avoid resistance. This requires 3 or more drugs which are potentially toxic.

Nervous system

- **Stroke:** ischaemic stroke. Exclude other causes. Easy to confuse subcortical lesions on CT with PML. Low threshold for MRI and CSF.
- **Cryptococcal meningitis:** CD4 <50. Headache, neck stiffness, fever, photophobia, cranial nerve palsies and papilloedema. Chronic meningitis. CT: may be normal or cryptococcomas, hydrocephalus. Serum cryptococcal neoformans antigen (CRAG) in serum and CSF (100% sensitivity for meningitis). CSF: raised WCC. Elevated or normal protein. Start ART and IV liposomal **amphotericin** B and **flucytosine** for 2 weeks followed by **fluconazole** for 8–12 weeks.
- **CMV encephalitis:** focal neurology and low GCS. CMV DNA in CST.
- **Cerebral toxoplasmosis:** host is cat. Ingestion of eggs. Reactivates when CD4 <50 cells/mm^3. Progressive symptoms over days. Seizures, fever and reduced GCS, hemiballismus/chorea. CT/MR shows multiple ring-enhancing lesions in cortex and basal ganglia. Capsule formation is poor due to reduced immune response so there is good antibiotic penetration. Positive IgG serology useful. Take advice. Good response to **pyrimethamine, sulfadiazine** and folinic acid. Repeat CT after 2 weeks shows improvement, if not then consider brain biopsy.
- **Progressive multifocal leucoencephalopathy:** onset can be over weeks. Usually CD4 <100 cells/mm^3. Can mimic white matter disease. Due to JC virus. One or more focal non-enhancing lesions of gradual onset. Fever, headache uncommon suggests toxoplasmosis. Can mimic stroke. CSF: PCR for JC virus. Optimise ART.
- **Tubercular meningitis:** cervical lymphadenopathy, headache, N&V, pyrexia, meningism. IIIrd and VIth cranial nerves. CSF: raised opening pressure and protein and low sugar and raised lymphocytes, CD4 <200 cells/mm^3. Needs 12+ months antitubercular therapy and ART.
- **Primary CNS lymphoma:** progressive symptoms. Headache and focal neurology. No fever. More likely if toxoplasma serology negative or failure to respond to treatment for toxoplasmosis. Multiple periventricular lesions. Irregular, weakly enhancing. CD4 <100 cells/mm^3. PCR of CSF shows EBV.
- **AIDS dementia complex:** progressive cognitive and functional decline. CSF normal. CT and MRI show atrophy.
- **Transverse myelitis:** sensory level with motor weakness, autonomic loss.
- **Guillain–Barré syndrome:** ▶Section 11.26.
- **Peripheral neuropathy:** typically, a sensory neuropathy.

Cardiopulmonary

- **Bacterial pneumonias:** fever, breathless, productive cough. Depends on degree of immunocompromise. 10 times commoner than in HIV negatives. Higher risks with IV drug abuse. Cover as well for PCP. Treat early. ▶Section 4.15.

- *Pneumocystis* **pneumonia:** CD4 <200 cells/mm^3. High LDH. Breathless, dry cough, fever, for 2 weeks, desaturation. If the CD4 >200 cells/mm^3 or on prophylaxis and compliant then PCP much less likely. ▸Section 4.15.
- **Tuberculosis:** test HIV in all those with evidence of TB. Assume infectious. Isolate and get sputum cultures and respiratory review once diagnosis confirmed. May be insidious and atypical and no cavitation and lower lobe involved. Anti-tuberculosis treatment should be started before ART or else may cause immune reconstitution inflammatory syndrome. ▸Section 9.33.
- **Cardiac:** may have a dilated cardiomyopathy and myocarditis. Needs echo. Manage heart failure and arrhythmias.
- **Disseminated** *Mycobacterium avium* **complex:** clarithromycin 500 mg twice daily plus ethambutol 15 mg/kg daily.

Gastroenterology – requires endoscopy and biopsy of lesions

- **Oro-oesophageal candidiasis:** painful swallowing. Red, painful bleeding mucosa. Can be candida. Treat with **Fluconazole** 200 mg daily for 14 d. Differential if ulcerated is CMV or HSV infection and OGD and swabs taken.
- **CMV colitis, oesophagitis, hepatitis:** owl's eye inclusion bodies. Consider IV **ganciclovir.** HSV then IV **aciclovir.**
- **Chronic diarrhoea:** some have an unknown cause. Others due to cryptosporidiosis infection. Also vulnerable to *Salmonella, Shigella, Campylobacter,* giardiasis and some may be mixed pathogens. Leads to dehydration, weight loss due to malabsorption. Send stool cultures.
- *Cystoisospora belli* **diarrhoea: Co-trimoxazole** 160/800 mg QDS for 10 d.
- **Others:** HIV enteropathy, gastrointestinal TB, sclerosing cholangitis.
- **Oral hairy leucoplakia:** corrugated white plaques running vertically on the side of the tongue. Diagnostic of HIV disease. Asymptomatic and is due to EBV.

Dermatology

- **Multi-dermatomal herpes zoster:** can be seen with CD4 >500 cells/mm^3. Treat with **Aciclovir** 800 mg 5 times a day PO for 5 d. Severe/immunocompromised **Aciclovir** 10 mg/kg TDS for 7–10 d. Alternative is **famciclovir.** Severe or ophthalmic involvement, switch to IV **aciclovir.**
- **Herpes simplex:** oral, mucosal disease, hands, face. Crusted vesicles. Treat with **Aciclovir** 400 mg TDS PO 10 days. Alternative is famciclovir.
- **Kaposi sarcoma:** purplish skin lesions. HHV8 infection. May be in skin or in lung and other organs. May respond to ART. Chemotherapy if ART fails or if poor prognostic features such as visceral involvement, oedema, ulcerated lesions and B symptoms.
- **Bacillary angiomatosis:** *Bartonella henselae* or *B. quintana*. Solitary superficial red–purple lesions resembling KS or pyogenic granuloma, to multiple subcutaneous nodules or plaques. Painful and may bleed or ulcerate. Can become disseminated with fevers, lymphadenopathy and hepatosplenomegaly. Biopsy and Warthin–Starry silver staining shows bacilli. Treatment with **doxycycline** or **azithromycin** is effective.

Haematology

- Thrombocytopenia: ▸Section 8.4.

Ophthalmic

- **CMV retinitis:** CD4 count <50 cells/mm^3 or as part of IRIS (see below). Ophthalmology consult. **Ganciclovir** may be given directly into the eye.

- **Varicella zoster:** can affect ophthalmic branch of V and so the cornea. It can also cause an acute retinal necrosis simultaneously. Look for vesicular tingling and then painful rash over V1 distribution or may be multi-dermatomal. IV **aciclovir** is given. ▶Section 9.22.

Pregnancy
- All pregnant women should have HIV testing at an early stage in pregnancy.
- ART has reduced the risk of mother-to-child transmission of HIV to <1%.
- Traditionally C-section preferred but less important if on ART.
- HIV may be transmitted by breastfeeding. Formula feeding recommended.
- **Co-trimoxazole primary prophylaxis** CD4 count < 200 cells/mm^3:
  Co-trimoxazole reduces the incidence of a number of opportunistic infections, e.g. *Pneumocystis jirovecii* pneumonia, cerebral toxoplasmosis, bacterial pneumonia, bacteraemia, cystoisosporiasis, malaria.
- **Co-trimoxazole** 960 mg OD but half this dose is as effective and less toxic. It may be continued in low-income countries with CD4 >200 cells/mm^3.

Antiretroviral drugs
- Combination therapy is key to avoid resistance. May also require prophylaxis, e.g. for pneumocystis. ART reduces viral load and improves survival. BHIVA recommends therapy-naïve patients start ART containing two nucleos(t)ide reverse transcriptase inhibitors (NRTIs) plus one of the following: a ritonavir-boosted protease inhibitor (PI/r), an NNRTI or an integrase inhibitor (INI).
- They recommend therapy-naïve patients start combination ART containing tenofovir (TDF) and emtricitabine (FTC) as the NRTI backbone combined with a third agent. This should be managed by experts in HIV medicine.

Different medications
- Nucleos(t)ide reverse transcriptase inhibitors (NRTIs): zidovudine, abacavir, lamivudine, didanosine, tenofovir.
- Protease inhibitors (PIs): e.g. ritonavir/saquinavir/indinavir.
- Non-nucleos(t)ide reverse transcriptase inhibitors (NNRTIs): active against HIV1, e.g. nevirapine/efavirenz.
- HIV cell fusion inhibitors, e.g. enfuvirtide.

Antiretroviral drugs side-effects
- **Lactic acidosis:** with NRTI. Increased mortality. N&V, raised lactate.
- **Pancreatitis:** seen with ddI, d4T and ddC drugs.
- **Lipodystrophy syndrome:** (insulin resistance/dyslipidaemia/fat redistribution), d4T.
- **Rhabdomyolysis:** protease inhibitors + statin. PIs are cytochrome p450 inhibitors: increased toxicity of drugs metabolised on this pathway. Check *BNF* or equivalent.
- **Toxic epidermal necrolysis/Stevens–Johnson syndrome:** nevirapine.

Immune reconstitution inflammatory syndrome (IRIS)
- Seen with introduction of ART. Rapid fall in viral load and raised CD4 count. More likely from a very low CD4 count.
- There is a rise in T cells and enhanced immune response to infections that had been subclinical. Certain infections involved are: *Mycobacterium avium* complex, CMV retinitis, worsening pulmonary TB, worsening cryptococcal meningitis.

CD4 count (per mm³) and opportunistic infections/malignancy
- **All:** Kaposi sarcoma, pulmonary TB, HZV, bacterial pneumonia, lymphoma.
- **CD4 <250:** PCP, oesophageal candidiasis, PML, HSV.
- **CD4 <100:** cerebral toxoplasmosis, HIV encephalopathy, cryptococcosis, miliary TB.
- **CD4 <50:** CMV retinitis, atypical mycobacterial infection.

9.35 Syphilis

- **About:** spirochete. *Treponema pallidum*. Sexual transmitted.
- **Clinical: primary:** painless oral, rectal or genital ulcer with painless nodes. **Secondary:** fever, malaise, rash. Maculopapular. Lymphadenopathy, nephritis, hepatitis, uveitis. **Tertiary:** skin, bone destructive lesions. **Quaternary:** aortic aneurysm, neurosyphilis, dementia, tabes dorsalis, Argyll Robertson pupils.
- **Investigations:** swab of ulcer dark ground microscopy. Serology: VDRL/TPPA/FTA. CSF testing when appropriate. Neurosyphilis WBC ≥20 cells/µl or a reactive CSF (VDRL) test result. HIV test.
- **Management:** primary: **Doxycycline** 100 mg BD × 10 d, **Benzathine penicillin** 2.4 MU IM × 2. Late: **Doxycycline** 100 mg BD × 28 d, **Benzathine penicillin** 2.4 MU IM × 3. Neurosyphilis **Procaine Penicillin G** 2 g (2.4 MU) IM OD plus **Probenecid** 500 mg QDS × 17 d or **Doxycycline** 200 mg BD × 28 d. Screen for other sexually transmitted infections and contact screen. Steroids may be given to prevent Jarisch–Herxheimer reaction, e.g. **Prednisolone** 40–60 mg daily for 3 d.

9.36 Oropharyngeal bacterial infections

- **Glandular fever:** CMV, EBV. Amoxicillin/ampicillin causes rash.
- **Common viral:** measles, mumps, rubella, coryza and many of the common viral illnesses may cause some throat pain and associated pharyngitis.
- **Acute pharyngitis:** avoid ampicillin/amoxicillin. Mainly viral (adenovirus, rhinovirus, RSV). Management is supportive. Bacterial (*Strep. pyogenes* – Group A beta-haemolytic streptococci) more likely if fever and purulent tonsillar exudate and cervical lymphadenopathy without significant cough. Can confirm with rapid antigen detection test (RADT) and throat culture. Local complications include peritonsillar abscess. Treat with **Phenoxymethylpenicillin (Pen V)** 500 mg QDS PO for 10 d or **Clarithromycin** 500 mg BD for 10 d. Complications: acute rheumatic fever, scarlet fever, post-streptococcal glomerulonephritis.
- **Acute epiglottitis:** see Stridor, ▶ Section 4.4.

9.37 Diphtheria

- **About:** *Corynebacterium diphtheria, C. ulcerans*. Fatality 5–10%.
- **Aetiology:** releases an exotoxin which blocks protein synthesis. Mild cases can go undiagnosed. Toxin acts as an RNA translational inhibitor. Local tissue necrosis. Toxaemia and paralysis due to demyelinating peripheral neuritis. Cardiac failure due to myocarditis.
- **Microbiology:** Gram-positive, aerobic, non-motile, rod-shaped bacteria. From direct physical contact or aerosolised from infected person.
- **Clinical:** produces a grey thick membrane in pharynx. Nasal, laryngeal and pharyngeal mucosa affected. Can lead to airway obstruction and stridor. Sore

throat, fever, malaise. Heart failure, heart block and arrhythmias. Cranial nerve palsies, diplopia, dysarthria, dysphagia. Sensorimotor polyneuropathy.

- **Investigations:** FBC, U&E, CRP, CXR. ECG: heart block and arrhythmias. NCS shows demyelination. Cultures from larynx/pharynx. Echocardiogram.
- **Management:** ABC, O_2. Bed rest and telemetry initially. Isolation and treatment of the index case. Prevention with diphtheria toxoid immunisation and is also given with suspected diphtheria infection. Give 2 weeks of **Benzylpenicillin** 1.2 g QDS IV/IM or **Amoxicillin** 500 mg TDS IV or **Erythromycin** 500 mg QDS IV/PO. **Clarithromycin** may be used. Oral antibiotics when able. **Horse serum-derived antitoxin** 10,000–100,000 units IM after initial test dose to exclude allergy. Be ready to manage anaphylaxis. Remove membrane by laryngoscopy or bronchoscopy to prevent airways obstruction. Also treat contacts. Seek expert help.

9.38 Lemierre's syndrome

- **About:** mortality 5%. Septic thrombosis of internal jugular vein (IJV).
- **Microbiology:** *Fusobacterium necrophorum* produces a lipopolysaccharide endotoxin (leukocidin) and haemolysin increases virulence. Also *Streptococcus* sp., *Bacteroides* sp., *Peptostreptococcus* sp., and *Eikenella corrodens*.
- **Aetiology:** disseminated abscesses. Septic thrombophlebitis of the internal jugular vein. Associated infection of the oropharynx due to G–ve anaerobic bacillus. Main sources of infection are tonsil, pharynx and chest.
- **Clinical:** sore throat, painful swollen neck, fever, rigors, haemoptysis, dyspnoea if lungs involved. Pus on tonsils. Thrombophlebitis of the IJV. Cranial palsies (IX to XII). Septic emboli, joints, liver, spleen, osteomyelitis, meningitis.
- **Investigation:** FBC raised WCC, CRP, ESR. Blood cultures. CXR: cavitatory abscesses from septic emboli, pleural effusions. CT thorax: may find septic pulmonary emboli and internal jugular venous thrombosis and lung cavitation from abscesses. Pleural fluid/empyema. USS of neck veins shows occluded IJV.
- **Differential:** infectious endocarditis. Granulomatosis with polyangiitis (WG) as lung lesions and ENT issues (check cANCA).
- **Management:** HDU/ITU level care. O_2. Supportive. Antibiotics: take microbiological advice. High dose IV antibiotics, e.g. **Tazocin** 4.5 g TDS IV (BD if renal dysfunction) + **Metronidazole** 1g TDS IV. Often sensitive to penicillin, clindamycin, chloramphenicol. Some beta-lactamase activity may be seen. **Anticoagulation** with IV heparin/LMWH: controversial and may speed recovery, though there may be worries about bleeding from septic emboli. Some reserve it only for evidence of clot progression towards cavernous sinuses, others for SVC thrombophlebitis. In those with uncontrolled sepsis and repeated septic emboli despite appropriate medical therapy, surgical ligation or excision of the IJV should be performed, although this treatment is rarely needed today.
- **Reference:** Golpe *et al.* (1999) Lemierre's syndrome. *Postgrad Med J*, 75:141.

9.39 Traveller's diarrhoea

- **About:** half of travellers in developing countries. Poor sanitation, use only boiled or bottled water, unpeeled fruit, avoid ice cubes, salads. Most bacterial spread faeco-oral. More common with acid suppression, e.g. PPI. Malaria can cause diarrhoea.
- **Cause:** *E. coli* (ETEC/EAEC below), salmonella, campylobacter, shigella, enteric fever, cholera, giardia, cryptosporidium, rotavirus, malaria.

- **Clinical:** loose watery diarrhoea, colic and dehydration. Severe: bloody diarrhoea, fever, abdominal pain and severely dehydrated.
- **Investigate:** U&E, LFTs, stools for ova, cysts, parasites and culture. HIV can be associated with *Cryptosporidium*.
- **Management:** limit spread, hand washing. Most self-limit with oral rehydration therapies. Some need medical care and IV hydration. Severe give **ciprofloxacin.** If amoebiasis suspected (bloody diarrhoea) then add **metronidazole** for 10 d. Caution with antimotility agents. Some later develop lactose intolerance. Need lactose hydrogen breath test. Hypovolaemia, ▶Section 2.20.

9.40 Gastroenteritis and similar infections

- **About:** usually a self-limiting bowel infection.
- **Risks:** dehydration. Elderly, pregnant, immunocompromised, comorbidities.
- **Causes:** viral: norovirus, rotavirus, adenovirus, etc. Bacterial: non-typhoidal *Salmonella, Campylobacter, Shigella* (blood dysentery stools), cholera (*Vibrio cholerae*, rice water stool).
- **Inflammatory diarrhoea:** abdominal pain, fever, small volume bloody stool. Involves the distal small bowel and colon with invasion and mucosal cell death. Similar to ulcerative colitis. Typical infection is with *Shigella*.
- **Secretory diarrhoea:** nausea, vomiting, high volume water stool with early dehydration and low BP, less fever, less bloody stools, e.g. cholera.
- **Clinical:** colicky abdominal pain, diarrhoea and dehydration are main symptoms, with low BP. Oliguria, syncope. Can be bloody diarrhoea.
- **Investigations:** FBC, U&E, LFT, CRP, stools for microscopy and culture. Prevention is key: avoid contact for 24–48 h after symptoms have stopped. Side room or home if can manage and hydrated. Hand washing with soap and water. Wear gloves and aprons where advised.
- **Management:** isolation and good hand washing and infection control. Oral rehydration therapy for mild cases. More severe need IV fluids. Most resolve without antibiotics. Severe cases consider antibiotics as below. Antibiotics: treat if >6 type unformed stools per day, fever, blood or significant comorbidities; beware that antibiotics should be restricted to the most severe cases and most will resolve naturally. **Ciprofloxacin** 500 mg BD PO is the antibiotic of choice in most infections. However, antibiotics best avoided if you suspect *E. coli* 0157:H7 as increases risk of HUS, see ▶Section 8.6. **Metronidazole** for giardiasis and amoebiasis. For *Campylobacter* **clarithromycin.** Can be associated with later development of Guillain–Barré syndrome and reactive arthritis.

9.41 *Campylobacter* infection

- **About:** *Campylobacter* is a common cause of bacterial infection of the gut.
- **Source:** *Campylobacter jejuni* and *C. coli*. From contaminated food, raw chicken, milk, cattle. Adequate cooking should eradicate infection in food.
- **Clinical:** fever, vomiting and diarrhoea 3–7 days after ingestion. More common during the summer months, and late in the autumn.
- **Investigations:** stool culture. Serology, FBC, U&E.
- **Complications:** Guillain–Barré syndrome, Miller Fisher syndrome, septicaemia, cholecystitis, UTI, appendicitis. Reiter's syndrome.

- **Management:** isolate. Good hand hygiene. Hydration. Antibiotics may be used in those with severe illness who are >65, pregnant women, and people with weakened immune systems, such as those with a blood disorder, with AIDS, or receiving chemotherapy. **Ciprofloxacin** 500 mg PO BD for 5 days.

9.42 Escherichia coli infections

- **About:** there are hundreds of strains of *Escherichia coli*. Most living in the gut are harmless. Can be differentiated by distinct somatic (O) and flagellar (H) antigens and has specific virulence characteristics that usually are plasmid-mediated. The invasive and haemorrhagic cause a bloody diarrhoea.
- **Enteropathogenic** (EPEC) mild–severe disease with watery diarrhoea.
- **Enterotoxigenic** (ETEC) causes marked watery diarrhoea and vomiting.
- **Enteroinvasive** (EIEC) damages colonic cells with watery (bloody) diarrhoea but no toxin, usually mild and self-limiting.
- **Enterohaemorrhagic** (EHEC) with verocytotoxin (VTEC) such as O157:H7 and others. Usually from poorly cooked food: milk and meat. Similar to *Shigella dysenteriae* type 1. Enterotoxins can affect kidneys, heart, brain and cause HUS/TTP. Avoid antibiotics. Cause watery/bloody diarrhoea, dehydration, AKI.
- **Management:** self-limiting so usually supportive and oral or IV rehydration as needed. Avoid antibiotics, especially if O157:H7 suspected.

9.43 Staphylococcal food poisoning

- **Source:** cheese, meats. Poor hygiene and storage.
- **Cause:** *Staphylococcus aureus* enterotoxins preformed in the food.
- **Clinical:** after 3–6 hrs severe vomiting and diarrhoea. Severe dehydration.
- **Investigations:** if needed FBC, U&E, RP, LFT.
- **Management:** needs oral/IV rehydration and anti-emetics. Avoid admission if possible. The illness cannot be passed from one person to another.

9.44 Shigella dysenteriae

- **About:** *Shigella dysenteriae, flexneri, boydii and sonnei*. Gram-negative.
- **Path:** infecting dose 10 bacilli. Invade colonic mucosa. Release Shiga toxin. Contaminated food, flies, men having sex with men. Institutions.
- **Clinical:** inflammatory bloody diarrhoea, colic, abdominal pain. Fever, dehydration. Later Reiter's syndrome (red eye, arthritis, urethritis).
- **Investigations:** FBC, U&E, CRP. Stool for culture.
- **Differential:** acute severe colitis.
- **Complications:** rectal prolapse, megacolon, Reiter's syndrome, HUS.
- **Management:** oral/IV rehydrate. **Ciprofloxacin** 500 mg BD × 5 d or **azithromycin** or **ceftriaxone.**

9.45 Enteric fever (typhoid/paratyphoid)

- **About:** *Salmonella typhi* causes typhoid fever (TF) and *Salmonella paratyphi* A and B cause paratyphoid fever. Can be life-threatening unless treated promptly.
- **Sources:** faeco-oral spread. 5% become chronic carriers in gallbladder.

- **Aetiology:** bacilli localise to lymphoid tissue of the small intestine. Infects Peyer's patches and follicles which swell and then ulcerate and usually heal. Spreads via thoracic duct to lymph nodes and reticuloendothelial system.
- **Clinical:** IP 5–21 d, 2–3 weeks of progressive symptoms. **Week one:** fever, headache, myalgia, bradycardia, constipation. **Week two:** rose spots, splenomegaly, dry cough. Abdominal distension and diarrhoea. Paratyphoid tends to be milder and shorter.
- **Complications:** bowel perforation and haemorrhage, bone infections, meningitis, cholecystitis, myocarditis, nephritis.
- **Investigations:** blood and stool cultures positive in first 2 weeks (stools positive in chronic carriers). FBC: fall in WCC and platelets. U&E: AKI, elevated LFTs. Serology is possible. Widal test detects antibodies to O and H antigens but not specific.
- **Management: Ciprofloxacin** 500 mg BD or **Ceftriaxone** 1–2 g OD or **Azithromycin** 500 mg – 1g OD. Treat severe cases for 14 d or where resistance suspected (Asia). Supportive care required. Surgery for any bowel perforation. Fever may take 5 d to resolve.
- **Reference:** Parry & Beeching (2009) Treatment of enteric fever. *BMJ*, 338:b1159.

9.46 *Bacillus cereus*

- **Source:** seen classically from fresh rice. Heat-stable exotoxin.
- **Micro:** toxin-producing organisms may have watery diarrhoea presentation.
- **Clinical:** severe vomiting or watery diarrhoea. Self-limiting <1 d.
- **Management:** needs oral rehydration. IV if severe and dehydrated.

9.47 Cholera

- **About:** faeco-oral or vomitus. Cholera survives in fresh and salt water.
- **Micro:** Gram-negative bacillus *Vibrio cholerae* serotype 01 releases toxin which activates acetylate cyclase in intestinal mucosa with active secretion of water and chloride.
- **Clinical:** IP hours to 6 d. Sudden acute painless secretory diarrhoea. Most mild. Some have severe volume loss. Others lose huge volume into bowel before diarrhoea 'sicca' and can die. Vomiting. Hypovolaemic shock.
- **Investigations:** U&E: AKI. Diagnosis: examination of a wet film with dark-field microscopy for darting motility.
- **Management:** mild give oral salt/water replacement. Others may need IV Ringer Lactate replacement. Can lose 10 L/d which needs to be replaced. Severe disease. Single dose **Doxycycline** 300 mg or **Ciprofloxacin** 1 g to shorten course.

9.48 Giardiasis

- **About:** *Giardia lamblia* also called *Giardia duodenalis or intestinalis*.
- **Source:** contaminated food, water or surfaces. Faeco-oral. Oro-anal sex.
- **Micro:** eukaryotic, flagellated, binucleated protozoan parasite. IP 9–15 d.
- **Clinical:** bloating, flatulence, foul-smelling stools, watery or fatty diarrhoea, malabsorption, weakness. Many asymptomatic.
- **Investigations:** send stool ova, cysts, parasites – motile trophozoites in stool. Giardia stool antigen and PCR tests may be available.
- **Management:** prevent by boiling water for 1 min. Oral or IV rehydration. **Metronidazole** 2 g OD for 3 d. Courses may need repeated.

9.49 Amoebiasis

- **About:** protozoan parasite *Entamoeba histolytica* cyst ingestion.
- **Pathology:** invades colonic epithelium with necrosis and flask-like ulcers.
- **Sources:** contaminated water, salads, ice cubes. Seen worldwide. Notifiable. Cysts can survive in the environment for 12 d and up to 30 d in water.
- **Clinical:** (1) Acute colitis with bloody diarrhoea, even perforation. Days to weeks. (2) Liver abscess: 2–5 months post ingestion, RUQ pain, weight loss, enlarged liver, positive serology. (3) Asymptomatic infection (90%).
- **Investigations:** *E. histolytica/dispar* stool microscopy OR a positive faecal *E. histolytica* PCR OR positive amoebic fluorescent antibody test (FAT). USS/CT liver. Aspirate non-foul smelling 'anchovy sauce'. Left lobe abscesses higher risk of rupture into critical sites (e.g. pericardium) so may need intervention. Cysts are commonly seen in faeces but not diagnostic. POCUS to look for abscess.
  NB: *E. histolytica* needs molecular tests to distinguish from non-pathogenic *E. dispar* which has no clinical relevance.
- **Prevent:** drink sealed bottled water, no ice. Avoid peeled fruit and unsealed food. Eat only food witnessed totally cooked on clean plates.
- **Management of colitis:** ABC, **Metronidazole** PO followed by **Diloxanide furoate** PO to clear cysts. **Liver abscess: Metronidazole** 500 mg TDS × 7–10 days. Those with diarrhoea should not return to work/other settings until 48 h after resolution of diarrhoea. Test household/sexual contacts for asymptomatic infection and treat.
- **Reference:** PHE (2017) Interim Public Health Operational Guidelines for Amoebiasis (*Entamoeba histolytica*).

9.50 Neurocysticercosis

- **About:** tapeworm (*Taenia solium*) infection ingested from infected food or water. Seen where pigs kept in close contact with human faeces. 2nd commonest infective cause of epilepsy worldwide (1st is TB).
- **Pathology:** in brain forms small non-purulent abscesses that can later calcify. Dying cysts in muscle, eye, brain elicit inflammatory reaction.
- **Types** are viable parenchymal NCC, single enhancing lesions, calcified parenchymal NCC, ventricular NCC and subarachnoid NCC.
- **Clinical:** most present with seizures or raised ICP. Cerebellar/brainstem signs, dementia, obstructive hydrocephalus. Headaches, backache if in spine. Eyes – blindness. All should have fundoscopy before starting treatment.
- **Investigations:** bloods: leucocytosis, eosinophilia, raised ESR. Plain X-rays of muscles show calcified cysts. Non-contrast brain CT calcified lesions. MR lesions different stages: vesicular, colloidal and nodular–granular stage. May show obstructive hydrocephalus. CSF: raised protein, oligoclonal bands, eosinophilia. Diagnosis with serologic testing with enzyme-linked immunotransfer blot.
- **Management:** neurosurgical shunting for hydrocephalus. Anticonvulsants, e.g. levetiracetam for seizures. **Steroids** and then **albendazole** or **praziquantel.** This dampens inflammatory response and cerebral oedema (but screen for TB first). Monitor LFTs/WCC. Repeat MRI at 6 months. Take expert opinion.
- **Reference:** Diagnosis and Treatment of Neurocysticercosis: 2017 Clinical Practice Guidelines by the Infectious Diseases Society of America (IDSA) and the American Society of Tropical Medicine and Hygiene (ASTMH).

9.51 *Clostridium tetani* (tetanus)

- **About:** a potent neurotoxin causes a spastic paralysis.
- **Sources:** tetanus spores in soil. Can survive hostile conditions for long time.
- **Aetiology:** anaerobe Gram-positive bacillus with drumstick spore, produces tetanospasmin affects motor neurons with severe spasms and lethality.
- **Prevent:** childhood DTaP vaccine series. Adults tetanus booster every 10 y.
- **Clinical:** IP 3–21 d, occasionally longer. Contaminated wound puncture, open fracture, burns, bites and scratches, injection drug use. Localised tetanus is rigidity, spasms around the site of the infection. Hypertonic muscles with rigidity, spasms, clonus, risus sardonicus, opisthotonus. Trismus 'lockjaw' (cephalic tetanus).
- **Grades: Grade 1** (mild): mild–moderate trismus. General spasticity, little or no dysphagia, no respiratory embarrassment. **Grade 2** (moderate): moderate trismus and general spasticity, some dysphagia and resp embarrassment, fleeting spasms occur. **Grade 3a** (severe): severe trismus and general spasticity, severe dysphagia and resp difficulties, severe/prolonged spasms (spontaneous and on stimulation). **Grade 3b** (very severe): above + autonomic dysfunction, sympathetic overdrive. **Poor prognosis:** short IP, rapid onset, acquired from burns, wound, umbilical stump, septic abortion, delayed treatment, head or neck lesion.
- **Investigations:** FBC, U&E, LFT, check FVC, ABG, ECG. Wound samples for culture/ PCR is the primary confirmatory laboratory test for the presence of tetanus toxin.
- **Management:** ABC. Admit to ITU. Quiet room. Avoid stimuli. Cardiac monitor. Start treatment before lab tests. Wound debridement. Tracheostomy. Start **Benzylpenicillin** 600 mg IV 4 h or **Metronidazole. Anti-tetanus antibodies** <50 kg, 5,000 IU; >50 kg, 10,000 IU. Skin care, physiotherapy, sedation. Manage any seizures/spasm with **Diazepam** 5–10 mg or **Lorazepam** 1–2 mg IV. Baclofen, muscle relaxants, magnesium. Monitor for autonomic complications use labetalol. Survival usually results in a full recovery over 6 weeks.
- **Reference:** PHE (2019) Tetanus: Guidance on the management of suspected tetanus cases and on the assessment and management of tetanus-prone wounds.

9.52 Lyme disease

- **About:** *Borrelia burgdorferi* transmitted by *Ixodes* ticks. Early treatment with **Doxycycline** can prevent infection and may be life-saving.
- **Clinical:** bull's eye target lesion erythema migrans (EM), headache, arthralgia. Later: heart (heart block), neuropathy, neuritis, arthritis, cranial neuropathy (bilateral VII), meningitis.
- **Diagnosis:** if no EM then check ELISA and if positive or symptoms beyond 12 weeks check immunoblot test and if positive treat.
- **Treatment:** remove ticks <24 h often prevents transmission. Check skin and scalp. If EM present or positive immunoblot start doxycycline earlier the better. However if there is a high clinical suspicion of Lyme disease consider starting treatment while waiting for test results as tests do not rule out Lyme disease even if results are negative. Treatment within 72 h of a tick bite is more than 80% effective in preventing Lyme disease. Suspected infection. EM only or cranial nerves: **Doxycycline** 200 mg PO OD × 21 d or **Amoxicillin** 1 g TDS × 21 d. Give 28 d for arthritis or acrodermatitis. CNS Lyme: IV **Ceftriaxone** 2 g BD or 4 g OD × 21 d. Cardiac Lyme disease: IV **Ceftriaxone** 2 g OD × 21 d.
- **Reference:** NICE (2018) *Lyme disease* [NG95].

9.53 Group B streptococcal infection (GBS)

- **About:** *Streptococcus agalactiae* asymptomatic coloniser and an invasive pathogen. In older adults associated with diabetes, cancer, liver disease.
- **Pathology:** serious illness in babies with meningitis, pneumonia, sepsis. Older adults osteomyelitis, urosepsis, pneumonia, peritonitis, infectious arthritis, meningitis, endocarditis. Found in 20% female genital tract.
- **Microbiology:** Gram-positive cocci in short chains. Beta (complete) haemolytic on blood agar. Catalase negative. CAMP test.
- **Clinical:** skin and soft tissue infections, often an asymptomatic bacteraemia. May cause often mitral valve endocarditis, cellulitis, abscesses, foot infection, or decubitus ulcers often worsened by diabetes mellitus. Also acute and chronic osteomyelitis and septic arthritis of multiple joints. Necrotising fasciitis and pyomyositis. Meningitis. Urinary tract infections.
- **Investigations:** FBC, CRP, U&E, cultures. Investigate if positive blood culture, e.g. echocardiogram, MRI. Predelivery mothers are treated with IV penicillin if positive rectovaginal culture, preterm, 37 weeks, prolonged rupture of membranes, fever at delivery.
- **Management:** IV **Benzylpenicillin** (Pen G) is first line for invasive disease. Also consider **levofloxacin, tazocin.** Treat 10 d for bacteraemia, pneumonia, pyelonephritis and skin/soft tissue infections. For meningitis (min 14 d) septic arthritis, osteomyelitis, endocarditis and ventriculitis (min 4 weeks). Adding **Gentamicin** for the initial 2 weeks of therapy is recommended for endocarditis. Increasing resistance to beta lactams.

9.54 Sexually transmitted infections

- **HIV:** see ▶ Section 9.34. **Syphilis:** see ▶ Section 9.35.
- **Herpes simplex:** see ▶ Section 9.24.
- **NB:** where relevant take a sexual history, get consent, check HIV, refer to GUM clinic for contact tracing, education and screening for other infections.
- **Gonorrhoea:** *Neisseria gonorrhoeae* Gram-neg diplococcus. Infects lower genital tract, rectum, pharynx and eyes. Transmission is usually the result of vaginal, anal or oral sex. IP 2–10 d. Dysuria, mucopurulent or purulent urethral discharge. Anal infection. PID. Cervix inflamed. Red eye in neonates. Can cause an acute aseptic arthritis. Treat IM **Ceftriaxone** 500 mg with **Azithromycin** 1 g PO which can be used if pregnant.
- **Chlamydia:** urethral symptoms. Epididymo-orchitis. **Azithromycin** 1 g PO single dose or **Doxycycline** 100 mg BD PO 7 d.
- **Lymphogranuloma venereum** (LGV): *Chlamydia trachomatis* types L1, 2, 3. Small, transient, painless ulcer, vesicle, and large groin nodes. **Doxycycline** BD PO for 21 d or **Erythromycin** 500 mg QDS PO.
- **Chancroid:** *Haemophilus ducreyi* (short Gram-neg bacillus). Single or multiple painful ulcers with ragged undermined edges. **Azithromycin** 1 g PO.
- **Granuloma inguinale:** *Klebsiella granulomatis.* Painless ulcers. Swollen inguinal nodes. **Azithromycin** 1 g weekly PO or **Doxycycline** 100 mg BD orally or **Ceftriaxone** 1 g IM daily.

9.55 Monkeypox

- **About:** discovered 1958. Monkeypox is a rare infection most commonly found in west or central Africa. Monkeypox virus. Fatality around 5%. Transmission by close contact, cough, sneezes, fomites, bedding. Children most vulnerable.
- **Virology:** virus is member of the *Orthopoxvirus* genus in family *Poxviridae*.
- **Clinical:** IP 7–21 days. Infectious 28 days. Days 0–5: fever, headache, muscle ache, lymphadenopathy distinctive. Rash days 1–2. Face and hands rather than trunk. Macules, papules, vesicles, and pustules. Resolves in 2–4 weeks. May resemble chickenpox. Complications: bronchopneumonia, sepsis, encephalitis, blindness from corneal damage.
- **Investigations:** send sample. PCR is useful. Serology and antigen detection methods are therefore not recommended.
- **Management:** supportive. Isolate. Needs full PPE and respirator. Prevent with smallpox vaccine. Reduce transmission. Smallpox vaccine, cidofovir, and tecovirimat can be used to control outbreaks of monkeypox. Speak with ID team.

9.56 Mucormycosis

- **About:** this black fungus is ubiquitous in nature. Spores transmitted in air.
- **At risk:** diabetic ketoacidosis, neutropenic patients, burn victims, haematological cancers, transplant, those on iron-chelating drugs.
- **Aetiology:** increased iron availability as a result of a change in tissue pH.
- **Pathology:** fungi grow along blood vessels and invade their walls. Protruding hyphae are highly thrombogenic, cause infraction and necrosis of tissues particularly the face and bony walls of the sinuses and the cribriform plate. Spread to orbit and brain (rhinocephalic form). Also pulmonary, gastrointestinal, cutaneous, and disseminated infection.
- **Clinical:** spreading facial infection in at-risk patient. Headache, pain, fever, black midline lesions. Chest and abdominal pain, nausea and vomiting.
- **Investigations:** biopsy and microscopy
- **Management:** early diagnosis and escalation is key. Surgical debridement of infected and necrotic tissue. Treat underlying condition. Consider Amphotericin B and take expert advice. Mortality is high.

9.57 Scrub typhus

- **About:** a rickettsial spotted fever.
- **Recent travel** in Eastern and Southern Asia, Northern Australia, India, Thailand, Tibet, Japan, Russia and mountainous regions of Nepal.
- **Cause:** *Orientia tsutsugamushi*. From bite of a trombiculid mite, 'chiggers'.
- **Clinical:** incubation period is 5–10 days. The illness starts abruptly with fever, headache, myalgia, nausea, vomiting and cough. Eschar at site of the bite. A rash appears on day 5–7 on the trunk and limbs.
- **Complications:** meningoencephalitis, myocarditis, shock & ARDS.
- **Investigations:** serological detection PCR in the blood.
- **Management: Doxycycline** 200 mg PO for 5 days. Fatality untreated 5–10%.

9.58   *Capnocytophaga canimorsus*

- **About:** fastidious, slow-growing, Gram-negative rod of the genus *Capnocytophaga*. Found in oral flora of cats and dogs.
- **Spread:** cat and dog bites, licks, or even close proximity with animals.
- **Risk:** immunodeficiency, asplenia.
- **Clinical:** sepsis, gangrene, bacteraemia, meningitis and endocarditis.
- **Management:** consider **Tazocin** 4.5 g TDS IV or **Meropenem** 1–2 g IV TDS.

9.59   Meticillin sensitive/resistant *Staph. aureus*

- **About:** acquired resistance to meticillin, flucloxacillin. The mec-A gene.
- **Clinical:** line infections, bone and soft tissue infections, pneumonias and septicaemia. MRSA is associated with higher mortality than MSSA.
- **Needs:** good asepsis, hand washing and eradication policies.
- **Investigations:** blood culture, skin swabs, nose and groin, IV lines.
- **Management:** any *Staph. aureus* bacteraemia 'always' gets at least 2 weeks of IV antibiotics and needs microbiological advice. *Staph. aureus* in the urine should also initiate concerns and blood cultures should be done. Look for cardiac or bone infections. Metastatic infections seen in those inadequately treated, to bone, spine and joint and heart. MRSA septicaemia should receive **vancomycin** or **teicoplanin**. **Doxycycline** used for soft tissue infections.

9.60   Bacterial resistance: VRE, ESBL, CRE/CRO

Vancomycin-resistant enterococcus (VRE)

- These are common commensals. VRE may be difficult to treat because of the limited range of effective antibiotics. May cause UTI, wounds and vascular catheter site infections. Many simply colonised and non-pathogenic.
- Limit spread. Single room isolation especially if diarrhoea and hand washing measures. Decolonisation generally unsuccessful and therefore not recommended.
- VRE are of limited virulence (unlike MRSA) and mostly colonise rather than infect. If detected in faeces needs no treatment. It rarely causes infection in the healthy. Take local microbiological advice. Uncomplicated cystitis due to VRE can usually be treated with nitrofurantoin.

Extended-spectrum beta-lactamases (ESBL)

- Bacteria that produce ESBLs are resistant to many penicillin and cephalosporin antibiotics. Usually *E. coli* and *Klebsiella* sp. *E. coli* produce CTX-M enzymes and may cause UTIs, more severe infections and septicaemia. Difficult to treat. In most fit and healthy individuals ESBL not a problem and they are well. Immunocompromised and elderly at greater risk. Management is based on isolation and limiting spread by hand washing and other means.

Carbapenem-resistant enterobacteriaceae/organisms (CRE/CRO)

- CRE are Enterobacteriaceae such as *E. coli*, *Klebsiella* resistant to carbapenems, e.g. meropenem. CRO are *Pseudomonas*, *Acinetobacter* with similar resistance. Organisms are endemic and often imported to those exposed to overseas healthcare.

- Infections with CRE/CRO have increased morbidity, mortality, prolonged hospital stay and expense. They are normal gut commensals. Can cause disease in the critically ill. Any recent inpatient in a hospital abroad needs isolated and screened <24 h of admission, usually by a rectal swab or stool sample, or from a wound, or urine if catheter, or sputum if productive.
- Most colonised patients have no symptoms. It takes two negative swabs to be clear. All positives must remain isolated. The aim is to prevent spread. Hand hygiene using soap and water is the only effective way of removing this organism from the hands. Visitors should wear disposable aprons and gloves.

10 Renal and urology

10.1 Pathophysiology

- The 2 kidneys lie retroperitoneally at level of T12–L3 vertebrae. Left kidney somewhat more superior than the right. On average 11 cm in length, 6 cm wide and 3 cm thick. Inner cortex, outer medulla, calyces, pelvis and ureter.
- Cortex: contains nephrons (1 M per kidney). Nephrons filter and drain and hang into the medulla: loops of Henle and collecting ducts. Reabsorbs water.
- They are supplied by renal arteries from aorta. 20% of cardiac output so 1 L blood (600 ml plasma) per min. 20% is filtered into Bowman's space.
- Normal GFR in men 130 ml/min/1.73 m^2; in women 120 ml/min/1.73 m^2.
- Drain into renal veins. GFR depends on BP, renal perfusion, afferent and efferent arteriole tone.

10.2 Haematuria

Taking referral/answering bleep
- When did it start? Quantity? Clots? Is patient passing urine or in retention? Is patient pyrexial, pain – cystitis/pyelonephritis? Recent catheterisation? Prostate disease?
- Pregnant? Known bladder malignancy? On any anticoagulants? 30% of patients with painless haematuria have a malignancy.

Definitions and causes
- **Microscopic haematuria:** non-visible haematuria. ≥2 red cells per high power field in MSU unrelated to exercise, menses or trauma.
- **Macroscopic haematuria:** visible haematuria.
- **Haematuria:** bleeding from glomerulus to urethra. Can be divided into glomerular and non-glomerular. **Glomerular haematuria:** usually with proteinuria, hypertension and renal dysfunction. Commonest is IgA nephropathy, type IV collagen nephropathy, Alport disease. **Non-glomerular haematuria:** stones, tumour, papillary necrosis.
- **Investigations:** FBC, U&E, CRP, urinalysis. Cystoscopy, intravenous urogram, renal USS. β-hCG. PSA and formal microscopy, culture and sensitivities. False positive dipstick for blood may be seen with menstruation or trauma (exercise or recent sex or local lesions – ulcers, warts). Haematuria, red cell casts, proteinuria – consider glomerulonephritis. CRP/echocardiogram/blood cultures if endocarditis considered (rare). Renal biopsy: to diagnose renal glomerular disease.
- **Red flags:** painless macroscopic haematuria, symptomatic microscopic haematuria in absence of UTI. Age >50, abdominal mass on examination, smokers.

Referral guidance for haematuria
- **Urology referral:** unexplained macroscopic (visible) haematuria at any age, microscopic haematuria (all ages), hesitancy, dysuria, frequency or urgency and absence of UTI, persisting asymptomatic microscopic haematuria age ≥40.
- **Nephrology referral:** microscopic haematuria and a low eGFR, haematuria and HTN >140/90 mmHg, proteinuria (ACR >30 mg/mmol or PCR >50 mg/mmol), macroscopic haematuria + infection, usually chest, family history of renal disease or haematuria.

Assessment

- **Indications for admission:** look for UTI and coagulopathy. Admit if clot retention, cardiovascular instability, uncontrolled pain, sepsis, AKI, coagulopathy, severe comorbidity, heavy haematuria or social restrictions.
- Those not needing admission should drink plenty of clear fluids and return for further medical attention if the following occur: clot retention or worsening haematuria despite adequate fluid intake, uncontrolled pain or fever, or inability to cope at home.
- Repeat observations and review medications and consider stopping anticoagulants depending on their need. Low BP or raised HR may suggest sepsis or haemorrhage.
- **Follow-up by a urological team** ideally <2 wk cancer referral target. Consider bladder and prostate cancer in males >40. In those <40 cystoscopy not mandatory if another cause found.
- **Significant macroscopic (visible) bleeding** can cause clot retention resulting in outflow obstruction and often a three-way catheter irrigation system should be used. In bleeding of this severity, reverse all anticoagulation and get urological advice. Ensure check Hb and replace blood. **Will need urgent cystoscopy** if persists and imaging of whole renal tract.
- **Microscopic haematuria** (not visible but positive dipstick) and protein consider as UTI. Lack of protein in dipstick could suggest tumour or stones.
- **Microscopic haematuria and proteinuria** nephrology review, e.g. glomerulonephritis.

Causes of haematuria	
Urinary tract infection (cystitis and pyelonephritis)	Commonest cause. Pain, dysuria, blood, protein, leucocytes in urine. Positive cultures. Confusion, suprapubic discomfort. Usually raised WCC and CRP. May present as delirium or 'off legs' in the elderly.
Traumatic bladder catheterisation	Often seen post-catheter or any form of instrumentation. Exacerbated by any antithrombotics. Bleed should settle, but if it persists investigate.
Bladder cancer	Common in older population and needs cystoscopy for diagnosis, biopsy and staging and treatment.
Renal cell cancer	Look for a renal mass, fever, USS or CT abdomen. Bladder cancer: persisting haematuria. Cystoscopy.
Prostate cancer	Raised PSA, bony metastases, prostatism, hard craggy prostate on PR. Urology referral.
Prostatitis	Pain and UTI-like symptoms.
Renal stones	Pain loin to groin. Passing grit in the urine. ▶ Section 10.8.
Thrombocytopenia	Check FBC and causes. ▶ Section 8.4.
Antithrombotics and anticoagulants	Warfarin, dabigatran and other DOAC, aspirin, clopidogrel and heparin can worsen bleeding and are not uncommon causes. Need risk assessed on temporary stopping or reduction of dose. ▶ Section 8.8.
Infective endocarditis	Murmur, fever, raised CRP, stigmata of endocarditis, needs echo.
Acute glomerulonephritis	Haematuria and proteinuria. May be RBC casts and dysmorphic RBCs. Check anti-GBM, ANCA, ASO titres and usual renal work-up.

Nephropathies causing microscopic haematuria	IgA nephropathy: commonest glomerulonephritis worldwide. Familial incidence. Younger patients than other causes. Proteinuria. Micro/macroscopic haematuria during respiratory infection, proteinuria and reduced eGFR. Follow-up needed. Some progress to end-stage renal failure.
Type IV collagen nephropathy	Causes a familial microscopic haematuria.
Alport syndrome	Seen in 1 in 50,000. Microscopic haematuria in children. Sensorineural deafness. Eye disease. Mutation COL4A5. Needs BP control, RAS blockade, renal replacement.
Thin basement membrane nephropathy	Family history of renal disease.
Tuberculosis	Weight loss, overseas, CXR, sterile pyuria classically.
Sickle cell anaemia	Usually known sickle cell anaemia. See ▶ Section 8.2.
Schistosomiasis	Overseas exposure due to *Schistosoma haematobium*. Also called bilharzia. Chronic bladder inflammation. Risk factor for bladder cancer.
False positive dipstick	Myoglobinuria, e.g., rhabdomyolysis.

10.3 ▶ Reduced urinary output (anuria/oliguria)

- **Taking referral/answering bleep/attending:** (attend quickly if low BP, hypoxic, pyrexia, raised HR, increased NEWS).
- **Resuscitate if needed:** ABC. O_2, check BP, HR, temperature. If low BP then get IV access, check bloods and manage as for shock. Cardiac monitor if AKI and hyperkalaemia. Ensure accurate fluid balance chart. Omit antihypertensive on drug chart. Correct any volume loss. If biochemical evidence of AKI then suspend nephrotoxic medications and ensure all drugs have been assessed for correct dose in AKI. In most cases simply increasing oral or IV fluids is sufficient. A cautious fluid challenge of 250–500 ml over 30 min and then repeated should cause some response.
- **Measure urine output:** determine exact urine output. Assess patient's hydration status. Quantify total (PO + IV) input and urine losses. Weight changes are useful: 1 kg = 1 L.
- **Reduced urine output:** oliguria: <500 ml/d urine output (which is about 20 ml/h). Oliguria is usually pre-renal but may be renal. If pre-renal and patient is dry then give fluids, e.g. 500 ml IV NS over 1 h and review. If the patient has poor intake and is not in heart failure then further fluids needed to improve urine output. Oliguria might suggest hypoperfusion and sepsis or other causes of shock. Attend quickly if low BP, raised temp, raised HR, raised EWS (could be subacute obstruction so consider bladder scan and catheter). If low BP assess as for low BP. If renal cause suspected ask about new drugs or IV contrast for an X-ray or angiogram that could precipitate or cause AKI. Is there rhabdomyolysis or severe infection? Check bloods and lactate and possible venous blood gases if AKI. Seek help.
- **No urine:** anuric think obstruction first. Has patient any suprapubic pain or is catheter blocked or is it acute retention? Clot? Ask staff to flush or change the catheter if one is in place. Bladder scan will tell you if bladder full or empty and then

catheterise. If obstruction still considered, then a renal USS is usually diagnostic. The question is at what level: is it urethra, prostate, bladder, ureters, renal? Those with post-renal causes need to be discussed with urology for surgical or radiologically placed drainage before definitive management.

- **Differential: recording error** – fluid balance underestimates urine output. **Pre-renal failure** – oliguria and recent low BP. Cardiogenic, haemorrhagic shock, sepsis, obstructive shock. Excessive antihypertensives. **Renal** – ischaemic, nephrotoxic drugs, nephritis. **Post-renal** – obstruction at renal pelvis, ureters, bladder, urethra. Stones, tumour, prostate.

10.4 Acute kidney injury

- **About:** AKI has replaced the term 'acute renal failure' to emphasis potential reversibility. AKI is a sudden rapid reduction in GFR and there may be oliguria and anuria. Mortality varies from 10 to 80% depending on population studied. Most resolve within 1 week, the remainder have a worse prognosis.
- **Causes:** many patients have a mixed aetiology. Sepsis, ischaemia and nephrotoxicity, hypoperfusion, obstruction often coexist and complicate recognition and treatment. Increases length of stay, mortality and expense. AKI is seen in 15% of hospital patients. A minority need a nephrologist. Most managed by generalists. Only 1% need dialysis. If vasculitis suspected, e.g. systemic illness, rash, fever, raised CRP, alveolar haemorrhage, send urgent ANCA/anti-GBM (talk to lab) and seek nephrology help immediately.
- **Aetiology:** reduced renal function: impaired control of water and electrolytes. Impaired excretion of drugs and other metabolites. Impaired acid–base control: need to excrete acid load. Impaired BP control, impaired EPO synthesis, impaired vitamin D hydroxylation.
- **Risk factors for AKI and poor outcome:** age >75, cardiac failure, liver disease CKD (eGFR <60 ml/min/1.73m²), DM. PVD, nephrotoxins, hypovolaemia, sepsis.

RIFLE and AKIN classification for AKI in adults		
Stage	Creatinine (μmol/L)	Urinary output
1: Risk	Creatinine >120, increased by >26 within 48 h or > ×1.5–1.99 baseline value <7 d	<0.5 ml/kg/h for >6 consecutive hours
2: Injury	Creatinine × 2 (creatinine >240) or > ×2.0–2.99 baseline value <7 d	<0.5 ml/kg/h for >12 consecutive hours
3: Failure	Creatinine increased ×3 or >354 mmol/L or dialysis needed	<0.3 ml/kg/h for >24 consecutive hours or anuria for 12 h
Loss	Complete loss of function needing RRT >4 weeks	

Measuring renal function in AKI

- **Serum creatinine** is a very useful test. Unless you have prior records it will not itself tell you if it is AKI or CKD. Those with muscles will have higher levels and a falsely low level is found in those with low muscle mass, e.g. frail.
- **Estimated glomerular filtration rate** varies according to age, sex, and body size, and declines with age. eGFR is therefore calculated using the CKD-EPI equation. NB: adjustment for race is no longer recommended by NICE (2022) in the calculation of eGFR using the CKD-EPI creatinine equation which is complex but takes age, serum

creatinine, race, gender and gives an estimate GFR. See online calculators. There is ongoing work to replace creatinine with a serum cystatin C test.

- **Creatinine clearance** (CrCl): useful for drug prescribing. Creatinine is a waste product and derived from muscle. It is filtered and not resorbed. Creatinine clearance is the amount of blood filtered by kidneys in each minute in order to make blood free of creatinine. It can be used to predict renal function. It can be done by a 24 h urine collection and blood sample. However more likely now to use formula to estimate CrCl. This is the Cockcroft–Gault equation. All tests that use a creatinine need to be alert that muscle mass is a key factor and may cause an elevated creatinine.

$$\text{Creatinine clearance (ml/min)} = \frac{(140 - \text{age [years]}) \times \text{weight [kg]}}{\text{serum creatinine [} \mu \text{mol/L]}} \quad \text{(Females)}$$

$$\frac{(140 - \text{age [years]}) \times \text{weight [kg]} \times 1.2}{\text{serum creatinine [} \mu \text{mol/L]}} \quad \text{(Males)}$$

Clinical assessment and initial management

- **ABCs:** O_2, IV access, bloods, urine, cultures, ECG (high K). Don't rush to catheterise unless retention / obstruction / oliguria / anuria / shock.
- **Assess hydration:** measure temp, BP and pulse, JVP and capillary refill (<3 sec) and GCS. A postural drop even lying to sitting may suggest hypovolaemia. Give 500 ml NS IV over 30 min and review.
- **Clinical:** determine if new or long-standing malaise, lethargy, delirium, N&V, generalised anorexia. **Chest:** breathless and haemoptysis – pulmonary oedema, consolidation, alveolar haemorrhage with vasculitis (granulomatosis with polyangiitis (WG) or Goodpasture's syndrome). **Cardiac:** pericardial rub due to uraemic pericarditis. A pericardial effusion may be seen on echo or CXR. Occasionally this may progress to tamponade. **Skin:** palpable purpura, neuropathy might suggest vasculitis. Skin pigmentation, pallor, itch, scratch marks are common. Impaired platelet function and bruising is seen.
- **Urine output:** oliguria helps define AKI but is non-specific. Anuria suggests post-renal obstruction.
- **Polyuria causes:** excess intake, CKD with impaired renal concentrating ability or high Ca/high glucose/low K, lithium, diuretics, interstitial nephritis, cranial or nephrogenic diabetes insipidus which may worsen hypovolaemia. A low volume concentrated urine with low Na suggests prerenal causes.
- **Drug chart:** always examine the drug chart – current and recent. Check each drug with *BNF* for renal advice. Aminoglycosides (gentamicin, etc.), vancomycin, cisplatin, lithium, NSAIDs, ACEi, ARBs, ciclosporin, radiocontrast, paracetamol OD. Myoglobin and haemoglobin are nephrotoxic.

Pre-renal failure (80%): commonest; patient needs volume

- Urine Na <20 mmol/L. High osmolality. Retention of Na and H_2O.
- **Causes:** shock, hypovolaemia, haemorrhage, severe sepsis, heart failure, cirrhosis, liver failure, renal artery stenosis.
- **Clinical:** low BP, shocked, raised HR. Acute setting. Burns, gastrointestinal losses, sepsis. Uraemia: drowsiness, poor appetite, itch, encephalopathy, pericardial rub. Late: seizures and coma.

Renal failure (10%): vasculitis / SLE / anti-GBM / GN / HUS / rhabdomyolysis

- Urine Na >40 mmol/L. Intrinsic renal disease: proteinuria and haematuria and red cell casts. Normal or low urine osmolality.
- Acute tubular necrosis (45%): acute fall in GFR: tubule cell damage and cell death. Ischaemia or toxin-driven. Ischaemia usually due to prolonged pre-renal failure. There can be recovery over 1–3 weeks with diuresis. May also be due to nephrotoxic drugs or DIC or myoglobinuria, radiocontrast. Glomerulonephritis (GN): neoplasia, autoimmune, drugs, genetic abnormalities and infections. Rapidly progressive GN: vascular/vasculitis (4%) – granulomatosis with polyangiitis (WG), HUS, TTP, hypertension, scleroderma, renal artery stenosis. Acute interstitial nephritis: hereditary, systemic, toxic and drug-induced. Acute on chronic renal failure (13%): mostly due to ATN and pre-renal disease. Haemolytic uraemic syndrome: microangiopathic anaemia, low Hb, raised LDH, raised bilirubin. Myeloma kidney: raised ESR, monoclonal band. Malignant hypertension: control BP.

Post-renal

- Urinary tract obstruction: stones, tumour, papillary necrosis, surgical ligation of ureters, extrinsic compression, retroperitoneal fibrosis. Catheterise if distended bladder. Admit to urology for relief of obstruction.

Chronic

- Renal USS: small kidneys usual. Normal/large kidneys if amyloid or diabetes or polycystic kidney disease. Normocytic normochromic anaemia, low Ca, raised P. Review old tests: raised creatinine. No signs or symptoms of acute illness.
- Progressive uraemic symptoms. Usually diabetes, HTN, APKD. Chronic fatigue. Multiple comorbidities. Polyuria and nocturia and low urine osmolality if concentrating defect.

Syndromic renal presentations to recognise

- **Nephrotic syndrome:** proteinuria (frothy urine) exceeding 3.5 g/24 h, hyperlipidaemia, lipiduria, oedema (puffy eyes in morning to generalised oedema/anasarca), hypoalbuminaemia <25 g/L, hypercoagulability. **Causes:** primary GN, minimal change disease (children), focal segmental glomerulosclerosis (most common cause in adults), membranous GN. Others: diabetic nephropathy, sarcoidosis, autoimmune: SLE, Sjögren's, infection: syphilis, hepatitis B, HIV, amyloidosis, multiple myeloma, vasculitis, cancer, drugs: gold, penicillamine, captopril, NSAIDs.
- **Nephritic syndrome:** haematuria/red cell casts, HTN, oliguria, uraemia, proteinuria (<3 g/24 h). **Causes:** post-infectious GN, primary, IgA nephropathy (Berger's disease), RPGN, proliferative GN, secondary GN, Henoch–Schönlein purpura, vasculitis.
- **Investigations:** urine dipstick, urine microscopy, CXR, U&E, LFTs, CRP, ESR, Ca, immunoglobulins, PPE, BJP, complement (C3, C4) autoantibodies (ANA, ANCA, anti-dsDNA, anti-GBM), renal ultrasound, renal biopsy.

Investigations

- **FBC and film:** low Hb not typical with AKI. High WCC, platelets? Haemolysis? Microangiopathic anaemia – check blood films.
- **Urinalysis** shows blood, protein and red cell casts on microscopy. Positive protein values of 3+ and 4+ on reagent strip testing of the urine suggest intrinsic glomerular disease and this is reinforced if there are a high number of red cells.

Increased white cells (>5 per high power field) are non-specific but are found more commonly with acute interstitial nephritis, renal or UTI and GN. If proteinuria do an urgent spot urine protein:creatinine ratio.

- **U&E:** raised urea/creatinine/K. **Lactate** >2 mmol/L: tissue hypoxia/sepsis.
- **Calcium/phosphate:** low Ca – CKD, high Ca – malignancy, myeloma, primary hyperparathyroidism. High phosphate.
- **LFTs:** low albumin with nephrotic syndrome. High blood glucose: with diabetes.
- **ABG:** low pH and low HCO_3 associated with AKI.
- **Coagulation tests:** can be abnormal if DIC associated with sepsis.
- **Blood cultures:** if sepsis is suspected.
- **Creatine kinase:** rise suggests rhabdomyolysis or acute MI.
- **CXR:** pulmonary oedema or alveolar haemorrhage. Cavitating lesions suggesting a pulmonary/renal syndrome. Pneumonia – sepsis.
- **ECG:** look for cardiac disease (LVH, STEMI/non-STEMI) or high K.
- **CT renal tracts:** exclude structural lesion or retroperitoneal fibrosis.
- **Renal USS:** within 24 h. Renal size, exclude obstruction.
- **Renal biopsy:** shows a crescentic type picture in RPGN. Biopsy if suspected GN/RPGN/tubulointerstitial nephritis or vasculitis. Raised ESR – myeloma or infection. Raised CRP if infection/vasculitis/autoimmune disorder.
- **PPE/urine Bence Jones:** always do both when looking for multiple myeloma.
- **Autoantibodies:** ANCA (MPO and PR3), anti-GBM, ANA, dsDNA.
- **Complement:** C3 and C4 and cryoglobulins. **HIV test:** where risk factors exist.
- **Magnetic resonance angiography** (MRA): if suspicion of renal artery stenosis.
- **Body weight:** measured daily gives a good idea of fluid balance.

Prevention

- Avoiding low BP and dehydration and reducing and stopping potentially nephrotoxic drugs. Some causes are predictable and preventable. If at risk of contrast-induced AKI (CI-AKI) give pre-procedure volume expansion with IV NS or isotonic **sodium bicarbonate.** No compelling evidence for the routine use of *N*-acetylcysteine to prevent CI-AKI. Manage rhabdomyolysis with IV volume expansion with IV N-saline and sodium bicarbonate.
- AKI following the administration of radiological contrast tends to occur within 72 h and often resolves after around 5 d.

Management: correct K, ensure euvolaemic, stop toxins, treat obstruction

- **Medical management: ABCs**, resuscitate, IV access, O_2. If non-obstructive liaise closely with renal physicians. The cause may be volume depletion or intravascular loss or nephrotoxic drugs or a mixed picture. Escalate early, use critical care outreach/nephrology if high NEWS or need advice.
- **PPI** can be considered to reduce the risk of upper gastrointestinal bleeding.
- **Manage vascular filling status:** determine using clinical signs and other results if under, normal or overfilled. Cautiously correct fluid balance, stop or adjust doses of all renally excreted or nephrotoxic drugs. In mild cases renal function will improve over several days with cautious fluid management. In those with impaired cardiac function small challenges with 250 ml IV NS over 10 min and then reassessment of urine output and fluid balance and pulse and postural BP is reasonable. More fluid may be given. In selected severe cases a CVP line may help guide fluid replacement. Once fluid balance is normal, then watch for an improvement in urine output suggesting pre-renal cause. If a hydrated patient is oliguric and non-obstructed, then a diuretic stimulus with **Furosemide** 100–120 mg may be given slowly IV

over 10–20 min. A failure to respond suggests that things have progressed beyond simple pre-renal failure, and we may be dealing with ATN. In those with ongoing oliguria and rising urea and creatinine consider renal referral.

- **Fluid balance and nutrition:** fluid replacement = output + 500 ml/d usually with NS. May need to replace more if diarrhoea. Normal enteral nutrition should be encouraged.
- **Drugs to stop:** ACEi, ARBs, NSAIDs, diuretics, metformin.
- **Protect antecubital veins:** in case haemodialysis will be needed at a later stage. Avoid non-dominant arm upper limb veins for future permanent access.
- **Exclude post-renal cause with USS:** if obstruction suspected (oliguria/anuria), then get a renal USS <24 h. A bladder catheter relieves lower urinary tract obstruction. If a urethral catheter cannot be placed due to an enlarged prostate or urethral stricture then a suprapubic catheter may be needed (ask urology for help). Imaging evidence of a dilated ureter and hydronephrosis will require **percutaneous nephrostomy.** A urinary catheter is a source of infection. If no obstruction and good output then assess need particularly in mild AKI. Trial without catheter as soon not needed. Once post-renal causes are treated there may be a marked diuresis which needs to be anticipated and compensated for in the fluid management plan. Frequent monitoring of I/O and U&E is required.
- **Stop nephrotoxic drugs:** stop/avoid drugs, e.g. ACE inhibitors, NSAIDs, AT2 blockers and reduce the dose of other drugs that are renally cleared. See *BNF.*
- **Specialist management:** escalate where creatinine >×3 baseline, or >354 µmol/L to critical care/nephrology or complications as below or where advice needed. Look for **autoimmune disease or GN** (if RPGN/granulomatosis with polyangiitis (WG) or Goodpasture's is suspected then quick card test for cANCA and anti-GBM), **myeloma kidney, HUS, TTP**, suspected poisoning. Further investigations such as renal biopsy are for the nephrologists to deal with. There may well be a return of function in the short term over the first few weeks, but in some patients cortical scarring means a progressive course into chronic renal failure and a need for life-long renal replacement therapy (RRT).

Complications
- **High K:** see ▶Section 5.3 for management of hyperkalaemia.
- **Metabolic acidosis:** as medical treatment for management of hyperkalaemia. A pH <7.15 requires critical care referral. May need dialysis. Consider administering sodium bicarbonate (100 mmol) to correct acidosis if H^+ is >100 nmol/L (pH <7.0). Chronic plasma bicarbonate concentrations should be maintained >22 mmol/L. Start dose of sodium bicarbonate 1 g 8-hourly.
- **Pulmonary oedema:** sit up, O_2 as per BTS guidance. If haemodynamically stable, try **Furosemide** 50–100 mg IV and then an infusion at 10 mg/h. Also consider if not low BP, 2 × **GTN spray** (800 mcg) and prepare **GTN:** 50 mg in 50 ml IV infusion. Start 1–10 ml/h. May need dialysis if cannot get rid of fluid.
- **Inotropes:** consider dopamine in improving outcome in AKI. Use of inotropes should be led by specialists. See Shock, ▶Section 2.13.

Renal replacement

- **Renal replacement management:** it may be that conservative measures are insufficient and urgent RRT is indicated. Usual indications are listed below. The patient will need either ITU for haemofiltration or renal unit transfer. Haemofiltration is most commonly used acutely as volume shifts are less and can be provided in an ITU set-up and can remove endotoxins in those who are septic. Be sure to talk to your intensivists and renal physicians early before this situation arises, if at all possible.
- **Indications for discussing urgent dialysis in AKI:** urea >35 mmol/L, high refractory K >6.5 mmol/L with ECG changes, acute pulmonary oedema, severe acidosis (pH <7.1–7.2, H^+ >79 nmol/L), HCO_3 <15, encephalopathy, bleeding due to uraemia and pericarditis. Ethylene glycol poisoning.
- **References:** www.renal.org/clinical/guidelinessection/AcuteKidneyInjury.aspx. KDIGO Group (2012) Clinical practice guideline for acute kidney injury. *Kidney Int Suppl*, 2:1.

10.5 Chronic kidney disease

- **About:** irreversible decline in kidney function over years. Asymptomatic until advanced. Glomerular filtration rate (GFR) is the best estimate of kidney function and is based on serum creatinine level, age, sex and race. Most will die from heart disease. eGFR/creatinine need to be stable to diagnose CKD. **NB: eGFR** = 60. Look for/treat causes, watch drugs. eGFR = 30 needs nephrology. eGFR = 15 needs dialysis or transplant.
- **Normal:** normal GFR is approximately 100 ml/min/1.73m². **G1:** GFR >59 ml/min. Managed in primary care. Annual assessment. **G2:** GFR 60–89 ml/min/1.73m² with proteinuria or haematuria or known renal pathology. Managed in primary care. Annual assessment. **G3a:** GFR 45–59 ml/min. Mild moderate **G3b:** GFR 30–44 ml/min: 6–12-month reviews. **G4:** GFR 15–29 ml/min/1.73m². **G5:** GFR <15 ml/min. End-stage renal failure.
- **Albumin creatinine ratio (ACR):** there is progressively more albumin in urine as CKD worsens. It needs an early morning urine. **A1:** <30 mg/g (<3 mg/mmol) or mild increase. **A2:** <30–300 mg/g (3–30 mg/mmol) moderately increased. **A3:** >300 mg/g (>30 mg/mmol) severely increased. It can also be elevated by fever, UTI, immune disorders, dehydration, drugs, haematuria, vigorous exercise.
- **Causes:** type 1/2 diabetes, HTN, glomerulonephritis, interstitial nephritis, APKD, obstructive nephropathy, VU reflux, recurrent kidney infection.
- **Clinical:** symptoms in stages 4/5. Low Hb (low EPO and platelet dysfunction bleeding). Fatigue, nausea, vomiting, fluid retention, hiccups, pericardial rub, cachexia. Look for sepsis, heart failure, hypovolaemia, examination for bladder enlargement. CKD causes HTN and HTN causes CKD, encephalopathy. Avoid non-dominant forearm veins with cannulas as may need AV fistula.

Classification of chronic kidney disease using GFR and ACR categories

GFR and ACR categories and risk of adverse outcomes			ACR categories (mg/mmol), description and range		
			<3 Normal to mildly increased	3–30 Moderately increased	>30 Severely increased
			A1	A2	A3
GFR categories (ml/min/1.73m²), description and range	≥90 Normal and high	G1	No CKD in the absence of markers of kidney damage		
	60–89 Mild reduction related to normal range for a young adult	G2			
	45–59 Mild–moderate reduction	G3a[1]			
	30–44 Moderate–severe reduction	G3b			
	15–29 Severe reduction	G4			
	<15 Kidney failure	G5			

Increasing risk →

[1] Consider using eGFRcystatinC for people with CKD G3aA1 (see recommendations 1.1.14 and 1.1.15)

Abbreviations: ACR, albumin:creatinine ratio; CKD, chronic kidney disease; GFR, glomerular filtration rate

Adapted with permission from Kidney Disease: Improving Global Outcomes (KDIGO) CKD Work Group (2013) KDIGO 2012 clinical practice guideline for the evaluation and management of chronic kidney disease. Kidney International (Suppl. 3): 1–150

- **Investigations: FBC:** if low Hb, exclude non-renal cause. Check haematinics. **U&E:** measure creatinine. Watch for high K. **CRP** – inflammation/infection. **Bone:** low Ca and high phosphate; high Ca: check myeloma. Oral phosphate binders will often be necessary. **Urinary protein is always renal:** albumin/creatinine or protein/creatinine ratio (ACR or PCR). Microalbuminuria predicts end-stage disease with diabetes. **USS renal tracts:** obstruction, cysts, asymmetrical, e.g. renal artery stenosis, small kidneys with CKD, tumours. **CT/MRA:** structural lesions, renal artery stenosis. **Renal biopsy:** when benefits outweigh risks, e.g. IgA nephropathy or focal glomerulosclerosis. **Serology:** ANCA/GBM when appropriate.

- **Management:** look for acute or chronic reversible causes and manage as AKI. **Anaemia:** develops with Stage 3B or 4 diseases. Check haematinics. Target 110–120 g/L. Consider iron oral or infusion ± erythropoiesis-stimulating agents. **Blood pressure:** aim for 130/80 mmHg for patients with proteinuria: urinary ACR >30 or PCR >50. **Urinary protein:** ACR >30 or PCR >50 suggests worsening renal function. Start ACEi/ARB if HTN: target BP 130/80 mmHg. ACR >70 or PCR >100 needs strict BP control and specialist referral/discussion. **Cardiovascular risk:** advice on smoking, exercise and lifestyle. Consider statins if macrovascular disease, or 10-y risk of events >20%. **Immunisation:** influenza and pneumococcal, hepatitis B if RRT contemplated. **Medication review:** stop nephrotoxic drugs (particularly NSAIDs) and ensure doses of others are appropriate to renal function.
- **Reference:** SIGN (2008) 103: Diagnosis and management of chronic kidney disease: a national clinical guideline.

10.6 ▶ Urinary tract infection

- **About:** UTI usually symptomatic bacterial infection of the urinary tract. Kidney (acute pyelonephritis) young females. Bladder (acute cystitis) young females. Prostate (prostatitis) – older males, due to urinary infection, in younger often an STI. Positive dipstick and no symptoms should not be treated in older pts.
- **Note:** asymptomatic bacteriuria (ABU) does not itself require treating in uncomplicated patients. UTI denotes symptomatic disease. However, ABU during pregnancy is associated with complications such as preterm birth and perinatal mortality for the fetus and with pyelonephritis for the mother. Treatment of ABU in pregnant women decreases the risk of pyelonephritis by 75%. Uncomplicated UTI refers to acute cystitis or pyelonephritis in non-pregnant outpatient women with a normal anatomy and no instrumentation of the urinary tract.
- **Risks:** catheters or instrumentation of urinary tract, pregnancy. Post-coital: void afterwards because organisms milked into bladder. Diabetes mellitus (women only), incontinence, lack of circumcision in men. Structural abnormalities, neurogenic bladder, dehydration.
- **Microbiology:** *E. coli* 85%. *Staph. saprophyticus* 10%. Others include *Klebsiella, Proteus, Citrobacter, Pseudomonas aeruginosa.* Gram-positive enterococci and *Staph. aureus* and even yeasts.
- **Clinical:** general malaise, fever, N&V, most often female. **Pyelonephritis:** classically unilateral loin pain, rarely bilateral, fever, rigors. **Cystitis:** suprapubic discomfort, frequency, dysuria. **Prostatitis:** dysuria, perineal pain, frequency. **Elderly:** delirium, falls, instability, agitation.
- **Investigations:** FBC, U&E raised WCC, high CRP. U&E typically normal unless underlying renal issues. **Urine dipstick:** protein and blood support infection but may have other causes. **Nitrites:** not all bacteria convert nitrate to nitrite, and a sufficient concentration must be present to be detectable. Positive test strongly supports infection. **Leucocyte esterase:** enzyme found in polymorphs in the urine. Either is a positive test when the clinical picture is suggestive. A negative dipstick test is not good enough to exclude bacteriuria in pregnant women – send a sample for culture. **Urine microscopy:** WCC can be a helpful marker before culture results available at 24 h. A lower diagnostic threshold is used in women than men. **Urine culture:** gold standard but contamination from poor sampling can complicate matters. USS renal can be considered in recurrent UTI to exclude anatomical issue.

Diagnostic criteria for UTI

- ≥100 CFU/ml + 2 samples WCC ≥10/mm³ in symptomatic women.
- ≥100 CFU/ml in symptomatic young females.
- ≥1000 CFU/ml in symptomatic male or catheterised patient.
- ≥10,000 CFU/ml on 2 occasions in asymptomatic individuals.

Management

- ABC, manage sepsis. Ensure adequate hydration, analgesia and nutrition and IV fluids. Look for and treat any causes. Start antibiotics once urine has been sent for culture unless sterile sampling difficult, where it can be prudent and pragmatic to treat empirically rather than wait for a contaminated sample that can never be obtained.
- **Complications:** bacteraemia and urosepsis. SIRS. Delirium. Falls. AKI. **Diabetic:** obstructive uropathy associated with acute papillary necrosis causing AKI if bilateral. Staghorn calculi if chronic infection develops, renal/perinephric abscess formation. Emphysematous pyelonephritis where gas-forming bacteria proliferate.
- **Cystitis/lower UTI** (simple cystitis without fever or loin pain): take advice if urosepsis or there has been a multi-resistant pattern in antibiotic sensitivity seen In previous isolates. Nitrofurantoin PO (avoid if eGFR <60 ml/min, G6PD deficiency, porphyria). Duration of treatment: 3 d in non-pregnant women/uncomplicated UTI, 7 d in men. **Prevention:** drink 2 L/d, regular complete emptying of bladder, good personal hygiene, empty bladder before and after sex, cranberry juice/tablets may be effective
- **Pregnant with cystitis/lower UTI:** as above but also pregnant. Approximately 2–10% of pregnancies are accompanied by asymptomatic bacteriuria and of these, 40% develop infection. Most *E. coli*. Screen at 12–16 weeks. Send a sample for culture and sensitivities. Amoxicillin and cephalosporins for 1 week are safe and effective. Avoid trimethoprim in pregnancy.
- **Acute pyelonephritis: Co-amoxiclav** 1.2 g TDS IV or 625 mg 8 h PO. Switch to oral when improving. If pyrexial after 48 h, consider renal USS to exclude renal abscess. Review with results of culture. Treat for 2 weeks. Gentamicin IV.
- **Indwelling urinary catheters:** antibiotic treatment is not required unless patient is systemically unwell. Treatment should follow antibiotic sensitivity test result with changing/removal of the catheter. For empirical management discuss with consultant microbiologist.
- **Catheter change:** urinary catheter insertion or change of antibiotics are no longer routinely recommended, unless previous catheter-related sepsis, or change/removal is likely to be traumatic, or history of recurrent UTIs or neutropenic. 30 mins before catheter change give **Gentamicin** 160 mg, even with renal impairment. If MRSA positive at any time in the past give a single dose of IV **Teicoplanin** 400 mg as well.

10.7 Renal obstruction (obstructive uropathy)

- **Cause of post-renal AKI:** complete obstruction causes anuria, partial causes oliguria. Early treatment (usually surgical/radiological) can restore renal function. Can occur at any level from renal calyces to the distal urethra. Admit under urology.
- **Aetiology:** normal sites of narrowing are junctions between renal pelvis and ureter, ureter and bladder, bladder and urethra (bladder neck) and urethral meatus. Acquired causes and congenital cases seen in children. Depends on degree of obstruction, whether obstruction is slow and progressive. Depends on if it affects both or a single kidney. Is there underlying renal disease?

- **Causes:** congenital narrowing usual at sites mentioned above; posterior urethral valves. Phimosis and meatal stenosis. Infection with oedema and scarring. Tumour – cervix, uterus, colorectal, bladder, prostate. Debris: blood clots, sloughed papillae, benign prostatic hypertrophy. Pregnant uterus pressure, retroperitoneal fibrosis. Malignancy extrinsic compression – cervical, ovarian, bowel. Abdominal aortic aneurysm. Trauma at any level. Neurological – diabetic neuropathy, spinal cord disease. Accidental ligation at abdominal surgery.
- **Clinical:** acute obstruction: pain due to build-up of hydrostatic pressure in kidney. Bilateral acute obstruction: anuria and AKI. Partial obstruction: polyuria and nocturia as concentrating ability impaired. Chronic picture: hypertension and polycythaemia. Look for phimosis or meatal stricture, full bladder, flank pain or abdominal masses. PR examination for prostate enlargement and rectal tumour. Gynaecological exam: uterine or cervical or ovarian disease.
- **Investigations: bloods:** FBC: raised WCC, U&E AKI, raised CRP. Check Ca. **Urinalysis:** protein, leucocytes, glucose. **Imaging: bladder scan:** urine in bladder, post-voiding volume. **USS renal tracts:** useful to see obstruction and a dilated system with hydronephrosis or hydroureter. **Non-contrast CT** is modality of choice for stones. **IVU:** can delineate level of stenosis. **Voiding cystourethrography.** Antegrade/retrograde urography for renal pelvis and ureter.
- **Management: supportive:** ABC, manage hydration, electrolytes and acid–base balance. May be AKI. Watch K. Treat any infection. **Imaging, usually USS or non-contrast CT,** should be done quickly and urological referral if signs of obstruction. Urgent relief of obstruction to restore function and reduce risk of urosepsis. May be simple urethral catheterisation or drainage by nephrostomy/ ureterostomy or suprapubic catheter as is appropriate.
- **Individualised treatment of particular cause.** There is often a post-obstruction diuresis (even 1 L/h) following treatment requiring appropriate fluid replacement to avoid pre-renal problems.

10.8 Nephrolithiasis (renal stones)

- **About:** calculi in kidney and/or ureters. Care in those with single kidney or CKD. Renal stones seen in 10% of adults at some time. Admit under urology. Most are men aged 20–50 and recurrence is common.
- **NB:** urological emergency if infection occurs in the stagnant urine proximal to the stone (pyonephrosis) or if patient has solitary kidney with anuria due to a stone in the ureter.
- **Stones:** reduced urine output leads to supersaturation and stone formation. Calcium oxalate and calcium phosphate in 80% (radio-opaque). Urate stones in 10% (radio-lucent). Cystine in 1% (radio-opaque). Struvite (magnesium ammonium phosphate) in 5% (radio-opaque).
- **Causes:** distal RTA, gout, T2DM, primary hyperparathyroidism, idiopathic hypercalcaemia, cystinuria, polycystic kidneys, dietary or internal hyperoxaluria. Hyperuricosuria. Stone formation exacerbated by hot climates with resultant oliguria.
- **Clinical:** excruciating back or abdominal or flank pain: 'loin to groin/labia'. Patient writhing around in agony, unlike peritonitis who lie still. The pain can last minutes or hours and there can be intervals of no pain. N&V, frequency, dysuria, oliguria and haematuria. Chronic distension may be painless. Fever suggests infection. Low BP may suggest sepsis or alternative diagnosis, e.g. AAA. Check testes to exclude torsion. Check hernia orifices. Renal angle tender pyelonephritis.

- **Investigation: FBC:** high WCC and CRP with infection. **β-hCG:** always if pregnancy possible. **Urinalysis:** nitrites suggest UTI. Red cells compatible with stone disease but not always seen. Culture if WCC/nitrites. Alkaline urine pH >7.6 seen with struvite stones. pH <5 suggests uric acid. **AXR (KUB):** sensitivity for stones 45–60%. **U&E** calcium and urate and PTH if raised calcium: ensure no stone-forming causes and renal function.
- **Non-contrast helical CT urogram:** sensitivity and specificity >95%. Detects radio-opaque and radio-lucent stones. No need for intravenous contrast medium. Impaction is usually at ureter/bladder junction or ureter/pelvis or pelvic brim. CT excludes differential which includes AAA. **Intravenous urography (IVU):** shows level of ureteric obstruction and defines pelvicalyceal anatomy. It can miss some radio-lucent ureteric or renal stones (10–20% of stones). It is about 70–90% accurate. **USS renal tracts:** use in pregnancy, in children, and in febrile people. A low 50% diagnostic accuracy for stone detection, but main use is to diagnose hydronephrosis in people with complicated renal colic.
- **Differentials:** appendicitis (pain is right-sided), diverticulitis (pain is left-sided). Ectopic pregnancy, pyelonephritis, salpingitis in women, ruptured AAA.
- **Complications:** urinary tract obstruction and upper UTI. Pyelonephritis, pyonephrosis, urosepsis can ensue. AKI.
- **Cautions:** special care must be taken with those with renal stones and pre-existing renal disease, single kidney, kidney transplant, bilateral renal obstruction, pregnancy. Stone >5 mm or larger where impaction likely. Any signs of infection. Unusual for stones to present age >60 so look for alternative diagnoses.
- **Management: conservative:** collect and sieve all urine to catch stones. Send for biochemical analysis. Encourage oral fluids and maintain hydration and urine flow. Most stones ≤5 mm in diameter pass in 90% of cases. Stones >8 mm impact in 95%. Management is conservative. Pain control and in uncomplicated cases care may be at home. Advise the discharged person to seek urgent medical assistance if fevers or rigors, pain worsens or abrupt recurrence of severe pain. **Caution:** admit under urology those with signs of infection, single or transplanted kidney, pre-existing renal impairment, bilateral obstructing stones are suspected, significant analgesic need, dehydration and unable to maintain oral intake, pregnancy, patient preference, diagnosis uncertain in older patient or ectopic pregnancy in younger female. Choices for analgesia include **Diclofenac** 100 mg PR or IM (max 150 mg/d). **Pethidine** 100 mg IM or **Morphine** 10 mg IM with **cyclizine** or IV/IM **metoclopramide** (avoid in those <20 y). Reduce the dose by 25–50% in moderate or severe renal impairment.
- **Medical expulsive therapy:** α1-adrenergic blockers are indicated for those with adequate renal function reserve with a newly diagnosed distal ureteric stone (<10 mm), whose symptoms are controlled, and who have no clinical evidence of sepsis. **Tamsulosin** 0.4 mg OD is the drug of choice and has been shown to reduce time to expulsion and need for intervention and increases the probability that larger 5–10 mm distal ureteric stones will pass. **Nifedipine XL** 30 mg daily can also increase stone expulsion rate from 35% to 79% when combined with a steroid. **Prednisolone** 10 mg BD in a 5-d burst can be added to both. This may help reduce the intense inflammatory reaction.
- **Surgical removal:** consider if stone does not pass with basket extraction, surgical removal or lithotripsy.

- **ESWL** (extracorporeal shock-wave lithotripsy): focused sound waves fracture stone. Non-invasive and can be done as outpatient.
- **Percutaneous nephrolithotomy:** for larger stones/staghorn calculi. Nephroscope inserted into renal pelvis and collecting system and stone broken up and extracted.
- **Ureteroscopy** can be done with a laser to break up the stone. Ureteric injury low in experienced hands.
- **Open surgery:** done with large stones, multiple stones, etc.
- **Discharge:** if pain settles and there is no stone or the stone is ≤5 mm on X-ray kidney–ureter–bladder, the patient may be discharged with an NSAID orally, e.g. **Diclofenac** 50 mg TDS. An urgent IVU should be requested and referral to urology. If the pain does not settle admit. Higher risk patients are those with a solitary or transplanted kidney, pre-existing renal impairment or where bilateral obstructing stones are suspected.
- **Prevention:** high fluid intake, urine volume 2 L/d, coffee, tea, beer, wine, orange juice reduces stone formation. Moderate not high protein, Avoid sugar-sweetened drinks. Calcium intake is fine and binds oxalate. Thiazides may help.

10.9 Acute interstitial nephritis

- **About:** immune disorder with acute inflammation in tubulointerstitium usually drug-induced, e.g. PPIs. As well as toxins and systemic illness.
- **Causes:** PPI, penicillin, NSAIDs, mesalazine, TB, hantavirus, leptospirosis, myeloma, mushrooms, SLE, Sjögren's, sulphonamides. Take full drug Hx.
- **Clinical:** oliguric AKI. Drug cause may cause fever, rash.
- **Investigations:** FBC: eosinophilia. Urine: sterile modest proteinuria (PCR <100 mg/mmol) and WBC and casts. Eosinophils in 70% of patients but this is a non-specific finding. Nephrotic syndrome seen with NSAIDs. Renal biopsy is diagnostic may have granulomas.
- **Management:** if drug cause then stop it. High-dose steroids **Prednisolone** 1 mg/kg/d may help. Treat specific causes if possible.

10.10 Ischaemic priapism

- **About:** unwanted/painful erection >4 h. 95% ischaemic with sluggish or non-existent blood flow. Due to sludging and obstruction to blood flow.
- **Causes:** sickle cell disease, leukaemia, neoplasia, drugs, e.g. cocaine, etc. and drugs injected to cause erection. Priapism also seen with spinal cord transection.
- **Clinical:** penis may be swollen, rigid and painful.
- **Investigations:** FBC, sickle test, blood film, U&E. Penile Doppler – no flow and penile blood gas – hypoxia.
- **Management:** cooling, rest, ice packs over penis, pain relief, discuss with urology. Irrigation with NS aspirate 20–50 ml usual dark hypoxic blood from corpus cavernosum with butterfly needle until bright red blood seen. Sympathomimetics: intracavernosal **Phenylephrine** 100–200 mcg every 5–10 min; maximum 1 mg in 1 h. Dilute to 100 mcg/ml and inject in 1–2 ml aliquots. Observe for palpitations, arrhythmias, headache. **Urology:** surgical shunts used only after a trial of intracavernous injection of sympathomimetics has failed.
- **Reference:** European Association of Urology (2015) Guidelines on priapism.

10.11 ▶ Contrast-induced nephropathy

- **About:** post-contrast peak effect on creatinine occurs between 48 and 72 h.
- **Aetiology:** toxic effect of iodinated radiocontrast agents. Patients often have coexistent issues, e.g. sepsis, shock, heart failure, diabetes.
- **Risk:** highest: Cr >200 μmol/L or CrCl <30 ml/min or eGFR <30 ml/min, dehydration, increasing age, CKD, anaemia, diabetes mellitus, myeloma, CCF, nephrotic, sepsis, NSAIDs, nephrotoxins. Using >300 ml of contrast.
- **Definition:** 24% increase or 44 μmol/L increase in serum creatinine within 72 h of contrast and no alternative explanation.
- **Mitigation:** use a different imaging modality. Stop nephrotoxins including metformin. Use lowest contrast load. IV NS up to 1 ml/kg/h for 12 h before and after procedure. *N-acetylcysteine* 600 mg PO BD before and day after procedure. Check creatinine baseline 48 h and 5 and 10 d.

11 Neurology

11.1 ▶ Basic science

- **Physiology:** brain is 1% of body weight but gets 10% of cardiac output for its high metabolic demand and is vulnerable to emboli and ischaemia. Any reduction in global cerebral perfusion for more than a few seconds causes coma and collapse. The brain is irrigated by four arteries: two internal carotid arteries anteriorly (anterior circulation) and the two vertebrals posteriorly which then join to form the basilar (posterior circulation). Vertebrals arise from ipsilateral subclavians. The branches of these arteries meet again with the circle of Willis with posterior communicating artery connecting ICA to PCA and the anterior communicating between R and L anterior cerebral arteries.

- **Pathophysiology:** the brain is contained within a bony box. If pressure increases the largest exit is the foramen magnum. Bony box contains, by volume, 80% brain, 10% blood, 10% CSF. Separate compartments due to the falx (right/left) and tentorium (supra/sub). These limit the scope of expansion but can focus pressure within contents.

- **Normal ICP** 7–17 mmHg. A high intracranial volume will cause a gradual and ultimately exponential rise in ICP which leads to brainstem compression and death. **High ICP** will reduce cerebral perfusion pressure, which is mean systemic arterial pressure (MAP) minus ICP. Normal 'opening' pressure is 10–25 cm CSF. Always measure opening pressure at LP. Rising ICP can result in focal signs and herniation syndromes. High CO_2 causes cerebral vasodilation and a low CO_2 causes vasoconstriction. Reducing CO_2 reduces ICP.

Motor

- **About:** cell bodies for the corticospinal/nuclear tracts lie in layer V of the primary motor cortex (PMC) in the precentral gyrus. Voluntary precise motor movements are decided within centres within the frontal lobe and relayed to the PMC. There are two neurons between PMC and muscle, the upper (UMN) and lower motor neurons (LMN).

- **Upper motor neuron:** myelinated motor axons exit the PMC and pass inferiorly as the corona radiata via the posterior limb of the internal capsule to form the cerebral peduncle in front of the midbrain. Corticonuclear fibres synapse with local cranial nerve motor nuclei to the eyes (III, IV, VI), face (X, VII), tongue (XII) and pharynx and larynx (IX, X). Corticospinal tracts pass to the spinal cord to innervate respiratory, trunk, arms and leg muscles. Within the brainstem the motor fibres lie ventrally. At the level of the medulla (pyramid) the motor fibres cross right to left and left to right, accounting for the contralaterality of the motor system. At the level of the foramen magnum the fibres pass laterally to form the lateral corticospinal tracts in the spinal cord. The axon descends until it reaches its corresponding nerve root level where it synapses with the anterior horn cell. Structural lesions cause a C/L UMN weakness. Structural lesions within the brainstem cause an ipsilateral cranial nerve palsy and C/L UMN weakness.

- **Lower motor neuron:** formed at the anterior horn cell. The axon exits the cord and fuses with the posterior nerve root to form a nerve root that passes down and eventually out via its spinal foramina. Motor (myotomes) to arms formed in brachial plexus and to legs in sacral plexus. Cutaneous and other sensation (dermatomes). Structural lesions will simply cause an ipsilateral LMN weakness and sensory loss respecting dermatomes/myotomes.

- **Neuromuscular junction:** action potential reaches the terminal bouton and if sufficient Ach is released there is then summation of the stimulus and the generation of an action potential that leads to muscular contraction. Ach is broken down by local cholinesterase. Weakness (myasthenia) can be caused by a lack of Ach – denervation or even excess Ach, e.g. organophosphates, or damage to the post-synaptic nicotinic Ach receptor – such that an action potential cannot form.

Brainstem

- Contains cranial nerve nuclei and descending motor and ascending sensory tracts, the reticular formation required for sleep and wakefulness. The important clinical anatomical facts are below. Brainstem has three levels. Neuroanatomy books show the images inverted compared with CT/MRI imaging.
- **Midbrain:** V-shaped on cross-sectional imaging. Corticospinal/nuclear anteriorly. Periaqueduct: IIIrd nerve and below IVth nerve nucleus. IIIrd nerve exits anteriorly. Close to the posterior communicating artery.
- **Pons:** bulbous appearance. Motor fibre bundles anteriorly. Packed with axons via pons to/from cerebellum. V, VI, VII and VIII nerve nuclei. VII/VI close together. Any ipsilateral VII/VI suggests pontine lesion affecting both nuclei. Posterior to pons 'bridge' IVth ventricle. In front of the pons lies the basilar artery.
- **Medulla:** butterfly-like shape. Motor fibres anteriorly decussate. Posterolateral aspect vulnerable to infarction due to posterior inferior cerebellar artery occlusion. Causes Horner's syndrome (sympathetic), swallowing loss (nucleus ambiguus (IX, X, XI) damage to the vestibular nuclei and inferior cerebellar peduncle and spinal trigeminal nucleus.

Cerebellum

- Coordinates motor function with other parts of the brain. Lies behind the IVth ventricle and pons. Sensory and motor input from motor/premotor cortex. Feedback to these same centres.
- Hemispheres deal with ipsilateral movement. Hemispheric damage causes ipsilateral cerebellar signs. Midline damage causes a truncal ataxia.
- Acute cerebellar dysfunction is a feature of acute and chronic alcohol and drug toxicities, e.g. anticonvulsants and stroke disease. Structural damage lateralises same side, toxic issues are generalised.

Patterns of motor/sensory/autonomic neurology

- **Large cortical lesion (stroke/tumour/trauma): C/L (contralateral) hemiparesis, C/L hemisensory loss, C/L hemianopia.** Lt: aphasia. Rt: neglect/anosognosia.
- **Brainstem:** ipsilateral cranial nerve lesion + C/L hemiparesis.
- **Cerebellum:** past pointing, dysarthric speech, nystagmus and dysdiadochokinesia. Unilateral suggests stroke.
- **Complete cord lesion:** above C5 diaphragm weak. C5–T1 upper limb. L1–S3 lower limb. UMN weakness, below lesion paraparesis – increased reflexes, clonus. Sensory level, bowel/bladder, autonomic dysfunction.
- **Cauda equina: (below L1)** back pain. LMN flaccid weakness legs, plantars down, reflexes reduced, saddle/genital anaesthesia (S3–S5), weak sphincters, lax anal tone. Eventual wasting, fasciculation.

- **Polyneuropathy:** progressive LMN weakness, distal glove/stocking sensory loss, sphincter loss, autonomic, wasting, fasciculations develop.
- **Muscle end-plate:** fatiguability, no wasting, reflexes reduced, plantar absent.
- **Myopathy:** proximal weakness, low tone, reduced reflexes, mild wasting.

Cranial nerves

- (I) **Olfactory:** loss of smell. Frontal meningiomas. ENT, PD, Covid.
- (II) **Optic nerve:** visual acuity, fields, pupil response, fundoscopy.
- (III) **Oculomotor** (midbrain): levator palpebrae superioris, superior, inferior and medial rectus, inferior oblique. Parasympathetic to constrict pupils for accommodation and light (Edinger–Westphal nucleus to ciliary ganglion).
- (IV) **Trochlear** (midbrain): superior oblique. Unable to look down and in.
- (V) **Trigeminal** (pons): muscles of mastication, sensory face (ophthalmic, maxillary, mandibular branches) dura mater, intracranial blood vessels, teeth.
- (VI) **Abducent** (pons): lateral rectus.
- (VII) **Facial** (pons): facial expression, closes eye, stapedius. Sensory external ear canal. Taste anterior 2/3rds tongue. Salivary/lacrimal glands.
- (VIII) **Vestibulocochlear** (pons): balance (vestibular) hearing (cochlea).
- (IX) **Glossopharyngeal** (medulla): sensory pharynx, middle ear, carotid sinus and body, posterior 1/3rd tongue. Salivary glands. Stylopharyngeus.
- (X) **Vagus** (medulla): sensory from pharynx, larynx, oesophagus, aortic bodies and arch. Parasympathetic to chest and abdominal organs.
- (XI) **Spinal accessory** (medulla): sternomastoid and trapezius.
- (XII) **Hypoglossal** (medulla): motor to ipsilateral tongue.

Autonomic

- **Sympathetic:** fight/flight responses. Adrenaline. Increase heart rate, inotropic, pupils dilate, bronchodilation, increase muscle blood flow, reduced skin flow, reduce lacrimation, reduced intestinal motility, salivation. Increased sweating. Internal urinary sphincter contraction. The sympathetic ganglion lies in the sympathetic chain close to the spinal cord. Sympathetic: Preganglionic: release Ach. Post-ganglionic: release noradrenaline to adrenergic receptor except releases Ach at sweat glands.
- **Parasympathetic:** bradycardia, increased lacrimal and salivary secretions, pupil constriction, bronchoconstriction, detrusor stimulation and urination and defecation. Parasympathetic ganglion lies close to the target organ. Para: Preganglionic releases Ach to nicotinic receptors. Post-ganglionic ACh to muscarinic receptor.
- **Autonomic dysfunction:** chronic: diabetes, amyloid. Acutely: GBS and drug toxicities. Can cause severe autonomic instability.
- **Anticholinergics** (antimuscarinics): e.g. atropine block parasympathetic muscarinic Ach receptors. It causes increased heart rate, dilates pupils, dry secretions, urinary retention, dilates pupils so they can't focus.
- **Adrenergic blockers:** block alpha/beta-adrenergic receptors. Lower BP and heart rate.
- **Adrenergic agonists:** can stimulate. These raise heart rate, heart contractility and BP and heart rate.

Vision

- **Optic nerve lesion:** mild will cause altered colour perception (red colour washed out), reduced acuity and even loss of vision. There may be nothing to find clinically. Later optic atrophy. Classically with optic neuritis/MS.
- **Optic chiasm:** central lesion e.g. pituitary macroadenoma ± haemorrhage or some other SOL can compress chiasm often causing an asymmetrical bitemporal hemianopia. Sudden acute onset with pituitary apoplexy.
- **Cortical vision:** left parietal, temporal and occipital except frontal cortex contain optic tracts. Damage to the left side causes a right partial or complete homonymous hemianopia and vice versa. Temporal lobe lesion causes a superior quadrantanopia, parietal an inferior quadrantanopia.

Sensory pathways (ascends to contralateral parietal lobe)

- **Cortical level sensory:** left parietal cortex receives the sensory input from the right – touch, vibration, and all sensation other than smell.
- **Anatomy ascending sensory function** (3 neurons and 3 synapses): sensation is more subjective sign. Different modalities are carried in different tracts, and this can help to localise a lesion and so different modalities are tested. All perceived sensation terminates eventually in the contralateral post central gyrus of the parietal lobe.
- **Posterior column/medial lemniscus pathway:** vibration and proprioception enter via the dorsal root and pass into the ipsilateral posterior columns (lower body sensation in the medial gracile fasciculus and upper body in the lateral cuneate fasciculus). This ascends to form the medial lemniscus tract within the brainstem which then crosses at the medulla to synapse in the contralateral thalamus higher up and then passes via the internal capsule up to terminate in the primary sensory cortex on the post central gyrus of the parietal lobe.
- **Spinothalamic:** pain and temperature enter via the dorsal root and pass to opposite side close to the central canal. They then pass up the cord to synapse in the ipsilateral thalamus and pass as axons via the internal capsule on the post central gyrus of the parietal lobe.

11.2   Clinical assessment

Determine pathology using duration and onset in history

- **Sudden and immediate:** dramatic. Usually vascular or electrical. Vascular (embolic stroke is sudden, thrombotic stroke tends to stutter in onset, haemorrhage can be sudden but usually slow and progressive), seizure, SAH, functional, migraine (usually over minutes).
- **Minutes to hours:** migrainous aura, seizure, thrombotic stroke rarely, an expanding haemorrhagic stroke, SDH, EDH.
- **Hours to days:** demyelination, inflammation, infections, e.g. viral encephalitis, meningitis.
- **Months:** Creutzfeldt–Jakob disease, aggressive tumours, e.g. glioblastomas or metastases, MND/ALS.
- **Years:** low-grade gliomas, progressive stroke disease, neurodegenerative diseases, e.g. Parkinson's, Alzheimer's, Huntington's. Primary progressive MS, secondary progressive MS. MND (ALS).
- **Recurrent:** migraine, epilepsy, demyelination, stroke, relapsing remitting MS. Primary headaches.

Determine pathology using positive vs. negative neurology
- **Positive:** tingling, flashing lights, allodynia, jerks and movements. Migrainous aura spreads over minutes (cortical spreading depression) or a focal seizure spread over seconds, usually due to an irritative focus.
- **Negative:** weakness, hemianopia, loss of sensation, incoordination, deafness. Suggests destructive pathology – inflammatory, vascular, demyelination, tumour, etc.

11.3 Patterns of weakness

Cortical damage C/L UMN weak and C/L sensory loss and C/L hemianopia
- **Acute stroke:** comes on over seconds/minutes. C/L weakness (face/arm/leg), C/L hemianopia and sensory loss. Aphasia/neglect. ▶Section 11.18.
- **Post seizure:** Todd's paralysis. Weakness post-seizure. ▶Section 11.15.
- **Tumour:** progressive contralateral weakness, seizures. ▶Section 17.4.
- **Cerebral abscess:** focal sub/cortical neurology, seizures. ▶Section 11.12.
- **Demyelination:** subacute progressive contralateral weakness over days. History of prior episodes. Consider MS or ADEM. ▶Section 11.33.
- **Subdural haematoma: C/L weakness,** head trauma, anticoagulants. ▶Section 11.24.
- **Epidural haematoma:** head trauma, lucid then coma. C/L weakness. ▶Section 11.25.
- **Motor neurone disease (MND):** UMN/LMN. No sensory or eye signs. ▶Section 11.35.
- **Parenchymal infection:** PML, HSV, neurocysticercosis, TB, syphilis.
- **Parasagittal meningioma:** bilateral UMN legs weak. Compresses both frontal motor strips. ▶Section 17.4.

Lesions in brainstem
- Ipsilateral cranial nerve palsy + C/L UMN above medulla.
- Also diplopia, INO, dizziness, hiccups, dysphagia, ataxia, nystagmus.
- Ipsilateral cerebellar signs, tongue weakness.
- Complete ptosis (IIIrd), partial (Horner's).

Lesions in the spinal cord
- **Clinical:** high tone, spasticity, hypertonic, hyperreflexia, upgoing plantar, loss of sensation below lesion. Priapism sphincters. Neurogenic shock.
- **Notes:** cord lesions – above lesion normal neurology, LMN at the level of lesion such as a reduced reflex and weakness and UMN below. Transection C1–4 quadriparesis, respiratory failure, C5–T1 arm and leg weakness, sensory level, below T1 paraparesis, sensory level. Lesions may be subtotal and asymmetrical. Cord damage may be complete. However, often it is incomplete, and this can lead to several syndromes:
- **Central cord syndrome:** significant traumatic cervical hyperextension can cause ischaemic central cord damage. Weakness and loss of sensation in both arms, intact motor and sensation in leg. Will need neurorehabilitation and usually seen on trauma ward.
- **Hemisection of cord:** loss of ipsilateral posterior columns (vibration and proprioception) and corticospinal (UMN weakness) and C/L spinothalamic (pain

and temperature). Also called Brown-Séquard syndrome. Any aetiology causing unilateral cord damage and dysfunction.

- **Subacute combined degeneration:** B12 deficiency, UMN weakness and dorsal column loss. May be peripheral neuropathy and loss of ankle jerks.
- **Transverse myelitis:** LMN at level and UMN weakness and sensory level below. Depends on level. Lhermitte's signs. Clumsy hand. Asymmetry. May be urinary retention. Autonomic dysfunction. Commonly due to multiple sclerosis and may find other signs of lesions. MS, ▶Section 11.33. Other causes are neuromyelitis optica (myelitis and optic neuritis and Ab to aquaporin 4; ▶Section 11.33), viral, e.g. HIV, CMV, HSV, post mycoplasma, vasculitis and even paraneoplastic. The CSF and MRI show inflammatory changes. Steroids, IVIg and PLEX for inflammatory causes.
- **Cervical spondylotic myelopathy:** canal stenosis can cause progressive damage to cord. Affects lower limbs first. Numb and clumsy hands. Progressive upper limb neurology. Nerve roots may be compressed with pain and weakness. Usually C5/6 or C4/5 or C6/7. Neck and pain down roots into shoulders and arms. C6/7 compresses C7 weak triceps and dermatomal sensory loss. C5/C6 lesion C6 affects biceps. Diagnosis with MRI. May settle conservatively. Surgical decompression for progressive neurological disability.
- **Functional 'block':** diagnosis of exclusion – can mimic any neurological disorder or none. The absence of hard signs helps. Normal tests. Expert review needed. Can occur and resolve quickly or slowly. Pattern of weakness/sensory loss can mimic true pathology. Paraplegia, stroke-like, seizure-like. Give-way weakness. Lots of extreme effort. A lifted leg can be held up against gravity but not lifted. Uneconomic gaits and postures. Contrast between exam findings and therapy findings. Positive Hoover's sign. Normal imaging. Give lots of positive support: 'you have a block'. Be supportive and sympathetic and especially reassuring. True malingerers are the exception. Poorly understood manifestation of non-structural illness.
- **Syringomyelia:** cape-like dissociated loss of pain and temperature. Syrinx on MRI often with Chiari malformation.
- **Physical injury to cord:** an acute cord lesion due to trauma or some space-occupying lesion will cause LMN at level of injury and UMN weakness below the level, sensory level, affect sphincters. Early on motor may be flaccid then replaced by a spastic paraparesis, affects arms if above T1. Pain is an important feature in conscious patients. Also retention. Priapism seen. Needs immobilisation of neck and back and appropriate care in transfers. Needs imaging and trauma management. ABC, labile BP as may be autonomic sympathetic damage so cautious with anaesthesia. Care of local trauma/orthopaedics team.
- **Vascular:** anterior cord infarction or haemorrhage 'spinal stroke', e.g. related to aortic aneurysm surgery or embolism/thrombosis, cavernomas and AVM or coagulopathies. Anterior cord syndrome: spastic bilateral weakness and spinothalamic loss. Preserved posterior columns (seen with anterior spinal artery infarction). Central cord syndrome: cervical level hyperextension can cause ischaemic central cord damage. Weakness and loss of sensation in both arms, intact motor and sensation in leg.
- **Malignant cord compression:** there is little space for lesions lying in the canal to expand without compressing neural structures. Spinal metastases can impinge the vascular supply to the cord as well as cause direct pressure. LMN at level affected and UMN and sensory loss below. Most are epidural and secondaries. Most commonly thoracic then lumbar then cervical. Give steroids. Image whole cord. ▶Section 17.8.

- **Metabolic:** B12 deficiency – posterior column and UMN corticospinal loss. Megaloblastic anaemia. High LDH, low B12. Check levels and replace.
- **Infections:** syphilis (tertiary): Tabes dorsalis–dorsal column loss. Pain variable can be severe. Immunosuppressed, HIV.
- **Spinal cord abscess:** pain, tender, swelling. Any level including below L1. Pott's disease of spine with kyphosis due to TB. High CRP. Blood cultures. CXR, plain films MRI.
- **Spinal cord AVM or haemorrhage:** tortuous vessels on surface of cord. May not be seen on MRI needs angiogram. It can bleed. Other causes of bleed hereditary haemorrhagic telangiectasia, cavernoma, coagulopathy.
- **Epidural haematoma/abscess** can cause sudden acute cord injury (on anticoagulants or bleed from AV malformation, post lumbar puncture/epidural). Epidural abscess, e.g. spinal tuberculosis or other infection. Reverse anticoagulants. Urgent neurosurgical consult.

Lesions below cord: weakness, reduced tone and reflexes
- **Poliomyelitis:** causes an acute flaccid paralysis. Usually asymmetrical. May be limbs, bulbar or respiratory. Non-vaccinated from endemic areas.
- **Acute myelopathy or cauda equina lesion:** sudden or subacute onset of quadriplegia or paraplegia and loss of sphincter control and sensory level. Need to identify if this is a compressive lesion or medical cause, e.g. spinal stroke or transverse myelitis. Urgent MRI indicated and if non-compression then LP for CSF. Cord lesions often cause initial flaccid weakness but becomes hypertonic within 24–48 h. Pain may help identify level and suggests a more surgical compressive cause. See ▶ Section 11.28.
- **Infections and abscess formation:** see above.
- **Disc prolapse:** soft central part of the disc, the nucleus pulposus, may rupture through the outer layers of the disc (annulus fibrosus). Most commonly posterolateral. If fragment of nucleus compresses nerve root patient experiences pain, e.g. sciatica. Also numbness and weakness in dermatome/myotome. Commonest discs to prolapse are the L4/5 on L5 root and the L5/S1 discs on S1 root. Causes pain (sciatica) with straight leg raise as nerve stretched. Others are possible including L3/4. There will be loss of corresponding reflex. A central disc protrusion can compress the central part of the canal. Effects depend on size and position of herniated disc and canal size. Central disc prolapses below L1 can cause the rare conus medullaris or cauda equina syndrome. Discs can also rarely herniate at cervical level with nerve root pain into arm and LMN signs in the region of the compressed root. A central cervical disc lesion may cause progressive spasticity and abnormal gait below as well as acute pain and needs urgent imaging.
- **Malignant cauda equina compression:** there will be pain, sphincters with reduced anal tone and incontinence and LMN leg weakness. Most are epidural and secondaries. Consider steroids and urgent imaging and referral to oncology and spinal team. ▶ Section 17.8.
- **Acute trauma injury to spine below L1 affecting cauda:** trauma team review. Back pain, saddle anaesthesia, loss anal tone, LMN weakness, atonic bladder, loss of vasomotor control, atonic bowel. May be asymmetrical and partial. Needs urgent imaging and surgical review.

Peripheral neuropathy (weakness, wasting, fasciculations, absent reflexes)
- **Ascending inflammatory demyelinating polyneuropathy (GBS/AIDP):** ascending usually symmetrical weakness of both legs over days with areflexia.

Sensory and autonomic symptoms. Raised CSF protein. Areflexia is a useful sign. Use NCS/EMG/LP to confirm. Needs IVIg. May follow illness. CIDP slower in onset and steroid responsive. ▶Section 11.26.

- **Polyneuropathy:** most commonly GBS with a progressive LMN weakness. No reflexes. Others are CIDP, HIV polyneuropathy GBS. ▶Section 11.26.
- **Symmetrical peripheral neuropathy:** can be motor, e.g. hereditary sensorimotor neuropathy (CMT and related conditions). ▶Section 11.34. Causes e.g. alcohol (peripheral symmetrical sensory), diabetes, lead toxicity, drugs, leprosy, paraneoplastic (lung cancer), etc.
- **Peripheral mononeuropathy:** median, ulnar, radial, common peroneal. Motor and sensory characteristics. Use NCS/EMG to confirm.
- **Multifocal motor neuropathy with conduction block:** middle-aged, slowly progressive weakness, wrist drop, foot drop, asymmetrical. Minimal wasting, fasciculations. Diagnose with NCS/EMG anti GM1 antibody. Responds to IVIg; can be confused with MND.
- **Critical illness polyneuropathy:** weakness post ITU. Can be face, arms, legs, respiratory muscles. Usually post ventilation. Similar critical illness myopathy may be seen. Needs NCS/EMG. CSF normal. Axonal. Intensive insulin therapy.
- **Diphtheria:** descending paralysis, unable to focus with vision, oropharyngeal weakness, limb weakness, quadriparesis. Sensorimotor. NCS show demyelination. Give diphtheria antitoxin as early as possible and supportive care.
- **Porphyria:** severe acute axonal polyradiculopathy or neuronopathy. Asymmetrical and proximal weakness and sensory loss. Motor of face, eyes, limbs, respiratory. Raised delta-aminolaevulinic acid. Can mimic GBS. See ▶Section 5.17.

Neuromuscular junction weakness, reduced tone and reflexes and fatiguability

- **Myasthenia gravis (MG):** progressive fatiguable weakness: proximal limbs and neck flexion are weak, face (bilateral ptosis) and diplopia and difficulty swallowing. Consider myasthenia. Check antibodies against acetylcholine receptors. Ice cube/tensilon test. See ▶Section 11.27.
- **Lambert–Eaton syndrome:** weakness and fatiguability. Exercise may improve strength then fatigues. Paraneoplastic in many. Get EMG. Treatment 3,4 diaminopyridine. PLEX and IVIg can be tried.
- **Botulism:** *Clostridium botulinum*. Progressive descending bulbar weakness and generalised flaccid paralysis. See ▶Section 9.18.
- **Tick paralysis:** seen in Australia and North America. Weakness 2–5 d after tick exposure. Usually children. Female tick releases a neurotoxin in saliva. Might find large engorged tick on skin (often scalp); when tick removed symptoms improve and resolve – grasp the tick as close to the skin as possible and pull in a firm steady manner ensuring all parts removed. Tick toxin blocks Ach release. Progressive ascending weakness like GBS.

Muscle (wasting/symmetrical proximal weakness) reduced reflexes and tone

- **Proximal myopathy:** proximal weakness, unable to raise hands above shoulders or sit to stand. Look for rash, cushingoid, osteomalacia, etc.
- **(Dermato/poly)myositis:** elderly. Insidious onset of weakness. Proximal arm weakness. Dysphagia, weak neck flexion. Skin lesions. Lung fibrosis, cardiac arrhythmias. Paraneoplastic in some. Raised CK/ESR helps. Positive ANA and EMG findings. Muscle biopsy. Needs Rheumatology/steroids.

- **Inclusion body myositis:** age >50. Progressive quad weakness. Unable to do stairs. Forearm wasting. Wasting. Foot drop. Diabetes. ESR/CK are normal. Get EMG and biopsy. Poor response to steroids and IVIg.

Transient/episodic weakness
- **Myasthenia gravis** and similar conditions above.
- **Sleep paralysis:** transient inability to move or speak on waking. Linked to narcolepsy. May have daytime sleepiness, cataplexy, hypnagogic hallucinations, sleep paralysis.
- **TIA:** will correspond with a transient arterial occlusion – see stroke.
- **Electrolytes:** low K, Ca, Mg all cause generalised weakness until recover.
- **Periodic paralysis:** onset usually childhood, low K and raised K levels, associated with thyroid disease. Seen more in Asians. Sudden episodic generalised weakness. Provoked by fasting or high carbohydrate meals or exercise. Measure electrolytes. Replace K if needed.
- **Post-ictal 'Todd's paralysis' weakness.**
- **Migraine with aura/hemiplegic migraine:** associated migrainous syndrome.
- **Multiple sclerosis** and worsening in warm environment.

11.4 ▶ Coma

- **Anatomy:** wakefulness is controlled by the reticular activating system (RAS), a fine net of nerves within the brainstem ascending as far as the thalamus and hypothalamus bilaterally. The RAS is closely associated with the cranial nerve nuclei for eye movement as well as the medial longitudinal fasciculus, so associated eye signs are commonly seen and help with localisation.
- **Causes:** compression, stroke, tumours and any other pathology can cause a rise in ICP with brainstem compression, ischaemia and dysfunction until respiration ceases.

Glasgow Coma Scale
- Developed by Glasgow neurosurgeons 1970s pre brain imaging. Aim to identify those with worsening neurology needing neurosurgical intervention. Always communicate the individual EVM456 rather than just the absolute score.
- Describe score as X out of 15 to ensure no misunderstanding but qualify it with individual components. Higher is better. Changes may be more important than actual values. Coma is generally defined as a GCS of 3–8. Dysphasic patients will score low for verbal even if no signs of coma.
- **Eye opening E1–4:** E1: nothing; E2: eye opens to pain (supraorbital, sternal pressure/rub); E3: eye opens to speech (wake patient if asleep); E4: eye opens spontaneously.
- **Best verbal V1–5:** V1: nothing; V2: incomprehensible sounds (moans); V3: inappropriate words (random words no conversation); V4: confused (disorientation and confusion); V5: normal (coherent and appropriate – month, age).
- **Best motor M1–6:** M1: no movement; M2: arm extends to pain (decerebrate response); M3: arm flexes to pain (decorticate response); M4: arm withdraws from pain (retracts when pinched; flexion OK); M5: hand localises to pain (gets above chin if supra-orbital pressure applied); M6: obeys commands (patient follows simple commands).

Clinical clues: always think hypoglycaemia

- **What is the GCS?** Look for clues – why in hospital? Any trauma? Medications – hypoglycaemics? Opiates/codeine? Anticoagulants? What is the temperature, pulse, BP, O_2 sats, respiratory rate? Look all over for a petechial rash, meningism, seizure-like episodes or known epilepsy. If reduced GCS, place patient in the recovery position. Get anaesthetic review. Look at drug chart. A single dose of codeine or Oramorph can be enough to reduce GCS. *Perform repeated top to toe assessment. Check back and perineum.* If new patient to look for any signs of trauma or any other signs, e.g. petechiae from meningococcaemia, Kernig's signs. If any concerns of spinal injury, then immobilise.
- **Check observations:** temp/HR/BP/O_2 sats, RR and ensure not hypothermic (exposure, hypothyroid) and if so treat. Check bedside CBG. See treatment below.
- **Opiate toxicity:** see treatment below. Search for and remove any opiate, fentanyl, buprenorphine patches. Consider naloxone. Take senior advice.
- **CT head** excludes structural problem: SAH, subdural, extradural, intracerebral or cerebellar bleed, tumour, oedema, herniation syndromes, hydrocephalus. If normal it is a medical coma.
- **Cerebral malaria: recent travel endemic area.** Haemolysis. Flu-like illness. Investigate/treat quickly. Thick/thin films. Talk to lab. Call ID.
- **Encephalitis/meningitis:** if CT shows no surgical cause then needs LP with opening CSF pressures to be performed – check no coagulopathy first.
- **Post-seizure or non-convulsive status: see below.**
- **Stroke:** usually obvious on scan, large bleed with coning or malignant MCA with oedema and midline shift. Bilateral thalamic and top of the basilar artery infarcts can give coma disproportionate to CT findings. MRI can help.
- **Toxicology screen:** ketones, ABG, blood cultures.
- **TCA overdose:** can cause coma and fixed dilated pupils, upgoing plantars.
- **Consider the coma cocktail** of management below.
- **Trauma and injury:** Battle's sign, panda eyes, skull lacerations or haematomas. If so consider immobilising the spine and CT head/spine.
- **Asymmetry:** an asymmetrical motor response to pain may suggest a lateralising structural lesion rather than toxic metabolic cause.
- **Post-ictal:** headache, incontinent, known epilepsy, alcohol (DTs), bitten (usually the side) tongue may suggest seizure and post-ictal drowsiness.
- **Eyes:** pupil response is important. IIIrd nerve close to the tentorium. Vulnerable to pressure from a posterior communicating/superior cerebellar aneurysm. Pupil constricting fibres lie on the surface of the nerve so pupil dilated with impaired response to light if the nerve is compressed. Isolated pontine lesions can have responsive but pinpoint pupils. Pupils useful in the comatose patient.
- **Meningism:** in the comatose patient look for meningism. Assuming no cervical injury then use passive neck flexion so that chin is almost touching chest. If there is any flexion of the knees then consider meningeal irritation and the need for CT/LP to exclude meningitis or SAH as a cause of coma. If the CT scan is normal then the coma is more likely drug-induced, metabolic or post-ictal – see further information below.
- **Dilated pupil:** cocaine use, atropine, pressure on ipsilateral IIIrd, Miller Fisher/botulism, AAC glaucoma. Suspect coning if sluggish to constrict or fixed and dilated. If progresses both pupils fixed and dilated. Ipratropium can cause dilation and TCA overdose – coma, dilated pupils, upgoing plantars.

- **Constricted pupil:** usually reactive but very hard to detect (consider opiates and a test dose of naloxone, Horner's syndrome). Rarely an isolated pontine bleed or infarct. Toxic conditions cause small symmetrical reactive pupils.
- **Bilateral fixed dilated:** massive brainstem injury with IIIrd nerve. Exclude hypothermia and drug toxicity/adrenergic syndrome/cocaine.
- **Dysconjugate gaze suggests brainstem pathology.** If the head can be safely turned (no cervical injury) then usually the eye moves relative to the orbit fixated at same position. If the eyes are static within the orbit this is abnormal loss of 'doll's eye movement'.
- **Averted gaze:** destructive cortical lesion on right, patient has hemianopia to left so ignores left and looks right. Irritative lesion on right causing seizure the patient's gaze turns to the left and vice versa for left cortical lesion.
- **Jaundiced:** hepatic encephalopathy, falciparum malaria, malignancy. Look for petechiae – meningococcaemia, DIC. Pyrexia, cold sores: HSV encephalitis.
- **Back:** turn patient and check back, including along spinal cord and orifices. Abdominal, chest and cardiac exam are needed.
- **Seizures:** treat for seizures acutely if suspected. IV anticonvulsant: (levetiracetam) if persisting seizures (always consider non-convulsive status).

Investigations

- **Bloods:** FBC, U&E CRP: WCC, glucose, TSH/FT_4 (myxoedema coma), infection. ABG: hypoxia, hypercarbia, acidosis. For metabolic acidosis calculate anion gap. Malaria – thick/thin films.
- **Urine:** blood, protein, WCC, toxicology screen if overdose suspected (check blood paracetamol/salicylates).
- **Non-contrast CT head:** often the most discriminating test in an unexplained coma and needs to be done immediately post-arrival in the emergency department. Neurosurgical consult if abnormal head CT and surgically amenable finding ± mannitol or steroids – see doses below. If coma and normal CT then treat vascular, infective, toxicology, metabolic causes. Consider LP, EEG, toxicology, etc. Rare 'stroke and normal CT' causes of coma are basilar artery thrombosis (bright basilar artery) or bilateral thalamic infarcts.
- **LP:** if no contraindications and suspected meningitis or encephalitis.
- **EEG:** done later.
- **MRI:** when there is strong suspicion that there is a bilateral thalamic (artery of Percheron) or top of the basilar artery infarct. May also show post seizure changes. Difficult to safely monitor sick restless patient in MRI scanner.

Coma with a normal/near normal (initial) CT head

- Head injury, hypoglycaemia, sepsis, low Na, myxoedema.
- Post-cardiac arrest, hypoxic brain damage.
- Drug toxicity – TCA overdose, anticonvulsants, benzodiazepines, TCA, opiates/codeine/sedation.
- Post seizure, non-convulsive status (EEG).
- Top of the basilar artery occlusion (bright basilar on CT).
- Bilateral thalamic ischaemic stroke (artery of Percheron).
- Encephalopathy, encephalitis, meningoencephalitis, cerebral malaria.
- Hypoactive delirium, malingering/psychiatric.

Differentials for coma

- **Post head injury:** head trauma which has been missed by emergency department? Look for injury. Blood in ear canal. Get CT head/neck for fractures, haemorrhage, oedema. CT may look normal if there is diffuse neuronal injury with perhaps signs of cerebral oedema.
- **Subarachnoid haemorrhage:** thunderclap headache, coma and recovery, nausea, vomiting. CTA: blood in subarachnoid space and aneurysm/AVM may be seen. Urgent neurosurgical consult. See ▶Section 11.22.
- **Ischaemic stroke:** malignant MCA or large cerebellar infarct or bleeding or basilar artery thrombosis. Get CT scan, take advice.
- **Non-convulsive SE:** may be few or no outward sign of ongoing seizures except perhaps eye flickering. Needs EEG. See below ▶Section 11.16.
- **Post cardiac arrest:** often urgent PCI and consider therapeutic hypothermia (cooled to 32–34°C for 12–24 h if rhythm was VF). Supportive management after PCI. May be significant hypoxic brain damage. ▶Section 1.11.
- **Severe renal failure:** uraemia can cause coma esp with opiates. ▶Section 10.4.
- **Drug overdose:** alcohol, ethylene glycol (specific antidote), benzodiazepines (flumazenil in selected cases), TCAs with coma and fixed dilated pupils, upgoing plantars. This list is not comprehensive.
- **Opiates/codeine:** miosis, respiratory depression. Oral/IV opiates, patches stop/give naloxone.
- **Post-ictal/non-convulsive status:** ABCs if fitting has stopped. May need anticonvulsant if status. Recovers gradually awaken within 2 h – if not then start to look for causes. ▶Sections 11.15 and 11.16.
- **Raised ICP:** ischaemic/haemorrhagic stroke, abscess, tumour, SDH, EDH, SAH, hydrocephalus, oedema/blood/obstructed CSF seen on CT.
- **Cerebral oedema:** post-hypoxic brain damage or malignant MCA stroke, tumour, metastases, abscess, vasogenic oedema, DKA, high altitude, Reye's syndrome, hypoxic injury, CO poisoning, SIADH.
- **Liver failure:** jaundice, abnormal LFTs, signs of liver failure; recent paracetamol overdose – N-acetylcysteine. ▶Section 7.2.
- **Encephalopathy:** drug-induced, metabolic, liver failure. Sodium valproate can cause coma and associated with high blood ammonia. ▶Section 7.11.
- **Endocrine:** hypothyroid: hypothyroid appearance, thyroidectomy scar, low HR, give thyroxine ± steroids. ▶Section 5.7.

Coma cocktail: consider where the cause of coma is uncertain

- **ABCDE** O_2 intubate, ventilation if hypoxic GCS <9. Airway.
- **Glucose** 20–50 ml of 50% IV or equivalent if hypoglycaemia is possible. Check CBG. In those with unexplained hypoglycaemia send lab glucose ± C-peptide.
- **Naloxone** 400 mcg IV repeated as needed up to 1.2 mg. Opiate toxicity, see ▶Section 14.26.
- **Pabrinex** IV paired vials 8 h for 2 d if suspected malnutrition/alcoholism.
- **Ceftriaxone** 2 g IV BD + steroids for bacterial meningitis.
- **Aciclovir** IV 10 mg/kg for any suspicion of HSV encephalitis.
- **Dexamethasone** 10 mg IV stat for tumour-related cerebral oedema.
- **Mannitol** 200 ml of 20% (20 g/100 ml) IV infusion for raised ICP/incipient coning as a bridge to surgery or shunting hydrocephalus.
- **Flumazenil** 0.2–0.5 mg slow IV for benzo overdose. Caution if risk of seizures.
- **NB:** Many of these can be stopped following a senior review if felt to be unnecessary and when the diagnosis and cause are more apparent.

Management

- **Suspected hypoglycaemia** all need rapid CBG. If low or unsure then 50 ml of 20–50% glucose IV if indicated or **Glucagon** 1 mg IM/SC. Look for cause. May need 10% infusion if ongoing.
- **Ischaemic stroke: admit HASU.** Discuss with stroke team. Thrombectomy may be considered if basilar thrombosis seen. Malignant MCA syndrome refer to neurosurgeons. Large cerebellar stroke with coma refer neurosurgeons for possible decompression.
- **Haemorrhagic stroke:** haemorrhage, raised ICP (cerebellar bleeds and some supratentorial superficial cortical bleeds benefit from surgery). Manage secondary hydrocephalus with external ventricular drainage. See ▶ Section 11.21.
- **Subdural haematoma:** stop/reverse anticoagulants. CT is diagnostic. Neurosurgical referral. See ▶ Section 11.24.
- **Alcoholism/nalnourished/anorexia** or any suggestion of dietary issues give Pabrinex IV paired vials TDS for 1–2 d.
- **Opiate overdose: Naloxone** 100–400 mcg IV (lower dose in chronic users) if opiate abuse/use suspected. Up to **naloxone** 2 mg may be needed.
- **Benzodiazepine: Flumazenil** 0.2–0.5 mg slow IV if benzodiazepine excess and compromised and no history of epilepsy. An infusion may be needed.
- **CNS infections:** meningitis: purpura, fever, neck stiffness. Meningism. CT/LP. Give **ceftriaxone, aciclovir ± amoxicillin.** See ▶ Section 11.10.
- **Encephalitis:** seizure, focal signs, fever, neck stiffness, delirium. Assume HSV and give IV **aciclovir.** Needs CT/LP. See ▶ Section 11.8.
- **Cerebral malaria:** travel in endemic area <6 months. Blood films to lab. Urgent expert advice. **Quinine** IV. See ▶ Section 9.3.
- **Epilepsy: if non-convulsive status suspected** consider **Lorazepam** 1–2 mg IV. Alternatively patient may be post-ictal from generalised seizure. See ▶ Section 11.15/11.16.
- **Hyperglycaemia:** DKA/HHS dehydration, ketones in urine/breath, high Na, cerebral oedema. See ▶ Section 5.18.
- **Addisonian crisis:** low BP, scar/general pigmentation, high K, low Na. Give **Hydrocortisone** 100 mg IV 6 h. See ▶ Section 5.1.
- **Pituitary apoplexy:** CT bleeding, visual loss. Give **Hydrocortisone** 100 mg IV 6 h. See ▶ Section 5.9. Urgent neurosurgical consult.
- **Myxoedema coma:** give T_3/T_4 and **Hydrocortisone** 100 mg IV 6 h. See ▶ Section 5.7.

Supportive measures

- **ABC:** O_2, cannula. HDU/ITU bed. Skin care, bowel, bladder care. Recovery position. Nasopharyngeal airway. If GCS <9 get anaesthetic review for assessment if they need intubation. GCS was designed for head trauma and not medical patients. Some have a GCS of <9 and have an open and patent airway/adequate ventilatory rate/sats >92%.
- **Intubation:** if there is poor respiratory effort then BVM ventilation manually whilst preparing for intubation. Check core temperature. Use critical care outreach team. ITU referral. Consultant to consultant referral if needed.
- **Medications:** these are often stopped. If they are vital then try other routes, e.g. PR for aspirin. An NG tube can be placed for vital medications. Some important medications to continue – steroids (may need to be increased) or immunosuppression, Parkinson's medications (rotigotine patch), anti-anginals,

antibiotic prophylaxis, warfarin or other anticoagulants where appropriate, rate-controlling medications, e.g. **digoxin** (give IV or NG) or beta-blockers, HAART therapies, anticonvulsants.
- **Coma cocktail** above. If rapidly worsening, apnoeic then arrest team.
- **Hydration:** can be difficult to assess. Fluid replacement 25–30 ml/kg per day in all comatose patients, to match normal losses. If coma persists then manage feeding and nutritional issues.
- **Urinary catheters:** patients can be padded. Suprapubic pressure can result in reflex bladder emptying. Use if retention or close output monitoring need.
- **Exposure:** avoid hypothermia. Blankets or 'space blankets' and warmers.
- **Stress ulcers:** prevent with PPI/H_2 blocker in selected patients.
- **Resuscitation status:** assess ceiling of care, MET calls, CPR, etc.
- **Management of** raised **ICP:** see below.
- **Palliation:** where appropriate.

11.5 Acute headache

- **Physiology:** the brain is insensitive to pain. Pain is from meningeal arteries, proximal portions of cerebral arteries, dura at the base of the brain, venous sinuses and cranial nerves 5, 7, 9 and 10, and cervical nerves 2 and 3.
- **About:** on referral if thunderclap (peak less than 5 min) and/or worst ever at onset then SAH is the immediate concern. What is the GCS and observations? How is the patient? Symptoms/signs other than headache? Has there been a head injury? Meningism, fever, rash or malaise? Meningitis/encephalitis. Medications causing headache: nitrates, dipyridamole, beta-blockers, sildenafil, calcium channel blockers, ACEi, alcohol, analgesia headaches with opiates, triptans, NSAIDs.
- **Discussion:** most will be benign (only 7% of suspected SAH are SAH) but all need to be taken seriously. The human and medicolegal cost of missing SAH is high. Keep a low threshold to CT/LP. Caution diagnosing 'new' migraine as nearly half of secondary headaches (SAH, tumours, raised ICP, etc.) respond to triptans. **Note:** when to worry: the old adage 'first, worst bad headache' or headache + weakness/confusion/meningism.
- **Expert review:** Forbes R. (2014) Acute headache. *Ulster Med J.* 83(1):3.

Immediate assessment

- **ABC, GCS.** Look for focal neurology. A low GCS or thunderclap headache or possible head injury or anticoagulants requires immediate CT brain. Exclude aneurysmal SAH. A classic thunderclap encompasses headaches which proceed from nil to maximal within 1 min and not just those that feel like being hit round the head with a baseball bat. Early CT <6 h very sensitive for SAH.
- **Headaches with eye signs:** cluster headache restless middle-aged patient responds to high flow O_2. All patients ask about recent LP or epidural with low-pressure headache. Horner's syndrome (small pupil, partial ptosis are the main signs) in carotid dissection or lateral medullary infarct (vertebral dissection), or lung tumour and cerebral metastases. Look for eye symptoms: red eye with injected conjunctiva consider acute angle closure glaucoma in older patient. Also consider GCA.
- **Investigations: ESR/CRP/temporal artery ultrasound or biopsy** if temporal arteritis (GCA) considered (age >50 y).

- **CT head:** will exclude bleeding and tumour. If CT negative and recent SAH suspected then LP may be needed; however, modern scanners very sensitive. LP risks other disabling headaches. If concerns of SAH (wait 12 h post max headache), meningitis or encephalitis and no contraindications. Measure opening pressure.
- **CTA/MRA arch to vertex:** carotid/vertebral dissection/aneurysm/RCVS suspected.

Red flags related to headache
- Sudden onset severe (max <4 min): exclude SAH. Needs CT/LP.
- Worse headache with cough or bending: MRI for posterior fossa lesion.
- Worse headache in morning with nausea/vomiting (exclude SOL).
- Increased severity over time: consider SOL/mass.
- Worse when standing low ICP, CSF leak, colloid cyst of IIIrd ventricle.
- Headache + confusion/delirium/altered mentation.
- Headache + neurological symptoms/signs need investigation.
- Headache + visual loss age >50 y: check ESR/CRP. GCA.
- Headache + immunosuppressed, HIV, TB, meningitis, lymphoma.
- Headache + cancer: exclude cerebral metastases.
- Headache + HTN >20 weeks of pregnancy consider pre-eclampsia. Proteinuria.

11.6 ▶ Primary headaches

- Primary headaches have no identifiable structural pathology and the outcome is good. Diagnose only after a secondary cause excluded especially in older patients with new headache or where there are red flags.
- They are by definition benign but can be severe and disabling at the time.
- Most structural causes can be identified on CT.

Causes
- **Migraine (no aura):** aura absent but severe often pulsating, often recurring unilateral headache may last 4–72 h. Shorter with effective treatment, longer than 72 h in others. Desire to be left alone, quiet, lie down and sleep. Severe attack looks ill, nauseated, grey pallor. Feels very miserable. Headache often worse than those with aura. Manage as migraine with aura.
- **Migraine (aura):** recurrent episodic headache with systemic symptoms. Comes on gradually, and there may be preceding aura such as tingling, weakness, and altered speech, word finding difficulties, flashing lights, scotomas or fortification spectra. Positive family history. Headache then comes on and lasts 4–72 h by definition but some are shorter and some longer. Patients feel awful; look grey, want to lie down and sleep. 1st-line: **Aspirin** 900 mg or **Ibuprofen** 600 mg PO if not vomiting or else **Diclofenac** 100 mg PR + **metoclopramide.** 2nd-line: triptans, e.g. **Sumatriptan** 50–100 mg PO or 6 mg SC (C/I with IHD/TIA, stroke). If severe vomiting, consider IV NS.
- **Cluster headaches** (commonest of the trigeminal autonomic cephalgias). Occur in repeated attacks. Men > women. Severe. Unilateral. Retro-orbital stabbing. Tearing, miosis, ptosis. Restless, pacing floor. Give **100% O$_2$** and **Sumatriptan** 6 mg SC for the relief of acute attacks of cluster headache. Prevent with **prednisolone** or **verapamil.**
- **Paroxysmal hemicranias:** severe, unilateral orbital, supraorbital, and/or temporal pain, always same side, lasting 2–45 min up to 5–10 times/d. With either conjunctival injection, lacrimation, nasal congestion, runny nose, ptosis, eyelid oedema. Dramatic effect of **Indometacin** 150 mg daily.

- **Short-lasting unilateral neuralgiform headache attacks with conjunctival injection and tearing (SUNCT) syndrome:** rare, males > females in middle age. Moderate headache lasts 1 min. Ipsilateral conjunctival injection, lacrimation. Nasal stuffiness/rhinorrhoea and increased intraocular pressure on the symptomatic side and swelling of the eyelids. Usually frontal and periocular. Intractable to medications.
- **Medication overuse headache:** must be excluded in all patients with chronic daily headache (headache >15 d per month for more than 3 m) and those using opioid-containing medications or overusing triptans. Resembles migraine or tension-type headache. Chronic analgesic e.g. codeine. Gradual withdrawal. Prevent with **amitriptyline** or **gabapentin.**
- **Tension headache:** chronic band-like headache but many variants. Rarely truly thunderclap. Often long history of similar episodes. No associated symptoms or signs beyond headache. Give NSAID or paracetamol.
- **Coital/post-coital headache:** diagnosis once SAH excluded. May occur with orgasm. For first/uninvestigated attacks exclude SAH with CT/LP/MRA. Multiple episodes with no harm likely benign cause. Consider NSAIDs prior to sex. Benign form is called orgasmic cephalgia.
- **Exploding head syndrome:** not a true headache but can be misunderstood with poor history. Auditory hallucination that occurs whilst falling asleep – sound like a gun going off in one's head. May be unable to speak or move. Benign condition – avoid extensive investigations or treatment.

11.7 ▶ Secondary headaches

- **About:** there is identifiable structural pathology on imaging that needs identified and managed. Primary and secondary headaches can coexist.

Causes

- **Subarachnoid haemorrhage:** 'red flags – worst ever headache, neck stiffness, meningism, vomited, onset with exercise'. Rupture of an aneurysm or AVM is usually catastrophic and presents with thunderclap headache and often collapse and coma. ▶Section 11.22.
- **Acute stroke:** ischaemic and acute haemorrhagic stroke can cause sudden headache but commoner with haemorrhage. CT scan diagnostic for bleed acutely. Worrying is patient on anticoagulation or with any focal neurology. In those with ischaemic stroke it is often on the affected side and is a vascular headache which represents shunted blood through collaterals due to a major arterial obstruction, e.g. MCA occlusion. ▶Section 11.20.
- **Cerebral venous thrombosis:** consider this within the differential of thunderclap presentation. CT head may be normal, show clot or venous infarction ± haemorrhage. Suspect if LP shows high red cells, high opening pressure and increased lymphocytes. Diagnose formally with CT venography or MR venography, whichever available. Anticoagulate. ▶Section 11.20.
- **Space-occupying lesion:** gradually increasing size or oedema or bleed into a focal lesion, e.g. tumour ▶Section 17.4 or abscess, ▶Section 11.12.
- **Acute infection:** bacterial meningitis: look for petechiae if meningococcaemia, neck stiffness, Kernig's sign, meningism. Acute delirium in elderly, pyrexia. Treat empirically if any suspicion. ▶Section 11.10.

- **Systemic illness headache:** many with fever of recent onset and headache will have a systemic illness headache usually self-limiting with good outcome, when the underlying infection resolves. Some, however, end up with a non-specific persistent headache for months.
- **Viral meningitis:** similar presentation to bacterial meningitis so investigate and treat as for bacterial meningitis until diagnosis excluded. ▶ Section 11.11.
- **Encephalitis:** fever, obtunded, seizures, focal neurology, cold sores. Needs LP and antivirals: IV **Aciclovir** if diagnosis considered. ▶ Section 11.8.
- **Pituitary apoplexy:** severe headache and IIIrd nerve palsy and visual loss as severe pressure around optic nerve from haematoma. CT/MRI may show infarction/bleeding. May have known pituitary tumour. Needs neurosurgical decompression if vision affected. Needs IV **Hydrocortisone** 100 mg IV because acute hypopituitarism is possible. Neurosurgical consult to save vision. ▶ Section 5.9.
- **Cervical (internal carotid or vertebral) arterial dissection:** neck, retro-orbital pain or occipital pain. Associated focal neurological signs. Horner's syndrome with ipsilateral carotid dissection. Brainstem signs with vertebral dissection and may also have a Horner's from PICA thrombosis and lateral medullary syndrome. ▶ Section 11.20.
- **Colloid cysts:** headache, syncope. CT IIIrd ventricle cyst, acute hydrocephalus.
- **Reversible cerebral vasoconstriction syndrome** (RCVS): ▶ Section 11.41.
- **Temporal (giant cell) arteritis:** subacute headache in older patient. Check ESR or CRP. Temporal artery tenderness or polymyalgia symptoms or transient or persistent visual loss. Needs TAB. ▶ Section 13.4.
- **Acute angle closure glaucoma:** consider in a patient with headache associated with eye pain, red eye, halos or unilateral visual symptoms. Urgent ophthalmology referral. ▶ Section 13.1.
- **Carbon monoxide poisoning:** CO from incomplete combustion of gas, oil, coal or wood. Cold weather. Consider if >1 person affected in shared tent, house, flat, boat or vehicle. Do not be fooled by falsely normal SaO_2. Check ABG and COHb levels. ▶ Section 14.10.
- **Spontaneous intracranial hypotension:** marked low pressure headache on standing. Can come on suddenly. Relieved by remaining supine. Post LP or spontaneous leak. Give fluids and simple caffeinated drinks. May need epidural blood patches (usually done by anaesthetist). Typical meningeal enhancement on MRI and cerebellar tonsillar descent and bilateral SDH. CSF opening pressure <10 cmH_2O.

11.8   Viral encephalitis

- **About:** high mortality. Most due to *herpes simplex 1* (HSV-1).
- **Aetiology:** acute inflammation of brain parenchyma ± spinal cord.
- **Travel:** recent exposure to ticks, travel where viral encephalitis endemic.
- **Clinical:** headache, fever, pyrexia, reduced GCS, hemiparesis, altered speech, psychosis/delirium, brainstem signs.

Causes of viral encephalitis

Agent	Clinical
Herpes simplex 1/2	Cold sores, high fever. Favours temporal lobes, frontal and limbic system. Can show haemorrhagic necrosis. Rarely HSV encephalitis (HSE) may later be complicated by autoimmune encephalitis. Increased risk of HSV if deficient in toll-like receptor 3. Younger. IV **Aciclovir**. Some may later develop anti-NMDAR encephalitis which may need IVIg. May mimic ischaemic stroke.
Herpes simplex 2	Relapsing meningitis/meningoencephalitis in adults.
Varicella zoster	Rash. All ages. May be shingles. Immunocompromised.
West Nile virus (WNV)	Arbovirus mosquito. Erythematous rash. Age >50. 10% fatality. Epidemic in USA. Often brainstem encephalitis with coma.
Japanese encephalitis	Arbovirus. General + movement disorder. Epidemics.
Enterovirus	Coxsackie/echovirus. Seen in summer/autumn.
Others	Measles, mumps, rubella, rabies, EBV, HIV JC virus.
Immunocompromised AIDS, transplant	Toxoplasmosis, CMV, TB, cryptococcus, primary CNS lymphoma, PML.

> **Cerebral malaria: should always be suspected with patients returning from malaria endemic areas with an encephalitis presentation.**

- **Non-infectious:** post-viral autoimmune. Most common is anti-NMDA receptor encephalitis associated with psychosis, seizures, dyskinesias, hypoventilation, and autonomic instability, attributed to antibodies against the GluN1 subunit of the NMDA receptor. Can be post HSV or associated with ovarian teratomas. Treat steroids/tumour removal, IVIg, PLEX.

Investigations

- **Bloods:** FBC: raised WCC, raised CRP. U&E: may see hyponatraemia.
- **CT/MR imaging:** urgent CT: to exclude abscess and to show asymmetric lesions in the temporal lobes with HSV. May be necrosis and haemorrhage. MRI: DWI is most sensitive. T2 changes in mesial temporal lobe/inferofrontal and insular cortex with oedema/necrosis with HSV (similar with autoimmune and HHV6). Thalamic changes with WNV.
- **CSF:** get LP and CSF as early as possible. WCC >5 white cells x 10^9/L mainly lymphocytes. Neutrophils can predominate early. WCC may be normal. Protein is normal to moderately raised and glucose is normal. Neutrophils more with WNV and CMV. Measure opening pressures. Anticoagulated patients may need it reversed to enable LP. All should have PCR for HSV (1 and 2), VZV and enteroviruses as this will identify 90% of cases due to viral pathogens. Early on PCR can be falsely negative so consider repeating LP and CSF PCR if there is a high index of suspicion. WNV virus if suspected. Bloody CSF may give falsely negative PCR.
- **Serology:** if PCR not sent then at Day 10 send CSF and serum HSV specific IgG antibody testing. A HIV test should be performed on all patients.
- **Immunocompromised:** HIV test. CD4 count. CSF PCR for HSV 1/2, VZV, enteroviruses, EBV, CMV. Culture for TB. Indian ink staining and/or cryptococcal antigen (CRAG) testing for *Cryptococcus neoformans*. Ab for toxoplasmosis and if

positive CSF PCR for *Toxoplasma gondii*. Serology for syphilis and CSF for syphilis. Also consider CSF PCR for HHV6 and 7 and JC/BK virus. CSF for *Coccidioides* sp. and *Histoplasma* sp.

- **EEG:** periodic high voltage sharp waves and slow wave complexes at 2–3 s intervals in temporal leads.
- **Autoimmune:** Ab to VGKC complex or NMDA receptor if considered.
- **Stereotactic brain biopsy:** rarely needed. HSV shows neuronal inclusion bodies called Cowdry Type A, found in the neuronal nucleus.
- **Poor prognostic indicators for HSV:** age >30. Coma, bilateral abnormal EEG. Raised CNS viral load, treatment delayed (4 d), abnormal CT/MR.
- **Differential:** autoimmune encephalitis (limbic with antibodies to VGKC, Hashimoto's with thyroid disease, antibodies to NMDA receptors), ADEM.

Management

- **ABC**, O_2. Get CT/MRI. Main concern is HSV. IV hydration. NG feeding. HDU bed if needed. VTE prophylaxis after LP. Analgesia. Skin care.
- **Suspected HSE or suspected VZV:** any suspicion even pre LP or imaging give **Aciclovir** 10 mg/kg 8 h IV × 14–21 d. Untreated HSV is a tragedy with disability and death. Treatment reduces mortality from 54% to 28%. Check CSF at day 14 to ensure PCR negative before ending treatment. Corticosteroids may be useful in HSE under specialist supervision, but we await the outcome of a current trial. Some may later worsen and need repeat CSF due to the development of anti-NMDAR encephalitis which may need IVIg.
- **Suspected VZV:** Aciclovir 10 mg/kg TDS IV × 14 d. No specific treatment is needed for VZV cerebellitis seen in younger pts. If there is a vasculitis component, there is a stronger case for using corticosteroids.
- **Suspected CMV infection:** encephalitis/retinitis. Untreated AIDS or transplant. Ganciclovir. Discuss with ID/HIV team.
- **Reference:** Ellul & Solomon (2018) Acute encephalitis – diagnosis and management. *Clinical Medicine*, 18(2):155.

11.9 Rabies (acute viral encephalomyelitis)

- **About:** causes a fatal encephalomyelitis. Found worldwide. Lyssavirus of rhabdovirus family. Disease has long IP. Worldwide 60,000 deaths/year.
- **Epidemiology:** usually Asia/Africa. UK free of rabies since 1922. However, European Bat Lyssavirus 1 found in serotine bats in southern England in 2018, European Bat Lyssavirus 2 (EBLV2), a rabies-like virus, has been found in Daubenton's bats across the UK.
- **Aetiology:** bite from dog, bat, fox, skunk or other animal introduces virus. Contact with mouth, eyes, nose, or fresh wound. Incubation period 1–3 months. Shorter if the wound is to patient's head and neck.
- **Clinical:** onset with fever, hydrophobia, laryngospasm, agitation, coma, tremor, muscle spasms. Ascending flaccid quadriparesis like GBS or polio. Associated encephalitis.
- **Investigations:** saliva, CSF <100/mm³ lymphocytes. Protein mildly elevated. MRI – brainstem T2 changes. Immunology may be negative so use PCR for virus. Negri bodies in cytoplasm of brain biopsy of dog if available.
- **Management:** try to manage exposure before disease develops with post-exposure prophylaxis (PEP) – those at risk will get rabies vaccine and human rabies immunoglobulin (HRIG). Symptomatic patients need ITU. No effective treatment.

Support. Milwaukee protocol (vaccination, HRIG, ribavirin, interferon gamma, ketamine) may be tried.
- **Reference:** UK Health Security Agency (2021) Guidelines on managing rabies post exposure.

11.10 ▶ Acute bacterial meningitis

- **About:** bacterial infection of meninges. Notifiable disease. Delay in treatment increases mortality and morbidity. Difficulty with atypical and subacute presentation. Treat on clinical suspicion alone.
- **Clinical clues:** consider if ANY of the following are present: headache, fever, altered consciousness, neck stiffness, rash, seizures, shock. Get CSF but give empirical therapy. This does not cover *Listeria* species. Suspect in older, diabetic or immunocompromised patients.
- **Aetiology:** pneumococcus/meningococcus/HiB all capsulated. They colonise nasopharynx and secrete IgA protease.
- **Pathology:** purulent exudate in the subarachnoid space. Loss of cerebral autoregulation. Localised thrombophlebitis and vasogenic oedema. Arterial/venous thrombosis and infarction. Raised protein levels.

Infectious agents causing meningitis

- ***Streptococcus pneumoniae:*** Gram-positive. From pneumococcal pneumonia, sinusitis, otitis media. Alcoholics, diabetics, post-splenectomy, complement deficiency, basal skull fractures, CSF leaks. Can cause CVST, hemiplegia, hydrocephalus, ventriculitis with 20–40% mortality. Prevent with pneumococcal vaccination. Increasing penicillin resistance.
- ***Neisseria meningitidis:*** Gram-negative diplococcus. Serotype B commonest (75%). Others A and C (reducing due to vaccination) commonest in developing world and W135. Children and adolescents. Petechial (non-blanching) rashes or purpura are vital to early diagnosis. Complement deficiencies, e.g. properdin, increase risk. Septicaemia – Waterhouse–Friderichsen syndrome with adrenal haemorrhage causing shock is seen. Also DIC. Haemorrhagic rash.
- ***Haemophilus influenzae:*** small Gram-negative. Children. Capsulated type B strains. Reduced due to HiB vaccination. Related to ENT infection in some. Develop deafness, CVST, SIADH, subdural collections.
- **Other Gram-negatives:** frail, debilitated, diabetics and cirrhotics often with head injuries and post-craniotomy.
- **Group B streptococci:** neonatal infection. Now all ages, including elderly.
- ***Listeria monocytogenes:*** age >50, pregnant, immunocompromised. Foods, soft cheese, patés, coleslaw, undercooked meats. Brainstem signs. Listeriosis, ▶ Section 9.17.
- ***Staphylococcus aureus:*** post-op neurosurgery, trauma, shunt-associated meningitis post invasive procedure with coagulase-negative *Staph.*
- **Viral meningitis:** HSV, VZV, EBV, CMV, mumps, HIV, echo-/enterovirus and Coxsackie. Usually benign. Suspected HSV meningitis give **Aciclovir** if severe. Headache and meningism consider encephalitis.
- **Cryptococcal (fungal):** immunosuppression, HIV/AIDS (▶ Section 9.34), steroids, lymphoma.
- **Tuberculosis:** insidious, cranial nerve palsies. Raised lymphocytes and protein, low glucose. Give steroids. TB, ▶ Section 9.33.

- **Cerebral malaria:** if recently in endemic area.
- *Naegleria fowleri:* rapidly fatal meningoencephalitis. Jumping into warm freshwater. Children/young adults. Enters via cribriform plate. Amoebas in CSF. Amphotericin B has been effective for a few survivors.

Clinical

- Headache, flu-like illness, drowsy, often young at college but all are at risk. Check for meningism – neck stiffness (unable chin to chest), meningeal irritation, resists passive neck flexion; Kernig's sign: patient supine with thigh flexed back to abdomen and knee flexed. Pain on straightening the knee; Brudzinski's sign: supine and flexing neck causes flexion of hips and knees. Signs muted in the young and elderly or immunocompromised.
- A stiff neck on physical examination has limited diagnostic value in the elderly, since nuchal rigidity may occur without meningitis (e.g. cervical arthritis) and meningitis may occur without nuchal rigidity.
- Recent chest infection, craniotomy, rhinorrhoea, petechiae (non-blanching), hands and feet and conjunctiva. Some present with delirium, stroke-like episodes, falls. Fever, N&V, photophobia, seizures, VI nerve palsy, papilloedema. Low GCS, decerebrate posturing, falling heart rate.
- **Complications:** seizures, stroke from arterial/venous thrombosis, low Na. Raised ICP, hydrocephalus, cerebral abscess/empyema, cerebral herniation.

Investigations

- **FBC, U&E,** raised **CRP, blood cultures, LP** and antibiotics commenced.
- **CT scan:** imaging not needed if fully conscious, no lateralising signs, no seizures and no HIV infection. In a fully conscious patient, a CT scan delays treatment and delays the LP.
- **Lumbar puncture:** aids diagnosis and treatment of bacterial meningitis and also avoiding antibiotics for aseptic meningitis. Most cases of headache and fever of recent onset will have a systemic illness headache. If LP delayed then antibiotics should be given. LP may be avoided if severe sepsis, rapidly evolving rash or severe cardiorespiratory compromise or coagulopathy. Blood cultures should be sent.
- **CSF:** opening pressure, check glucose (with concurrent blood glucose), protein, microscopy and culture, lactate, meningococcal and pneumococcal.
- **CSF PCR:** *Neisseria meningitidis, Streptococcus pneumoniae,* Herpes simplex virus (HSV), Enterovirus. HSV PCR if features of encephalitis. It may be falsely negative in the first 36–72 hours of the illness. Consider repeating LP and CSF PCR if there is a high index of suspicion.
- **Bacterial antigens:** CSF bacterial antigen tests have low sensitivity and specificity and so should be interpreted with caution.
- **NB:** *bloody tap you can allow 1 white cell for 500–1000 red cells.*

CSF analysis: discuss with ID or neurology if unsure; correlate clinically

- **Normal:** pressure 10–20 cmH$_2$O. Clear and colourless CSF. Negative Gram stain. <5 WCC/mm^3. <10 RBC/μl. Protein <0.4 g/L. Glucose 3.3–4.4 mmol/L.
- **Bacterial meningitis:** pressure 10–30 cmH$_2$O. CSF cloudy, turbid and Gram stain is 60–90% positive. 100–1000 neutrophils/mm^3 (early) and >1000 neutrophils/mm^3 (late). <10 RBC/μl. CSF protein high >1 g/L. CSF glucose low.
- **Viral meningitis:** pressure 10–25 cmH$_2$O. CSF clear. Send viral PCR. Normal protein. <10 RBC/μl. Lymphocytes 50–1000/mm^3 and can have neutrophils. Normal glucose.

- **Tuberculosis meningitis:** pressure 10–30 cmH$_2$O. CSF opaque, if left to settle it forms a fibrin web. Elevated WBC, early neutrophils then lymphocytes. Look for AFB. Glucose low. Protein elevated (1–5 g/L).
- **Fungal meningitis:** pressure 10–30 cmH$_2$O. CSF may be yellow, fibrin web, viscous. Indian ink stain or Gram stain for cryptococcus and antigen in CSF or blood. <10 RBC/µl. Raised lymphocytes 100–500/mm^3. Fungal 5–2000 lymphocytes/mm^3.

Other investigations
- **Skin biopsy** of petechial skin lesions can reveal organisms.
- **Differential:** viral meningitis, HSV encephalitis, Rocky Mountain spotted fever in USA. SAH, ADEM, cerebral abscess, cerebral malaria. HIV/AIDS.

Management (ABC, antibiotics + steroids)
- **Supportive:** ABCs, O$_2$. Antibiotics as below. Send samples. Urgent senior review ± critical care input: rapidly progressive rash, poor peripheral perfusion, capillary refill time >4 s, oliguria or SBP <90 mmHg, respiratory rate <8 or >30 /min, pulse rate <40 or >140 /min, acidosis (pH <7.3) or base excess worse than −5, WBC <4 × 10^9/L, lactate >4 mmol/L, GCS <12 or a drop of 2 points, poor response to initial fluid resuscitation.
- **Antibiotics (adjust when CSF results available and take advice):** penetration of antibiotics aided by meningeal inflammation. Send blood cultures, LP/CSF before antibiotics if possible. Treat meningococcal for 5 days, pneumococcal for 10 days and listeria for 21 days. No pathogen 10 days. Aciclovir 10–14 days. IV **Ceftriaxone** 2 g BD + IV **Steroids** for 4 days. If penicillin-resistant pneumococcus suspected add **vancomycin.** If listeria suspected: IV **Amoxicillin** 2 g 4 h or if pen allergy and not pregnant or breast-feeding **Co-trimoxazole** 120 mg/kg/day in 2–4 divided doses. Suspect listeria if age >50, pregnant, immunocompromised. Meningitis post-head injury/neurosurgery/brain abscess: **Meropenem** 2 g BD IV.
- **Steroids:** adults with suspected pneumococcal or *H. influenzae* meningitis, give IV **Dexamethasone** 10 mg 6 hourly with first dose of antibiotics (continue for 4 days). Steroids reduce complications but do not reduce overall mortality with *H. influenzae*, TB, pneumococcus. Not given if shown to be listerial meningitis. Avoid dexamethasone in septic shock, meningococcal septicaemia, or if immunocompromised, or in meningitis following surgery.
- **Antifungals:** cryptococcal meningitis needs **Liposomal amphotericin B** 3 mg/kg IV/d and **flucytosine** and then **Fluconazole** 400 mg OD. Discuss with infectious diseases experts.
- **Antivirals:** consider **Aciclovir** 10 mg/kg 8 h IV if HSV meningoencephalitis is within the differential. Low threshold for treatment whilst awaiting CSF PCR. Usually given for 14 days.
- **Notifiable disease and managing close contacts.** Inform local public health. Take local advice. **Ciprofloxacin** 500 mg PO stat is now preferred over **rifampicin.** Take microbiological advice if unsure. Staff do not need prophylaxis unless they gave mouth to mouth resuscitation.
- **Reference:** Cochrane Review (2016) Corticosteroids for acute bacterial meningitis. British Infection Society, Early Management of Suspected Meningitis and Meningococcal Sepsis in Immunocompetent Adults. 3rd ed.

11.11 ▸ Acute viral (aseptic) meningitis

- **About:** meningeal inflammation but a more benign and self-limited illness than bacterial meningitis. There may be a microencephalitis.
- **Causes:** enteroviruses 80%, mumps, HSV2, CMV, measles, influenza, HH6.
- **Clinical:** nausea, vomiting, irritability, delirium, headache, neck stiffness, photophobia, malaise. No focal neurology or seizures, etc.
- **Investigations:** FBC, WCC and CRP may show inflammatory response. HIV test advised. CT/MRI usually normal. Severe cases T1-weighted MRI may show diffuse enhancement of the meninges. LP and CSF: elevated lymphocytes. Virology: PCR to HSV, CMV, HIV. Toxoplasma serology if needed. Send blood, faeces, throat swabs for viral serology and cultures.
- **Differential:** partially treated bacterial meningitis so ask about prior antibiotic usage, other inflammatory and granulomatous or malignant conditions.
- **Management:** supportive usually recovery in 7–10 d with excellent prognosis. Manage headache and fever with analgesics and paracetamol. Ensure hydrated. Usually benign and self-limited and self-caring can be managed at home. Consider treating those with immunodeficiency. **HSV meningitis** treatment with **aciclovir** should be only for those with evidence of associated encephalitis. Take advice if unsure. **CMV meningitis:** use ganciclovir/foscarnet in immunocompromised hosts.

11.12 ▸ Cerebral abscess

- **Types:** differentiate intracerebral and subdural pus collections. An abscess has pus in the parenchyma and the other pus in subdural space (empyema).
- **Risk factors:** alcoholism, immunosuppression, e.g. post-transplant, skull fracture, associated mastoiditis or localised infection. Dental abscess, bronchiectasis, TB, AIDS, bacterial endocarditis. All commoner in men.
- **Aetiology:** local spread, e.g. *Staph. aureus* from penetrating skull trauma. From sinus ENT infections. *Pseudomonas* from ears, anaerobes and streptococci from oral cavity. Systemic blood spread from lung abscess, bronchiectasis, congenital cyanotic heart disease (Fallot's), PFO, pulmonary AV fistula, endocarditis. Immunocompromised/HIV – toxoplasma and nocardia and fungal infections.
- **Pathology:** early cerebritis (local infection and infiltration) → late cerebritis (central necrosis) → collagen capsule formation with central necrosis takes 2 weeks. Steroids slow time course. Abscess capsule can impede antibiotic penetration. Can be bacterial, fungal, or parasitic. Can be single or multiple.
- **Clinical:** focal symptoms of space-occupying lesion. Headache, focal seizure. Delirium. Raised ICP – general malaise, drowsiness, progressive coma, hemianopia with temporal lobe abscess, movement disorder. Neurological signs, poor dentition. Evidence of neglect/alcoholism. Clubbing, murmurs, dental abscess, jaundice, ear disease. Patients can appear well if pus is well walled off.
- **Differential:** malignant glioma (also has ring enhancement but does not show DWI changes on MRI). Needle aspiration (may be only way to differentiate), metastatic tumour (look for primary), toxoplasmosis (HIV, positive serology, response to treatment), nocardia (brain biopsy, treat).
- **Investigations:** bloods: elevated ESR/CRP/WCC. May be normal. Blood cultures, HIV serology. Echocardiogram: endocarditis. CXR: bronchiectasis, exclude lung tumour. CT brain with contrast/MRI brain with gadolinium shows ring-enhancing lesion with extensive surrounding oedema. Necrotic centre in early stages can

show restricted diffusion on DWI. Look for hydrocephalus and signs of raised ICP or signs of local sepsis, CT sinuses for sinusitis, mastoiditis. There may be a subdural collection. LP avoided if raised ICP and imminent herniation syndrome – take advice. A brainstem abscess should raise concerns over *Listeria* but there is no capsule and antibiotics should be given. Stereotactic biopsy and culture to confirm diagnosis and identify organism to direct antibiotic therapy may be needed.

- **Management:** take neurosurgical advice. Drainage may be by needle aspiration or excision and drainage if superficial and non-eloquent area. Multiple small abscesses managed medically. A short course of steroids (Dexamethasone 16–24 mg/d) may have a role if significant oedema until definitive drainage. Take advice.
- **Antibiotics:** empirical IV **Ceftriaxone** 2 g BD + IV **Metronidazole** 500 mg TDS for 6–8 weeks and review. A capsule can prevent antibiotic penetration with low levels in the core. Take microbiology advice. Anticonvulsants may be needed for seizures. Occasionally abscess can rupture causing a ventriculitis with very poor prognosis. Neurorehabilitation. Follow up radiologically until abscess resolved.

11.13 ▶ Septic cavernous sinus thrombosis

- **About:** intracranial sinuses have no valves so infection from central face can spread back to infect blood-filled cavernous sinuses which lie on either side of pituitary fossa with the internal carotid artery and III, IV and VI nerves. Can cause local cavernous sinus thrombosis.
- **Microbiology:** *Staph. aureus* 70%, streptococci, pneumococci, Gram-negatives. Spread from facial cellulitis/sinusitis of sphenoid/ethmoid sinuses.
- **Clinical:** fever, periorbital oedema, headache, photophobia, proptosis, ptosis, III/IV/VI nerve palsy, diplopia, papilloedema, retinal haemorrhage, visual loss. Spread can be rapid (hours) to deep veins causing thrombosis.
- **Investigations:** FBC, WCC, CRP, CT brain to exclude another diagnosis. MRI and MRV/CTV is definitive for diagnosis.
- **Differential: orbital cellulitis:** periorbital swelling, proptosis, chemosis, ophthalmoplegia, fever, decreased vision, and pain. Usually unilateral. CSF normal. **Preseptal cellulitis:** no proptosis or ophthalmoplegia. **Orbital apex syndrome:** infection in the posterior orbit causes visual loss and ophthalmoplegia out of proportion to proptosis and periorbital oedema which may be minimal. Also local malignancy and Inflammatory diseases.
- **Management:** IV antibiotics with anti-staphylococcal cover. Surgery is rare other than to drain co-terminous sinus infections. Anticoagulation may be considered to prevent extension of venous thrombosis.

11.14 ▶ Idiopathic intracranial hypertension

- **About:** risk is permanent visual loss if not treated in time.
- **Risks:** weight gain, tetracycline, steroids, amiodarone, tamoxifen, minocycline, isotretinoin, all-*trans* retinoic acid for APML, ciclosporin.
- **Clinical:** females > males. BMI >30 kg/m². Headache in morning, wakes patient, worse with coughing, straining, pulsatile tinnitus. Dizziness, back pain 50%. Papilloedema, enlarged blind spot/field loss, unilateral or bilateral VIth nerve palsy with horizontal diplopia.
- **Investigations:** FBC, U&E, CRP, ESR. CT to exclude SOL. Formal perimetry by Ophthalmology. CTV/MRV to exclude cerebral venous sinus thrombosis.

Classical MRI signs: empty sella, flattened posterior aspect of globe, transverse venous sinus stenosis and distension of perioptic SA space ± tortuous optic nerve. LP opening pressures >25 cm CSF. CSF normal composition. Removing 20 ml helps headache/vision.

- **Management:** stop causative drugs, weight loss. **Acetazolamide** (if pressure >28 cm CSF) may be started. Refer Neurology/Ophthalmology for visual field follow-up. Those with fulminant IIH and rapid deterioration of vision over weeks can have lumbar drain and optic nerve sheath fenestration or CSF shunting can be helpful.

11.15 ▸ Seizures: status epilepticus

- **NB:** treat if seizure is abnormally prolonged >5 min or repeats within less than 1 h. Increased risks of short/long-term consequences if persists more than 30 min. Close monitoring and be ready to protect airway and breathing if sedated.
- **About:** epilepsy is an ongoing tendency to have seizures. One needs at least two seizures to diagnose and start treatment, though one event with a clear recurring structural cause can suffice. Few single seizures last >5 min. Status epilepticus (SE) is a medical emergency with mortality 17–26% (by older definition). 10–23% of those who survive are left with new or disabling CNS deficits. Status applies to all seizure types, but convulsive status epilepticus is most important. Half have chronic epilepsy. Seizures usually temporal or frontal lobe in origin. Stopping anti-epilepsy drugs (AED) is commonest cause. Recommencing is the treatment. Convulsive SE causes severe metabolic and physiological damage as well as raised ICP. Damage may be permanent. Non-convulsive status dealt in next section.
- **Causes and precipitants:** failure to take usual AEDs, sleep deprivation, tiredness, alcohol, stress, fever, infection. Primary epilepsy, pre-eclampsia (pregnant >20 weeks, BP >140/90, proteinuria). Hypoglycaemia, encephalitis, meningitis, space-occupying lesion – tumour, abscess, haematoma. Stroke. Cerebral vasculitis, severe low Na, severe low Ca, head trauma. Cocaine, opiates, overdose of TCA or phenothiazines. Idiopathic, pseudoseizures, cerebral malaria.
- **Clinical:** chest muscles contract generalised cry and then fall, rhythmic contraction of limbs, unresponsive. In SE the fit-like movement and unresponsiveness remains or recurs. A witnessed account of a first fit is vital to making the diagnosis. All efforts must be made to get this information if diagnosis uncertain. Patients may recall have a preceding aura: smells, tastes, especially with a focal temporal lobe focus. Tongue biting and urinary incontinence all suggest a generalised seizure as a differential. Most seizures are followed by a post-ictal phase of several hours for complete recovery which is useful in differentiating from other causes of collapse, which recover quickly, e.g. vasovagal and Stokes–Adams attacks. Nocturnal seizures – wake up with headache, wet bed, bruises, confused. A fertile fitting female with an abdominal mass may be pregnant with eclampsia.

Seizure classification (ILAE 2017)

- **Focal onset** (lateralises and commences one side of brain) + impaired awareness or aware (knows self and environment); both may also have motor onset (twitching, jerking, stiffening, jerking) OR non-motor (sensation, emotion, thinking, experiences) OR if spreads to both sides then called 'focal to bilateral seizure'.
- **Generalised onset** (bilateral widespread from start) and either motor (tonic clonic, tonic, clonic, myoclonic, atonic) OR non-motor (absence, no physical movement) OR:

- **Unknown onset** with motor or non-motor or unclassified as not enough information.

Assessment
- **Focal may suggest a structural lesion. Generalised:** originating at some point within and rapidly engaging bilaterally distributed networks. There is loss of consciousness.
- **Motor:** tonic–clonic ('grand mal' seizures, generalised from onset, lose consciousness, muscles stiffen, then jerking movements), absence ('petit mal') with loss of awareness. May appear to be staring, atonic (characterised by an abrupt loss of muscle tone), tonic (stiffening), clonic (repeated jerking) and myoclonic (brief shock-like jerks of a muscle or muscles).
- **Semiological features:** 'tingling' or 'numbness' C/L primary sensory cortex. Bilateral/unpleasant sensations: second somatosensory area (S2) superior bank of the Sylvian fissure and/or the posterior insula. Lateralising flashing lights: C/L occipital cortex. Visual hallucinations C/L Brodmann's area 17/18. Complex visual hallucinations C/L association cortex (parieto-temporal). Auditory auras Heschl's gyrus in the superior temporal gyrus. Olfactory auras mesial temporal lobe or amygdala. Gustatory auras the insula. Autonomic auras palpitations, sweating, 'goose bumps' the insular cortex. Abdominal auras temporal lobe/insula. Elation/fear: mesial temporal structures. Motor: motor cortex. Gelastic (uncontrolled laughing) and dacrystic (crying) seizures. From a hypothalamic lesion.

Differential of seizures
- **Non-epileptic attack disorder (NEAD):** not true seizures. Also known as 'pseudoseizures'. Easily mistaken for epilepsy. Eyes usually closed, resist eye opening. Seizures come on gradually and usually last longer than epilepsy seizures. Can be incontinent/violent. Lateral tongue bite uncommon. Increased respiratory rate. They persist and may be very demonstrative. Easily end up on the ITU. They do so more than normal seizures. EEG monitoring and expert input invaluable. May be seen in those with epilepsy. Management difficult. Often not malingering. Mechanism unknown. Be supportive and empathetic.
- **Generalised convulsive movements:** (pre) syncope/fainting with jerking movements especially if held up, severe rigors in obtunded patient, cardiorespiratory compromise with anoxic seizures, NEAD.
- **Drop attacks:** cardiac syncope, cataplexy, vertebrobasilar ischaemia.
- **Transient motor attacks:** tics, TIA, spasms, movement disorders.
- **Confusion or fugue states:** TGA, hysteria, intermittent psychosis, encephalopathy.

Investigations (never miss hypoglycaemia)
- **Bloods:** FBC, U&E (low/high Na), Ca and Mg. **LFTs:** alcohol withdrawal.
- **Glucose:** hypoglycaemia must always be tested for.
- **Check anticonvulsant levels:** seizures may be due to lack of compliance.
- **High raised CRP:** infection, inflammation, vasculitis, malignancy.
- **ECG and CXR** should be done.
- **Pregnancy test:** urine/serum β-hCG in all fertile females (eclampsia).
- **Brain imaging:** low threshold to CT brain acutely in a first-time seizure or where new neurology or trauma has occurred. MRI when stable if needed. Those with a clear seizure history who wake up quickly without deficit may not need imaging. In new patients MRI is the imaging modality of choice, but acutely CT is more available, quicker and allows monitoring. MRI can be done post discharge to look

for structural lesions, developmental abnormalities, and also for medial temporal sclerosis, a cause of temporal lobe epilepsy due to paediatric febrile convulsions.

- **EEG:** may show spike and wave patterns suggesting high risk of recurrence. It may be done as outpatient. It is very useful acutely to help diagnose NEADs.
- **Lumbar puncture:** if encephalitis/meningitis or SAH or HIV suspected. Have a low threshold if there is no obvious acceptable explanation for the seizure. Check opening pressure, WCC count, protein, glucose, Gram stain, smear for acid-fast bacilli, cryptococcus, viral and bacterial cultures. PCR for herpesvirus.
- **Toxicology screen:** for cocaine or other drugs if suspected. Anticonvulsant levels should be taken for later assessment.
- **Prolactin level (PRL):** goes up with generalised and some focal seizures but not with NEAD. Take within 30 min of post-ictal period. If elevated may be useful at a later date to determine baseline PRL level as mild hyperprolactinaemia is not uncommon in the general population for various reasons.

Management – watch the clock 0–10 min

- ABC and O_2. Monitor time of onset. Temp, BP, pulse, capillary blood glucose, GCS and pupils. Place in safe recovery position. Protect airway and head. Get IV access (send bloods: U&E, glucose, Ca, Mg, anticonvulsant level, toxicology if needed). Monitor closely. O_2 sats, HR, BP, respiratory rate, GCS.
- Manage in an appropriate area with monitoring and staff. Do not insert anything in the mouth. Fits usually terminate in 2–4 min. Eyes often open, lateral tongue bite, may be incontinent. Often no need to give any medications keep safe, recovery position. Consider nasopharyngeal airway.
- If at any time seizure has terminated then manage supportively and allow to wake up after post-ictal period. Continue to monitor for further seizures. Look for precipitant. Check and manage any hypoglycaemia.

10–30 min (be ready to manage respiratory depression)

- With all these drugs be ready to manage respiratory depression.
- **Seizure persists >5 min or further seizure. Get IV access: Lorazepam** 4 mg IV given at 2 mg/min and may be repeated once after 10 min if needed or **diazepam** (Diazemuls) 5–10 mg IV or **Diazepam** 10–20 mg PR if no IV access. Prehospital or no IV access: **buccal Midazolam** 10 mg buccal is preferred if no IV access. Given by oral syringe between gum and cheek divided between both sides of mouth. Good efficacy and safety.
- **Suspicion of excess opiates** give naloxone (0.2–2.0 mg slow IV).
- **Start fluids,** e.g. 1 L NS over 4–6 h.
- **Possible hypoglycaemia:** glucose (25 g) 30–50 ml of 50% solution. If confirmed start 10% glucose infusion. Give **Glucagon** 1 mg IM/SC if delay with glucose.
- **Alcoholism or malnutrition:** Pabrinex IV paired vials TDS for 2 d if any suggestion of alcohol abuse or impaired nutrition.

Consider second-line agents

- Reasonable to give the drug they take if you suspect poor adherence as the cause. The doses of these agents have been increased in guidelines.
- **Levetiracetam** loading dose 60 mg/kg in 100 ml NS given over 10 min. Max 4500 mg.
- **Valproate** loading dose 40 mg/kg in 100 ml NS over 5–10 min. Max 3000 mg. Can be given over 10 min. Avoid in females aged 8–55 y.

- **Phenytoin** 20 mg/kg over 60 min loading dose (max 2000 mg) with cardiac monitoring and large cannula. Older patients more prone to side-effects and cardiac toxicity so levetiracetam is first choice. If already on phenytoin, then send level and consider maintenance dose only or consider another agents. Phenytoin has zero order (saturation) kinetics, resulting in a large exponential rise in serum concentration as the dose increases. Watch levels (therapeutic range 10–20 mg/L or 40–80 µmol/L).

30–90 min: seizure fails to terminate or recurs

- **ITU/CCOT:** get ITU help if airway unsafe or GCS <9 and not quickly improving. If fits continuing, then discuss transfer to ITU. Will need EEG monitoring. Some need monitoring of ICP. Revise anti-epileptic drug therapy. Avoid opiates.
- **Refractory seizures after 30–40 min:** consider transfer to ITU for intubation and GA. Intensivists can consider loading dose of **propofol** and infusion or **midazolam** or **thiopental sodium** titrated to effect (the dose regimen is beyond this text and the patient will be under ITU care); after 2–3 d infusion rate needs reduction as fat stores are saturated. Continued for 12–24 h after the last clinical or electrographic seizure, then dose tapered.
- **EEG monitoring:** necessary for refractory status. Consider the possibility of non-epileptic status. In refractory convulsive SE, the primary end-point is suppression of epileptic activity on the EEG, with a secondary end-point of burst-suppression pattern (that is, short intervals of up to 1 s between bursts of background rhythm). EEG monitoring is vital.

Other considerations

- **Ask why.** Exclude meningoencephalitis (▶ Sections 11.8 and 11.10). If suspected, give IV **Aciclovir** 10 mg/kg 8 h and **ceftriaxone** 2 g 12 h. Get an LP when possible after a CT has shown no contraindications. Exclude drug toxicity, metabolic causes, sepsis (check WCC, lactate), alcohol or other drug withdrawal. Look for head injury. **Have a low threshold to MRI when settled.** Obtain collateral history and context. Is there head injury, drugs, history of epilepsy, medications taken? If the patient is pregnant, then always consider eclampsia, meningitis due to listeria or CVST or other stroke cause.
- **Suspected vasculitis or vasogenic oedema (tumour):** should be evidence on imaging and in the right clinical context take expert advice and consider **Dexamethasone** 10 mg IV after senior consult. No role for steroids for acute ischaemic or haemorrhagic stroke or head injury.
- **Complications:** aspiration pneumonia, rhabdomyolysis, AKI, trauma, dislocated shoulder, cardiorespiratory depression from seizure/sedation.
- **Recovery: most** awaken gradually. If GCS does not improve by 20 min after cessation of movements, or the mental status remains abnormal 30–60 min after the convulsions cease, non-convulsive status must be considered (do EEG) or some other explanation should be sought.
- **Non-epileptic attack disorder (NEAD): see comments above.**
- **Isoniazid-related seizures:** take advice. Need large doses of pyridoxine.
- **Post stroke epilepsy:** large cortical infarcts or haemorrhage. Increased risk if parahippocampal gyrus that surrounds the hippocampus is affected. Usually comes on several months after the stroke. Consider valproate or levetiracetam.

Simple uncomplicated seizure

- **Discharge:** consider discharge if known epilepsy, full recovery to baseline, well, self-caring independent patient, seizure was short-lasting and terminated without sedation. Prefer patient to be under supervision or a responsible adult to check up on patient and on normal adequate anticonvulsant therapy.
- **Driving:** YOU MUST advise patient not to drive AND DOCUMENT IT. You should advise patient to inform DVLA in Swansea. The responsibility is theirs. It is yours to inform and document it. DVLA will send you or GP a form to complete. Usually licence withdrawn for 6–12 months but that is a DVLA decision.
- **Follow-up:** arrange neurological follow-up with first fit clinic and in the meantime book an outpatient EEG and MRI. Starting long-term anticonvulsants.
- **Management of epilepsy is three-fold:** (1) Prevention: avoid precipitants – tiredness, alcohol, drugs. (2) AEDs: compliance is vital. (3) Surgery in a small number to either resect the seizure focus or pathways that allow generalisation or deep brain stimulation. Refer first fit clinic.
- **For first seizure** the need for ongoing anti-epileptic drugs depends upon the presence of an ongoing precipitant and the ability to avoid precipitants. In most cases medication is not commenced after a single seizure. There is a 45% risk of a further seizure in 2 years. Where there is an active ongoing precipitant, e.g. a tumour or a structural abnormality, then it may be reasonable to start an anticonvulsant with the first seizure. Efficacy varies little between drugs and choice is more limited by side-effects and interactions and pregnancy, and now there is probably a trend to use the newer agents. All patients with first seizure should have a specialist neurology review. Pregnant patients, in fact fertile females who may become pregnant, require neurological consult before starting any agent which should be at the first fit clinic within weeks of diagnosis or discuss directly with Neurology before discharge. Generally any of the following agents are used: **Phenytoin** 150–300 mg OD PO, **Valproate** 300 mg BD PO, **Levetiracetam** 250 mg BD PO. Follow *BNF* advice.
- **General advice:** further refinement should be left to the neurologist. In the meantime advice regarding no driving, avoiding machinery or situations where unexpected loss of consciousness would cause significant harm, e.g. using hazardous machinery, cycling in traffic, climbing ladders, or swimming unaccompanied (this list is not exhaustive), then advice to curtail the activity should be given until more specialist assessment. Document driving advice in notes.
- **Sudden unexpected death in epilepsy** (SUDEP). Rare. May occur after a generalised tonic–clonic seizure (commoner if over 3 fits/y), those not on AEDs or sub-therapeutic levels, early adulthood, and epilepsy of long duration and mental retardation. May be related to central apnoea. Related to nocturnal seizures and possibly poor control.
- **St John's wort:** avoid with AEDs as can affect drug levels of many of them.
- **Juvenile myoclonic epilepsy:** 'cornflake epilepsy' myoclonic jerks in morning, tonic–clonic seizures, often after waking. First line are valproate and lamotrigine. Avoid valproate in fertile females as teratogenic. JME needs lifelong drug therapy.
- **Catamenial epilepsy:** associated with menstruation, usually worsens mid-cycle at ovulation. May be treated with clobazam midcycle with AEDs.
- **Pregnancy and epilepsy,** ▶ Section 16.18.
- **Anti-epileptic hypersensitivity syndrome:** rare but potentially fatal syndrome. Seen with some anti-epileptic drugs (carbamazepine, lamotrigine, phenytoin and others (see *BNF*)). Starts within 8 weeks of commencement with fever, rash,

and lymphadenopathy, liver dysfunction, haematological, renal and pulmonary abnormalities, vasculitis, and multi-organ failure. STOP DRUG immediately and never restart. Take expert advice.
- **References:** Arif *et al.* (2008) Treatment of status epilepticus. *Semin Neurol,* 28:342. NICE (2013) CG137: Epilepsy.

11.16 Non-convulsive status epilepticus

- **About:** coma or delirium due to ongoing seizures. May be misdiagnosed. Cause of hypoactive delirium. Treatment with benzodiazepine. EEG is the gold standard test. Consider this diagnosis in all comatose patients.
- **Aetiology:** all age groups – infants to elderly. May follow benzodiazepine withdrawal. May follow a generalised seizure in a patient who fails to recover quickly. Less metabolic derangement. Risk of sustaining focal damage.
- **Different forms: focal:** without motor features. **Absence:** inappropriate treatment of idiopathic generalised epilepsy (e.g. carbamazepine). Try low dose **lorazepam.** Focal with secondary generalisation: EEG can be helpful but diagnosis is very much clinical in nature. Confusional state with variable clinical symptoms and absence of coma. Treat with benzodiazepines or oral clobazam.
- **Clinical** (confirm with EEG where uncertain and possible): generalised tonic–clonic seizure and a long post-ictal period. Reduced GCS with mild subtle twitching or blinking and fluctuating mental status and behaviour. Reduced GCS with a history of a previous seizure. Elderly patients with hypoactive delirium or low GCS especially if on neuroleptic medications. Stroke patients who look clinically worse than expected.
- **Investigations:** FBC, U&E, LFT, Ca, ALP, CRP: as for SE. CT brain scan: may show underlying pathology, e.g. tumour, stroke, haemorrhage, abscess, encephalitis. EEG: diagnostic generalised spike and slow wave discharges.
- **Management:** minimal evidence of lasting neurologic deficits due to non-convulsive SE. There are various types as shown above with some differentials. Low dose **Lorazepam** 1–2 mg IM or equivalent. Assess for clinical or EEG improvement and respiratory depression, low BP, or other adverse effect. Consider **levetiracetam** or **phenytoin** as for status and assess clinical response. Investigations and management are much the same as status epilepticus (▶ Section 11.16).
- **Reference:** NICE (2013) CG137: *Epilepsy.*

11.17 Neuroleptic malignant syndrome

- **About:** 1 in 200 individuals taking antipsychotic drugs. Mortality 10%. Usually soon after starting antipsychotics/lithium or metoclopramide or domperidone. Withdrawal of L-dopa and dopamine agonists.
- **Aetiology:** central inhibition of dopaminergic transmission giving rise to autonomic instability and dysregulation. Neurotransmitter depletion.
- **Clinical:** patient on antipsychotics. High CK and fever often >40°C. Drowsy, young, Parkinson's disease. Extrapyramidal symptoms, exhaustion, dehydration, low Na, catatonic, tachycardia, low BP, autonomic instability, severe lead pipe rigidity, trismus, sweating, salivation, urinary incontinence.
- **Investigations:** FBC, U&E: elevated WCC, CRP. AKI: high creatinine. High CK 200–100,000 mmol/L with rhabdomyolysis. Check Ca, Mg, TFTs. Monitor for AKI, ARDS, DIC, aspiration.
- **Differential:** serotonin syndrome: post serotonergic drug, diarrhoea, reflexes ++. Malignant hyperthermia – anaesthesia, trismus.

- **Management:** ABC: O_2. Stop causative agent. Consider ITU if GCS <9. Ensure cooling and hydration. Consider **Dantrolene** 1 mg/kg IV (up to 10 mg/kg) or **bromocriptine**. Also consider levodopa, pergolide, benzodiazepines. Reintroduction of antipsychotics by senior staff later.

11.18 Stroke disease

- **About:** the stroke physician's job is challenging – prevent strokes but when they happen to first reliably diagnose stroke and then identify the most likely underlying stroke aetiology and then develop a strategy to prevent a recurrence.
- **Epidemiology:** 3rd commonest cause of death. 80% are ischaemic and the remaining are 15% haemorrhagic with 5% SAH. Similar pathologies can cause both – venous infarction famously can cause haemorrhage, dissections can lead to SAH, SAH can lead to delayed cerebral ischaemia, septic emboli from endocarditis can cause obstruction and bleeding. In the vast majority the cause is simple. In selected cases (beyond the scope of this book) one needs to think beyond the obvious.
- **Physiology:** the brain is 1–2% body weight but gets 10–15% of flow. Normal blood flow is 50 ml/100 g/min. Reversible damage is possible at flows of 8–23 ml/100 g/min. Irreversible damage is seen at flows <8 ml/100 g/min. Grey matter has a higher metabolic demand than white matter. Ischaemic stroke is a dead core within minutes and a potentially salvageable penumbra (within a few hours) via lysis and thrombectomy.
- **Atypical or young stroke,** consider asking yourself the VIVID list: is this **vasculitis, infective, venous, and inflammatory or dissection?** If you never consider an unusual aetiology you will never diagnose it. However, avoid over-investigation and false positives. The management, for example, of PFOs and certain thrombophilias and other 'risk factors' is unclear and potentially hazardous therapies must be evidence-based. Association does not always mean causation.

11.19 Transient ischaemic attacks

- **Definition:** focal transient ischaemia of the brain or retina lasting <24 h (actually in reality <20 min). TIAs are a risk factor for large disabling strokes. Risk is greatest in the days following the TIA. Patients should be seen urgently in a stroke prevention (TIA) clinic in order to confirm diagnosis, rapid screening and manage/reduce risk factors. An accurate diagnosis of TIA should only be, with few exceptions, made if all the symptoms can be ascribed to the transient occlusion of a single arterial vessel.

TIA differentials
- Have caution in diagnosing TIA where all the symptoms cannot be blamed on a single transient arterial occlusion. Stereotypical TIAs rarely recur more than 3–4 times and these are possibly migraine, seizure or functional. If unsure take expert advice. Repeated identical attacks are not cardioembolic. If the patient still has persisting neurology at point of referral then treat as stroke. This is important as persisting neurology can be haemorrhage and so anti-platelets would not be wise and these patients need urgent stroke referral and CT brain.
- **Migraine with aura:** usually the aura part is confused with TIA. May be positive flashing lights, fortification spectra, a moving scotoma with a bright margin, word-finding difficulties, stuttering expressive dysphasia-like episode (never receptive in my experience), tingling and paraesthesia. The headache usually comes on later. Common in young and females but may commence in later years.

Migraine aura and no headache is acephalgic migraine. Stereotypical repeated episodes likely migraine.

- **Hypoglycaemia:** always exclude. Diabetics on hypoglycaemic agents. Acute alcohol. Quinine. Insulinoma, Addison's, liver failure.
- **Hypocalcaemia:** hypoparathyroidism, renal failure, post parathyroidectomy. Tingling. Twitching mouth. Carpopedal spasm. Chvostek's sign.
- **Anxiety attack:** hyperventilation, tingling, generalised weakness, enquire about triggers.
- **Focal seizure with motor/non-motor:** sensory symptoms, tingling, slow progression over a minute moving over face and arm. Unwanted movements in face, hand or leg have been reported with TIA. Needs EEG and MRI to exclude irritative focus. Ask about other seizure-like activity (Seizures/epilepsy, ▶ Section 11.16). Difficulty with speech associated with focal seizure 'speech arrest'.
- **Pre/syncope:** often easy as there is a global deficit. TIA does not cause presyncope or syncope. A vasovagal/faint may cause tingling and twitching with TLOC.
- **Transient global amnesia:** historical diagnosis. Needs history from witness. Aetiology unclear. Benign. During episode patient, often middle-aged, keeps repeating questions about current status. No focal deficit. Language, vision, motor normal. Recognises family. "Why am I here?" repeatedly. Upset. Often sleeps and recovers with no memory at all of episode. **Criteria:** episode witnessed and reported. Anterograde amnesia during attack. No clouding of consciousness. No focal neurological deficits during or after the attack. No features of epilepsy. Duration <24 h. No recent head injury or active epilepsy. MRI can show dot of restricted diffusion in hippocampus. Reassurance. Not TIA. No further investigations.
- **Optic neuritis:** a visual loss/change in colour perception from optic neuritis. Sensory or motor symptoms. Usually coming on over hours rather than seconds. Young female.
- **Pressure neuropathy:** a radial, common peroneal nerve, median nerve, ulnar nerve. Usually in setting where nerve compressed.
- **Within the bounds of normal experience:** we all can experience tingling, paraesthesia, drop a cup, say the wrong word and many other symptoms which we would not regard as significant. Need to define significance and avoid overdiagnosis.
- **Others:** anything can be referred to a TIA clinic from dizziness caused by a PE, to SDH, to known brain metastases and anxiety states. A large SDH with midline shift can give recurrent transient focal neurology.

Clinical assessment

- **Clinical:** unilateral weakness of face/arm/leg. Variable hemisensory loss – face/arm/leg. Transient dysphasia, transient ataxia, transient hemianopia, or transient monocular blindness. Ask about headache – can suggest haemorrhage/stroke/migraine/temporal arteritis. Look for AF, residual neurology, and temporal artery tenderness. Residual weakness, mild or subtle dysphasia, ataxia. Look for pronator drift. Difficulty heel/toe walking. Look for hemisensory loss. Listening for bruits is useful but the decision for carotid imaging depends on symptoms of ipsilateral carotid territory ischaemia.
- **Clinical TIA less likely: positive** phenomena, e.g. flashing lights, fortification spectra. Isolated vertigo without other brainstem symptoms. Bilateral symptoms. Syncope or presyncope or altered consciousness. Memory loss. Repeated stereotypical episodes for weeks/months would seem to be unusual

for TIA – focal seizure. Unlikely to be cardioembolic if same neurological deficit each time. A complex progressive story.

ABCD² scoring

- ABCD² is not encouraged now. But included for historical purposes and to highlight risk factors. All patients should be seen as quickly as possible.
- **Age:** >60 (+ 1).
- **BP:** SBP >140 and/or DBP >90 mmHg (+ 1).
- **Clinical:** unilateral weakness (+2), dysphasia/dysarthria, no weakness (+1).
- **Duration:** 10–59 min (+1), >60 min (+2).
- **Diabetes** (+1).

Assessment: repeated episodes in 1 week gives an automatic score of 4 (high risk). For those with repeated episode, a carotid bruit or AF are a high-risk priority. Score of 6–7 gives 2-d stroke risk of 8% and 7-d risk of 12%. Score of <4 gives 2-d risk of 1% and 7-d risk of 1% [*Lancet* 2007;369:283]. However, new RCP guidance (2016) recommends that all TIA should be seen <24 h and that scoring system such as ABCD² not needed. Telephone triage may help to select those with a convincing history as true TIAs are seen in less than half of all referrals. Patients with suspected TIA that happened over a week ago can be seen within 7 d.

Investigations

- **FBC, U&E, ESR/CRP** (GCA) headache or amaurosis fugax, age >50. Fasting blood glucose and lipids.
- **CXR:** especially in smokers (lung cancer + brain metastases).
- **ECG, echocardiogram** (age <50, abnormal ECG, murmur, recent MI).
- **Carotid Doppler** scan in those with TIA and symptomatic carotid stenosis over 50% and a potential candidate for endarterectomy.
- **CT brain:** can help exclude TIA mimics or infarction/haemorrhage.
- **MRI with diffusion weighted imaging:** modality of choice (the more prolonged the episode the more likely to see changes).
- **Comments:** TIA can be a soft diagnosis – by definition there are no residual signs or symptoms, and imaging may be entirely normal. With stroke and imaging the diagnosis is far more solid. The stroke physician must weigh up the history in the context of *a priori* risk and the likely probability of a TIA that could suggest imminent stroke. Avoid labelling unexplained 'odd spells' as TIA. Remember if you cannot ascribe all the symptoms to the transient blockage of a cerebral blood vessel then the diagnosis of TIA is unsafe and needs to be reviewed. Repeated stereotypical transient neurological episodes are migraine or focal seizures or consider another diagnosis. If very frequent a trial of an AED may be useful. Consider neurological opinion. Transient neurological symptoms immediately post syncope or seizure are unlikely to be TIA but due to the syncope or seizure. Take advice if unsure.
- **Management: Clopidogrel** 300 mg then 75 mg OD plus **Aspirin** 300 mg then 75 mg OD for 21 days then monotherapy with clopidogrel 75 mg OD. **Ticagrelor** may be used instead of Clopidogrel. Consider PPI. **Atorvastatin** 20–80 mg ON.
- **Admission:** we rarely admit high risk TIA referrals unless very concerned (most are not TIAs, take advice if unsure) but see in TIA clinic same day with carotid Doppler/CT or MRI, or next morning after commencing antiplatelet and statin. Some presenting after hours I do keep overnight if I am concerned and if that's the

quickest and safest way to get earliest imaging and duplex for the patient next morning. Take expert advice if unsure.

- **Driving:** not to drive for 28 d (UK DVLA). No need to involve DVLA if complete resolution but should inform motor insurance. Exception is if the patient drives a lorry, bus, coach or taxi, when DVLA need to be informed and approval needed to drive. If unsure refer.
- **Carotid surgery:** refer to vascular if symptomatic stenosis >50% and good operative candidate. Stenting may be considered in some.
- **Atrial fibrillation:** consider starting a DOAC immediately in the clinic following conversation on risks and benefits.
- **Risks:** smoking cessation and hypertension management. Diet advice. Exercise.
- **Other tests:** depending on age and strength of diagnosis other tests such as echo/trans-oesophageal echo and thrombophilia screens may be undertaken.
- **Repeated TIAs:** many are not TIA but migraine, focal seizures, anxiety, syncope and some remain unexplained. Repeated stereotypical episodes improve with anticonvulsants. May be useful to get MRI to exclude focal lesion and/or EEG. It would be unusual for AF or cardioembolism to cause identical TIAs.

11.20 ▶ Acute ischaemic stroke (AIS)

- **About:** sudden onset of focal negative neurological symptoms and signs due to focal brain ischaemia and infarction. 80% of strokes are ischaemic. Try to predict vessel occluded as almost all ischaemic strokes have vessel-specific clinical syndromes. Occur at all ages. See RCP 2023 Guidelines at www.strokeguideline.org.
- **Definitions:** WHO definition: neurological deficit of cerebrovascular cause that persists beyond 24 h or is interrupted by death within 24 h. Includes brain, retinal and spinal ischaemia. Imaging definition: early CT changes but often delayed 2–3 h but thrombus can be seen. MRI DWI changes seen within minutes.
- **Time of stroke onset is key:** strokes may be symptomless until an activity is attempted, e.g. movement, speech, etc., therefore onset is really from when patient last known to be well and fully functional with no deficit.

Differentials

- **Focal/generalised seizure:** motor or sensory. Todd's paresis. Usually as part of a generalised seizure which may not be witnessed or nocturnal. Weakness resolves. Patient obtunded. May be an epilepsy history. Nocturnal seizure: suspect if patient wakes up with sore head, incontinent, tongue bitten, feels unwell. Post-stroke seizures tend to be seen months after the stroke with a focus in the territory of the previous stroke.
- **Migraine with unilateral motor symptoms (MUMS):** younger patient with known history of stroke-like symptoms as part of migraine with aura. If this is first ever presentation then treat as stroke. Positive symptoms: flashing lights, scotomas, complete visual loss, speech disturbance/dysphasia, headache. Care needed as some strokes seem to be accompanied by migraine-like episodes. Consider thrombolysis if first presentation and stroke is real possibility. If possible, rapid DWI can help. If recurrent stereotypical then migraine more likely.
- **Old stroke systemic illness** ('Ozzies'): CT shows old stroke, history of a stroke with a sudden worsening of same symptomatology on same side. Usually precipitated by fatigue, infection or metabolic cause. Once treated neurology resolves. May need MRI to be certain.

- **Functional:** younger patient, challenging life, often smokers and risk factors but atypical signs. Arms drift down, no pronation. Give way weakness. Excessive effort. Power stronger when limbs tested separately. Incongruent abilities with therapists. Bizarre gaits. Normal imaging. Need positive stroke team support with full expectation of recovery.
- **Bell's palsy/Ramsay Hunt syndrome:** facial weakness. ▶Section 11.32.

Causes once stroke diagnosed

- **Large artery disease:** atherosclerosis within aortic arch and its branches, ICA especially at its bifurcation within carotid siphon and within large intracranial vessels. Same is seen in the vertebral artery and basilar artery. Disease is caused by progressive increase in plaque size and obstruction. Plaque rupture and thrombosis or even distal embolisation of thrombus and debris (artery to artery stroke). If stenosis comes on gradually over time there is a chance of development of collaterals making subsequent occlusion less severe, even symptomless. Atherosclerosis common within the aortic arch or its branches and can lead to obstruction or embolisation of thrombus. Arterial dissection of carotid or vertebral can cause local acute occlusion or thromboembolism into its area of perfusion.
- **Cardio-embolism (30%):** look for AF particularly when associated with valvular heart disease. Also endocarditis, MI and apical thrombus, atrial myxoma and paradoxical emboli across a patent foramen ovale (PFO)/atrial septal aneurysm. There is an increased incidence of PFO in young cryptogenic strokes, but association does not prove causality and evidence for closure is poor. Cardiac echo (TTE and TOE) is indicated. 24-h tape may pick up paroxysmal AF. 7-d tape even better.
- **Small artery disease (40%):** there is localised stenosis and thrombosis usually of deep perforating arteries of the cerebral hemisphere and brainstem. The driver behind this is diabetes and hypertension. These are end arteries with little collateralisation. The result is lacunar infarction. These are small deep lesions usually <1.5 cm in diameter. Over time the cumulative effect of multiple lacunar infarcts is a subcortical vascular encephalopathy.
- **Venous thrombosis:** atypical, crosses arterial boundaries and may be bilateral parietal. Seizures, headache, stroke. Suspect infarct or haemorrhage in a prothrombotic state or local infection. Request an MR venography or CT venography.
- **Low flow:** low BP causes watershed infarction between ACA/MCA and MCA/PCA and deep/superficial vessels.
- **Alternative: rarely** consider are they microbleeds? May not show up on CT. Needs specific MRI sequences.

Risk factors for acute ischaemic stroke

- Atherosclerosis – age, hypertension, DM, hyperlipidaemia, smoking.
- Arterial dissection – hypertension, trauma.
- Connective tissue disease, fibromuscular dysplasia.
- Vasculitis – temporal arteritis.
- Polyarteritis nodosa, Behçet's, arterial spasm – migraine, SAH.
- Embolic: AF, valve disease, myxoma, PFO, LV dysfunction, mural thrombus.
- Thrombophilia – prothrombin, factor V Leiden, protein C and S deficiency, malignancy. Oestrogens, antiphospholipid syndrome, hyperviscosity.

Clinical syndromes (ischaemic stroke)

Artery	Clinical – think 'which is the culprit vessel?'
Anterior cerebral artery	C/L hemiplegia leg >> face and arm. Gait disturbance. Urinary incontinence. Primitive reflexes. Abulia.
Middle cerebral artery	C/L hemiplegia face, arm >> leg. C/L hemisensory loss. C/L homonymous hemianopia. Aphasia if dominant side affected. Anosognosia/ neglect if non-dominant.
Posterior cerebral artery	C/L homonymous hemianopia with macular sparing. Memory loss, somnolescence, cognitive changes.
Vertebral and PICA	Lateral medullary syndrome, pontine and midbrain infarcts, Horner's syndrome, ipsilateral cerebellar signs, spinothalamic loss, dysphagia, hiccups, vertigo. PICA=posterior inferior cerebellar artery
Lacunar strokes **Small penetrating vessels**	**Medial and lateral lenticulostriate:** (from MCA/ACA) cause C/L lacunar syndromes involving internal capsule. Pure motor, pure sensory, dysarthria + clumsy hand, ataxic hemiplegia. **Pontine perforators:** pontine lacunar-type motor/ataxic syndromes. Cranial nerve syndromes. Also focal thalamic and cerebellar infarcts.
Top of basilar artery occlusion	Diplopia, hemianopia, vertigo, progressive coma, ophthalmoplegia.

Initial investigations
- **Bloods:** FBC, CRP, ESR, U&E, LFT, glucose, lipids.
- **ECG:** primarily to find AF or MI/LVH/cardiomyopathy.
- **CXR:** cardiomegaly, lung tumours with brain metastases mimicking stroke.
- **Non-contrast CT head** may initially be normal and may take 6–12 h for hypodensity to show. Earlier signs include subtle signs such as loss of grey/ white matter, cortical differentiation, thrombus in MCA or basilar arteries, sulcal effacement, loss of insular ribbon. Cortical and subcortical atrophy and small vessel disease may be seen.
- **CTA:** from aortic arch to the vertex will show the culprit vessel and any *in situ* thrombus. Consider in those for possible thrombectomy.
- **CT perfusion:** this helps in difficult cases to identify a mismatch suggesting a small cortex and large penumbra which is needed for thrombectomy. Infarct core has marked reduced cerebral blood flow (CBF) and cerebral blood volume (CBV). Penumbra has reduced CBF but normal CBV. This can be displayed and can aid decision-making. Useful in those presenting after 6 h to see how much brain is still viable in the penumbra.
- **MRI:** some may use DWI-FLAIR mismatch especially in wake up strokes. Do within 1 h of arrival.
- **7-d tape:** done in most patients where PAF suspected, e.g. cardioembolic strokes on different sides/anterior and posterior circulations strokes.

Additional tests in selected patients
- **Carotid Doppler:** mild non-disabling anterior circulation stroke/TIA and fit and willing enough for a carotid endarterectomy if a symptomatic stenosis is found.
- **Echocardiogram:** age <50, significant murmur, ECG changes, cardiac symptoms.

- **CT angiogram:** can show up circle of Willis demonstrating acute occlusion of a major branch, e.g. MCA. It can also show neck vessel stenosis of occlusion (carotid and vertebral). However, only done as initial work-up in selected centres. It needs to be considered if there is a plan to refer for vascular intervention. May be done as option to look for AVM or dissection but most centres use MR angiography.
- **CT + contrast:** when a tumour is suspected. Looking for enhancement.
- **MRI:** DWI for infarction, gradient echo/T2* for haemorrhage. Selected patients where diagnosis uncertain, location of stroke needed.
- **MR/CT venography:** if cerebral venous/sinus thrombosis suspected.
- **MR angiography:** if carotid stenosis or intracranial stenosis or aneurysm or dissection or vascular anomaly considered.
- **Troponin:** ACS suspected. **BNP** if heart failure suspected.
- **Vasculitis screen: raised** CRP. Younger, seizure, headache, multiple infarcts/bleed. Angiography changes.
- **Sickle test:** if sickle cell anaemia suspected. See ▶Section 8.2.
- **Thrombophilia** screen in those <45 with history of venous/arterial thrombosis or family history of VTE or venous thrombosis in unusual site, e.g. cerebral/portal/hepatic vein. Other than anti-cardiolipin there is a very poor correlation with arterial strokes and these thrombophilias. Most useful for venous infarcts.

Hyperacute management
- **Stroke unit:** regular neurological observations – temperature, pulse, BP, GCS, pupillary responses. Stroke unit admission reduces mortality.
- **Reperfusion therapies for ischaemic stroke:** intravenous thrombolysis (IVT) and mechanical thrombectomy: see guidance below if indicated.
- **General care:** IV hydration and swallowing assessment before eating, skin care, nutrition. Consider NG tube if unsafe swallow after 12 h.
- **VTE prevention:** for immobile patients, intermittent pneumatic calf compression for 30 d is preferred, as well as early mobilisation. UFH/LMWH should be avoided.
- **Medical:** if not for thrombolysis and non-haemorrhagic, start **Aspirin** 300 mg stat PO/PR for 2 weeks.
- **Hypertension** not treated acutely unless SBP persistently over 200 mmHg for ischaemic stroke and 180 mmHg for haemorrhage. Reductions in BP should be very gradual or can severely reduce cerebral perfusion.

Ongoing management
- **Antiplatelet: Aspirin** 300 mg PO/PR × 2 weeks. Add a PPI if history of dyspepsia. Then convert **Aspirin** 300 mg to **Clopidogrel** 75 mg OD (1st-line therapy). Use combined **Aspirin** 75 mg + **Dipyridamole** 200 mg BD if unable to take clopidogrel.
- **Hypertension:** it is usual to delay treatment up to 1 week unless severe, i.e. BP >185/110 mmHg and if so then consider thiazide + ACEi/AT2 blocker or calcium channel blocker via NG or PO may be given. Lower BP slowly over hours and days.
- **Cholesterol: Atorvastatin** 20–80 mg start after 48 h if new, or continue if already on statin. Aim for total cholesterol <4.0 mmol/L or LDL <2 mmol/L.
- **Anticoagulant:** DOAC or warfarin for those with AF or PAF with no C/I, after patient consent commence low dose warfarin 3–4 mg/d around day 10. Aim for INR of 2–3 by day 14. Use CHA_2DS_2VaSc and **HAS-BLED** or **ORBIT** score (▶Section 3.15) to assess relative risks of anticoagulation. Those with a stroke or TIA with AF must be anticoagulated at 10–14 d unless contraindication.
- **Diabetes:** maintain blood glucose 5–15 mmol/L and avoid hypoglycaemia.

- **Oxygen:** give as per BTS guidelines.
- **Fluids/nutrition:** bedside swallow assessment ('SIP test') and if normal then allow normal intake but keep under review. Get speech and language therapy review if unsure. If nil orally start IV fluids, preferably IV NS at 100 ml/h initially. If swallow remains poor then start NG feeding if indicated after assessment at 24–48 h. Do not place NG immediately unless vital oral meds required, e.g. L-dopa medications, etc. Take expert advice on PEG tube usage.
- **Carotid stenosis:** Doppler or CTA to screen for symptomatic carotid stenosis in those who would be candidates for urgent carotid endarterectomy, i.e. **TIA and mild non-disabling strokes.**
- **Top of the basilar occlusion:** acute comatose, eye signs, extensor plantars. Bright basilar dot on CT. If suspected, then consider CTA to confirm thrombus. If no good other explanation and no other C/Is, then consider IVT <4.5 h and/or MT within 24 h of onset. Prognosis usually grim so may be worth attempting. Outcome may leave patient locked in and quadriparetic. Get consent. Specialist decision. What would patient wish?
- **Artery of Percheron occlusion:** subtle coma/somnolescence and eye signs (full or partial IIIrd nerve) and normal CT. MRI may show bilateral thalamic infarction ± midbrain. Might consider alteplase off-licence but rapid diagnosis difficult within time window, difficult with coma differentials. May need urgent DWI to confirm. Specialist decision.
- **Cerebral venous/sinus thrombosis:** infarction, oedema and haemorrhage seen. Does not respect arterial boundaries. May be bilateral about the midline. Bleeding due to RBC diapedesis and not vessel rupture. Anticoagulation can be given. Look for prothrombotic state, puerperium or local sepsis. Cerebral deep vein thrombosis worse prognosis. CT dense vein and cord sign. Delta sign if thrombus occupies the superior sagittal sinus. Needs CT venography or MR angiography/venography. Anticoagulate for at least 3 months. Use full-dose heparin and then warfarin with a target INR of 2–3 for at least 3 months if possible.

Acute stroke complications

- **Malignant MCA syndrome and hemicraniectomy:** analysis has shown that mortality is reduced from 70 to 30%; survival with good functional outcome is doubled from 20 to 40%. One-third survive with substantial disability. There is no age cut-off. **Consider** if: pre-stroke ranking <2, imaging evidence of >50% MCA infarction (involving deep and superficial MCA territory), >145 cm³ volume of infarction, within 48 h of stroke onset. Patients will usually have an NIHSS >15, particularly if dominant hemisphere infarct. Patients with dominant as well as non-dominant hemisphere infarcts are suitable for decompression. **The following may not be suitable:** older patients, significant comorbidity that would hinder survival or rehabilitation, bilateral fixed dilated pupils, time >48 h after stroke onset, PCA/ACA involved. Referral tends to go via tertiary centre stroke physicians who arrange neurosurgical consult.
- **Haemorrhagic transformation:** withhold antiplatelets, LMWH, DOAC, or other anticoagulation. Usually conservative management.
- **Pulmonary embolism/DVT:** CTPA confirm radiologically. Consider anticoagulation for at least 3 months.

Reperfusion strategies for acute ischaemic stroke

- **If NIHSS = ≥6 and time <5h: recommend thrombectomy** if proven LAO and able to do arterial puncture <5 h after known onset and there are no contraindications such as pre-stroke modified Rankin Score (mRS) of ≥2, issues with accessibility of clot on CT-A, extensive early infarction changes on CT (>1/3 MCA area or ASPECTS <6), poor collateral supply.
- **If NIHSS = ≥6 and time >5h:** consider late thrombectomy after 5 h if (1) LAO is in the posterior circulation and <24 h of onset, or (2) LAO and evidence of salvageable brain tissue and onset <12 h and none of the listed contraindications.
- **If NIHSS = 4/5 and time <4.5h:** recommend IV thrombolysis if no contraindications.

Thrombolysis eligibility up to 9 h/wake up stroke

- Wake up stroke >4.5 h. Treat if DWI lesion + no FLAIR lesion.
- Wake up or onset unknown: perfusion study mismatch ratio >1.2, a mismatch volume >10 ml, and an ischaemic core volume <70 ml.
- 4.5 to 9 h. CT or MRI core-perfusion mismatch suggested: mismatch ratio >1.2, a mismatch volume >10 ml, and an ischaemic core volume <70 ml.

Clinical exclusion criteria to IV thrombolysis

- GCS <9, rapidly resolving symptoms.
- NIH score <4 or >25 (caution >22).
- SBP >185 mmHg, DBP >110 mmHg despite treatment.
- Fixed head or eye deviation.
- Seizure at stroke onset and residual deficit is post-ictal weakness.
- Pathology other than stroke is more likely.
- Thunderclap headache suggestive of SAH (should show blood on CT).

CT exclusion criteria for IV thrombolysis (IVT)

- CT hypodensity or sulcal effacement in >1/3 of MCA territory.
- CT shows bleeding, tumour, abscess, AVM or aneurysm.
- CT shows a developed stroke.

Lab results exclusion criteria (do not wait for these unless specific concerns)

- Blood glucose <3 mmol/L or >22 mmol/L.
- Platelet count <100 × 10^9/L.
- Hb <10 g/dl or haematocrit <25%.
- Abnormal INR >1.7 or APTT >36 sec.

Historical exclusion criteria to IV thrombolysis (IVT)

- **Anticoagulants: IV heparin or treatment dose SC** within 48 h. Recent dose of DOAC. On warfarin INR >1.7. Take advice.
- **Trauma:** recent puncture of non-compressible blood vessel, LP <7 d or traumatic CPR <10 d, surgery or visceral biopsy <4 weeks, major surgery <3 months, recent head injury, significant trauma (fracture or internal injuries) <3 months.
- **Bleeding:** history of recent bleeding (PR/PO/PU/gynae/epistaxis), any neoplasm with increased bleeding risk including intracranial neoplasm, endocarditis, pericarditis, arterial aneurysm, arteriovenous malformations: aortic aneurysm or ventricular aneurysm. Any known bleeding problem or blood disorder. Haemorrhagic retinopathy (untreated proliferative diabetic retinopathy).
- **Pregnancy:** pregnant (discuss) or childbirth <4 weeks ago, desire to breastfeed after treatment. Pregnancy is not a contraindication.

- **Stroke:** ischaemic stroke in past 3 months, haemorrhagic stroke any time in the past, arteriovenous malformation or aneurysm.
- **Gastrointestinal:** ulcerative GI disease <3 months, varices, active peptic ulcer disease, severe liver disease, coagulopathy or suspected varices.

Management pre and post IV thrombolysis (IVT)
- **Monitor BP every 15 min to ensure <185/110 mmHg.** If BP >185/110 mmHg and within pre-treatment thrombolysis window, then give **Labetalol** 10–20 mg IV unless C/I. It may be repeated. 2nd-line is **GTN** infusion 20 mg in 50 ml to run at 2–10 ml/h. If despite this BP >185/110 mmHg then do not give alteplase, especially if BP resistant and not confident that you can maintain BP <185/110 mmHg for the next 12–24 h.
- **Alteplase: 0.9 mg/kg body weight** (max 90 mg) infused IV over 60 min. Give 10% of the total dose administered as an initial IV bolus.
- **Monitor closely before, during and after thrombolysis** for at least 24 h. Watch for potential side-effects and complications. Should be prescribed by, and administration supervised by, a doctor once the approval has been obtained from the stroke/neurology consultant. In the first 24 h immediately after stroke thrombolysis try to avoid urinary catheter unless in retention. Avoid IM injection. Discuss with stroke team. Do not give any aspirin, NSAID, antiplatelet or anticoagulant. It is reasonable to give paracetamol IV/oral/PR; safe for analgesia or pyrexia.
- **Admission to a hyperacute stroke unit:** is key for good outcome and reduces disability and mortality.

Potential complications of IV thrombolysis
- **Anaphylaxis/angioedema (<1%):** as for anaphylaxis. Oral and tongue oedema may be seen and this can require expert airway management so involve anaesthetists early. Seen more so in those on ACEi and so should be monitored for during alteplase. Stop alteplase. Summon help. **Chlorpheniramine** 10 mg IV, **Hydrocortisone** 200 mg IV. Bleeding into tongue is differential (CT will show it). If swelling is due to haematoma secure airway and reverse anticoagulation. True anaphylaxis consider adrenaline 0.5 mg IM.
- **Neurological deterioration** (13%). May be due to bleeding, infarct extension, seizure, sepsis, malignant MCA.
- **Intracranial bleed:** suspect if fall in GCS, headache, new seizure, raised NIHSS, acute hypertension, N&V, pupillary changes stop alteplase and CT scan. **Bleeding on/after thrombolysis:** ▶ Section 8.12.
- **Extracranial haemorrhage:** signs of bleeding or shock. Stop alteplase. Control bleeding. **Bleeding on/after thrombolysis:** ▶ Section 8.12.
- **Reperfusion cerebral oedema:** ▶ Section 11.23.

Complications of thrombectomy
- Arterial dissection; distal embolisation of the plaque/thrombus, detachment of any stent, formation of a caroticocavernous fistula and reocclusion.
- Problems at puncture (usually at the femoral artery) such as haemorrhage, local infection and formation of pseudo-aneurysms.
- Eye: sclera oedema on treated side due to increased flow down the ophthalmic artery. Usually self-limiting but monitor for redness or painful swelling which may reflect more serious damage to the corneal surface.

11.21 Haemorrhagic stroke

- **About:** many different causes and patterns. Up to 15–20% of strokes are haemorrhagic. Intracerebral haemorrhage (ICH) is an important cause of stroke with a 30-d mortality rate of 20–30%. Leading causes include chronic hypertensive vasculopathy, cerebral amyloid angiopathy and anticoagulant-related haemorrhage.
- **Types:** lobar cortical haemorrhages, deep subcortical bleeds. Putaminal, thalamic, brainstem bleeds. SAH.
- **Haemorrhagic stroke mimics:** head trauma – look for soft tissue injury. Did patient fall and hit head and bled or did the bleed come first? Tumours, e.g. melanoma. Infarct with haemorrhagic transformation. Endocarditis with haemorrhage from septic emboli. Cerebral venous sinus thrombosis and secondary haemorrhage.
- **Pathology:** haematoma formation usually splits white fibre bundles. Secondary oedema exacerbates increased ICP and coma/coning. Progressive bleeding not uncommon, especially if anticoagulated. Older atrophied brain may allow more room for expansion. Some bleeds may be low pressure, e.g. cavernomas from venous side. Bleeding into ventricular system. Obstructive hydrocephalus.
- **Prognosis:** 15% of strokes ICH. 5% due to SAH. 30–50% death within 30 d.

Causes of haemorrhagic stroke
- **Hypertension:** lobar/deep bleeds basal ganglia, thalamus, cerebellum, pons.
- **Arteriovenous malformations:** seizures, younger patients. SAH.
- **Cavernoma (cavernous angioma):** seizures, bleeds younger patients. ICH.
- **Cerebral amyloid angiopathy:** causes lobar more than deep haemorrhages in those >70 usually without hypertension. Convexity SAH and ICH.
- **Warfarin, haemophilia, thrombolysis, DIC, warfarin, coagulopathy.**
- **Embolic stroke:** higher rate of haemorrhagic transformation seen with embolic strokes and any large stroke especially if hypertensive.
- **Cerebral venous sinus thrombosis:** haemorrhage and infarction seen. Prothrombotic.
- **Endocarditis:** bleed from mycotic aneurysms from septic emboli.
- **Sickle cell disease:** ischaemic and haemorrhagic stroke. See ▸ Section 8.2.
- **Malignancy:** primary or metastatic cancer.
- **Vasculitis:** PAN, SLE, granulomatosis with polyangiitis, Takayasu's, GCA.
- **Systemic:** sarcoid, Behçet's disease.
- **Trauma:** history. Signs of head injury. Not stroke.

Investigations
- **Bloods:** FBC: low platelets, raised INR if warfarin/liver disease, CRP, ESR, glucose. U&E: (low Na with SAH). LFTs.
- **Non-contrast CT:** sensitive for blood and shows haematoma in brain substance ± oedema, ± extension into ventricles, ± hydrocephalus and signs of raised ICP. Intraventricular blood is a poor prognostic indicator.
- **Contrast CT:** contrast may be given if tumour suspected or SAH to locate an aneurysm. A 'spot sign' in PICH suggests an area of active dynamic bleeding and marks a poorer prognosis. Contrast is rarely given acutely.
- **MRI:** T2* and gradient echo (GRE) black blood sequences detect bleeding. Helpful acutely and later when the haematoma has resolved. Old bleeds slit-like appearance

with signs of haemosiderin. Interval scan at 6 weeks can help exclude an underlying vascular lesion, e.g. tumour, AVM, cavernoma, aneurysms.
- **MR venography:** if any suspicion of venous thrombosis with haemorrhage.
- **MRA/CTA:** allows imaging of aneurysms and dissections and vascular malformations. Also see vessel outline and signs of vasculitis or spasm.
- **Digital subtraction cerebral angiography:** for selected cases in tertiary centres with aSAH or AVM. 1% stroke risk associated with the procedure. Involves selective catheterisation of carotids and subclavian arteries.
- **Echocardiography:** TTE/TOE and CRP and multiple cultures if endocarditis suspected. Septic emboli bleed and mimic ICH.
- **Lumbar puncture** for red cells and xanthochromia if SAH suspected.

Management: see RCP Guidelines 2023 at www.strokeguideline.org
- **Supportive:** ABC, IV fluids, ITU review if GCS <9 and high EWS.
- **Admit to stroke unit.** Monitor temperature, pulse, BP, GCS, pupillary responses. Swallow assessment, NG tube if needed. Multidisciplinary care and rehabilitation.

Managing bleeding due to drugs and other causes
- **Warfarin/VKA** give vitamin K 5–10 mg IV stat if INR elevated along with 4-factor prothrombin complex concentrates (PCC), e.g. **Octaplex/Beriplex or FFP.** Stop Warfarin and reverse in the short term even with metal prosthetic cardiac valves.
- **Low platelets:** Give platelets if <80–100 × 10^9/L. Most risk <50 × 10^9/L.
- **Antiplatelets:** if on antiplatelet therapy, platelet transfusion should be avoided and can worsen outcome unless thrombocytopenic. Take advice.
- **DOAC and bleeding** ▶ See Section 8.11.
- **Protamine** should be considered if heparin has been administered within 4 h of the onset of bleeding ▶ See Section 8.10.
- **Hypertension:** RCP (2023) recommends that those with primary ICH who present <6 h of onset with a SBP >150 mmHg should be treated urgently using a locally agreed protocol for SBP lowering to <140 mmHg for at least 7 d, unless: GCS <5, haematoma is very large and death is expected; a structural cause for the haematoma is identified; immediate surgery to evacuate the haematoma is planned.
- **Surgery (after clotting normalised):** refer to neurosurgeons, especially if cerebellar haematoma >3 cm diameter and/or developing hydrocephalus and falling GCS for **external ventricular drainage (EVD) and shunting,** or sub-occipital craniectomy for evacuation of the clot. Little evidence to suggest neurosurgical benefit in supratentorial bleeds, the exception being young patient with a superficial bleed close to the cortex and easily accessed. Deep hypertensive bleeds rarely benefit from surgery.
- **IV steroids** have no evidence base and may raise BP and glucose.
- **Mannitol** may be used to lower high ICP whilst en route for neurosurgery.
- **Stop statins:** controversial. Some evidence to stop them. Statins may be beneficial post bleed (*Int J Stroke* 2015;10:10). Follow local advice.
- **VTE prevention:** early mobility, intermittent pneumatic calf compression is the method of choice in all. LMWH/UFH should be avoided. For PE consider IVC filter insertion.
- **Manage diabetes:** (target BG 5–15 mmol/L) avoid hypoglycaemia.
- **Seizures:** anticonvulsants: e.g. IV Levetiracetam, valproate may be needed.

- **End of life care:** the decision may be for palliation, though some patients can make surprising recovery. Take advice. May be reasonable to postpone DNACPR decisions for the first 24 h. See DNACPR, ▶Section 15.9.
- **Reference:** National Clinical Guideline for Stroke for the UK and Ireland (2023) www.strokeguideline.org.

11.22 Subarachnoid haemorrhage

- **About:** it is a form of stroke. A common challenge for the acute physician. Background knowledge helps manage the risks. Mortality rates are 30–45% for aneurysmal SAH. Approx. 20–50% of aneurysms rupture over a patient's life. Symptomatic aneurysms need clipping or coiling; asymptomatic aneurysms need an expert assessment of risks. 'Red flags – worst ever headache, neck stiffness, vomited, onset with exercise' – however, only 7% of those screened will have had SAH. Always ask, is this RCVS? ▶Section 11.41.
- **Main early risks** are rebleeding, vasospasm, arrhythmias, hydrocephalus, seizures. Traumatic SAH due to head injury is not covered here. Unruptured aneurysms seen in 3% of population. Annual rupture rate 0.5–1% per annum.
- **Note:** CT scan alone can rule out SAH in patients presenting with lone acute severe headache, GCS = 15, no neurological features or neck pain, if performed <6 h of onset with a 3rd generation CT scanner with thin slices, reported by a radiologist experienced in reporting CT brain scans.
- **Pathophysiology:** spontaneous bleeding from aneurysm/AVM which lie in the subarachnoid space. Subarachnoid space surrounds the brain and spinal cord. Blood needs to reach below L1/2 to be detectable by LP. The pressures may cause bleeding into local brain parenchyma. Blood tends to track into sulci and ventricles and basal cisterns. Blood then pools around cisterns and circle of Willis and later can elicit vasospasm. *In vivo* conversion of Hb over 12 h to bilirubin detectable as xanthochromia. Seizures occur in 5–15% of patients. Cerebral vasospasm seen in 20–40% of patients and half die or suffer delayed cerebral ischaemia with infarction. The risk of developing hydrocephalus depends on volume of blood within the subarachnoid space and ventricles. Aneurysms can rebleed which can be catastrophic.
- Rebleeding is increased by measures that rapidly lower intracranial pressure. Aim to treat before this happens. 90% of aneurysms lie in the anterior circulation, usually on the anterior communicating artery (ACOMM 30%), and posterior communicating artery (PCOMM 25%), the MCA bifurcation (20%), the ICA bifurcation (8%) and other locations (7%); 10% of aneurysms arise from the posterior circulation usually at the basilar tip but also PICA/AICA and SCA. 10–15% of patients presenting with SAH have multiple aneurysms. Occasionally an aneurysm on the ICA in the cavernous sinus can rupture and be contained, causing a caroticocavernous fistula with pulsatile whooshing sound and an audible skull bruit. May follow thunderclap headache.

Causes of SAH

- **Aneurysmal SAH** (aSAH) (80%): aneurysms 5–7 mm diameter in the anterior circulation lowest risk of rupture, risk higher for those in posterior circulation. In contrast to sporadic aneurysms, familial aneurysms often larger (>10 mm) and multiple. Intracranial aneurysms develop with increasing age and usually arise at areas of vessel branching. Rupture rate increases with size. Small aneurysms are commoner, and so bleeds are seen more in smaller aneurysms. Related to smoking and excessive alcohol, connective tissue diseases. 1st-degree relative with SAH. Smoking, binge drinking, illicit drugs. Increased incidence with adult polycystic kidney disease (10%). SLE. Marfan and Ehlers–Danlos syndromes, pseudoxanthoma elasticum and sickle cell disease (See ▶Section 8.2).

- **Arteriovenous malformations** (10%): vascular anomalies which consist of a plexiform network of abnormal high pressure arteries and low pressure veins linked by one or more fistulae. They lack the typical capillary bed interposed between the arteriole and venule and have arterioles with a thinner than normal muscularis. Bleeding is about 2/100 per year amongst patients with no history of bleeding. Annual rate of repeat haemorrhage is 18%. Can present initially as bleeding or seizures.
- **Perimesencephalic:** SAH on CT, blood in the cisterns around the brainstem and suprasellar cistern. LP confirms SAH but DSA/CTA normal. Do well with rebleeding uncommon. Possibly venous tear or rupture with bleeding.
- **Trauma:** SAH with head injury. Treat as per traumatic brain injury.
- **Vasculitis** (rare): bleed from intracranial cervical arterial dissections.
- **Cerebral amyloid angiopathy:** age >70, convexity SAH, cortical bleeding.
- **Reversible cerebral vasoconstriction syndrome:** thunderclap headache, focal deficits, convexity SAH. Needs MR/CT/DSA. ▶Section 11.41.
- **Cerebral venous sinus thrombosis:** thunderclap headache, convexity SAH.
- **Dural arteriovenous fistula:** convexity SAH, diagnosed with DS angiography with bilateral external carotid injections.
- **Pituitary apoplexy** (see ▶Section 5.9).
- **Posterior reversible encephalopathy syndrome** (PRES) convexity SAH. (see ▶Section 11.40).
- **Cortical or meningeal tumours:** convexity SAH.
- **Children:** sickle cell disease (see ▶Section 8.2), Moyamoya disease.

Clinical

- **Headache:** prior headaches may be experienced in 30–50% due to warning 'sentinel' bleeds or due to pressure from expansion of the aneurysm prior to rupture. Often described as 'worst ever headache' which comes on very acutely – 'hit around back of head'. The headache usually persists in some form. Some cases less acute. Definitions range from any with maximal headache onset <10 min. Headache may be occipital or cervical and bleeding from a cervical AVM may be missed on CT. Blood tracking down may cause some neck stiffness from meningeal irritation. Vomiting, syncope and seizure may accompany onset. Triptans and other anti-migraine therapies can improve the headache from SAH so be cautious. In an acute headache 1 in 10 are SAH but if there are additional signs then this becomes 1 in 4.
- **Timing:** comes on at rest or exertion, during sleep, coitus and straining. Enquire after associated collapse/syncope and then recovery, photophobia and neck stiffness, vomiting, diplopia. Think SAH if sore stiff neck and meningism.
- **Reduced GCS:** progressive bleeding leads to coma, coning and sudden death.
- **Localisation clues:** may be found but CT anyway. Some signs are useful. Headache and IIIrd nerve palsy suggest an ipsilateral PCOMM/superior cerebellar artery aneurysm. Leg weakness and extensor plantars suggest ACOMM aneurysm. Hemiparesis suggests MCA aneurysm. If there are signs and one suspects SAH there really should be blood on the CT. If there are lateralising sign and a normal CT within

6 h of headache, then SAH is very unlikely. Arterial or venous infarction both cause headache. Take urgent expert advice. Arrhythmias and myocardial dysfunction and even pulmonary oedema and cardiac arrest – aggressive resuscitation is warranted as outcome can be reasonable. 1 in 7 will have intraocular haemorrhages.

- **Differential of thunderclap headache:** primary thunderclap headache: when all tests are negative this is the presumed diagnosis. Cerebral venous thrombosis, benign orgasmic cephalgia. Migraine or cluster headache, reversible cerebral vasoconstriction syndrome. Primary parenchymal haemorrhage, tumour with bleed, carotid/vertebral dissection.
- **Grading of subarachnoid bleeds:** World Federation of Neurosurgeons: I. GCS 15 no focal deficits. II. GCS 13–14 no focal deficits. III. GCS 13–14 focal deficits present. IV. GCS 7–12 irrespective of deficits. V. GCS 3–6 irrespective of deficits.

Ottawa SAH rule

- The Ottawa SAH rule contains 6 clinical variables to consider: (1) Age 40+ (2) Neck pain or stiffness (3) Witnessed loss of consciousness (4) Onset during exertion (5) Thunderclap headache (instantly peaking pain) (6) Limited neck flexion on examination. Consider CT in anyone with 1 or more findings present. Very sensitive (100%) but not specific.

Investigations

- **Bloods:** FBC, U&E: low Na (natriuresis or SIADH) low Hb/low Hct – more difficult to see a small SAH on CT if moderately to severely anaemic.
- **Coagulation screen:** on anticoagulants, bleeding disorder, low platelets.
- **ECG:** arrhythmias and pulmonary oedema possible. Dynamic T wave and ST changes may be seen but don't necessarily suggest ACS. Measure troponin and cardiology review if concerns. Obviously do not anticoagulate.
- **Non-contrast CT head:** thin cuts through base of brain shows high signal attenuation of fresh blood in the basal cisterns. MCA aneurysm blood in the Sylvian fissure. ACOMM aneurysm causes blood in intrahemispheric fissure and frontal lobe. PCOMM/superior cerebellar artery aneurysm can cause a IIIrd nerve palsy and blood in mesial temporal lobe and basilar cistern. Blood also seen around the brainstem in prepontine, premedullary and interpeduncular cisterns as well as within ventricles. CT is 98% sensitive in the first 12 h and is over 99% in the first 6 h. **NB:** Three recent studies show that 3rd-generation brain CT scans performed within 6 h after onset of acute headache in patients with suspected aSAH reliably excludes SAH in both academic and non-academic centres, where scans are read by non-neuroradiologists. Evidence suggests that LP is not needed in these patients. Those with low GCS or unknown time of onset, where symptoms are atypical, e.g. neck pain (one case with neck pain turned out to have a cervical AVM), or >6 h from onset should be considered for LP and local expert advice taken if unsure. Blood on CT less clear if low Hb or Hct. Sensitivity approaches 100% within 6 h of onset and 85% beyond 6 h. Sensitivity improves with modern scanners. Convexity SAH where blood is only seen on the convex surface is usually related to venous bleeding or venous infarction, amyloid angiopathy in elderly, PRES, vasculitis and reversible cerebral vasoconstriction syndrome. Fisher classification based on CT: Grade 1 – no blood seen. Grade 2 – <1 mm thick. Grade 3 – >1 mm thick. Grade 4 – diffuse or intraventricular bleed or parenchymal extension.
- **Lumbar puncture with opening pressure:** (see above as CT can exclude SAH if normal in first 6 h of acute headache) if required, e.g. presentation after 6 h

or atypical presentation and normal CT, then LP needs to be done at 12 h after onset (NOT BEFORE): SAH causes uniformly bloody CSF on LP with xanthochromia due to yellow bilirubin pigment from haemoglobin breakdown which is present for up to 3–4 weeks. **Bilirubin** is degraded by light and only forms *in vivo*. Can be seen if sample held against white background such that any yellow pigment is positive test. Interpretation is variable. **Spectrophotometry** can be used to differentiate between a bloody tap and 'true' xanthochromia more objectively. Pure oxyhaemoglobin which is non-diagnostic will have a single early peak, followed closely by a small bilirubin continuation and fall called the 'bilirubin shoulder'. **Red cells:** a traumatic tap may be suggested by a fall in red cell numbers in successive bottles; however, caution must be taken and this is not an absolute rule and traumatic taps can occur in those with SAH. The absolute level of RBCs must be taken and a high baseline level should still raise some suspicion of SAH. A count of <10 RBCs/mm^3 constitutes a negative tap, RBC >100/mm^3 in all tubes should be considered positive, especially if xanthochromia (bilirubin) is present. Opening pressure should be measured routinely in all LPs and if elevated one diagnosis to consider is cerebral venous sinus thrombosis and next step is CT venography or MR venography. NB: an LP is not benign and can result in a disabling low-pressure headache and so should not be undertaken without reasonable suspicion despite normal CT.

- **CSF xanthochromia** (breakdown product of haem) suggests recent bleed with haemolysis and so not a bloody tap. In some centres there is restricted access as samples now go to reference laboratories. Xanthochromia can be determined visually or by spectrophotometry which is not available in some hospitals. CSF, especially if bloody, should be spun down immediately and if the supernatant is yellow (compared with water against a white background), the diagnosis of SAH is practically certain. The specimen should be stored in darkness, preferably wrapped in aluminium foil because the ultraviolet components of daylight can break down bilirubin. Xanthochromia is present 3 weeks after the bleed in 70% of patients, and it is still detectable at 4 weeks in 40% of patients, so there may be an argument for a late LP.
- **CT/MR angiography:** CT angiography is easily accessible, available and relatively quick and can detect aneurysms down to 1 mm (MR angiography to about 3 mm). MR angiography is more difficult in those who are unwell in terms of monitoring. Catheter angiography only needed if aneurysm not seen or more anatomical definition is needed.
- **CT/MR venography:** if cerebral venous sinus thrombosis is considered usually with a convexity bleed.
- **Catheter cerebral angiography:** gold standard. Most sensitive test to identify bleeding source and usually done by the tertiary neuroscience centre.
- **Transcranial Doppler:** can detect vasospasm and delayed cerebral ischaemia in the MCA in the ITU.

Early complications of SAH

- **Rebleeding:** seen in 20% with high mortality. All interventions aim to prevent this by coiling/clipping. Rebleeding is a risk of aneurysmal SAH and much less so with AVMs or perimesencephalic bleeds.
- **Delayed cerebral ischaemia/vasospasm can cause ischaemic stroke:** likely due to blood breakdown products swilling around the branches of the circle of Willis.

Causes acute ischaemia/infarction. Site may be distant to bleeding aneurysm even opposite side. Seen in about 30%.

- **Obstructive hydrocephalus:** detected by CT (temporal horns dilated, blood in 4th ventricle). Refer to neurosurgeons for EVD.
- **Arrhythmias and myocardial dysfunction:** ECG telemetry.
- **Hyponatraemia** can be due to renal sodium loss or SIADH. Determine which using serum/urine osmolality as management differential.
- **Seizures:** manage as below.
- **Death:** from raised ICP and coning seen from haematoma/hydrocephalus. 10–15% die before hospital: 40% in week 1. 50% die in first 6 months.
- **Cognitive impairment:** long-term cognitive/functional issues may be seen.

Management

- **Prehospital care:** ABCs and rapid triage and transport to hospital and urgent CT. An early CT within 6 h is more sensitive than delayed imaging and is a reason to justify immediate imaging in all such patients. ITU assessment if GCS <9. Resuscitation. IV fluids usually NS. Avoid hypotonic fluids. If clearly a traumatic SAH from head injury (see topic above) then manage as per head injury and neurosurgical review for clot evacuation and monitoring for development of complications such as hydrocephalus and neurosurgical referral.
- **Bed rest.** Codeine and laxative/stool softener. Anti-emetics. Hydration and slight hypervolaemia suggested with 3 L/day. Low Na may well be due to renal Na loss rather than SIADH unless SIADH proven. Avoid fluid restriction. Avoid hypotonic fluids. Use N-Saline as fluid of choice.
- **Initial:** once diagnosis of aSAH then start all patients on **Nimodipine** 60 mg PO/NG 4 h for 21 d as early as possible. It reduces vasospasm and delayed cerebral ischaemic (below) neurologic deficit, cerebral infarction and mortality.
- **Rebleeding:** early intervention and management of aneurysm. In total 40% will rebleed if untreated within 4 weeks. Commonest within first 2 weeks of the SAH. A bimodal peak of the first 24–48 h and between days 7 and 10. Prevent with early angiography and aneurysm coiling or clipping.
- **Aneurysmal coiling:** preferred option with better outcomes. Interventional neuroradiologists can pack small platinum coils within the aneurysm to induce thrombosis. Note 10–15% of patients have more than one aneurysm.
- **Aneurysmal clipping:** perform a craniotomy and perform microsurgical clipping of aneurysm, or management of AVM in order to prevent rebleeding.
- **Delayed cerebral ischaemia/vasospasm:** reduced flow in branches of the circle of Willis usually occurs from day 2–3 to day 14 post SAH and can lead to ischaemic stroke which may be distant to the aneurysm. It can be detected by neurological signs or by transcranial Doppler showing increased velocities in circle of Willis/branches or angiography. Start **nimodipine** early as above. Evidence for magnesium usage to prevent vasospasm is controversial. May need ITU if comatose and needs airway protection. Orotracheal intubation and mechanical ventilation if falling GCS <9 or progressive neurology. Traditionally managed also with haemodilution (target Hct 30–35%), hypertension (using vasopressors) and hypervolaemia to optimise cerebral perfusion.
- **Hydrocephalus (10%):** if acute hydrocephalus on CT due to ventricular blood then refer for EVD and maintain ICP at <20 mmHg and CPP >60 mmHg.
- **Intracranial hypertension:** hyperventilate to maintain $PaCO_2$ of 30–35 mmHg to reduce elevated ICP. **Mannitol** 200 ml of 20% (20g/100ml) IV infusion over

20–30 min reduces ICP 50% peaks in effect after 90 min, and lasts 4 h. Used in ITU setting with ICP monitoring.
- **Seizures:** if occur (anticonvulsants may be given as prophylaxis) then start levetiracetam. Primary prophylaxis not usually warranted.
- **Telemetry:** risk of cardiac arrhythmias/cardiac dysfunction.
- **Troponin: SAH may elevate troponin.**
- **Hypertension:** manage BP with **Labetalol** 10–20 mg IV bolus which can be repeated if BP >180/110 mmHg. Target SBP <140 mmHg. However, to treat and avoid ischaemia related to vasospasm a higher BP may be preferable to improve cerebral blood flow once the aneurysm has been treated.
- **BP control and smoking cessation improve outcomes.**
- Neurological rehabilitation for any resultant brain injury.
- Take advice on screening family members for silent aneurysms.
- **Reference:** Gray & Foëx (2015) BET 2: does a normal CT scan within 6 h rule out subarachnoid haemorrhage? *Emerg Med J*, 32:898.

11.23 Cerebral hyperperfusion syndrome

- **About:** rare complication following a major increase in ipsilateral cerebral blood flow (CBF) usually seen 1–7 d following carotid reperfusion by endarterectomy or stenting. May even be seen post thrombolysis in stroke.
- **Aetiology:** damage to blood–brain barrier, severe oedema ± haemorrhage.
- **Risks:** post-op HTN, recent contralateral carotid endarterectomy, high-grade stenosis with poor collateral flow.
- **Clinical:** deterioration days after CEA/stroke reperfusion. Patient is more drowsy, agitated, stroke-like signs, seizure.
- **Investigations:** CT shows ipsilateral oedema ± haemorrhage.
- **Management:** ABC, elevate the head to 30°. Correct hyperthermia, hypoxia, hyperglycaemia, hypotension. If there is haemorrhagic transformation prognosis is poor with mortality about 50%. Consider ITU/HASU bed, lower BP e.g. labetalol. Target unclear but a MAP of 110 mmHg may be considered. Consider **mannitol** and **Dexamethasone** 4 mg IV 6 h & **Furosemide** 20–40 mg IV. Consider decompressive hemicraniectomy once clotting corrected.

11.24 Subdural haematoma

- **About:** acceleration–deceleration injury. Can cause vague neurology due to pressure until adaption fails and there is a large rise in ICP. If any concern then a CT head is needed especially if on any antithrombotic therapy.
- **Aetiology:** rupture/tearing of bridging veins crossing subdural space. Increased shear with larger subdural space in elderly. Mild to severe trauma. Worsened by coagulopathy or antiplatelets.
- **Risks:** falls and trauma, anticoagulants, elderly patients, dementia, alcohol abuse. Chronic persisting SDH seen males, older, cerebral atrophy.
- **Clinical:** confusion, headache, minimal signs, reduced GCS, IIIrd nerve palsy, coning, delirium, seizure, unsteadiness. C/L hemiparesis or hemisensory loss, dysphasia, Cheyne–Stokes respiration. Can even cause transient pseudo TIA-like symptoms, e.g. tingling, dysphasia, focal seizure.
- **Investigation:** FBC, U&E: ensure normal – low Na. Coagulation: check INR, platelets or coagulation screen if on warfarin or liver disease.

Non-contrast CT: day 0–5: rim of hyperdense 'bright' crescent-shaped extra-axial blood. Day 6–20: isodense to brain can be missed so look for midline shift or get MRI which shows it well. A quarter are bilateral. Day 21+: darkens to that of CSF. Look for midline shift, obliterated IIIrd ventricle, dilation of contralateral ventricle, obstructive hydrocephalus and signs of raised ICP. Avoid LP as risks of coning. SDH acts as a space-occupying lesion.

- **Management:** supportive: ABC. O_2 as per BTS guidelines, IV fluids if swallow unsafe. Manage any coagulopathy. Stop all anticoagulants or antiplatelets (take advice if high risk). Consider ITU if GCS <9.
- **Neurosurgery:** small subdurals managed conservatively. Larger acute haematomas with neurology need craniectomy. Evacuate all with a rim >10 mm or midline shift >5 mm regardless of GCS. If GCS <9 and SDH <10 mm thick and midline shift <5 mm, then surgery indicated if GCS has dropped 2 or more points since time of injury or there are asymmetric or fixed dilated pupils and/or ICP >20 mmHg.
- **Subacute SDH** with neurology may be aspirated under local anaesthetic as clot has liquefied into a 'motor oil' consistency by burr-hole craniotomy.
- **Chronic SDH:** over time, acute SDH can become chronic and bleeding may recur. May take months for things to settle.
- **Post-surgical complications:** seizures, subdural empyema, aspiration, sepsis, haemorrhagic stroke, SIADH, pneumonia.
- **Reference:** Bullock *et al.* (2006) Surgical management of acute subdural hematomas. *Neurosurgery*, 58:S2–16.

11.25 Epidural haematoma/head trauma

- **About:** usually seen by trauma and orthopaedics rather than physicians because head injury related. Rarely non-traumatic with bleeding disorders.
- **Aetiology:** usually a tear of middle meningeal artery which bleeds rapidly. May have skull fracture. Also bleeding from veins and fractured bone. May have rapid expansion and seen often in young where there is little room for any increase in intracranial volume. ICP rises quickly with devastating results.
- **Clinical:** trauma patients need a full top to toe survey to look for other injuries. Classically a head injury (perhaps with LOC) followed by lucid period and then sudden decline. Signs of raised ICP. Reduced GCS, IIIrd nerve palsy, coning, delirium, seizure, headache, unsteadiness. C/L hemiparesis or hemisensory loss, Cheyne–Stokes respiration. CSF leaks: rhinorrhoea and otorrhoea can suggest skull fracture. Signs of trauma and injury: Battle's sign, panda eyes, skull lacerations or haematomas.
- **Investigation:** FBC, U&E, LFT, coagulation, ABG, group and cross-match. Lactate. **Non-contrast CT:** there is a hyperdense lens-shaped convexity of blood on the inner surface of the skull restricted by the suture lines of the skull. Look for midline shift and signs of raised ICP. May be contrecoup injuries seen and subarachnoid and intraparenchymal haemorrhage. Look at bony windows for fracture. Plain X-ray/CT scan C-spine and full trauma assessment.
- **CSF leak:** elevated glucose on dipstick. If unsure send for β_2 transferrin which is found in CSF but not in tears, saliva or nasal secretions.

Management
- ABC stabilisation and urgent imaging. Caution with nasopharyngeal airway if suspected basal skull fractures. IV fluids. Resuscitation if needed. Close monitoring

of GCS and pupils. If GCS <9 then ITU referral. Trauma team review. Discuss with neurosurgeons. Asymmetrical pupils and coma needs IV **Mannitol** 200 ml of 20% and urgent shipping to neurosurgeons for clot evacuation to lower ICP. Single or bilateral fixed dilated pupils suggests an imminent herniation syndrome and coning. Needs surgical drainage combined with drugs, hypothermia and ventilation to lower ICP and neurocritical care. Pupillary abnormalities and GCS <9 should be evacuated as quickly as possible. Small stable bleeds may be managed conservatively following a period of monitoring in a neurosurgical unit with immediate access to intervention. Bleeding and haematoma expansion can occur. Ensure any other injuries are managed, e.g. long bone fractures, C-spine injuries, abdominal injuries, etc. In those rare cases of bleeding disorder being involved this needs urgent correction.

- **Neurosurgery:** recommended to evacuate the epidural haematomas with volume >30 cm^2 irrespective of GCS (www.braintrauma.org). Evacuation of clot is straightforward but ligating the middle meningeal artery can be difficult.
- **CSF leaks:** may settle conservatively but risk of bacterial meningitis. Steroids: avoid in traumatic brain injury. Anticonvulsants: No evidence for prophylactic use of AEDs without seizures.
- **Reference:** Bullock *et al.* (2006) Surgical management of acute epidural hematomas. *Neurosurgery*, 58:S7–15.

11.26 Guillain–Barré syndrome

- **About:** acute onset over days of weakness with areflexia and respiratory failure in some cases. Worse prognosis if *Campylobacter jejuni* infection.
- **NB:** be ready to intubate. Check VC 6 h (caution if VC <1.5 L); intubate if VC is <20 ml/kg. ABG to look for a rise in $PaCO_2$ which occurs before any hypoxia. Bedside assessment – can they count to 20 in one breath hold?
- **Aetiology:** possible cross-reacting autoimmune-reactive T cells mediate response instigated by infectious antigen. Seen usually 7 d post *C. jejuni* infection, CMV, HIV, EBV, mycoplasma, Lyme disease, Zika fever.
- **Pathology:** most show multifocal demyelination and raised CSF protein. Slowed conduction. Axonal variants have axonal disruption and Wallerian degeneration.

Different forms (most are demyelinating)
- **Acute inflammatory demyelinating polyneuropathy** (AIDP) (90%): various antibodies. Mortality 5%.
- **Acute motor and sensory axonal neuropathy** (AMSAN) (5%): similar to AMAN but also affects sensory roots. Mortality 10–15%.
- **Acute motor axonal neuropathy** (AMAN): anti-GD1a/GM1 antibodies. Seen more commonly in China. Post diarrhoeal *Campylobacter*, Zika virus, hepatitis viruses, IV ganglioside, vaccination, surgery.
- **Miller Fisher syndrome (5%):** diplopia and then ataxia, areflexia: anti-GQ1b and anti-GT1a. Needs IVIg if cannot walk.
- **Pure sensory/autonomic neuropathy.** Rarest form. May have an encephalopathy. Widespread symp/parasympathetic failure.

Clinical
- Progressive weakness in legs and arms and even bilateral facial muscles often 'ascending' comes on over hours/days with areflexia in weak limbs.

- Progressive phase lasts days to 4 weeks (often 2 weeks). Relative symmetry. Mild sensory symptoms or signs (not present in acute motor axonal neuropathy). Weakness of facial muscles.
- Bulbar, IIIrd nerve, autonomic dysfunction. Pain (common).
- Severe back pain, respiratory and swallowing weakness. Distal sensory loss. Loss of distal reflexes. Papilloedema due to high CSF protein.
- Hypertension, arrhythmias, ptosis, ophthalmoplegia.
- Assess power of neck flexion/extension/shoulder abduction – correlates with diaphragmatic weakness. Some presentations may however be atypical.
- Reflexes may be present in early 1–2 days. Wide spectrum from short illness to quadriplegia and ventilator dependent for months.
- It can occur with those with back pain and mild tingling and weakness

Findings that make GBS less likely
- CSF: raised WCC (mononuclear cells or polymorphonuclear cells >50/µl).
- Severe pulmonary dysfunction with little or no limb weakness at onset.
- Severe sensory signs with little or no weakness at onset.
- Bladder/bowel dysfunction at onset. Fever at onset.
- Sharp spinal cord sensory level. Marked, persistent asymmetry of weakness.
- Slow progression without respiratory involvement.

Hughes functional grading scale
- Grade 0: healthy, Grade 1: able to run, Grade 2: can walk 5 m independently, Grade 3: can walk 5 m with help, Grade 4: chair/bed-bound, Grade 5: ventilated, Grade 6: death. Slow steady recovery over weeks up to 6 months is typical.

Differentials (exclude cord or cauda equina syndrome)
- **Poliomyelitis:** LMN weakness. Rare where immunisation is used.
- **Botulism: descending** flaccid paralysis, bilateral cranial neuropathies, blurred vision, diplopia, bulbar weakness, dry mouth, hypotension. ▶ Section 9.18.
- **Tick paralysis:** toxin within the tick. Children. Remove tick with improvement within hours. Some can worsen. Consider if recent tick exposure.
- **Acute spinal cord compression:** when signs still remain flaccid before tone increases. Sensory level, early bladder involved, pain.
- **Chronic inflammatory demyelinating polyneuropathy:** slowly progressive. Very slow velocity on NCS.
- **Acute myelopathy:** HIV, paraneoplastic. May be flaccid weakness early. But usually UMN. MRI useful.
- **Cauda equina lesion:** flaccid weakness. Pain, incontinence and saddle anaesthesia and back pain. Consider MRI.
- **Acute neuropathy:** porphyria, arsenic, thallium, organophosphates, lead.
- **Lyme disease:** tick bite, rash, endemic area.

Investigations
- **Bloods:** FBC, U&E to check K. Low Na due to SIADH can be seen.
- **ECG:** autonomic neuropathy so arrhythmias and ST/T wave changes.
- **CSF:** protein >1 g by 2nd week (caution as 50% normal in week 1), 'acellular' WCC <10/mm^3. Glucose normal. If WCC >50 consider HIV, Lyme disease, polio.
- **MRI spine:** if any diagnostic doubt exclude a cord/cauda equina lesion. Will depend on pattern of weakness. GBS can cause spinal nerve root enhancement with gadolinium but this is non-specific.

- **Nerve conduction studies:** most (90%) show demyelination (slowed nerve conduction velocities and prolonged or absent F wave). May show axonal degeneration with AMAN/AMSAN – worse prognosis. If very slow consider CIDP.
- **Antibody measurements** rarely useful except prognostically, e.g. anti-GD1a or anti-GQ1b found in Miller Fisher variant.

Management

- **ABC and O$_2$** as per BTS guidelines. Respiratory support where required. Tracheal suction can cause low BP due to autonomic instability and so ongoing telemetry and BP monitoring, for autonomic difficulties which can lead to dysrhythmia, are required. Probability of respiratory insufficiency can be assessed with the Erasmus GBS Respiratory Insufficiency Score (EGRIS) – see online calculators. It uses days between onset and hospital admission, facial weakness and MRC sum of weakness.
- **Monitor FVC to guide need for intubation.** FVC is better than negative inspiratory force or maximal expiratory pressure (*never PEFR*) at least 6-hourly for worsening, but none predict intubation need well and bedside clinical review is vital. Normal FVC is 4.5 L or 70 ml/kg. HDU monitoring if FVC <1.5 L. Consider intubation FVC <1.2 L for a 65 kg person. Seen more so in those with bulbar or neck or shoulder weakness. Blood gases can be reassuringly normal until late. Other factors supporting intubation are bulbar dysfunction with a need for airway protection and significant hypoxaemia due to ongoing aspiration or atelectasis. Dysautonomia is a concern in the peri-intubation period with profound hypotension.
- **Neurology consult:** usually given in those who have impaired mobility or rapidly progressive weakness or bulbar or autonomic or respiratory issues. Close liaison with ITU and outreach teams should be maintained. Rapid deterioration can be seen 24–48 h. Treatment is IVIg which is easier than PLEX. Steroids not effective. In cases where response is poor a second course may be considered or PLEX tried. At least one quarter deteriorate during or just after IVIg or PLEX. This suggests they may be worse without therapy.
- **IVIg** 400 mg/kg/d for 5 d. Expensive. Give within first 2 weeks in those unable to walk unaided. As with any blood-derived product there are issues of allergy and infection such as HIV and viral hepatitis and concerns over prions. Can give headache, malaise. C/I with AKI and IgA deficiency. Check IgA level first is advised but some specialists don't. Be ready to treat anaphylaxis. Take local advice. Relapse is possible in 10%. Written consent suggested.
- **Plasma exchange (PLEX):** as effective as IVIg. Preferred if IgA deficiency or renal failure. Needs central venous access. Give four alternate-day exchanges over 7–10 d for a total of 200–250 ml/kg. Steroids have no benefit in GBS.
- **Outcome:** 85% may have a good recovery, others are left with a degree of disability, usually monophasic but can recur and may even become progressive resembling CIDP.
- **Worse outcome** post-diarrhoea, ventilated, older patient, rapid onset <7 d, muscle wasting. Not given IVIg. Serum albumin <35 g/L at 2 weeks.
- **VTE prophylaxis:** prevent VTE with LMWH and early mobilisation or IPC.
- **Ongoing rehabilitation** over weeks and months.
- **Speech and language therapy** to assess swallow safety and speech.
- **NG feeding** in the interim and PEG if delayed return of bulbar function.
- **Neuropathic pain:** carbamazepine and gabapentin and opiates as required. Amitriptyline avoided as can theoretically cause arrhythmias.
- **Laxatives** to avoid constipation from opiates and immobility.
- **Reference:** Willison *et al.* (2016) Guillain–Barré syndrome. *Lancet*, 388:717.

11.27 Myasthenia gravis

- **About:** suspected or confirmed myasthenia avoid drugs that can increase weakness by checking all suitable in the *BNF* or equivalent. Myasthenic crisis can cause severe respiratory compromise. Precipitated by acute infection other illness or medications. Avoid: aminoglycosides, penicillamine, quinolones.
- **Aetiology:** abs to nicotinic Ach receptor or muscle-specific protein kinase (musk) protein. Complement-mediated damage of receptors and post-synaptic Ach receptor.
- **Associations:** rheumatoid arthritis, pernicious anaemia, SLE. Sarcoidosis. Sjögren's disease, polymyositis, ulcerative colitis, pemphigus.
- **Clinical:** fatiguable weakness of skeletal, ocular and respiratory and bulbar musculature. Fluctuating proximal weakness worsens with exercise – fatiguability. Sustained upward gaze causes diplopia and symmetrical ptosis. Eyelid twitch response (Cogan's lid twitch) is characteristic. Normal pupils. Respiratory muscle weakness with weak cough and weak neck flexion. Poor swallow, abnormal smile, dysarthria common. Bulbar nasal speech, risk of aspiration. Pregnancy: MG worsens in 1st trimester of pregnancy and then improves. Myasthenic crises: profound weakness leads to respiratory failure.
- **Drugs and events exacerbating weakness:** steroids, antibiotics, phenytoin, quinidine, quinolones, chloroquine, penicillamine, verapamil, magnesium, imipenem, chlorpromazine. Anaesthetic agents/neuromuscular blockers: care must be taken before any anaesthesia (check *BNF*). Cardiac: beta-blockers, calcium channel blockers, some anti-arrhythmic, statins. Other: anticholinergic, anticonvulsants, antipsychotics, lithium. Events: acute illness, surgery or infections can worsen symptoms.
- **Differential:** cholinergic crisis: due to excessive meds for MG causing lacrimation, vomiting, bradycardia, salivation, pulmonary oedema, miosis. Lambert–Eaton syndrome: paraneoplastic, non-fatiguable. Botulism: bacterial toxin, tinned foods, mydriasis. Drug-induced myasthenia (penicillamine, aminoglycosides). Chronic progressive external ophthalmoplegia. GBS: protein and WCC LP findings. MND and myopathies.
- **Investigations:** bloods: FBC, U&E, ESR, TFTs: check K, Ca, Mg levels. Autoantibodies: acetylcholine receptor (90%), muscle-specific receptor tyrosine kinase. Thymoma patients 15%: antibody to muscle proteins ryanodine and titin. In myasthenia 10% are negative for autoantibodies. **Tensilon test:** edrophonium chloride (Tensilon). Cardiac monitor and resuscitation equipment in case of low HR/asystole needing atropine. **Edrophonium** 1 mg IV test dose given and if no problems then 2 mg IV given with determination of clinical improvement in motor power. Further **Edrophonium** 2–10 mg IV in total may be given. Particularly useful in MG patients with ocular symptoms. Onset <1 min and lasts for 5 min. Also give placebo. Ice cube test: placed over eyelid with ptosis for 1–2 min and improves ptosis. Cold reduces activity of cholinesterase. **Repetitive nerve stimulation and single fibre electromyography** is the most sensitive test (>95%) for diagnosing MG. When a motor unit is activated, the action potentials reaching muscle fibres are not all synchronous. It is highly accurate in confirming MG by detecting 'jitter'. **MRI/CT thorax:** detect anterior mediastinum thymoma (found in 12% of patients with MG). All should be considered for thymectomy.
- **Management:** myasthenic crisis: monitor respiration: fall in vital capacity <1 L (may be difficult if significant facial weakness), a rise in CO_2 or weak neck flexion

suggests respiratory muscle weakness. A fall in PO_2 may be late. May be exacerbated by bulbar weakness. Non-invasive ventilation may be trialled but needs immediate access to mechanical ventilation if deteriorating. Elective intubation of a myasthenic patient with impending respiratory failure is favoured over emergent intubation.

- **Prednisolone** 40–80 mg/d as a single slow reducing dose may be used but can cause initial worsening so some start at smaller but less effective dose, e.g. prednisolone 20 mg OD. Usually started under inpatient supervision. Be ready to deal with increased weakness.
- **Immune modulation:** acute crisis use plasma exchange (PLEX) or IVIg. PLEX: 5 sessions over 1–2 weeks works faster than IVIg. A fall in acetylcholinesterase receptor antibody levels correlates to clinical response. **IVIg** 400 mg/kg/day *over 5 days*. Check for IgA deficiency. Close liaison with neurologists. Other agents include azathioprine, mycophenolate and ciclosporin.
- **Cholinergic crisis:** patients taking an excess of acetylcholinesterase inhibitors treatment. Muscle weakness, fasciculation, paralysis, pallor, salivation, brady, sweating, small pupils. Acetylcholinesterase inhibitors should be significantly lowered or discontinued to avoid excessive pulmonary secretions in the setting of respiratory distress in all MG patients.
- **Pyridostigmine** 30–60 mg PO 4 h initially has an onset of effect in 30 min and a duration of 4 h. Long-acting formulations for overnight. Side-effects: cholinergic crisis, severe weakness, low HR, and low BP.
- **Thymectomy** remains part of treatment in patients with thymic tumours.
- **Reference:** Wendell & Levine (2011) Myasthenic crisis. *Neurohospitalist*, 1(1):16–22.

11.28 Acute cord/cauda injury

- **About: identify** acute spinal cord or cauda equina pathology early and act quickly to prevent long-term consequences. Surgical causes might be missed despite trauma assessment in the emergency department and the patient may be admitted medically. Bilateral leg weakness can be flaccid with reduced reflexes and loss of sphincters early in both spinal and cauda equina lesion.
- MRI of the whole spine in those with malignant disease as other subclinical lesions may be present. Clinical pathways vary regionally so be sure to follow local protocols and referral pathways to the appropriate spinal teams where needed.

Functional anatomy: UMN becomes LMN at anterior horn cell

- UMN spinal cord starts at foramen magnum and descends within the spinal canal to lower border of L1 vertebra. There are 30 vertebrae. It carries 31 pairs of spinal nerves on either side (8 cervical nerves (but 7 vertebrae), 12 thoracic, 5 lumbar, 5 sacral, 1 coccygeal). The cord carries efferent motor and autonomic fibres to sweat glands and sphincters and afferent sensory. Cord lesions are UMN with sensory level signs and can be partial. A lesion in the cord gives weakness, increased tone, spasticity, upgoing plantars and hyperreflexia.
- LMN nerve roots exit cord and descend alongside cord in spinal canal to pass out via corresponding vertebral foramina. The cord ends as the conus medullaris with LMN spinal nerves forming the cauda equina. Cauda equina lesions are LMN mainly sensory from perianal region, saddle area and backs of legs as well as weakness, reduced tone, absent or downgoing plantars and reduced reflexes. Lesions may be bilateral or unilateral often with radicular pain. Urinary retention occurs late.

Sensory dermatomes/myotomes for lowest intact level localisation

- **Cervical:** C2 – occiput, C3 – thyroid cartilage, C4 – suprasternal notch and spontaneous breathing, C5 – infraclavicular with shoulder shrug and biceps, C6 – thumb and elbow flexion with biceps, C7 – index finger, elbow extension triceps, C8 – little finger and finger flexion.
- **Thoracic:** T4 – nipple, T10 – umbilicus.
- **Lumbar:** L1 – inguinal region and hip flexion, L2 – medial thigh and hip flexion, L3 – medial thigh and hip adduction/knee extension, L4 – medial thigh and hip abduction/ankle dorsiflexion, L5 – web space 1st, 2nd toes and big toe extension.
- **Sacral:** S1 – lateral foot and plantar flexion, S2 – perianal and plantar flexion, S3–5 – perianal with rectal tone.

Pathology to spinal cord and cauda

- Key facts: pathology at vertebral level above L1 to vertebral canal contents will cause UMN cord damage with a sensory level and LMN damage to the few roots that are waiting to exit canal lying alongside.
- Lesions below L1 vertebral level will affect cauda equina and roots and cause LMN and saddle distribution sensory loss.

Physical damage to vertebral column and cord

- This can be by any significant trauma, bullet, knife, shrapnel or by a tumour or haematoma or a centrally prolapsed lumbar disc. The management may be surgical decompression. Pain will usually be a key and obvious finding. A more subacute presentation with a tumour or inflammatory mass. Any lesion above L1 will damage cord and UMN, below will damage cauda and be LMN.
- Diagnostically obvious, RTA: 50%, especially if thrown from vehicle. Falls: 25% even from standing in elderly, especially at C2. Violence (especially gunshot wounds): 15%. Sports accidents: 10%, e.g. diving, rugby. Others: 5%. Increased risk: ankylosing spondylitis, cervical spondylosis, narrow spinal canal. Key issues will be to immobilise an unstable spine and ABC. If a physical cause which may need a surgical remedy then urgent imaging is needed.

Investigations

- **Trauma:** simple radiology is vital but in non-traumatic cases or where possible go straight to MRI when cord/cauda equina pathology suspected. The whole of the spine should be visualised and symptoms and signs correlated with findings. Lateral/anteroposterior and odontoid peg views of spine. Lateral view must show C7/T1 junction. CT scan head and cervical spine (especially C1/2 lesions) and may be done instead of plain films. Fractures may exist at multiple levels. MRI is better for showing bone and ligamentous injury.
- **Medical/oncological:** urgent MRI is required to diagnose and assess or exclude a mechanical cause. Infarction of the cord may show up as may inflammatory lesions and different levels of cancer involvement. Also consider FBC, ESR/CRP, ALP, myeloma screen, U&E, LFTs, HIV test, ECG (AF with vascular lesion), INR (warfarin), CXR (lung cancer/metastases/TB), B12/folate, syphilis serology, lumbar puncture.

Management (image and referral to spinal pathway)

- **General:** ABCs. Manage BP, O_2, IV fluids. Skin care with 2-hourly turns to prevent pressure or neuropathic ulcers, intermittent or temporary urinary catheterisation to prevent over-distension of bladder and infection. If trauma and spine may be unstable, then spine must be immobilised using a hard collar initially and additional with sandbags. High cord lesions (above C5) with diaphragmatic paralysis may necessitate rapid sequence induction protecting C-spine.

- **MRI shows cord non-metastatic compression:** discuss with surgeons who may advise **Dexamethasone** 10 mg IV and transfer for decompression. An extradural haematoma or abscess needs surgical review and reversal of anticoagulation or antibiotics, respectively.
- **Metastatic spinal cord compression (MSCC):** ▶ Section 17.8.
- **If MRI is normal then look for a medical cause:** exclude spinal stroke – MRI DWI and gadolinium contrast, especially if AVM is in the differential. Needs LP to look for cells and protein, oligoclonal bands, HIV and consider neurology referral. Consider MRI brain if MS suspected to look for additional evidence of disseminated lesions.
- **Cauda equina lesion:** is also a surgical decompression emergency often due to a central disc prolapse below L1. Low back pain, weak legs and reduced reflexes. Saddle anaesthesia. Urgent MRI of lumbar spine and referral for surgical review. Oncology also if malignant.
- **Autonomic dysreflexia:** risk of provoking acute, uncontrolled hypertension leading to LVF, AKI, MI and cerebral haemorrhage. Spinal cord injury at or above T6. Precipitated by a strong sensory afferent input to the spinal cord. May be from bladder and bowel. Massive reflex sympathetic surge with widespread vasoconstriction below diaphragm. There is a reflex bradycardia. Pale skin with vasoconstriction and 'goose bumps' below lesion and vasodilation and sweating and nasal congestion and flushing above. Stimuli are varied from UTI to rectal exam to coitus, DVT and PE or local trauma. Treat by sitting patient up, give oral antihypertensives, IV or transdermal nitrates or oral amlodipine and lower BP gradually. Consider catheter if retention. Manage pressure ulcers. Main issue is recognising and so take expert advice.

11.29 Acute transverse myelitis

- **About:** acute inflammation of spinal cord. Often at thoracic level. 10–20%. Some will develop MS. Urgent MRI to exclude compression.
- **Causes:** multiple sclerosis, neuromyelitis optica, infections, autoimmune or post-infectious/vaccine inflammation, vasculitis.
- **Clinical:** progressive UMN weakness over hours or days in both legs ± hands. Back pain, sensory level, motor and sphincter deficits – urinary retention. MS often incomplete and asymmetric. Neuromyelitis optica involves 3+ cord segments with associated optic neuritis.
- **Investigations:** MRI brain and spinal cord with gadolinium, CSF analysis. Neuromyelitis optica IgG, CXR, CRP, ESR, serum and CSF oligoclonal bands, ANA, B12, copper, HIV, Lyme disease, mycoplasma.
- **Management:** ABC, nursing care, bladder and bowels, rehabilitation, skin care. **Methylprednisolone** 1g/d for 5 d. PLEX may be considered. About 1/3 recover fully, third have some weakness and the rest no recovery.

11.30 Acute dystonic reactions

- **About:** can be quite dramatic/bizarre. Often seen in those on antipsychotics. Stop the causative drug. Commoner in males, family history of dystonia, young and with alcohol.

- **Drugs:** erythromycin, haloperidol, metoclopramide, prochlorperazine, SSRIs, cocaine, sumatriptan, ranitidine, carbamazepine.
- **Aetiology:** nigrostriatal D2 receptor blockade, excess striatal cholinergic output. Seen within 7 d of drug.
- **Clinical:** oculogyric crises – sustained upward gaze, torticollis, tongue protrusion, trismus. Sustained contractions of facial muscles, neck, trunk, pelvis, extremities, larynx. Everything else is normal, e.g. cognition, consciousness, vital signs. Can very rarely compromise airway with laryngeal/pharyngeal dystonia.
- **Differential:** tetanus, strychnine poisoning, hyperventilation (carpopedal spasm). Low Ca/Mg and tetany, Wilson's disease.
- **Management:** identify and stop causative drug. Reassure. Drug advice. May use anticholinergics. Consider **Procyclidine** 5–10 mg IV if severe or give orally as 2.5–5 mg TDS PO until resolves. **Benzatropine** 1–2 mg slow IV. **Diazepam** 2–5 mg PO/IV has been used. Give drugs up to 30 min to work.
- **Reference:** Campbell (2001) The management of acute dystonic reactions. *Aust Prescr*, 24:19.

11.31 ▶ Acute vertigo

- Vertigo is the sensory illusion of the world moving when you are still and is caused by peripheral vestibular, and possibly central neurological, dysfunction. Sit on a chair and spin around several times with care. You will sense an unpleasant feeling of movement when you are stationary. That is vertigo and the exact historical experience you need to elicit from the patient. It is very distinct from presyncope or simple unsteadiness/disequilibrium. You need to be able to diagnose accurately to reduce unnecessary tests and referrals.
- Differentials are shown below and most cause recurrent vertigo. As with all recurrent episodic disorders, the first ever episode is the most challenging diagnostically. Stroke is a rare cause usually of a monophasic episode often with other focal lateralising neurology. Recurrent identical episodes of acute vertigo are very rarely vascular and other diagnoses should be considered first.
- Red flags suggesting central cause are a normal head impulse test, new onset (occipital) headache, any central neurological symptoms or signs, acute deafness need urgent stroke team referral. Positionally provoked vertigo is usually BPPV. Movement often makes any vertiginous symptoms worse, but in BPPV there is a very clear relationship between movement and abrupt onset.

Examination
- **ENT and neurology:** check tympanic membranes, no new onset deafness (rub fingers to each ear), no facial weakness, dysphagia, or dysphonia.
- **Hearing loss:** most suggest a peripheral cause. Very rare exception is an acute anterior inferior cerebellar artery infarct with vertigo and hearing loss.
- **Gait:** central disease impairs gait such that patient cannot walk unaided. Peripheral can walk unaided but with some unsteadiness and anxiety.
- **Neurology:** face/limb weakness, diplopia, objective ataxia, or sensory loss, cerebellar signs, Horner's syndrome. Check Romberg's sign. These suggest brainstem disease such as lateral medullary or cerebellar stroke or demyelination.
- **Vertigo:** peripheral disease tends to be a unidirectional nystagmus in all positions of gaze. With central the fast phase can be bidirectional or vertical.

- **Head impulse/thrust test:** positive for peripheral disease – the side to which patient turns head and there is a corrective saccade in the affected side. Sit face to face with the patient and hold the patient's head from the front. Ask patient to fixate on examiner's nose and the head is rapidly turned 10° to one side and then to the other side while watching the eyes for presence or absence of any corrective movements. If turned normally the vestibular ocular reflex remains intact and eyes continue to fixate on the visual target. On affected side, the reflex fails and the eyes make a corrective saccade to re-fixate on the visual target. Sometimes the corrective saccade is easily missed so sometimes can be useful for a 3rd person to film the movements, e.g. with a smartphone for instant re-analysis. I would not do this test if there is neck pain or any suggestion of a cervical dissection. Can follow a positive test with Unterberger test.
- **Dix–Hallpike test:** positive in BPPV. Check for ototoxic medications.
- **Unterberger stepping test:** shows which labyrinth may be dysfunctional in a peripheral vertigo. Patient stands and steps in one position for 1 min with their eyes closed. Test positive if patient rotates towards the side of the lesion. Useful only when peripheral cause suspected.

Differentials

- **Acute vestibular/labyrinthitis neuronitis:** episodic symptoms of severe vertigo and nausea lasting several days. Subacute onset. Hearing spared. No tinnitus. May be viral illness. No other neurology. Self-limiting but can take months. May need vestibular sedatives for a few days. Head impulse test positive. No evidence that steroids or antivirals are useful. See below for management.
- **Vestibular migraine:** vertigo may be part of a developing aura in migraine and may be followed classically by headache as well as other features of N&V which can make the diagnosis difficult. Usual precipitants. Headache is the main feature. Treat with NSAIDs. Initial episode may require imaging to exclude intracranial pathology. May require migraine prophylaxis.
- **Benign paroxysmal positional vertigo (BPPV):** transient rotatory vertigo lasts seconds to a minute precipitated by a change in head position relative to gravity (offending ear down, e.g. turning over in bed, and looking up at a high shelf). Patients experience movement sensation with nausea, vomiting and imbalance. Symptoms occur on and off over days or weeks, usually resolves in months, but may recur. Often idiopathic or post-head injury or infection. Diagnosis by Dix–Hallpike test detects posterior canal pathology. The three step (20 sec each) Epley manoeuvre or Daroff manoeuvre can be used as repositioning technique with 90% success. ENT review.
- **Ménière's disease:** older patients. Sense of fullness in ear, attacks of disabling episodic vertigo last an hour (at least 20 min). Progressive tinnitus and low frequency hearing loss. It is progressive over years. Vestibular sedatives for acute attacks. Try a low salt diet and betahistine for prophylaxis. May consider prochlorperazine. Bendroflumethiazide. ENT referral for diagnosis, audiogram and possible surgery or other measures.
- **Brainstem/cerebellar stroke/MS:** typically cerebellar, pontine, medullary pathology. Needs MRI. Vascular syndromes, MS and such can cause a severe central vertigo. May be haemorrhagic or ischaemic stroke. Lateral medullary syndrome (PICA), labyrinthine stroke (AICA infarct) with hearing loss, brainstem lacunar stroke from pontine perforators. Refer to stroke team. Cerebellar syndrome may be found with ipsilateral signs. Feeling of disequilibrium. Ataxic.

Midline lesions cause a more truncal ataxia. 'Vertebrobasilar insufficiency' is a deprecated diagnosis. Most patients with severe vertebrobasilar stenosis have few persisting symptoms.

- **Drug toxicity:** use of gentamicin, furosemide, quinine, aspirin, erythromycin or other ototoxic medications. Structures affected bilaterally so vertigo less pronounced.
- **Acoustic neuroma** (schwannoma) is a very rare cause of acute vertigo as there is some central compensation. Cerebellopontine angle tumour. Cranial nerve palsy. Seen with neurofibromatosis. Grow 1 mm/year.
- **Presyncope/faint:** feeling of disconnection, darkening of vision, feel about to pass out, usually standing, situational, provocation – fear, anxiety. No true vertigo or minimal and never the dominant symptom. Needs a cardiovascular work-up – ECG, tilt table, lying standing BP.
- **Tullio phenomenon:** sound-induced vertigo and nystagmus. Hyperacusis. Can hear eyeballs move. Caused by superior semicircular canal dehiscence (SCCD). ENT referral.

Management

- General management of acute vertigo includes correct diagnosis and management as above as well as bed rest, fluids (oral or IV if needed) and reassurance. Head movements can be particularly distressing especially with peripheral vestibular dysfunction. Vestibular sedatives, e.g. **Prochlorperazine** 5–10 mg TDS PO can help acutely and the sedative side-effects can also promote rest. Occasionally **diazepam** IV or PO can be used which can suppress vestibular nucleus activity. Things tend to improve after several days with gradual return to normal function, which may take weeks for vestibular neuronitis. Activity should be promoted and helps adaptive recovery of the vestibular system. Vestibular sedatives should be weaned off as they may impair the normal compensatory mechanisms.
- Acute and chronic vertigo can lead to reduced productivity, quality of life, depression and falls/injuries.
- **Reference:** Barraclough & Bronstein (2009) Vertigo. *BMJ*, 339:b3493.

11.32 Bell's palsy/Ramsay Hunt syndrome

- **About: facial weakness** can mimic stroke but with care the diagnosis should be straightforward. Usual age 15–45 years, diabetes, post viral, immunocompromised, pregnancy.
- **Aetiology:** inflammation/demyelination of the facial nerve within the canal. Supplies muscles of facial expression, taste anterior tongue and stapedius. Likely viral (HSV-1) but mechanism poorly understood. Bilateral weakness: sarcoid, Lyme disease, botulism, GBS – refer to neurology. Slowly progressing and worsening needs malignancy excluded.
- **Clinical:** classically wake up with facial weakness and 'numbness'. Full progression peaks at 72 h. Pain behind ear, tinnitus, weak upper and lower face with weakened eye closure, difficulty raising eyebrows. Corner of mouth lower. Sensory symptoms – numb/tingling feeling though touch sensation is intact (mechanism unclear). Eye elevates on attempted eye closure (Bell's sign), hyperacusis, loss of taste on ipsilateral tongue. If any additional neurology e.g. VIth nerve or arm/leg sensory motor or ataxia/nystagmus/diplopia then consider MRI head for MS, stroke, tumour.
- **Ramsay Hunt syndrome:** Bell's palsy + painful vesicles in ear canal (HZV)

House–Brackmann facial nerve grading system
1. Normal: normal facial function in all areas.
2. Mild dysfunction: slight weakness on close inspection.
3. Moderate: obvious, but not disfiguring difference between two sides.
4. Moderately severe dysfunction: obvious weakness/disfigurement.
5. Severe dysfunction: only barely perceptible motion.
6. Total paralysis: loss of tone, asymmetry, no motion.

Additional
- **Complications:** eye injury, facial pain, dry mouth, intolerance to loud noises, abnormal facial muscle contraction during voluntary movements, and psychological sequelae.
- **Investigations:** none usually. May do FBC, U&E, glucose, ACE/Ca if sarcoid. MRI brain if pontine lesion or other CNS pathology suspected. Neurophysiological studies in selected patients with delayed resolution.
- **Management:** steroids recommended if within 72 h of onset. Balance risks of hyperglycaemia and psychosis in mild cases, lower doses/shorter courses may be given pragmatically – 25 mg BD for 10 d or 30 mg BD for 5 d, followed by a taper down 50/40/30/20/10 mg/d for a total of 10 d. No evidence for antivirals unless suspect Ramsay Hunt but some give. Exceptions to steroids may be diabetes, morbid obesity, previous steroid intolerance and psychiatric disorders. Pregnant women should be treated on an individualised basis.
- **Eye care is key:** if eye closure affected refer Ophthalmology for advice. Wear glasses, artificial tears (Lacri-lube) applied frequently, tape lid and eye patch at night, ask patient to physically close eyelids with fingers during day at times. Give eye lubricating drops, Ophthalmology may consider tarsorrhaphy and Botox to upper lid to aid closure. 70% full recovery, 15% partial, 15% residual signs. If at 6 weeks poor resolution ENT referral.
- **Ramsay Hunt syndrome:** oral **aciclovir** ± prednisolone. Prognosis worse.
- **Red flag to refer:** worsening, other neurologic findings, UMN facial weakness, possible cancer. Systemic or severe local infection. Trauma.
- **Reference:** NICE (2019) CKS: Bell's palsy.

11.33 Acute demyelination/multiple sclerosis

- **About:** usually seen as part of multiple sclerosis. Rarer types include acute disseminated encephalomyelitis (ADEM), neuromyelitis optica (NMO).
- **Aetiology:** flare-up of existing MS or *de novo* presentation. Effects depend upon how much myelin involved and if partial or total. Stress, fatigue, infection and heat can exacerbate neurology.

Clinical
- **Clinically isolated syndrome** (CIS): a first episode of neurologic symptoms that lasts at least 24 h and is caused by inflammation or demyelination. In itself it cannot substantiate a diagnosis of MS.
- **Optic neuritis:** altered colour vision, blind spots, some visual loss.
- **Cerebellum/connections:** vertigo, nystagmus, ipsilateral cerebellar signs.
- **Brainstem:** ataxia, rubral tremor, VI nerve palsy or INO with diplopia, vertigo, nausea, vomiting, hiccup (area postrema), difficulty swallowing.

- **Subcortical white matter:** C/L weakness and sensory signs, dysarthria. Rarely dysphasia.
- **Cord:** transverse myelitis. Shock-like sensation on flexing neck (Lhermitte's symptom), tingling, weakness, sphincter disturbance.

Differentials

- **ADEM:** single episode, multiple lesions, seizures, reduced GCS. Post vaccination/ viral. MRI – multiple enhancing CNS lesions.
- **MS:** single CIS and later relapsing recurring lesions. May be primary or secondarily progressive.
- **Progressive multifocal leucoencephalopathy:** JC virus in immunosuppressed, AIDS (CD4 50–100), natalizumab, rituximab.
- **Stroke disease:** multiple subcortical lesions, diabetic, HTN – consider CADASIL.
- **Rare:** other rarer leucodystrophies. **NMO** – transverse myelitis affecting 3+ levels with optic neuritis. High cervical lesions can affect respiration. Needs steroids. NMO (aquaporin 4) antibody.

Investigations

- **Bloods:** FBC, U&E, CRP. Urinalysis. CXR. HIV test. NMO AQP4-IgG.
- **CT scan:** May show subcortical hypodensity. Excludes some differentials. MRI is the modality of choice.
- **MRI head and spine:** defines size, location, number and acuteness and aetiology of lesions (e.g. MS patients do have strokes). MS shows round or ovoid lesions in the periventricular and corpus callosum, which may have been clinically silent. Best seen on T2 and FLAIR sequences. Acute plaques enhance with gadolinium as rings. Linear Dawson's fingers perpendicular to ventricles. Older lesions in brainstem and cerebellum or cervical cord.
- **CSF:** increased IgG and oligoclonal bands in CSF not found in serum. CSF analysis to exclude any infective cause particularly before considering steroids if diagnostic uncertainty.

Management

- Any individual who experiences an acute episode (including optic neuritis) sufficient to cause distressing symptoms or an increased limitation on activities should be offered steroids. Consider IV **Methylprednisolone** 1 g daily for 3–5 d or **Methylprednisolone** 500 mg OD PO for 5 d within 14 d of the onset of relapse symptoms. NICE recommends no more than 3 courses/year and steroids should last no longer than 3 weeks. Those not treated should improve and admission needed only if unable to manage at home. Steroids do not reduce disability and can have adverse effects on weight, BP, bones and diabetes.
- **Neurology review** needed for disease-modifying therapies (DMTs). **ADEM** treated with steroids and potentially PLEX. **NMO: Eculizumab** adults with neuromyelitis spectrum disorder (NMO) who have the AQP4 antibody.
- Rehabilitation and specialist MS neurologist review (now 13+ agents available) and neurorehabilitation and advice on catheters and other issues.
- **MS prognosis** worse if motor rather than sensory symptoms and high number and volume of lesions on brain MRI and younger age of onset.
- **Reference:** NICE (2014) CG186: Multiple sclerosis in adults: management.

11.34 ▶ Acute peripheral mononeuropathy

- **About:** usually either vascular or pressure. Occasionally toxic. Weakness is LMN with fasciculations, wasting, areflexia.
- **Patterns: mononeuropathy:** flaccid weakness or sensory loss in distribution of a single peripheral nerve. **Mononeuritis multiplex:** multiple mononeuropathies. **Polyneuropathy:** often length related and so start distally. GBS, AIDP, CIDP.
- **Aetiology:** deficient B12, folate. Alcohol. Chemotherapeutic agents, amiodarone, lead. Metabolic: diabetes.

Causes
- **Trauma:** pressure impairs vascular supply and damages nerve.
- **Vascular:** HTN, DM, acute onset.
- **Motor:** porphyria, lead, diphtheria, GBS/CIDP, drugs.
- **Sensory:** alcohol, DM, hypothyroid, uraemia, sarcoid, paraneoplastic, B12 deficiency, amyloid.

Investigations
- None needed if clear cause, e.g. trauma or compression.
- FBC, U&E, ESR, B12, folate, TFT, glucose, ferritin iron, PPE, HIV.

Acute peripheral neuropathies
- **Radial nerve:** wrist drop. Pressure on nerve as wraps around humerus and often lies between skin and bone and can be damaged and awareness reduced, e.g. anaesthetised by alcohol excess or perioperative with arm resting on edge. Median and ulnar nerve intact.
- **Median nerve:** carpal tunnel syndrome pain in hand and arm worst at night.
- **Ulnar nerve:** commonly entrapped at the elbow (medial epicondyle) and can be exacerbated by repetitive or prolonged use of the elbow. Causes weakness of small muscles of the hand. Differential is C8 lesion.
- **Common peroneal nerve:** high stepping gait. Look for a history of extrinsic compression at neck of fibula. Sensory to lateral calf. Sensation to space between 1st and 2nd toe. Spares the 5th toe. Reflexes, plantars and ankle jerk normal. Differentiate from L5 lesion (back pain with sensory loss outer thigh to buttocks with prolapse at L4/5). If unsure get spine imaging. Worldwide commonest cause is leprosy. Also diabetes.
- **Facial nerve** (VII): Bell's palsy, Ramsay Hunt syndrome, ▶Section 11.32.
- **III/IV/VI:** causes diplopia. Painful IIIrd nerve suggests SOL/aneurysm. Emergency CTA. CT/MRI as needed to exclude brainstem stroke.

Management
- Often conservative. Treat any pressure palsy. Manage any diabetes. Often resolves after several weeks. Consider splinting in neutral position, ensuring mobility passively continued to prevent stiffness.

11.35 ▶ Motor neurone disease

- **About:** slow insidious onset with UMN/LMN signs. May present acutely with weakness or aspiration. In USA called amyotrophic lateral sclerosis.
- **Clinical:** aged 40+ (sometimes younger). Progressive weakness over weeks or longer. Mixed UMN/LMN in arms and legs in the same areas with florid

fasciculations, wasting, hyperreflexia, **no diplopia or sensory loss or sphincter involvement.** Bulbar palsy. Sphincters preserved. Wasting fasciculation especially in hands, legs and tongue. Muscle wasting causes weight loss. Look in the mouth! Wasted fasciculating tongue. Exaggerated jaw jerk.

- **Investigations:** EMG. May need MRI head and spine.
- **Differential:** multifocal motor neuropathy with conduction block affecting males in 40s, cervical spondylosis.
- **Management:** supportive. Ventilatory assistance in some. PEG tube can help. Palliation. **Riluzole** adds 2–3 months to life expectancy of 2 years from diagnosis. Course can be unpredictable. Death average 2 years from diagnosis.

11.36 Acute hydrocephalus and shunts

- **About:** hydrocephalus is an excessive accumulation of cerebrospinal fluid (CSF) within the head caused by a disturbance of formation, flow or absorption. CSF volume 120–150 ml. Body produces 500 ml/d from choroid plexus. Travels from lateral ventricles via 3rd ventricle via aqueduct into 4th ventricle and out via foramina of Magendie and Luschka. Into subarachnoid space. CSF production falls as ICP rises and compensation (stabilisation of hydrocephalus at a new steady state) may occur through transventricular absorption of CSF.
- **Types: communicating:** CSF flow is unimpeded due to obstruction to CSF reabsorption. **Obstructive:** there is a partial or total occlusion to CSF flow somewhere in the normal pathway. The proximal cavities are distended. There is a pressure differential. LP can result in herniation and should be avoided. **Normal pressure hydrocephalus:** enlarged ventricles on CT. ICP seems normal.
- **Acute causes in adults: communicating:** haemorrhage, meningitis, SAH, head injury, idiopathic, cerebral venous sinus thrombosis. **Non-communicating:** tumour, colloid cyst, mass, haemorrhage, posterior fossa infarct/bleed/tumour.
- **Clinical:** symptoms of raised ICP (▶ Section 11.37), slowing of mental capacity, unsteadiness, incontinence, drowsiness, headaches. Gait dyspraxia, dementia, rarely papilloedema. May also be symptoms of causes, e.g. sarcoid, TB, meningitis, malignancy.
- **Investigations:** CT: shows distended ventricles proximal to obstructed system. Enlargement of the temporal horns (best indicator). The temporal and frontal horns dilate first, often asymmetrically. CT also can show periventricular oedema or 'lucency'. If 3rd ventricle dilated there will be outward bowing of the lateral walls. Assess the size of the fourth ventricle – if large, this suggests a communicating hydrocephalus, whereas a relatively small 4th ventricle implies obstructive hydrocephalus that might be best treated by endoscopic 3rd ventriculostomy rather than a ventriculo-peritoneal shunt. MRI shows distended system and oedema around the ventricles. MRI may also show the site and cause of blockage if not apparent on CT. Transependymal oedema, or periventricular oozing, may be visible as high T2. **NB:** LPs if needed can be performed only in cases of communicating hydrocephalus.
- **Management: medical: acetazolamide** reduces CSF. **Mannitol** *in extremis.* Consider urgent neurosurgical referral for ventriculo-peritoneal (VP) shunt. Alternatives for obstruction are endoscopic 3rd ventriculostomy. Shunts have a valve which drains if CSF pressure >10 mmHg. The shunt is normally inserted through a burr hole in the right parieto-occipital region and the valve will usually sit behind the right ear.

- **Shunt blockage:** drowsiness is by far the best clinical predictor of VP shunt block. Headache and vomiting are less predictive of acute shunt block. Other symptoms reported are seizures, abdominal pseudocyst, syringomyelia, cranial nerve palsies and hemiparesis. Causes include choroid plexus, red cells, tumour cells or a high CSF protein concentration. Infection is always a concern. Wherever possible CT scan findings should be interpreted in the context of previous imaging. NB: not all cases of proven shunt blockage present with an increase in ventricle size. Take neurosurgical advice.
- **Reference:** Pople (2002) Hydrocephalus and shunts: what the neurologist should know. *J Neurol Neurosurg Psychiatry*, 73:i17.

11.37 Managing raised intracranial pressure

- **About: raised** ICP can lead to coning and death. Needs rapid diagnosis and treatment. CPP = MAP – ICP (or CVP if greater). Remember pressure on the diencephalon and consciousness structures only to rise to that which impairs venous drainage before symptoms of coma are caused.
- **Aetiology:** the brain and CSF and blood are all contained within a rigid bony box. ICP will increase linearly with added volume with some compensation until a point where ICP rise becomes exponential.
- **Causes are excess soft tissue:** benign/malignant/primary/metastatic tumour, cerebral oedema (vasogenic/cytotoxic), brain (DKA, the non-ketotic hyperosmolar state, and low Na), abscess. **Excess CSF:** hydrocephalus (obstructive or communicating), e.g. idiopathic intracranial hypertension, cerebral venous thrombosis, SAH with impaired ventricular drainage. **Excess blood:** haematoma (ICH/SDH/EDH/SAH), vasodilation (raised PCO_2).
- **Clinical:** triad: headache, papilloedema and vomiting often after waking is considered indicative of raised ICP. The headache is worse with coughing, sneezing, recumbency or exertion. Papilloedema: if fundi can be seen. Mydriatics can confuse eye signs and best avoided. Papilloedema usually indicates raised pressure. However, raised ICP may fail to cause papilloedema if the subarachnoid sleeve around the optic nerve does not communicate with the subarachnoid space. Progressive coma: fall in GCS, pupillary dilation, Cheyne–Stokes respiration, low HR, hypertension and additional signs with herniation syndromes. If you see a SOL don't stop there because metastases can be multiple so look at all the slices pre- and post-contrast, always look for an SDH, subarachnoid blood and check no early signs of hydrocephalus.
- **Investigations:** FBC, U&E: may show anaemia and suggest pathology. LFTs – liver failure, alcoholism. CXR: may show a lung tumour or sarcoidosis or TB. Lactate, ABG – sepsis, acidosis. CT brain ± contrast: IV contrast is usually given (ensure IV access) if radiology identify a SOL during initial CT. CT may show haemorrhage or tumour and vasogenic or cytotoxic oedema. May be signs of herniation. Cerebral oedema alone may be due to DKA, traumatic injury, Reye's syndrome, low Na, fulminant hepatic encephalopathy, encephalitis and other toxic/metabolic insults.
- **Non-contrast CT** may show obstructive hydrocephalus with enlarged temporal horns and trans-ependymal oedema as low density margins of the ventricles which can resemble small vessel disease. Measurement of ICP can be by direct invasive measures in a neurological ICU by inserting a probe into ventricles. ▶Section 11.39.

Herniation syndromes

- **Anterior/sub-falcine herniation:** unilateral pressure from above and laterally pushing down and medially pushes the cingulate gyrus under the falx and can nip the contralateral anterior cerebral artery and cause infarction. Usually a superior frontoparietal cortical space-occupying lesion or SDH/EDH. Coma usually, leg weakness, abulia.
- **Trans-tentorial herniation:** compresses IIIrd nerve (ipsilateral), stretching VIth nerve. Posterior cerebral artery (C/L hemianopia), cerebral peduncle (C/L hemiparesis); posterior midbrain: bilateral ptosis, upward gaze; reticular activating system: coma, medulla: HTN and low HR.
- **Uncal herniation:** uncus is displaced medially and inferiorly over the free edge of the tentorium cerebelli. Usually due to a mass inferiorly in the cerebral hemisphere in the temporal lobe. Indentation of the contralateral cerebral peduncle, known as Kernohan's notch, causes ipsilateral hemiparesis, which falsely localises the symptoms to the other side. Clinical: coma, ipsilateral IIIrd nerve palsy, ipsilateral hemiparesis.
- **Kernohan's notch weakness:** fascinatingly rare but does occur. A high cerebral SOL forces the brain down and laterally and compresses the opposite motor fibres in the cerebral peduncle against the tentorium causing a notch and this pressure therefore causes an ipsilateral rather than contralateral weakness to the SOL, e.g. R SDH with R hemiparesis.
- **Tonsillar herniation:** compression of the medulla (apnoea and death), compressed PICA (lateral medullary syndrome). Cushing reflex – raised BP + bradycardia.

Emergency management of raised ICP (take early expert advice)

- **Decide whether treatment is appropriate:** with a massive cerebral injury (infarct or haemorrhage or tumour) and clear evidence of raised ICP then outcome is likely to be poor and palliation may be more appropriate.
- **ABC:** ensure SaO_2 >90%, treat fever, SBP >100 mmHg and elevate the head of the bed by 15–30°. Hypothermia is sometimes used. Monitor blood sugar and attempt glucose control of 5–15 mmol/L. Avoid hypoglycaemia. Manage seizures. Treat anaemia. Treat an ICP >22 mmHg.
- **Surgical:** external ventricular drainage for hydrocephalus, burr holes or craniectomy for large SDH/EDH, hemicraniectomy for malignant MCA, and sub-occipital craniectomy for cerebellar bleed, tumour debulking by surgery or radiotherapy. Use medical measures to buy time to allow transfer to a neurosurgical centre and surgery where useful.
- **Mechanical hyperventilation** to lower $PaCO_2$ <4.0 kPa reduces ICP. Use **propofol, midazolam** and **morphine.**
- **Mannitol** 1 g/kg. Give 100 ml of a 20% solution (20 g) over 15 min. Then give the remainder over 45 min.
- **Dexamethasone 8 mg stat IV and 4 mg QDS PO/IV** if tumour with vasogenic oedema. Steroids also for suspected bacterial or TB meningitis with antimicrobials. Avoid steroids with acute stroke or head trauma.
- **Keep SBP >100 mmHg** consider inotropes/vasopressors to maintain brain perfusion. Autoregulation is impaired and so BP needs to be supported.
- **Infections:** treat if any suspicion of meningitis, encephalitis. Get an LP if safe.
- **Lumbar puncture:** removal of CSF may be dangerous if, for example, there is a large supratentorial mass lesion or hydrocephalus but it can be diagnostic and therapeutic (e.g. idiopathic intracranial hypertension) if there is communicating

hydrocephalus but must only be done after imaging excludes a lesion that could precipitate a herniation syndrome. Take expert advice if unsure.

11.38 Cerebral oedema

- **Vasogenic:** vascular permeability of blood–brain barrier, e.g. tumour (steroids potentially useful). Increased permeability of capillary endothelial cells, tumour, abscess, around a haemorrhage, contusion, meningitis. The neurons and glia are relatively normal in appearance. May respond to steroids. On CT the grey–white matter differentiation is maintained and the oedema involves white matter, extending in finger-like fashion.
- **Cytotoxic:** 'cell death', e.g. ischaemic stroke. Failure of the normal homeostatic mechanisms that maintain cell size: neurons, glia and endothelial cells swell. Due to cellular energy (ATP) failure. Hypoxic ischaemic/infarction, osmolar injury, some toxins; part of the secondary injury sequence following head trauma. Does not respond to steroids. BBB remains intact.
- **Interstitial or transependymal:** characterised by an increase in the water content of the periventricular white matter. Seen with obstruction of CSF flow, e.g. hydrocephalus.

11.39 Neurosurgical options

Procedures
- **Burr holes:** hole through skull which may be done under local anaesthetic to drain extradural haematoma or chronic SDH. Can allow placement of drains or monitoring equipment.
- **Craniectomy:** removal of part of the skull, e.g. hemicraniectomy for malignant MCA syndrome or sub-occipital craniectomy for cerebellar strokes or SOLs. Needs general anaesthesia.
- **Clipping aneurysms:** clip across the base of aneurysm. Requires craniotomy. Hospital stay at least 2–3 d. More complications than coiling.
- **Coiling aneurysms:** neuro-interventionalist (neuroradiologist or neurosurgeon or neurologist) packs detachable platinum coils into the aneurysms to induce thrombosis. Usually done via catheters inserted via femoral artery. Studies have shown that patients with a ruptured aneurysm tend to do better in the long term after a coiling procedure. Hospital stay shorter.
- **Biopsy:** indicated to get tissue samples of areas within the brain suspicious for tumours or infections. A simple biopsy may be done for easy to access lesions. Stereotactic biopsy may be needed for deep-seated lesions, multiple lesions, or lesions in a surgically poor candidate who cannot tolerate anaesthesia.
- **Debulking tumours:** those that cannot be resected completely a palliative debulking can take place to slow progression and symptoms.

11.40 Posterior reversible encephalopathy syndrome

- **About:** PRES is associated with many scenarios, e.g. hypertension, eclampsia, autoimmune conditions, renal failure, sepsis, immunocompromised/suppressed state, HIV, transplants., SLE, Covid-19.
- **Aetiology:** HTN and endothelial injury seem to be almost always present. Vasoconstriction resulting in vasogenic and cytotoxic oedema is found.

- **Clinical:** sudden visual disturbances, headache, vomits, seizures, reduced GCS.
- **Investigations:** FBC, U&E, CRP. CXR. CT/MRI head: symmetrical bilateral white matter lesions suggest oedema are seen usually but not exclusively in the posterior parieto-occipital regions of the cerebral hemispheres. LP/CSF to exclude infectious/inflammatory process. Toxicology screen.
- **Management:** supportive. Treat BP and remove or treat any underlying cause. May need ITU. Manage seizures. Mortality up to 19%. **Obstetric cases:** may be seen with pre-eclampsia. O_2, ABC, obstetric emergency IV **Magnesium sulfate**. Fetal monitoring and delivery planning: recommended but timing depends on gestational age and fetal maturity and risk to mother of continuing the pregnancy. Obstetrician may give steroids to improve lung maturity if delivery planned within 1 week. Commence labetalol.

11.41 Reversible cerebral vasoconstriction syndrome

- **About:** only occurs postpartum and is associated with severe hypertension and recurrent thunderclap headaches. Most patients do well. Must be considered in any thunderclap headache presentation. Likely underdiagnosed.
- **Common precipitants:** cannabis, binge alcohol consumption, cocaine, postpartum, vascular dissection, surgical manipulation, SSRI, SNRI, steroids, ergots, triptans, epinephrine, interferon alpha, ciclosporin, sulprostone.
- **Clinical:** single or repeated thunderclap headache. Max intensity <1 min. The issue is to differentiate from aSAH. Seizures, focal neurological deficits, ischaemic stroke and non-aneurysmal convexity SAH.
- **Investigations:** MRA/CTA/DSA: 'beads on a string' due to multifocal segmental cerebral artery vasoconstriction on cerebral angiography. Oedema is an early manifestation of RCVS and is usually diagnosed within a few days of clinical onset. It is better seen on MRI than on CT scans, with symmetrical FLAIR hyperintensities showing a distribution similar to that of posterior reversible encephalopathy syndrome. Oedema usually reverses within 1 month, much earlier than does vasoconstriction. May be convexity SAH. LP – increased blood and protein. Repeat angiography at or before 3 months to show resolution.
- **Complications:** PRES, convexity SAH, ICH, ischaemic infarction, seizure.
- **Management:** verapamil/nimodipine may be given. Multiple suggested causes – idiopathic, pregnancy, vasoactive drugs, hypertensive crisis, etc.
- **Reference:** Burton & Bushnell (2019) Reversible cerebral vasoconstriction syndrome. *Stroke*, 50(8):2253.

12 Rheumatology

Introduction
- Always aspirate any red-hot painful joint to exclude septic arthritis, send Gram stain, culture and microscopy for crystals. Involve orthopaedics first if the joint has a prosthesis.

12.1 Septic arthritis

- **About:** infected joint can become a permanently painful and destroyed joint. Involve orthopaedic team and microbiology immediately.
- **Aetiology:** destruction of cartilage begins within 48 h due to pressure, proteases and cytokines from macrophages, bacteria and inflammatory cells.
- **Microbiology:** *Staph. aureus*, streptococci, gonococci, Gram-negatives, Lyme disease, salmonella (sickle cell). Viral – hepatitis B, parvovirus B19, and lymphocytic choriomeningitis viruses. *Cutibacterium acnes* can cause post-op shoulder septic arthritis.
- **Risks:** immunosuppressed, RA, age >80, prosthetic joints, recent steroid joint injections. Sickle cell, IV drug user, gonococcus, cellulitis, ulcers. diabetes.
- **Clinical:** new joint pain/swelling or increase in usual pain, erythema. Immobility (held in maximal position of comfort), systemic fever. Knee 50%, hip 22% and shoulder. Also ankles, wrists, elbow, and PIPs and DIPs. Also sternoclavicular and sacroiliac joints in generally decreasing frequency. Note that concurrent immunosuppression can dampen clinical findings.
- **Differential:** gout, pseudogout, fracture, reactive arthritis, osteoarthritis. RA itself does not give this presentation but it can have secondary infection. Crystal deposition uncommon in RA affected joints. Gonococcus – rash, sexually active. Lyme disease affects knee. Polyarticular – *Haemophilus*, gonococcus, meningococcus.
- **Investigations:** FBC: raised WCC, ESR and CRP, U&E, LFT, bone, urate, glucose, blood culture, CXR. Joint aspiration: relieves pressure and pain in tense effusion. Turbid pus with high WBC, predominantly neutrophils. Send aspirate for Gram stain, microscopy for crystals and culture. Consider urethral culture for gonococcus or skin lesion if STD likely. Plain X-rays to look for bony changes. Ultrasonography: can detect effusions and synovial changes. MRI can show bone and joint destruction and osteomyelitis. Radionuclide leucocyte scans can detect inflammation.
- **Management:** urgent consult with Orthopaedics as requires joint aspiration especially if prosthesis. This will relieve pressure and pain and provide microbiological information. **Flucloxacillin** 1–2 g QDS IV. MRSA-positive consider **vancomycin** or **teicoplanin** IV penicillin allergic. Add **Gentamicin** IV if coliforms are likely. If *N. gonorrhoea* then **Ceftriaxone** IV/IM OD. High risk MRSA consider **vancomycin** IV (adjusted to renal function).
- **Contact consultant microbiologist** if risk factors for, or evidence of, MRSA colonisation or infection or HIV-positive patient. Orthopaedic review as arthroscopy or open surgery may be required. Prosthetic joint infections: needs urgent microbiologist and orthopaedic review. Empirical therapy is usually not indicated unless patient is septic. Later physiotherapy and rehabilitation may be required.

12.2 Osteomyelitis

- **About:** infection of bone. Leads to pain, deformity and chronic disease. Differing picture in adults and children. Sickle cell disease and salmonella infection. Infection either haematogenous or direct from local wound sepsis.
- **Adult disease:** most due to *Staph. aureus*, enterobacter or streptococcus. In older adults the vertebral bodies are more likely to be infected, due to changes in blood flow with spinal osteomyelitis. TB remains prevalent in certain groups.
- **Risks:** compound fractures, prostheses, diabetes, alcoholism, AIDS, immunosuppression. Sickle cell, IV drug abuse (vertebrae), chronic steroids.
- **Clinical:** toxic, febrile and rigors, localised bone pain – long bone or spine, foot, tenderness, warmth and swelling. Children can have vague symptoms for weeks.
- **Investigations:** FBC: raised ESR, WCC and CRP. Plain X-ray: unreliable (will take 2–4 weeks for demineralisation of bone). Periosteal elevation is often found on plain film radiography. This finding, however, can lag up to 2 weeks behind the onset of the infection. MRI is sensitive but not specific as it cannot distinguish osteomyelitis from other causes of marrow oedema, such as normal post-surgical changes. Negative MRI findings essentially exclude osteomyelitis. Blood cultures positive in 50% of cases of acute osteomyelitis. Obtain pus by open surgery or needle aspiration. Bone biopsy for culture and histology.
- **Differential:** synovitis, trauma and fracture, bone cancer, sickle cell crisis.
- **Management:** rapid diagnosis and orthopaedic and microbiology liaison to choose optimal antimicrobial therapy. Acute osteomyelitis: **Flucloxacillin** 1–2g QDS IV ± **Fusidic acid** PO. Penicillin allergy: **Teicoplanin** IV + **Fusidic acid** PO. Duration of therapy: usually 4–6 weeks (minimum 2 weeks IV). High risk of MRSA add **Vancomycin** IV. Discuss with microbiology. Surgical: debridement and removal of necrotic tissue and drainage of any abscess or collections. Replacement of dead space with tissue flaps or bone grafts. Internal/external fixation. Amputation may be needed. Sickle cell disease: *Staph. aureus* and salmonella often involved organisms.

12.3 Reactive arthritis

- **About:** inflamed joint but sterile joint aspirate. Infection may be a trigger.
- **Aetiology:** salmonella, chlamydial, shigella, campylobacter. Others may be post viral, e.g. hepatitis B, parvovirus B19, hepatitis C, rubella, HIV, EBV. Post streptococcal with glomerulonephritis and vasculitis.
- **Clinical:** coexisting urethritis, conjunctivitis, diarrhoeal illness, males > females. Balanitis, keratoderma blennorrhagica (soles of feet). Large joints, knee, sacroiliitis, fever, malaise.
- **Investigations:** joint aspirate excludes infection and crystals. Raised WCC, ESR and CRP. Urethral swab. Stool for culture. Consider HIV test.
- **Management:** rest joint, NSAIDs, intra-articular steroids. Treat urethritis. Rheumatology review.

12.4 Acute gout and pseudogout

Never use allopurinol or febuxostat if on azathioprine or ciclosporin as may result in fatal pancytopenia.

- **About:** 20% population raised uric acid, 20% develop gout. Uric acid is product of purine metabolism. Humans lack uricase. 90% of the uric acid filtered at the glomerulus is taken up in proximal convoluted tubule. Pseudogout due to calcium pyrophosphate deposits (CPPDs).
- **Aetiology:** monosodium urate (MSU) crystallises in joint. Causes local inflammatory response.
- **Risks:** obese, thiazides, low dose aspirin (<3 g/d), ciclosporin. Fructose syrup. Renal disease, myelo-/lymphoproliferative, psoriasis, alcohol, red meat. Rare purine enzyme defects (Lesch–Nyhan syndrome), glycogen storage disease. Pseudogout seen with haemochromatosis, hyperparathyroidism, Wilson's disease, alkaptonuria.
- **Clinical:** red hot swollen painful joint, often 1st toe (podagra), ankle or knee onset age 40–60 usually. Pain often overnight. Fever, malaise. Attack usually lasts 1–2 weeks. Over time develops gouty tophi and microtophi in joints. Gout affects men more and in older women affects joints damaged by OA, e.g. knees or DIP joints with Heberden nodes. Clinically similar. Pseudogout common in elderly women and affects the knee or wrist.
- **Differential:** bacterial infection, soft tissue injury or fracture, sarcoidosis and CPPD arthropathy (pseudogout).
- **Investigations:** U&E, LFTs, FBC, raised ESR and CRP, TFT, calcium. Glucose, lipid. **Urate:** elevated level. Levels may fall during a flare. Upper limit is 420 μmol/L in males; 360 μmol/L in females. Gout rare if levels <360 μmol/L. **Joint aspiration:** MSU crystals – intracellular needle-shaped crystals with strong negative birefringence is diagnostic. Taken from aspiration of joint, bursa or tophus. CPPD crystals show rhomboidal, weakly positively birefringent crystals. Always send for Gram stain and culture of the fluid. May be elevated WCC. **Plain films** may be needed if fracture is a concern or erosive arthritis in chronic gout. **Haemochromatosis:** transferrin saturation is increased (50–100%) and serum ferritin is substantially elevated (>1.1 to 7.4 μmol/L (90–600 mg/dl or 900–6000 mcg/L).
- **Management:** lifestyle: hydration, obesity. Reduce red meat and alcohol, high fructose corn syrup. **Acute gout/pseudogout:** joint aspiration can reduce pain. NSAIDs may be tried first if no contraindication. Early active mobilisation is important. **Colchicine** 1 mg stat PO then 500 mcg QDS (max dose of 6 mg taken or diarrhoea). A low dose **Colchicine** 500 mcg BD may be given for weeks with allopurinol. Lastly a short course of **Prednisolone** 10–20 mg OD may be considered for a week or more.
- **Prevention:** urate-lowering therapy for repeated severe gout attacks with target urate <300–360 μmol/L. Do not start until 1 month after acute attack has settled and give along with NSAID/colchicine for 2–4 weeks. **Allopurinol** 100 mg/d increasing slowly over weeks to 300–600 mg/d to lower urate. Alternatives: **Febuxostat** 40–80 mg OD. Continue urate-lowering therapy for 6 months at least. Losartan may help to lower uric acid.

12.5 ▸ Rheumatoid arthritis

- **About:** known patient with RA and acute flare-up. In older patients can cause immobility – 'off legs'.
- **Clinical:** painful joint(s). Usually warm and tender to touch or squeeze. Involves wrists, MCP, PIP, ankles, etc. Morning stiffness. Rarely red hot joint. Active synovitis. Specialists may assess disease activity score.

- **Investigations:** raised WCC/ESR/CRP. U&E. Aspirate joint for infection/crystals. Exclude infection before steroids. Rheumatoid factor, anti-CCP rise may come years before clinical manifestations.
- **Management:** rest but maintain some mobility. NSAIDs and other methods such as applying heat/cold can ease stiffness or pain. Consider low dose **Prednisolone** 20 mg OD and assessment of other DMARDs, e.g. methotrexate, sulfasalazine. May consider IM depot of steroids. Very severe flares with systemic complications may need IV **methylprednisolone.** Rheumatological review when possible. Steroids often used to bridge the onset of action of DMARD to suppress disease progression. Consider bisphosphonate and calcium 1 g/d and vitamin D 800 U/d.

12.6 Shoulder pain

- **About:** glenohumeral is a ball-and-socket joint which gives shoulder a wide range of movement. It is held together by the rotator cuff. Inside the capsule is the synovium, which lubricates the joint. Above the shoulder joint is a smaller acromioclavicular joint which helps the shoulder to move through its full range, particularly when you're raising your arm, lifting or throwing.

Shouder pain: trauma often a precipitant

- **Osteoarthritis:** common. Often previous injury. Cartilage thin with osteophytes. Can be very painful. Limits arm and shoulder. Physiotherapy can help. Painkillers. NSAIDs. A steroid injection may be helpful. Discuss pros and cons of joint replacement surgery.
- **Polymyalgia rheumatica:** pain and stiffness shoulders and pelvis. Worse in morning. Responds to oral steroids.
- **Rheumatoid arthritis:** stiffness, pain and swelling. Joint replacement.
- **Calcific tendonitis:** pain, swelling and difficulty moving shoulder. Calcium crystals form inside tendon. Steroids may help. Keyhole surgery.
- **Frozen shoulder (adhesive capsulitis):** tight capsule around the joint. Seen after an injury, MI, stroke, diabetes. Can take 2–3 years to settle. Pains often at night. Steroids may help. Physiotherapy and exercise. Most recover.
- **Shoulder impingement or painful arc syndrome:** Pain from rotator cuff. Causes swelling, pain or damage to the tendons. Painful and difficult to move arm. Arm may feel weak. Needs rest and physiotherapy and analgesia. If the pain persists or recurs may need keyhole surgery.
- **Subacromial bursitis:** pain and swelling. Difficulty to raise arm above your head. Inflamed bursa. Seen post fall. Needs rest, physiotherapy and NSAID tablets or creams. Surgery is rarely needed.
- **A torn rotator cuff:** may be no history of trauma. Painful and difficult to raise arm above shoulder height. Diagnosed by MRI.

Management

- Simple analgesia, hot or cold therapies.
- Physiotherapy to improve usage and muscle function.
- Surgery in selected cases.

13 Ophthalmology

Introduction

- Ophthalmological problems are best dealt with by ophthalmic urgent care. They have the skills and equipment to perform a comprehensive eye examination. The most important part of any eye exam is detecting reversible reductions in vision. An assessment of acuity must always be made. The red eye and the blind eye are easy enough to diagnose. It is surprising how patients with structural brain lesions do not appreciate their hemianopia even when gross. Occasionally a red eye can be associated with systemic disease. The headache and painful IIIrd nerve signifying an expanding saccular aneurysm about to rupture is an important diagnosis not to miss. Horner's syndrome is a useful sign in stroke medicine and apical lung tumours. Those with suspected amaurosis fugax (transient monocular blindness) need an antiplatelet and referral to TIA services. Giant cell arteritis (GCA) mustn't be missed – steroids must be started to preserve vision in the unaffected eye to prevent complete blindness.
- Consider urgent ophthalmic referral for severe ocular pain, photophobia, sudden reduction in vision, coloured halos around point of light, proptosis or smaller pupil in affected eye. Any involvement of cornea or visual loss or glaucoma or orbital cellulitis or severe symptoms needs ophthalmic review.

13.1 ▶ Acute visual loss

- **About:** always assess and document acuity. Check ESR and CRP if GCA suspected and consider starting high dose steroids and urgent referral for temporal artery biopsy or ultrasound and expert assessment.

Causes

- **Arteritic anterior ischaemic optic neuropathy:** arteritic 'inflammatory' AION usually due to GCA. Occlusion of posterior ciliary artery which supplies optic nerve. Usually painless. Raised ESR/CRP. Aged >50. Temporal artery tenderness. Headache, jaw claudication. Usually unilateral but may proceed to complete visual loss in both eyes. Afferent pupillary defect. Start steroids: **Prednisolone** 1 mg/kg if suspected. ▶Section 13.4 on GCA below. Consider PPI with steroids.
- **Non-arteritic anterior ischaemic optic neuropathy:** atherosclerotic or thromboembolic occlusion of posterior ciliary artery which supplies optic nerve. Usually painless, associated with arteriosclerotic vascular disease, older males. Usually unilateral but may proceed to complete visual loss in both eyes. Atrial fibrillation. Main issue is differential from GCA. Afferent pupillary defect. Treat as for stroke disease. Echo for embolic source. ECG for AF. Carotid Doppler may show plaques or stenosis on affected side; assess and manage vascular risk factors.
- **Central retinal artery occlusion:** sudden severe visual loss in seconds. Afferent pupillary defect. May be complete or affect branches. Retina is pale and white with a cherry-coloured spot at macula. Associated with vascular risk factors. If seen within first hour, sudden pressure and release to the globe may dislodge embolism or propel it peripherally. Refer all patients who present with retinal artery occlusion within 24 h of the symptoms to ophthalmologist to attempt dislodging the embolus causing the occlusion. After 24 h from onset refer them to an ophthalmologist

within 1 week who may refer on to TIA clinic. Should have carotid Dopplers and ESR/CRP to exclude GCA. Give steroids immediately if GCA suspected. IV thrombolysis has been trialled and looks promising but awaits further evidence. A recent review suggests that a clinical trial of early systemic fibrinolytic therapy for CRAO is warranted within a 4.5 h window and that conservative treatments are futile and may be harmful [*JAMA Neurol* 2015;72:1148].

- **Central/branch retinal vein occlusion** (CRVO/BRVO): sudden or gradual painless visual loss in seconds. Afferent pupillary defect. May be complete or affect branches. Fundi – retina is red with haemorrhage with bloody venous infarction and engorged dilated retinal veins. HTN, DM, atherosclerosis, and glaucoma are major risk factors for the development of CRVO/BRVO in older patients. Others are vasculitis and thrombophilia. If seen within first hour sudden pressure and release to the globe may dislodge embolism or propel it peripherally. Several trials support the use of vascular endothelial growth factor (VEGF) inhibitors and intravitreal corticosteroids for the treatment of macular oedema in CRVO and BRVO. A fluorescein angiogram shows delayed filling in venous phase. Rare causes: Behçet's syndrome, antiphospholipid syndrome, and protein C deficiency, sarcoidosis.
- **Retinal detachment:** painless progressive visual loss depending on retinal area detached. If macula affected then central vision is lost. May see floaters and describe flashes of light. Fundoscopy shows pigmented cells in vitreous. Retinal detachment or break. In retinal detachment, the inner sensory retina detaches from the underlying pigmented epithelium of the retina. Patients also describe a shadow or curtain that comes across their field of vision. The most common cause of retinal detachment is a tear or hole in the retina that may be secondary to a posterior vitreous detachment or an ocular trauma.
- **Corneal ulcer:** severe pain, red eye and visual loss (see Red eye, ▶ Section 13.2).
- **Acute angle closure glaucoma:** pain + red eye + visual loss (see Red eye, ▶ Section 13.2).
- **Occipital stroke:** may give only clinical finding as visual loss. Haemorrhagic or infarction. May give homonymous hemianopia but bilateral strokes may occur depending on aetiology. ▶ Section 11.19. Bilateral occipital lesions. Anton's syndrome: blind patient maintains they can see. A form of visual anosognosia.
- **Occipital/parietal/temporal tumour:** visual loss and hemianopia progressive ± headache.
- **Optic neurltis:** eye movements may be painful. May be seen as a first presentation of multiple sclerosis or NMO. Often young and more commonly female. Monocular blindness comes on over hours so more subacute than acute. Afferent pupillary defect. Vision worse with heat. Variable defects and scotomas. Altered colour perception initially. Optic disc may be normal or swollen. Some recovery over 2–6 weeks with residual temporal pallor. Discuss high dose IV **methylprednisolone** with Neurology.
- **Vitreous haemorrhage:** may be due to proliferative retinopathy. Blood may obscure retina and loss of red reflex and afferent pupillary defect.
- **Pituitary apoplexy:** sudden headache and visual loss and possible IIIrd nerve palsy. Steroids for acute pituitary insufficiency and urgent neurosurgical decompression if vision affected (▶ Section 5.9).

13.2 Red eye

- **About:** patients with a red eye should go straight to eye casualty but may be misdirected to the general take. Watch for acute angle closure glaucoma in older patients where the presentation can be unclear.

Differentials

- **Allergic conjunctivitis:** allergic (history and other features of atopy). Conjunctiva is red and injected and there may be a discharge and anything from tingling to pain. Vision is normal. Cornea normal. Consider local steroids.
- **Bacterial conjunctivitis:** vision is normal. Cornea normal. Red conjunctiva, swollen eyelids, more purulent discharge. Vision may be reduced. Gritty eye. Good hand hygiene. Treat with **Chloramphenicol** 0.5% one drop at least 2 h. Continue for 48 h post resolution. Occasionally due to gonorrhoea where it is very severe with discharge and chemosis, preauricular node enlargement. Needs topical penicillin.
- **Viral conjunctivitis:** epidemics common. Painful red eye with watery exudate and conjunctiva can be bilateral. Vision is normal. Cornea normal. Eyelids can be swollen. Preauricular node. Good hand hygiene. May consider treatment with **Chloramphenicol** 0.5% if bacterial infection in differential. Can also be due to chlamydia.
- **Acute anterior uveitis** (iritis): red eye + pain + visual loss. Both redness, tearing and ocular pain on palpation over the sclera and involvement of the anterior chamber which can blur vision. Vessels dilated around the cornea. Pupil constricted, keratic precipitates and hypopyon in anterior chamber. Ophthalmic referral. Check CRP/ ESR, ANA, RF, etc. Associated with ankylosing spondylitis (HLA-B27), inflammatory bowel disease, sarcoid, tuberculosis, syphilis, toxoplasmosis, Behçet's syndrome, etc. Management for inflammatory causes is topical steroids with cyclopentolate 1%.
- **Corneal ulcer/abrasion:** red eye + intense pain + visual loss. Corneal defect on fluorescein staining. Needs ophthalmology and **Aciclovir** ointment 5/d for 2 weeks if HSV considered.
- **Acute angle closure glaucoma:** unilateral red eye + pain + visual loss. Halos around lights. Emergency and patients have an acute elevation in intraocular pressure. Mid dilated pupil. IOP >45 mmHg. Aged >50. May have systemic symptoms of N&V even abdominal symptoms. Seen later in day/evening as pupils dilate. Exam shows narrow anterior chamber and needs urgent ophthalmic referral. Give **Acetazolamide** 250–500 mg IV over 10 min (check for contraindications) and pilocarpine 4% drops to constrict pupil.
- **Subconjunctival haemorrhage:** common, painless, may be associated with trauma or simple coughing and exacerbated by anticoagulants (check INR if on warfarin). Conservative management.
- **Orbital cellulitis:** needs a low threshold for IV antibiotics. Take expert help. Monitor visual acuity. (▶Section 19.3).
- **Ophthalmic herpes zoster or simplex:** inflammation of the cornea. May be due to HSV. Pain, foreign body sensation and photophobia and lacrimation. HSV ulcer shows up with fluorescein zoster rash over eye. Can affect cornea. Needs ophthalmic review. **Aciclovir** 800 mg 5/d + **Aciclovir** 3% ointment applied 5/d.

13.3 ▶ Neuro-ophthalmology

- **Advice:** CT is excellent for detecting bleed. MRI can positively confirm stroke or other lesion, e.g. plaque. MR angiography for aneurysms. Always check visual acuity with some form of quantitative assessment that can be repeated. Snellen chart if available. Take expert advice early if unsure.
- Much acute neurology is vascular and stroke or neurology team may be helpful. Important diagnoses are raised ICP, acute hydrocephalus, large SOLs, pituitary apoplexy and expanding aneurysms. Large posterior communicating aneurysms may not be seen on non-contrast CT.

Differentials

- **Horner's syndrome:** disruption of sympathetic tract from ipsilateral thalamus through brainstem, cervical cord, thorax and lung apex along carotid artery to the eye. Small miosed pupil with mild ptosis. Three main diagnoses are lateral medullary syndrome, apical lung tumour and carotid dissection. Needs MRI/MR angiography brain ± CT chest.
- **Surgical IIIrd nerve lesion:** ptosis with dilated pupil down and out. Can be incomplete and milder versions. Concern is a posterior communicating aneurysmal expansion with pressure on IIIrd nerve as a sign of impending rupture and catastrophic SAH. Urgent CTA/MRA and neurosurgical consult.
- **Stroke IIIrd nerve lesion:** ptosis with dilated pupil down and C/L hemiparesis seen with Weber's syndrome and medial midbrain infarction often affects thalamus too. Needs MRI/MRA.
- **Medical IIIrd nerve:** ptosis with non-dilated pupil down and out and less severe variants. Damage to vasa nervorum supplying core of nerve. Pupillary fibres on nerve surface and unaffected. Needs work-up for vascular disease. Diabetes, HTN and rarer causes of ischaemic neuropathy. Manage as outpatient. MRI and vascular work up, start antiplatelet. Ophthalmic support.
- **Parinaud's syndrome:** lesion dorsal midbrain affecting IVth nerve with inability to look up. Confirm with MRI.
- **Internuclear ophthalmoplegia:** damage to the medial longitudinal fasciculus and the connections that yoke the eyes together between IIIrd and VIth nerve nuclei for lateral gaze. Failure to adduct with nystagmus in abducting eye. Usually seen in MS and stroke. Needs MRI. 'Can't add'.
- **Diplopia:** monocular diplopia is an eye rather than neurology issue. Binocular diplopia always consider orbital and intracranial issues affecting III/IV and VI and their connections with MLF. Exclude compressive lesion and orbital pathology, e.g. Graves' disease. Look for other localising signs to help, e.g. VI and VII suggests pontine lesion. C/L hemiparesis and IIIrd is midbrain. MRI is test of most use and if normal may simply be a cranial neuropathy which can be worked up with risk factors – DM, HTN and sarcoid, B12, folate etc., but can be often idiopathic and settle conservatively. Consider also Wernicke–Korsakoff syndrome and **Pabrinex** IV × 2 vials TDS for 3–5 d if suspected.
- **Intermittent diplopia:** suggests myasthenia gravis with fatiguability. Associated ptosis. Needs Tensilon test and Neurology follow-up.
- **Bitemporal visual loss:** may be asymmetrical. Always consider pituitary apoplexy and/or tumour. Will need IV **hydrocortisone** + neurosurgical referral.
- **Homonymous hemianopia:** will be a stroke or SOL. Needs CT/MRI brain.

- **Ophthalmoplegic migraine:** recurrent episodes of headache and associated symptoms and diplopia which resolves. Initial events need full work-up.
- **Retinal migraine:** recurrent episodes of headache and associated visual symptoms – fortification spectra, scotomas, bright lights, monocular blindness. Initial events need full work-up to exclude occipital lobe lesion, e.g. MRI.
- **Papilloedema:** optic nerve oedema. Raised ICP, idiopathic intracranial hypertension, SOL, tumours, SDH, EDH, SAH, AVM, hydrocephalus. Needs CT head.
- **Optic neuritis:** acute visual loss. Idiopathic, MS, viral, TB, sarcoid, visual loss over hours/days. (▶ Section 13.1).

13.4 Giant cell (temporal) arteritis

- **About:** inflammation of small and mid-sized arteries with occlusion/infarction. Occluded posterior ciliary arteries causing an anterior ischaemic optic neuropathy (AION). Atypical cases occur and can be a diagnostic challenge. Treat first and get TAB/USS and expert opinion later. Delayed treatment can result in complete blindness.
- **Aetiology:** commoner in females. Superficial temporal, posterior ciliary and ophthalmic arteries. Immune attack to the internal elastic lamina of the vessel wall. Large vessel disease can show aortic inflammation on PET scanning.
- **Pathology:** granulomatous infiltration, disruption of the internal elastic lamina, proliferation of the intima, occlusion of the lumen.
- **Clinical:** headache, jaw, tongue claudication (pain when chewing). Temporal artery tenderness and loss of pulse. Transient or permanent monocular visual loss. Systemic symptoms, e.g. weight loss, malaise, fever. PMR – pain over shoulders, proximal weakness. Fundoscopy: white optic disc oedema with splinter haemorrhages at disc margin.
- **Differentials:** migraine, TIA, non-arteritic AION. Optic neuritis, causes of sudden monocular blindness, PMR see Polymyalgia rheumatica, ▶ Section 15.7.
- **Investigations: FBC:** normocytic normochromic anaemia. **B12 folate ferritin:** normal (or ferritin elevated with CRP). **ALP:** elevated. **ESR:** elevated >50 mm/h (classically >100 mm/h). **CRP:** elevated. **Temporal artery biopsy** (TAB): needed within 7–14 d of starting steroids. **MRI:** T1 + gadolinium show increased wall thickness and mural inflammation. **Temporal artery ultrasound:** shows increased diameter of the TA and hypoechoic wall thickening (halo). Resolves with corticosteroid treatment. May be an alternative to TAB.
- **American College of Rheumatology classification criteria:** 3/5 criteria for diagnosis of GCA: sensitivity of 93.5% specificity of 91.2% (1) Age ≥50 y. (2) New onset localised headache. (3) Temporal artery tenderness or decreased temporal artery pulse. (4) ESR >50 mm/h. (5) TAB showing mononuclear infiltration or granulomatous inflammation.
- **Management:** if suspicion then high dose steroids started immediately to avoid any residual visual loss: **Prednisolone** 1 mg/kg usually. Consider PPI with steroids. **Steroids:** reduce slowly over 18 months titrated to clinical response and ESR/CRP. Steroid-sparing agents may be used. Start bone protection. TAB organised urgently and may help adjust therapy. A negative biopsy does not entirely exclude GCA as 'skip lesions'. Consider **Aspirin** 75 mg OD and PPI as well as good BP and vascular risk factor management. TIA/stroke seen in these patients.

14 Toxicology

Introduction

- In the UK, up-to-date and expert online support is available at **Toxbase** which can be accessed from NHS computers. Advice can be sought at the National Poisons Information Service. Also consult local guidelines and experts for help. Similar local and national systems exist in other countries.
- Most overdoses have stabilised by 12 h; however, delayed toxicity may be seen with aspirin, paracetamol, iron, paraquat, TCAs, co-phenotrope and overdoses of modified release preparations. All need admission.
- Death following overdose is rare but can be further reduced with ABC management, early access to ITU if needed and airway protection, ventilatory support, arrhythmias, electrolyte, acid–base, seizure and psychosis management and sedation as needed. Some will need antidotes, bowel irrigation and dialysis. Identify these.

14.1 Interventions to reduce toxicity

Action	Comments
Gastric lavage *Only if highly toxic overdose taken within last hour and airway protected*	Rare now. Airway protection needed to avoid aspiration. Intubated with anaesthetist at hand. Ensure O_2 and suction at hand. Place patient in left lateral head-down position. Raise foot of bed. **Not if corrosive agents or petroleum products** which can cause a chemical pneumonitis and ARDS if aspirated. Lubricated size 36–40 FG stomach tube inserted and attached to a funnel. Listen over stomach for injected air or aspirate gastric juices. If intubated then concerns about being in the trachea are unwarranted. Pour in 300 ml aliquots and then allow aspirate to come out. Massage over stomach to help tablets out. Finish with 50 g of activated charcoal.
Activated charcoal *Binds materials by van der Waal's forces or London dispersion force*	High degree of microporosity; 1 g surface area >500 m². Consider when <2 h since tablets taken. Tablets are toxic and can bind. Can reduce absorption of some substances by up to 60%. It remains within the GI tract and eliminates the toxin in faeces. May require laxative to aid passage. Best taken by cooperative patient or if not then consider administration via NG tube. For drug overdose or poisoning: 50–100 g of activated charcoal is given at first (usually 1 g/kg). Does not bind *iron, lithium, ethanol, methanol or ethylene glycol, mercury, acids, alkalis.*
Multi-dose activated charcoal	Give 50 g 4-hourly to adults. Interrupts enteroenteric, enterogastric, enterohepatic circulation of drugs, e.g. carbamazepine, dapsone, phenobarbital, quinine or theophylline toxicity. Give laxative.
Whole bowel irrigation (WBI)	Non-absorbable polyethylene glycol (PEG) is given via NG tube. About 1–2 L/h for adults. For body packers, sustained release formulations. Does not cause fluid shifts. Watch U&E. Administer until clear effluent from bowels.

Action	Comments
Haemodialysis	For substances **not heavily protein-bound:** alcohol, dabigatran, salicylates, lithium, ethanol, ethylene glycol, valproate, methanol, theophylline, carbamazepine.
Haemoperfusion	Carbamazepine, phenytoin, theophylline, paraquat, theophylline, barbiturates, lipid-soluble drugs.
Urinary alkalinisation	Used in salicylate toxicity. Give 1.5 L of 1.26% sodium bicarbonate over 2 h. Aim is to alkalinise blood and urine to 'trap' ionised salicylate or methotrexate, keep it out of the brain, and enhance urinary elimination. Salicylate toxicity, ▶ Section 14.31 for more. Hypokalaemia, ▶ Section 5.4 is the most common complication. Alkalotic tetany occurs occasionally, but hypocalcaemia is rare.
Intralipid therapy Intravenous fat emulsion (IFE), in the form of Intralipid 20%	Cardiac arrest due to local anaesthetic e.g. bupivacaine and any lipid-soluble drugs. IV fat emulsion (IFE) is given as Intralipid 20%. Treat toxicity from CCBs, haloperidol, TCAs, lipophilic BB, e.g. propranolol, lipid-soluble drugs especially local anaesthetics. Lipid emulsion 20% given at 1.5 ml/kg IV in 1 min as load dose followed by an infusion of 0.25 ml/kg/min for 30–60 min. **In a 70 kg patient** – take a 500 ml bag of Intralipid 20% and a 50 ml syringe, draw up 100 ml and give stat. Attach the Intralipid bag to an IV administration set (macrodrip) and run it IV over the next 15 min. Repeat 100 ml bolus if spontaneous circulation has not returned. Maximum total dose of 10 ml/kg is recommended in first 30 min, i.e. 700 ml. Continue CPR to aid circulation. Further information at www.lipidrescue.org. SE: hyperlipidaemia, pancreatitis, hyperviscosity.
(High dose) insulin–glucose euglycaemic therapy	May be used for beta-blocker and CCB toxicity. Monitored closely HIET is safe, and adverse events are predictable, uncommon and easily managed. Insulin increases glucose and lactate uptake by myocardial cells. It improves function without increased O_2 demand. Insulin promotes excitation–contraction coupling and contractility and acts as an inotrope which is not catecholamine-mediated, or affected by beta-blockers. It appears to improve myocardial contractility. No chronotropic effect. May cause vasodilation. SE: hypoglycaemia, low K, low Mg, low phosphate. **Give** 10% IV glucose with loading bolus of 0.5–1 U/kg Insulin then 1–10 U/kg/h (higher doses may be given according to clinical response). Used in an ITU/HDU setting with close monitoring. Large doses of insulin have been given with few side-effects as long as blood glucose and other electrolytes maintained.

14.2 Toxidromes and supportive management

Anti-cholinergic syndrome deficit of Ach 'dry, dilated and delirious'

Causes: antihistamines, TCA, antipsychotics, antidepressants, atropine and atropine-like drugs, belladonna and other plant-derived agents. Central/peripheral acetylcholine blockade. **Signs:** dry flushed skin and mouth, mydriasis, delirium, high HR, high temp, high resp rate, high BP, reduced bowel sounds, functional ileus, urinary retention, hypertension, hyperthermia, tremulousness and myoclonic jerking. **Management:** supportive, IV diazepam for seizures. IV fluids, ECG monitoring. Beta-blockers for raised HR. Catheterisation for retention.

Cholinergic syndrome excess Ach 'wet and weak' Saliva/urine/resp fluid/diarrhoea

Cause: organophosphates, carbamate insecticides, nerve agents, nicotine, edrophonium. **Excess acetylcholine** at central and peripheral Ach receptors. Low HR, low temp, low resp rate, low BP. May be due to reduced breakdown of Ach by acetylcholinesterase. Seen with sarin/organophosphate poisoning and carbamate pesticides. Excess medications for myasthenia or dementia. Flaccid paralysis, respiratory failure, increased sweating, hypertension, urination, diarrhoea, salivation, low HR, copious bronchial secretions, seizures. **DUMPSS:** diarrhoea, urination, miosis, paralysis, seizure, secretion. **Management:** ABCs. O_2 give antimuscarinic drugs like IV **atropine** and **pralidoxime.** Mechanical ventilation if not improving. Atropine blocks muscarinic sites. Pralidoxime blocks muscarinic and nicotinic sites. Supportive.

Opioid syndrome excess opiates: heroin, morphine, methadone, oxycodone

Clinical: pinpoint pupils, coma, low HR, low BP, constipation, itch. Respiratory depression. **Management:** supportive. **Naloxone.** O_2 as per BTS guidelines. Watch ABG. May need intubation.

Hallucinogenic: phencyclidine, LSD, MDMA

Hallucination, agitation, nystagmus. High HR, RR, high temp.

Serotonin syndrome excess 5HT/serotonin

Causes: MAOI ± SSRIs, neuroleptics. About: excess CNS serotonin, raised HR, BP, resp rate, shivering, sweating, mydriasis, diarrhoea, myoclonic jerks, increased reflexes, clonus, raised temp. Agitation, metabolic acidosis, rhabdomyolysis. DIC, AKI, seizures. **Cause:** antidepressants (SSRIs and SNRIs) and opioids, TCAs, MAOIs, lithium. **Management: diazepam** IV for seizures/agitation and can affect muscle tone. IV fluids. Supportive. Cyproheptadine. Should settle once causative drug stopped. Give O_2 as per BTS guidelines.

Adrenergic syndrome

Agitation, sweating, HTN, raised temp, dilated pupils, seizures, raised HR.

Sedative hypnotics: low HR, low BP, low RR, low temp.

Causes: benzodiazepines, barbiturates, alcohol. Supportive management.

Problems	Management (BB, beta-blockers; CCB, Ca channel blockers)
Acute anxiety or agitation	If symptoms placing patient at risk of harm. Causes include cannabis, alcohol, psychoactive drugs, antimuscarinics. Consider **diazepam IV 5–20 mg, lorazepam 0.5–4 mg IV/IM, haloperidol 0.5–5 mg IM** (not if seizure). Use smallest dose in elderly IM.
Airway	Recovery position (lowermost leg straight and the upper leg flexed) nasopharyngeal airway if comatose. Assess for intubation and ventilation if loss of gag/cough reflex or drop in GCS <9. Pulse oximetry and ABG.
Arrhythmias: *treat any hypoxia, acidosis or hypokalaemia*	**Bradycardia: atropine** 0.5–1 mg IV (max 3 mg), adrenaline, isoprenaline, external/transvenous pacing, calcium (not with digoxin). **High dose insulin–glucose therapy:** BBs, CCB. Give **Glucagon. Digibind** for digoxin overdose. **Sinus tachy:** treat cause. Beta-blockade. **TdP: (drugs):** IV **magnesium sulfate** 2 g (8 mmol) in 100 ml NS over 5 min, cardiac review. **VT:** IV 50 ml 8.4% $NaHCO_3$ for TCA/MAOI. Overdrive pacing, DC shock. Hypokalaemia, ▶ Section 5.4.

Problems	Management (BB, beta-blockers; CCB, Ca channel blockers)
Coma and respiratory depression Due to sedative agents	ABC is key concern. Look for anticonvulsants, antimuscarinics, benzodiazepines, alcohols, opiates, TCAs and consider **naloxone** or **flumazenil** (not if risk of seizure). Enlist help of ITU especially if GCS <9 or any airway compromise, e.g. angioedema or loss of gag reflex or cough. Place in recovery position – lower leg straight, upper flexed. Low threshold to CT head/LP if any concerns of other intracranial pathology. Coma worsened by any drug combined with alcohol/other sedatives. Give **thiamine** and **naloxone** for obtunded.
Delayed toxicity	Paracetamol: day 3: liver/renal failure. Also iron and paraquat.
Hypertension	May respond to **diazepam** if agitated. Treat pain, catheter for acute urinary retention. Consider IV labetalol, IV nitrates or nitroprusside or PO amlodipine. ▶ Section 3.21.
Hyperthermia	Fans, IV fluids and NG fluids, iced baths, **Dantrolene** 1 mg/kg IV. **Chlorpromazine** stops shivering. Intubate/ventilate.
Hypocalcaemia	Ethylene glycol, CCB overdose, 10–20 ml **10% Calcium gluconate** in 100 ml of G5W over 10 min.
Hypoglycaemia	Excluded in all patients with confusion, coma, delirium, by rapid bedside glucose testing. Consider **Glucagon** 1 mg IM/SC but if no response within minutes then 20–50 ml 50% **Glucose** IV or equivalent must be given. Longer-acting insulins/sulfonylureas treat for 24–48 h with 10% glucose. **Octreotide** for sulfonylurea-induced hypoglycaemia.
Hypotension	Raise foot of bed, get patient supine. Fluid resuscitation and/or inotropes/vasopressors depending on cause, e.g. CCB/TCA/BB with negative inotropic effect, ACEi with vasodilation, hypovolaemia needs IV fluids.
Hypothermia	Rewarming blankets. Watch for vasodilation-induced low BP. Give warmed IV and NG/PO fluids at 37°C. Warmed humidified O_2 by face mask.
Hypoxia	Give O_2 as per BTS guidelines; target 94–98% in most and 88–92% in COPD. (Sats do not detect CO poisoning.)
Metabolic acidosis	Look for cause. Check lactate, glucose, ABG, anion gap and osmolar gap if high anion gap. May need IV $NaHCO_3$.
Nausea/vomiting	Check patient has no signs of bowel obstruction. Exclude constipation, infection. Check U&E, FBC, Ca. Consider **metoclopramide, cyclizine, ondansetron.** IV fluids. Pabrinex IV paired vials TDS for 1–2 d if chronic, e.g. hyperemesis, etc.
Oliguria	Often pre-renal so hydrate to aim for urine output (aiming for 35–50 ml/h). Exclude urinary obstruction. Catheter.
Rhabdomyolysis	Pressure necrosis of muscle on hard surface in sedated patient or due to drugs or heat or muscle spasm. Raised CK, muscle pain. Compartment syndrome needing fasciotomy. AKI seen high CK >6000 U but sometimes lower. Good hydration, e.g. NS IV 500 ml/h initially to encourage urine output titrated to avoid overload. Alkalinise urine with $NaHCO_3$ infusion. Diuretics, e.g. furosemide or mannitol may enhance urine output. Treat any hyperkalaemia. Treat severe symptomatic hypocalcaemia.

Problems	Management (BB, beta-blockers; CCB, Ca channel blockers)
Seizures	Due to NSAIDs, AEDs, TCAs, theophylline, alcohol. Needs ABC, **lorazepam** 1–4 mg IV, **diazepam** 5–20 mg IV/PR.
Acute dystonia	Antipsychotics/metoclopramide. Treat with procyclidine, benzatropine, diazepam.

Specific clinical signs

Clinical signs and possible causes

- **Pink, rosy colour:** cyanide, carbon monoxide.
- **Breath:** bitter almonds with cyanide, acetone DKA, peanut smell with certain rodenticides, pear drops smell with chloral hydrate.
- **Nausea, vomiting:** paracetamol, opiates, NSAIDs, iron, salicylates.
- **Bullae:** TCAs, barbiturates.
- **Small pupils:** opiates, GHB, pontine bleed, cholinergic syndrome (insecticides), organophosphates.
- **Mouth: excess salivation:** cholinergics, buprenorphine, clonazepam, haloperidol, risperidone and venlafaxine.
- **Mouth: dry:** antidepressants, antihistamines and diuretics, hyperventilation.
- **Large pupils:** cocaine, TCAs, amphetamines, anticholinergic, adrenergic syndrome, atropine, 'belladonna', phenothiazines, hypoxia, hypothermia.
- **Nystagmus:** anticonvulsants, needle tracks, heroin.
- **Tinnitus:** salicylates.
- **Severe HTN:** cocaine, amphetamines, adrenergic syndrome.
- **Bradycardia:** digoxin, beta-blockers, CCBs, amiodarone, organophosphates, TCA, cyanide.
- **Tachycardia:** anticholinergic, salicylates, theophylline, sympathomimetics, anxiety, adrenergic syndrome.
- **Arrhythmias:** digoxin, TCAs, phenothiazines, anticholinergics.
- **Hypoglycaemia:** insulin, sulfonylurea, meglitinides, alcohol, quinine, salicylates. (Not metformin.)
- **Hyperglycaemia:** organophosphates, theophyllines, MAOIs.
- **Hyperventilation:** salicylates, metabolic acidosis (alcohols), renal failure.
- **Renal failure:** salicylates, paraquat, ethylene glycol.
- **Hyperthermia:** serotonin syndrome, cocaine, Ecstasy, salicylates, MAOIs, TCAs, theophylline, strychnine, malignant hyperthermia, neuroleptic malignant syndrome.
- **Hypothermia:** sedation/alcohol, phenothiazines, barbiturates.
- **RUQ pain/jaundice:** paracetamol poisoning, organic solvents, iron toxicity.
- **Abdominal pain:** iron poisoning, lead toxicity, NSAIDs.
- **Seizures:** mefenamic acid, TCAs, opioids, theophylline, cocaine, alcohol, amphetamines.
- **Rhabdomyolysis:** amphetamines, neuroleptics.
- **Acute hearing loss:** aminoglycosides, chloroquine, loop diuretics, chemotherapeutic agents.
- **Chest pain:** cocaine, carbon monoxide.
- **Oral ulcers:** corrosives, paraquat.
- **Elevated osmolar gap:** acetone, mannitol, methanol, ethanol, ethylene glycol.
- **Metabolic acidosis:** cyanide, hydrogen sulphide, isoniazid, metformin, NRTIs, iron.
- **Raised anion gap metabolic acidosis:** ethylene glycol, diethylene glycol, methanol, NSAIDs, toluene, salicylates.
- **Lactic acidosis:** ethylene glycol, cyanide, carbon monoxide, toluene, salicylates.
- **Dystonia:** metoclopramide, neuroleptics.
- **Blindness:** methanol, quinine.
- **Polyuria:** lithium toxicity, high glucose, low K, high Ca.

14.3 Investigations for overdose

Problems	Comments
Basic	FBC, U&E, LFT, Mg, Ca, glucose – all should have these.
Toxins	Salicylate, paracetamol levels on all deliberate overdoses. Can measure digoxin, theophylline, alcohol, ethylene glycol, lithium, TCA, barbiturates, benzodiazepine, paraquat, cocaine, opiates, amphetamine, cannabinoids as needed.
Coagulation screen	Any bleeding, petechiae, DIC. Warfarin – INR, heparin – APTT, prothrombin time.
ECG	All – especially tachycardia, bradycardia, digoxin. Look for long QT.
CXR	Any breathlessness or suspected lung disease.
Urine	Ethylene glycol toxicity with calcium oxalate crystalluria.
CT head ± LP	History unclear or coma, meningitis, encephalitis, SAH.
ABG (VBG)	Metabolic acidosis with ethylene glycol, methanol – salicylates. Renal/liver/RF. ABG for suspected RF.
Anion gap metabolic acidosis	$(Na) - (Cl + HCO_3)$ If >12 (or 16 if K included) consider toxicity due to ethanol, methanol, ethylene glycol, metformin, cyanide, isoniazid, salicylates.
Lactate	Metformin, iron, cyanide, valproate, carbon monoxide.
Osmolar gap	Calculate lab measured osmolality = $2 \times (Na + K) +$ glucose + urea. Normal <10. If >10 then consider ethanol, methanol, ethylene glycol.

14.4 General approach

- **ABC.** Determine what was taken and how much and what route. Paramedics may know. Empty packets. Rarely some patients need decontamination. Removal of clothes. Staff to wear protective clothes. Need irrigation of skin and eyes with saline for 15 min. Look for burns, smoke inhalation. Assess obs. Most can be started on 100% O_2 initially. Get IV access, start IV fluids. Assess GCS. If coma, consider CT head ± LP and don't simply blame toxin for a low GCS. Look for physical harm, trauma.
- **Burns victims:** Initially suspect CO/cyanide inhalation and check baseline arterial gas (COHb) and O_2 saturations and administer 100% FiO_2.
- **Be sceptical:** patients can over/underestimate what was taken or simply lie. Get paracetamol/salicylate levels. All patients suspected of taking a deliberate overdose need a psychiatric evaluation before being discharged; if they abscond or attempt to discharge against advice seek urgent help from your senior and/or psychiatric service.

14.5 Amphetamine and 3,4 MDMA toxicity

- **Various types:** methamphetamine ('crystal meth' or 'ice') and 3,4 methylene-dioxymethamphetamine ('Ecstasy') all cause increased presynaptic noradrenaline, dopamine. Increased serotonin release.
- **Clinical:** euphoria, psychosis, violence, dilated pupils, raised HR, raised BP, raised temp, anorexia, bruxism, sweating. Can cause: seizures, cerebral oedema, DIC, liver failure, AKI and rhabdomyolysis.
- **Investigations:** FBC, U&E low Na (MDMA due to SIADH), LFT, Mg, Ca, high CK, glucose, lactate. ECG. CT head ± LP if fever, meningism, coma, confusion, suspected cerebral oedema, infection.

- **Management:** if ingestion recent then **activated charcoal** may be used. Huge amounts, e.g. body packing for drug trafficking, consider whole bowel irrigation. **Supportive:** ITU review if GCS <9. ABC, O_2 as per BTS guidelines. ECG monitoring. **Hyperthermia:** external cooling. Consider **Dantrolene** 1 mg/kg IV (max 10 mg/kg). If **low BP:** give IV crystalloid if normonatraemic and euvolaemic or hypovolaemic. Fluids may be delayed until results back where Ecstasy-reduced SIADH may be suspected. MDMA-associated SIADH usually responds to fluid restriction. If comatose these patients should receive hypertonic saline solution to correct a portion of the metabolic imbalance rapidly. **Associated agitation: Diazepam** 10–20 mg IV. **Seizures:** IV **Lorazepam** 2–4 mg.

14.6 ▶ Beta-blocker toxicity

- **About:** widely used drugs. Competitively blocks β1 and β2 adrenoceptors. Some block Na channels and can cause seizures (propranolol/carvedilol).
- **Clinical:** bradycardia, low BP. Bronchospasm. LVF, shock. Seizures.
- **Investigations:** FBC, U&E, LFT, Mg, Ca, glucose, lactate. ECG: heart blocks, low HR, QT changes.
- **Management:** supportive: ABC/O_2, HDU if severe. IV crystalloid, telemetry. Gastric lavage if very early presentation. Bronchospasm **salbutamol** neb. Severe bradycardia: **Atropine** 0.5–1 mg up to 3 mg IV and/or temporary pacing may be needed. **If low BP/shock then consider** inotropes **adrenaline.** If response poor consider **Glucagon** 5–10 mg over 1–2 min, followed by IV infusion) 50–150 mcg/kg/h. (Glucagon activates adenyl cyclase and bypasses beta adrenoceptor). Also **insulin–glucose euglycaemic therapy:** ▶ Section 14.4. **Intralipid therapy** consider if fat soluble beta-blocker (propranolol/carvedilol), ▶ Section 14.3. **Intraaortic balloon pumping** has been used for circulatory support.
- **References:** Engebretsen *et al.* (2011) High-dose insulin therapy in beta-blocker and calcium channel-blocker poisoning. *Clin Toxicol*, 49:277. Shepherd (2006) Treatment of poisoning caused by beta-adrenergic and calcium-channel blockers. *Am J Health Pharmacy*, 63:1828.

14.7 ▶ Benzodiazepine toxicity

- **About:** diazepam, clonazepam, temazepam. Used as sedatives and anxiolytics. Accidental overdose with IV procedural sedation. Exacerbated with alcohol or other sedatives.
- **Clinical:** drowsiness and coma. If coma (GCS <10) look for other drugs or pathology. Pupils may be partially dilated, ataxia, dysarthria. Higher risk when combined with sedation, alcohol, underlying chest disease and elderly.
- **Investigations:** FBC, U&E, LFT, Mg, Ca, glucose, lactate. ECG. ABG if coma or low saturations or breathless.
- **Management:** ABC. Within 1 h 50–100 g of activated charcoal. Most overdoses are 'slept off'. Give O_2 as per BTS guidelines. Recovery position (lower leg straight, upper leg flexed) and nasopharyngeal airway if needed. IV fluids. ITU review if severe respiratory depression or GCS <9 or concerns about airway/cough/gag reflex: **Flumazenil** 200 mcg (0.2 mg) over 15 sec which may be repeated (max dose of 3 mg). There is a risk of lowering seizure threshold, especially in a mixed overdose with other drugs that also lower seizure threshold, e.g. alcohol, TCAs. Lone overdoses will rarely need ITU. Most are stable <24 h depending on severity of overdose.

14.8 Calcium channel blocker (CCB) toxicity

- **About:** L-type channel blockers potentially lethal. Give IV calcium.
- **Aetiology:** CCB block Ca influx into myocardial/vascular tissues via L-type channels. Amlodipine/nifedipine overdose cause high HR and low BP. Verapamil/diltiazem low HR/BP, cardiac arrest, cardiogenic shock.
- **Investigations:** FBC, U&E high K, LFT, Mg, Ca. ECG: low HR. Metabolic acidosis, high glucose.
- **Management:** give calcium (see below), supportive: ABC, O_2, ECG monitoring. Best on CCU or ITU/HDU. Give 500–1000 ml IV **crystalloids.** Treat low HR with IV **atropine** 0.5–1 mg (max 3 mg). Cardiac pacing if needed. Whole bowel irrigation with PEG and activated charcoal can reduce absorption of sustained-release verapamil.
- 30 ml 10% **Calcium gluconate** IV over 5–10 min (less irritant) or 10 ml 10% **Calcium chloride** IV over 5–10 min for low BP. Aim for mild high Ca – monitor for 12 h+ with modified release preparations. Persisting low BP/shock. Consider **Adrenaline** 2–10 mcg/min or **isoprenaline** 5 mcg/min or **Glucagon** 5–10 mg over 1–2 min, then 50–150 mcg/kg/h IV. If this fails consider **insulin–glucose euglycaemic therapy** (▶ Section 14.4). **Intra-aortic balloon pumping** has been used for circulatory support. Cardiac pacing may be considered for persisting significant low HR-induced hypotension. **Intralipid therapy:** may help verapamil/diltiazem, unclear for dihydropyridines. **Cardiac pacing** for severe bradycardia. If there is severe acidosis consider IV $NaHCO_3$.
- **References:** Engebretsen *et al.* (2011) High-dose insulin therapy in beta-blocker and calcium channel-blocker poisoning. *Clin Toxicol*, 49:277. Shepherd (2006) Treatment of poisoning caused by beta-adrenergic and calcium-channel blockers. *Am J Health Pharmacy*, 63:1828.

14.9 Sodium valproate toxicity

- **About:** commonly used. Generally safe AED. Valproate-induced hyperammonaemic encephalopathy (VIHE) may be seen without overdose.
- **Clinical:** delirium, coma, low BP, resp depression, seizure risk.
- **Investigations:** as for coma. FBC, U&E, LFTs, glucose, ECG, CT head, serum valproate, EEG continuous generalised slowing, theta and delta activity, triphasic waves. Blood ammonia elevated.
- **Management:** ABC, stop valproate, supportive. Multidose activated charcoal ± WBI may be considered if early. Try **naloxone**. IV **L-carnitine** may be helpful when there is high blood ammonia, hepatotoxicity, and coma. Treat until improves. Consider haemodialysis.

14.10 Carbon monoxide toxicity

- **NB:** Pulse oximetry will be falsely normal and fail to report severe hypoxia.
- **About:** if CO toxicity suspected check ABG and CO-Hb levels. CO is odourless, colourless formed by the incomplete combustion of fossil fuels. Poorly ventilated faulty home heating. Low dose toxicity may be subtle in its presentation, e.g. flu-like illness. Cold spell where gas/solid fuel home/water heating used, changes to home heating or ventilation. Watch for cyanide toxicity which may be seen in house fires.

- **Aetiology:** CO binds avidly to Hb with × 240 more affinity than does O_2. Saturation probes see CO-Hb as O_2-Hb giving a false normal SaO_2. Causes tissue hypoxia. The result is leftward shift in O_2-Hb dissociation curve. Causes myocardial and cerebral hypoxia and cerebral oedema.
- **Clinical:** drowsiness, delirium, syncope, flu-like illness, chest tightness, headache, fatigue, breathlessness, coma and death. Pink, rosy colouration.
- **Investigations:** FBC, U&E, LFT, lactate. Only an ABG will show hypoxia. Troponin. ECG. CXR. Measure CO-Hb specifically if diagnosis considered. Patients get O_2 en route and so hospital CO-Hb may not represent prior levels or the extent and severity of any hypoxia. Normal CO-Hb is 3–5%. Up to 10% in smokers. CO-Hb 10–20% causes nausea, headache. ECG changes. Severe >25% arrhythmias, cardiac ischaemia, resp failure and seizures.
- **Differential:** excess opiates, sedatives, alcohol. Stroke/SDH/SOL.
- **Management:** remove source: open windows, switch off heating/car engine. Supportive: O_2 sat unreliable. Get ABG. Start 100% O_2 via tight-fitting mask. If COPD/risk of type 2 RF consider mechanical ventilation. 100% O_2 reduces $T_{1/2}$ of CO from 4 h to 40 min. Treat until CO-Hb <5%; may be needed for 12–24 h. Severe cases with coma/neurology/delirium/ECG changes/arrhythmias/MI/pregnancy/CO-Hb >30% all needed **hyperbaric O_2** (3.0 atm pressure 60 min). Transporting to distant site can be hazardous and improved outcomes have not been proven. Take early expert advice. Mannitol may be considered for cerebral oedema. Treat if suspected cyanide toxicity (hydroxocobalamin).
- **Aim is to prevent:** cortical dysfunction, Parkinson's syndrome/disease, dementia, cardiac complications, long-term mortality, diabetes.

14.11 Cocaine toxicity

- **Always:** ask about usage if considered as a factor with HTN, chest pain, stroke. It is a CNS stimulant derived from the leaves of the coca plant.
- **Aetiology:** blocks reuptake of dopamine, serotonin, noradrenaline. Chronic usage may actually accelerate atherosclerosis. Pleasure from raising dopamine levels in the mesolimbic reward centres.
- **Administration:** snorted and absorbed via well-vascularised tissues lining the nose. Causes localised vasoconstriction. Damage to the nasal mucosa. Smoked or taken IV give a rapid response but a shorter high than snorting. Rubbed on gums or small amounts taken orally, or as a suppository. Cocaine-induced chest pain usually soon after taking due to spasm and generally not treated with thrombolysis. Users often have coexisting atherosclerotic disease and so are actually more prone to spasm.
- **Clinical:** chest pain, neurology from ischaemic or haemorrhagic stroke (esp. if underlying berry aneurysm), aortic dissection, high BP, tachycardia, pyrexia, euphoria/psychotic, mydriasis. Chronic myocarditis, atherosclerosis.
- **Investigations:** FBC, U&E, LFT, troponin. CXR cardiomegaly. ECG: ischaemia or look for STEMI, LVH. CT head if any neurology.
- **Management:** O_2 as per BTS guidance. IV fluids. Suspected ACS with ST elevation necessitates primary PCI. Thrombolysis avoided especially where hypertensive. Consider **GTN** 2 sprays (800 mcg) or **GTN** 500 mcg tablet SL. If chest pain persists then **GTN** 50 mg in 50 ml IV infusion. Start 1–10 ml/h prior to PCI. Avoid beta-blockade, which will cause HTN due to unopposed alpha effects. Alternative consider **Verapamil** 240–480 mg daily in divided doses. Hyperthermia is a side-effect of cocaine and should be treated with fluids, cooling and **Dantrolene:** 1 mg/kg body weight IV should be given. Agitation: **Diazepam** 1–5 mg PO/IV. Avoid haloperidol and phenothiazines which lower fit threshold.

14.12 Local anaesthetic toxicity

- **Source:** usage of lidocaine, bupivacaine overdose (accidental or deliberate).
- **Aetiology:** local anaesthetics block open Na channels.
- **Clinical:** tingling lips, blurred vision, tinnitus, respiratory depression, seizure, coma, arrhythmias, hypotension, cardiac arrest.
- **Management:** ABC. Severe toxicity: **Intralipid therapy** (▶ Section 14.1).

14.13 Cyanide toxicity

- **Source:** inhaled smoke contains hydrogen cyanide (HCN) and CO which can kill. Confirmation takes time. Treat empirically with hydroxocobalamin.
- **Aetiology:** mitochondrial dysfunction blocks ATP production. High lactate. Cyanides inhibit cytochrome oxidase. Blocks reversibly mitochondrial ATP production. High lactate.
- **Suspect:** smoke-inhalation victims if exposure to fire or smoke in an enclosed area, soot round the mouth/nose/back of mouth. Altered mental status, delirium, drowsy. Lactate >10 mmol/L. Check for CO poisoning.
- **Clinical:** in lethal overdoses death is in minutes usually pre-hospital. Survival to hospital bodes well. Evidence of smoke inhalation, cherry-red skin colour, smell of bitter almonds. Chest pain, dyspnoea, seizures, coma.
- **Investigation:** FBC, U&E, LFT, CXR, ECG. Lactate >10 mmol/L. ABG: RAG metabolic acidosis, high venous O_2 saturation. Check CO-Hb.
- **Management:** decontamination. ABC 100% O_2. ITU if high EWS. Get the cyanide antidote kit (Cyanokit): **Hydroxocobalamin** 5 g over 15 min IV in 200 ml NS which may be repeated (max 10 g). $NaHCO_3$ for severe acidosis. Other treatments: **Sodium nitrite** 300 mg IV (SE methaemoglobinaemia and NO-induced vasodilation). **Sodium thiosulphate** 50 ml of a 25% solution (12.5 g) infused 20 min. Converts cyanide to thiocyanate.
- **Reference:** https://www.atsdr.cdc.gov/MHMI/mmg8.pdf

14.14 Digoxin and oleander toxicity

- **About:** deliberate or accidental overdose. Lethal dose over 50 times daily dose 10 mg (adult). Well absorbed orally. Do not give calcium. Oleander contains a glycoside and is used in overdose in Asia.
- **Pharmacology:** half-life 30–40 h, peak toxicity at 6 h death at 6–12 h post ingestion. Digoxin blocks Na/K ATPase pump: high intracellular Ca reduces AV conduction. Causes low HR, raised vagal tone, automaticity high K.
- **Clinical:** nausea, vomiting, yellow vision, abdominal pain. Low HR, AV block, SVT (with AV block), AF, VT and even VF.
- **Investigations:** bloods: FBC, U&E, calcium, digoxin level. U&E: K >5.5 mmol/L suggests 90% untreated fatal toxicity. Serial ECGs: monitor for symptomatic low HR, CHB, VT, VF, AF, MAT.
- **Management:** ABC. Those with high K need Fab. K >5.5 mmol/L suggests fatal toxicity. Correct K and Mg. CCU monitoring for low BP, arrhythmias, cardiac arrest. Give **Atropine** 0.5–1 mg IV (max 3 mg) for brady/AV block. **Pacing** may be needed. Gastric lavage if seen within 1 h. Give activated charcoal if <1 h of ingestion in cooperative patient. Repeated dosing may be helpful. Manage low K with replacement. Manage high K with **$NaHCO_3$** and/or **insulin/glucose.** *Traditional*

advice has been to avoid calcium gluconate for hyperkalaemia with digoxin toxicity but evidence of harm unclear. See Toxbase. Bidirectional VT/VT/VF: give **Magnesium sulfate** 2 g (8 mmol) in 100 ml NS over 10 min IV and consider **Lidocaine** 50–100 mg IV. **Digoxin-immune Fab:** given where adult dose >10 mg ingested, life-threatening arrhythmias, digoxin level >15 nmol/ml (12 ng/ml), K >5 mmol/L. Note: 1 **Digibind** vial binds 0.5 mg of digoxin. It also works with oleander toxicity. Multiple vials needed in large overdose. Expensive, may not be stocked. Contact Pharmacy and Poisons Advisory Service for stores. If renal failure, then plasmapheresis may help clear digoxin–Fab complexes. In a cardiac arrest continue to give multiple vials of this for up to 30 min as resuscitation continues.

- **NB:** traditional advice had been to avoid calcium for hyperkalaemia with digoxin toxicity but evidence of harm unclear and depending on local advice may be ignored. Follow local hyperkalaemia guidance.

14.15 Ethanol (C_2H_5OH) toxicity

- **About:** significant toxicity in overdose and when mixed with other sedatives. Ethanol in some mouthwashes, hand-washes, antiseptics. Clarify if the alcohol ingested is a toxic alcohol (e.g. methanol, ethylene glycol).
- **Aetiology:** ethanol metabolised to acetaldehyde by alcohol dehydrogenase and then to acetate. Ingested alcohol almost totally absorbed within 1 h.
- **Clinical:** small amounts cause incoordination, euphoria. Slow reaction time. Moderate amounts – ataxia, dysarthria and even diplopia, sweating, tachycardia. Disinhibition, aggression, violence and accidents. Overdose: coma, resp depression, aspiration and death.
- **Investigations:** FBC, U&E, LFTs, GGT, PTT. Chronic: high GGT and raised MCV. Falls high CK. *CT head if coma/head injury.* Cannot assume alcohol. ABG: metabolic acidosis. Ethanol levels: mild: <150 mg/dl, mod: 150–300 mg/dl, severe: 300–500 mg/dl. Peak blood alcohol is at 90 min. Zero order elimination.
- **Complications:** coma, aspiration, head injury, low glucose. Alcoholic ketoacidosis, lactic acidosis, AKI, rhabdomyolysis, Korsakoff's psychosis.
- **Management:** supportive: ABC, O_2 as per BTS guidance. ITU review if GCS <9 or high EWS. Hydrate for good diuresis. Most are slept off in recovery position with close monitoring ± NP or other airway device. Some need mechanical ventilation for severe respiratory depression/airway management. Pabrinex IV paired vials 8 h for 1–2 d in chronic alcoholics. Hypoglycaemia may be seen. Give 10% glucose IV. **Lorazepam** 2–4 mg IV for seizures. Haemodialysis with blood ethanol levels >400 mg/dl or severe metabolic acidosis pH <7.0. Most patients have stabilised by 12 h. Consider then initiating alcohol withdrawal regimen with **Chlordiazepoxide** or **Diazepam** as needed. See Delirium tremens (▶Section 7.8). Later referral to community addiction teams.

14.16 Ethylene glycol / diethylene glycol toxicity

- **About:** antifreeze used to bulk alcohol drinks. Taken with alcohol may reduce toxicity. For inebriation or for suicide.
- **Aetiology:** EG forms glycolate (met acidosis) and oxalate which forms calcium oxalate crystals which are renal toxic. DEG is metabolised to 2-hydroxyethoxyacetate (met acidosis) and diglycolic acid which is renal toxic.
- **Clinical:** progression *Stage 1*: 0–12 h 'drunk' CNS depression/coma, ataxia, ophthalmoplegia, Kussmaul breathing, hypotonia, aspiration, seizures, cerebral

oedema; *Stage 2*: 12–24 h low BP, tachycardia, CCF, ARDS, lethal multi-organ failure; *Stage 3*: AKI. Flank pain, ATN. Oxalate crystals. High K and low Ca/low Mg. DEG causes N&V, headache, abdominal pain, coma, seizures, acidosis, AKI, pancreatitis, hepatitis and neurotoxicity.

- **Investigations:** ABG: raised anion gap (RAG) osmolar gap metabolic acidosis (MA). U&E: severe AKI high K, pH <7.3. Low Ca/Mg. Osmolar gap >10 mOsm/L. Lactate/ketones mildly elevated. Urine: Calcium oxalate crystals. Measure ethylene glycol levels: >500 mg/L (8 mmol/L) severe.
- **Management:** ABC, O_2. IV fluids. Absorption too quick for activated charcoal or gastric lavage. ITU if GCS <9 or multi-organ failure or dialysis. Treat if symptoms and RAG/MA and suspicion of ingestion. **Antidotes: Fomepizole** 15 mg/kg body wt stat followed by 4 × 12-h doses of 10 mg/kg, then 15 mg/kg every 12 h until glycol concentrations are not detectable. Also consider haemodialysis or haemodiafiltration. Alternative is **Ethanol** loading dose 50 g followed by an IV ethanol 10–12 g/h to produce blood ethanol concentrations of 500–1000 mg/L (11–22 mmol/L). Continue until the glycol is no longer detectable in the blood. Take advice from National Poisons Information Service. **Calcium gluconate** IV for severe symptomatic hypocalcaemia. **Acidosis:** IV $NaHCO_3$. **Seizures:** standard treatment. **Haemodialysis:** if pH <7.25, AKI, ethylene glycol levels >500 mg/L. Continue until acidosis corrected, EG levels fall. Watch for cerebral oedema.
- **Reference:** Brent (2009) Fomepizole for ethylene glycol and methanol poisoning. *New Engl J Med*, 360:2216.

14.17 ▶ Methanol toxicity

- **About:** 10 ml methanol (CH_3OH) can cause blindness, 30 ml death.
- **Aetiology:** toxic metabolite formate. Less toxic with alcohol.
- **Clinical:** latent period 0–12 h 'drunk'. Toxicity symptoms >12 h. Coma, abdominal pain, acidotic breathing, tachycardia, death, dilated pupils, early optic disc oedema/blindness. Later polyneuropathy, tremors, rigidity, spasticity. Parkinsonism with mild dementia.
- **Investigations:** U&E: AKI ABG: raised anion gap Metabolic acidosis (low HCO_3). LFT, FBC, Ca, glucose. pH <7.3. Low HCO_3 high osmolar gap >10 mOsm/L. AKI. Serum methanol >500 mg/L severe poisoning. Serum formate >12 mmol/L associated with visual/CNS sequelae. CT/MRI head: bilateral basal ganglia bleeds, high amylase.
- **Management:** ABC, O_2. IV fluids. Airways protection. ITU if GCS <9. Treat when: evidence of ingestion or suspicion + metabolic disturbance – osmolar gap >10 mmol/dl, arterial pH <7.3, raised anion gap metabolic acidosis. **Antidotes:** start fomepizole or ethanol. Both inhibit alcohol dehydrogenase. **Fomepizole** preferred. See Ethylene glycol. Take advice from National Poisons Information Service. Alcohol will cause inebriation. **Folinic acid (leucovorin)** 1 mg/kg then folic acid 1 mg/kg 6 h until acidosis resolves. May reduce ocular toxicity. **Acidosis:** correct with IV $NaHCO_3$. **Seizures:** standard treatment. **Haemodialysis:** removes formate/methanol. Use if pH <7.25, AKI until metabolism corrected and serum levels of methanol undetectable. Monitor for cerebral oedema.
- **Reference:** Brent (2009) Fomepizole for ethylene glycol and methanol poisoning. *New Engl J Med*, 360:2216.

14.18 Gamma hydroxybutyrate (GHB) toxicity

- **About:** white powder, forms an odourless, colourless liquid in water.
- **Uses:** date rape, sleep aid, bodybuilders. Exacerbated by alcohol/other drugs. Gamma butyrolactone (GBL) is similar.
- **Aetiology:** release of GH. GABA agonist.
- **Clinical:** euphoria, miosis, agitation, violence, amnesia, low BP, low HR, myoclonus. Rapid LOC with coma then recovery after 2–4 h. Unpredictable.
- **Investigations:** FBC, U&E, ABG as needed. Toxicology screen.
- **Management:** supportive: ABC and O_2 as per BTS guidelines. ITU GCS <9 or high EWS. IV fluids, mechanical ventilation 6–8 h then recovers rapidly.

14.19 Insulin toxicity

- **About:** deliberate or accidental. Insulin given IV/SC/IM causes hypoglycaemia (no effect orally). Long-acting insulins last >24 h.
- **Clinical:** hypoglycaemic causes confusion, tremor, hunger, panic, altered behaviour, confusion, coma, violence, agitation, amnesia, death.
- **Investigations:** CBG every 10–20 min with symptoms. Check FBC, U&E (K falls) LFTs. Check C-peptide (normal if endogenous insulin).
- **Management:** ABC, consider IV glucose 10–20% (with 20 mmol/L K) infusion, keep blood glucose >4 mmol/L. Long-acting insulins need an ongoing infusion. Surgical removal of insulin injection site has been used for overdose of long-acting insulin.
- **Reference:** Eldred *et al.* (2013). Problem based review: the patient who has taken an overdose of long-acting insulin analogue. *Acute Med*, 12:167.

14.20 Iron toxicity

- **About:** doses <60 mg/kg, e.g. 4.2 g for 70 kg unlikely to be toxic. Children vulnerable for toxicity. Delayed presentation can be fatal.
- **Clinical:** minor: nausea, vomiting, dyspepsia. Haematemesis, rectal bleeding, melaena, black stools. Major: hypotension, Kussmaul's breathing, hepatorenal failure. 48 h: hepatocellular necrosis can occur, liver fibrosis, scarring.
- **Investigations:** iron level at 4 h, lactate, ECG, FBC, U&E – AKI, LFTs. Abdominal X-ray – KUB: radio-opaque iron tablets seen suggest trying WBI. ABG: RAG metabolic acidosis. Monitor high ALT, PTT, low CBG.
- **Management:** supportive: ABCs, resuscitate, IV crystalloids. ITU if high EWS. **Assess risk:** ingested dose 20–60 mg/kg will give GI effects, 60–120 mg/kg systemic toxicity. Dose >120 mg/kg is potentially lethal. Act quickly.
- **Perform whole bowel irrigation:** those with radio-opacities on KUB until the opacities clear or for amounts taken >60 mg/kg. Surgical or endoscopic removal for significant overdoses. If coma or shock or iron level >5 mg/L or 90 μmol/L then start IV **desferrioxamine** 15 mg/kg/h (up to 80 mg/kg in 24 h). It can cause low BP and allergic reactions. If severe toxicity expected from amount ingested then treat before the result of the serum-iron measurement.

14.21 Lithium toxicity

- **About:** for bipolar affective disorders. No protein binding. Toxicity if dehydrated or diuretics. Usually due to reduced drug excretion. Precipitated by dehydration, AKI/CKD, infections, diuretics or NSAIDs, deliberate overdoses can have delayed effects.

- **Clinical:** acute: tremor, dysarthria, confusion, delirium, seizures, coma, death. Polyuria, polydipsia due to nephrogenic diabetes insipidus (NDI). Chronic toxicity: encephalopathy/coma, neuropathy, cerebellar dysfunction.
- **Investigations:** FBC, U&E: high Na due to NDI. ECG: T wave flattening, U waves, long QT, sepsis screen. Lithium levels 6 h: usual range 0.6–1.2 mmol/L. Toxic >2.0 mmol/L, coma >3.0 mmol/L, lethal >5.0 mmol/L. CT head if diagnosis unclear.
- **Complications:** truncal/gait ataxia, nystagmus, memory loss, dementia. SILENT syndrome of irreversible lithium-effectuated neurotoxicity.
- **Management:** ABC, IV NS 3–4 L/d to cause a good diuresis, measure I/O, avoid diuretics and NSAIDs. Supportive: rehydrate to manage NDI which can take weeks to recover. WBI: consider oral PEG solution if <2 h from acute ingestion in sustained release drug. **Haemodialysis:** important as can significantly lower lithium levels but may need repeated. Consider if comatose, ataxia, seizures.

14.22 Monoamine oxidase inhibitors toxicity

- **About:** caution as severe toxicity in overdose and risk of drug interactions.
- **Clinical:** euphoria, restless, pyrexia, seizures, opisthotonos, rhabdomyolysis and coma. May be delayed 12–24 h. BP can be high or low.
- **Investigations:** watch FBC, U&E, CRP, CK.
- **Management:** IV crystalloid for low BP. **Diazepam** 5–20 mg IV for agitation. **Dantrolene** 1 mg/kg IV for malignant hyperpyrexia.

14.23 Neuroleptics toxicity

- **About:** block dopamine D2 receptors. Haloperidol, sulpiride, or new agents: amisulpiride, olanzapine, quetiapine, risperidone.
- **Clinical:** low BP, low GCS, respiratory depression, hyper/hypothermia, seizures, rhabdomyolysis, acute dystonias. **Investigations:** FBC, U&E, CK. **ECG:** long QT, TdP.
- **Management:** stop drug. IV fluids, pressor agents for low BP. Treat acidosis with IV NaHCO$_3$. IV **Magnesium** 2 g (8 mmol) in 100 ml NS over 10 min or overdrive pacing for TdP. Torsades de pointes, ▶ Section 3.13.

14.24 Warfarin/direct oral anticoagulants toxicity

- **About:** bleeding is the main risk.
- **Management:** DOAC, ▶ Section 8.11. Warfarin/VKA, ▶ Section 8.9.

14.25 Non-steroidal anti-inflammatory drugs toxicity

- **About:** accidental and deliberate overdose. Ibuprofen and mefenamic acid.
- **Clinical:** gastric irritation. Abdominal pain. Mefenamic acid causes seizures. AKI and metabolic acidosis. Low GCS, nystagmus, tachycardia rarely seen.
- **Investigations:** FBC: anaemia with gastritis, U&E: AKI. ABG: metabolic acidosis (associated with ibuprofen overdoses).
- **Management:** give ABC, supportive, **activated charcoal** 50 g PO if more than 10 tablets <1 h. **Seizures:** ABC, O$_2$. See status epilepticus (▶ Section 11.16). **Gastritis:** oral PPI if symptoms. Manage upper GI haemorrhage (▶ Section 6.4). **Discharge:** most medically fit for discharge by 12 h if stable except in significant mefenamic acid or phenylbutazone poisoning, a 24-h post ingestion observation is advised. Needs psychiatric review.

14.26 Opioid/opiate toxicity

- **About:** toxicity from accidental or deliberate heroin (diamorphine) overdose. Seen with codeine, diamorphine and morphine.
- **Aetiology:** opiates bind to kappa and mu CNS opioid receptors.
- **Clinical:** coma, resp depression. Small pupils. Needle marks. Cardiac effects, e.g. look for transdermal skin patches of opiate medications.
- **Investigations:** check paracetamol/salicylate levels, toxicology screen. Blood glucose, U&E, FBC, ABG, LFTs, CXR. CT head if coma diagnosis unclear. ECG: QRS widening, arrhythmias, heart block.
- **Management:** ABC, O_2. HDU area. Recovery position. If airway unsafe consider intubation and ventilation especially if GCS <8 and not rapidly responsive to **naloxone**. Always check glucose and consider CT head. Remove opiate or other patches. Monitor for return of symptoms, e.g. pain.
- **Opiate overdose in opiate-naïve patient: Naloxone** 0.4 mg (400 mcg) IV in 10 ml 0.9% NS IV. Repeat up to 2 mg in total then give 66% of the dose needed to wake the patient as an infusion over 1 hr. Doses up to 10 mg have been given. IM **naloxone** has been used as an alternative. Drug abusers become agitated. If no response such as enlarging pupils, improving respiratory rate and GCS then seek other cause.
- **Opiate overdose with chronic opiate dependence** (terminal care, long-term usage or addiction): reverse opiate-induced resp depression without causing pain or harmful cytokine release. Give **Naloxone** 40–100 mcg. Make up 100 mcg in 10 ml NS and give slowly. Repeated up to 400 mcg (0.4 mg) then review. Note: tramadol and naloxone: excess tramadol can cause respiratory depression and seizure. Naloxone will give some improvement.
- **Reference:** Stage One: Warning risk of distress and death from inappropriate doses of Naloxone in patients on long-term opioid/opiate treatment (2014). NHS/PSA/W/2014/016. NHS England.

14.27 Organophosphate/carbamates toxicity

- **About:** organophosphate used as agricultural chemicals. Similar to nerve agent sarin. Carbamates have similar effects.
- **Aetiology:** they bind to an active site of acetylcholinesterase and inhibit the functionality of this enzyme by means of steric inhibition. Cannot break down Ach leads to excess Ach at synapses/neuromuscular junctions. Excess bronchial secretions and muscle weakness causes respiratory failure. They also bind erythrocyte cholinesterase which can be measured.
- **Clinical** ('wet and weak'): acute: bradycardia may be missing, N&V, colic, diarrhoea, sweating, rhinorrhoea, bronchorrhoea, miosis, generalised weakness, fasciculation, weak respiratory muscles, respiratory failure.
- **Intermediate syndrome:** within 96 h with all-over weakness needing respiratory support. Recovers within 3 weeks. OP-induced delayed polyneuropathy (OPIDN): at 1–3 weeks with distal symmetrical flaccid weakness and tingling wrist and foot drop.
- **Investigations:** low erythrocyte cholinesterase activity (better guide than serum cholinesterase activity). FBC, U&E, CXR: oedema, consolidation. ABG: type I RF. ECG: prolonged QTc interval.
- **Management:** decontamination. Protective clothing. ABC. Remove their clothes and wash skin with soap and water. Irrigate eyes, remove contact lenses. OPs can penetrate latex – use locally advised kit. Contaminated clothing is hazardous waste.

- **Supportive:** ABC. O_2. High dependency area. If doubtful then **Atropine** 1 mg IV with skin flushing and marked increased HR makes OP toxicity unlikely. Intubate and ventilate if hypoxia despite high FIO_2. Give adequate **Atropine** 2–3 mg IV and repeat doubling dose every 5 min (3 mg, 6 mg, 12 mg and so on) until drying of bronchial secretions and hypoxia improves, HR >80 beats/min, SBP >80 mmHg. Consider **Atropine** infusion at about 5 mg/h. Watch for development of intermediate syndrome with progressive weakness over 72 h with respiratory muscle weakness. TDP should be treated (▶Section 3.13). IV **$MgSO_4$** may be beneficial. **Pralidoxime (2-PAM)** 1–2 g slow IV in 30 min reactivates acetylcholinesterase and is given for nicotinic (weakness) symptoms. **Seizures:** managed with **Lorazepam** 2–4 mg IV/IM or **Diazepam** 5–10 mg IV as per seizure section; ▶Section 11.16.

14.28 Paracetamol (acetaminophen) toxicity

- **About:** liver failure/death in those who present late or are inadequately treated. Hepatotoxicity unlikely if *N*-acetylcysteine (NAC) started within 8 h of ingestion.
- **Pathophysiology:** paracetamol converted to highly toxic metabolite (*N*-acetyl-*p*-benzoquinone imine (NAPQI)) by hepatic cytochrome P450 2E1 (CYP2E1). Causes liver/renal failure. NAPQI inactivated by glutathione but rapidly consumed in overdose. Low glutathione: chronic alcoholics, starvation/fasting. Enzyme-inducing drugs (e.g. carbamazepine, phenytoin, barbiturates, St John's wort, isoniazid and rifampicin), AIDS, cystic fibrosis and other liver disease. Low BMI, urinalysis positive for ketones, low serum urea concentration. These factors no longer play a part in dosing algorithm.
- **Clinical history 1–24 h:** no symptoms. Nausea, vomiting. **24–72 h:** RUQ pain/discomfort. raised AST, raised PTT. **72–96 h:** hepatic necrosis and fulminant liver failure, jaundice, coagulopathy, delirium, encephalopathy, death. Consideration for transplantation. **4 days – 2 weeks:** resolution or death. Post-transplant recovery.
- **Investigations:** paracetamol (and salicylate) level: 4 h or later post ingestion. FBC, VBG, U&E, LFTs, INR(PT) then daily. ALT >1000 IU/L. Severe liver damage. Raised lactate, raised PT useful prognostically. Watch for AKI.

Management (MHRA (UK) Guidance 2014)
- **<1 h from ingestion:** if thought to have taken >12g or 150 mg/kg give activated charcoal 50 g (1 g/kg for children) PO or NG (for those >110 kg use 110 kg as weight).

Indications for acetylcysteine

- Patient whose PPC (plasma paracetamol concentration) falls on or above the treatment line.
- Patient who presents <8 h of ingestion of >150 mg/kg of paracetamol if there is going to be a delay from when OD taken of ≥8 h in obtaining the PPCs.
- Patient who presents 8–24 h after ingestion of >150 mg/kg of paracetamol even if the PPC is not yet available.
- Patient who presents >24 h after overdose if they are jaundiced/hepatic tenderness, their ALT is above the ULN, their INR >1.3, or PPC is detectable.
- Patient who presents <24 h of an OD if ALT/PT abnormal, even if PPC below nomogram.
- Where timing of OD uncertain or a staggered overdose. Check PPC levels.

- **No need to** treat if: not at risk of liver toxicity, PPC is below the treatment line or undetectable, INR and ALT are normal, patient is asymptomatic: no treatment is indicated and NAC may be discontinued if it has been started.
- **Acetylcysteine:** rash, angioedema, wheeze, low BP in 15% usually in first 2 h. *Harm recorded if NAC withheld if side-effects interpreted as anaphylaxis.* Acetylcysteine is more likely to cause adverse effects if paracetamol concentrations are low

or absent. Adverse effects are also more likely in women, asthmatics and in patients with a family history of allergy. Give at a slower rate such as first bag over 2 h. Give **Chlorphenamine** 10 mg IV/IM. **Salbutamol** 5 mg if needed. Rarely IM **adrenaline** and IV **hydrocortisone**. If cannot take NAC then take advice consider oral **methionine**. This can be hard to obtain out of hours and may not be in stock. If NAC or methionine cannot be given, then consider haemodialysis. In the USA oral NAC is used: consists of a loading dose of 140 mg/kg orally and maintenance dose of 70 mg/kg every 4 h for 17 doses. Induces nausea or vomiting in more than 50% of patients but is inexpensive and easier to give. Safer than IV administration. There is no evidence of any difference in efficacy (Green *et al.*, 2013). Take expert advice if unable to take NAC.

- *N*-acetylcysteine (NAC) administration:

  - Bag ONE 150 mg/kg in 200 ml 5% glucose over 1 h.
  - Bag TWO 50 mg/kg in 500 ml 5% glucose over 4 h.
  - Bag THREE 100 mg/kg in 1 L 5% glucose over 16 h.

- **Acute liver failure:** escalate any significant sign of liver failure as early as possible with the regional liver centres. Monitor for bleeding, encephalopathy, hypoglycaemia, oliguria, thrombocytopenia, acidosis, cerebral oedema.
- **Orthotopic liver transplant:** may be the only hope of survival with hyperacute liver failure following paracetamol. Criteria below are used in UK. Do not wait for criteria to be met before picking up telephone. Some are transferred and may settle. Post recovery: ensure psychiatry review prior to discharge.
- **Pregnant:** should be treated same as non-pregnant. Paracetamol and NAC cross placenta. No evidence of teratogenicity. Fetus protected by treating mother.
- **King's College criteria for liver transplant:** paracetamol-induced liver failure: an arterial pH <7.3 at 24 h after ingestion OR a PT >100 sec OR creatinine >300 μmol/L. Grade III/IV hepatic encephalopathy. Discuss with local liver centre long before this stage is reached.

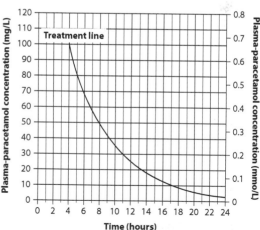

Nomogram for paracetamol overdose. Treat those lying to the right of the treatment line.
Reproduced from the MHRA 2014 under the Open Government Licence v3.0.

- **References:** Bateman (2011) Management of paracetamol poisoning. *BMJ*, 342:d2218. Green *et al.* (2013) Oral and IV acetylcysteine for treatment of acetaminophen toxicity: a systematic review and meta-analysis. *West J Emerg Med*, 14:218.

14.29 Paraquat toxicity

- **Aetiology:** pulmonary–renal syndrome. Superoxides and free radicals.
- **Prognosis:** dose >6 g fatal, 1.5–6 g mortality 60–70%, <1.5 g is rarely fatal.
- **Clinical:** mucosal ulceration, vomiting, diarrhoea, alveolitis, AKI. Oesophageal perforation, mediastinitis. CCF, RF. Lung fibrosis. LVF.
- **Investigations:** U&E: AKI. CXR: ARDS with oedema and fibrosis. ABG: type 1 RF and metabolic acidosis. Check paraquat levels.
- **Management:** prehospital. Immediately remove contaminated clothing. Wash from skin or mucous membranes soap and water. Medical: ABC, O_2 target sats of 92%. High FiO_2 may be harmful. Eventually type 1 RF occurs. **Activated charcoal** 50 g PO/NG and get early expert advice. Extracorporeal removal by prolonged haemodialysis or haemoperfusion has been used until paraquat levels are undetected. IV fluids to force diuresis. Consider cyclophosphamide and steroids or salicylates. Lung transplantation has failed whenever used.

14.30 Chloroquine/quinine toxicity

- **About:** quinine used to treat malaria and nocturnal cramps.
- **Aetiology:** sodium channel blocker. Toxic to retinal photoreceptor cells.
- **Clinical: Quinine:** partial/complete blindness, tinnitus, nausea, headache, tremor, ataxia, coma, resp depression, arrhythmias, low BP, cardiac arrest. **Chloroquine:** low BP, CCF, agitation, seizures, arrhythmias, cardiac arrest.
- **Investigation:** ECG: wide QRS. Prolonged QTc. Risk of VT, TdP and VF.
- **Management:** ABC, **Multidose activated charcoal** 50 g PO/NG. Gastric lavage if early presentation. Correct K. Low HR: **Atropine** 0.5–1 mg slow IV (max 3 mg). May be repeated. External/transvenous pacing. IV $NaHCO_3$ if QRS >120 msec for a pH of 7.45–7.55. Early ventilation and diazepam may help. Overdrive pacing for VT (TdP). Magnesium not useful. Torsades de pointes, ▶ Section 3.13.

14.31 Salicylate toxicity

- **Aetiology:** weak acid uncouples oxidative phosphorylation to cause hyperthermia. Calculate toxic doses per bodyweight of patient: mild >150 mg/kg, moderate >250 mg/kg, severe >500 mg/kg taken.
- **Clinical:** dehydration, low K and a progressive metabolic acidosis occur late. N&V and tinnitus, vertigo, hyperventilation, tachycardia, delirium, hallucinations, convulsions, lethargy. Hyperthermia suggests severe toxicity, especially in young children. Dyspnoea due to 'non-cardiogenic' pulmonary oedema.
- **Risks:** elderly and young, CNS involvement, metabolic acidosis, hyperpyrexia, pulmonary oedema, salicylate >700 mg/L (5.1 mmol/L).
- **Investigations:** U&E: low K and AKI, FBC, coagulopathy, LFT, high lactate, ABG: mixed resp alkalosis/metabolic acidosis. Low glucose, CXR if breathless. Salicylate level at 2 h post ingestion if symptoms and at 4 h if no symptoms. Level >500 mg/L is severe; level >700 mg/L (5.1 mmol/L) life-threatening. ECG arrhythmias.

- **Management:** gastric lavage if >500 mg/kg taken (with airway protection). If <1 h from ingestion ± then MDAC 50 g PO/NG stat repeated within 2–3 h of ingestion. Consider WBI with PEG if significant overdose. Promote diuresis with IV fluids 3–4 L/d. 10% glucose IV if hypoglycaemia. Replace K to ensure normokalaemia to allow acid–base correction.
- **Urinary alkalinisation:** *may be used for salicylates >500 mg/L (3.6 mmol/L): aim is to achieve urine pH 7.5–8.5:* IV 1 L **1.26% NaHCO₃** with 40 mmol KCl over 4 h repeated as needed up to 4 L/d. Consider haemodialysis with salicylate levels >700 mg/L (5.1 mmol/L) or with seizures, severe acidosis pH <7.2, AKI, ARDS, coma, CCF, non-cardiogenic pulmonary oedema. Watch for hypokalaemia. Alkalotic tetany may occur but hypocalcaemia is rare.

14.32 SSRI/SNRI toxicity

- **About:** selective serotonin (noradrenaline) reuptake inhibitor drugs. Increase CNS serotonin. Less toxic than TCAs. Fluoxetine, citalopram, venlafaxine.
- **Clinical: SSRI:** N&V, tremor, prolonged QTc, serotonergic syndromes. **SNRI:** tachycardia, tremor, agitation, wide QRS and QTc duration, arrhythmia, seizures, coma. **Mirtazapine:** drowsiness, nausea and vomiting.
- **Investigations:** U&E, LFT, FBC, CK, glucose. ECG: long QT, TdP arrhythmias.
- **Management:** ABC, IV fluids, respiratory support if needed. Agitation/seizures: IV **lorazepam/diazepam.** Manage hyperthermia. **Activated charcoal** 50 g PO if <1 h from overdose and >10 tablets taken. Manage TdP with IV **Magnesium sulfate** 2 g (8 mmol) in 100 ml NS over 10 min. Long QT/wide QRS give 250 ml 1.26% NaHCO₃, monitor CK for rhabdomyolysis, DIC, ARDS. Severe serotonin syndrome: usually medically stable by 12 h. Torsades de pointes, ▶ Section 3.13.

14.33 Tricyclic antidepressant toxicity

- **About:** amitriptyline and dosulepin very toxic. These antidepressants may be available to those at high risk of suicide. Anticholinergic toxidrome.
- **Aetiology:** alpha blockers, increases NA and 5HT. Block cardiac Na channels, anticholinergics, block K channels. Histamine receptor blockers.
- **Clinical:** tachycardia, dry skin, dry mouth, jerky, dilated pupils, urinary retention, hyperreflexia, low BP, seizures, coma, arrhythmias.
- **Investigations:** FBC, U&E, ABG: respiratory failure, metabolic acidosis. Paracetamol, salicylate levels. ECG changes suggest toxicity and Na channel blockade with QRS >120 msec, R wave >3 mm in aVr, prolonged QT, Brugada appearance LBBB/RBBB. CT head if seizure/coma exclude SOL.
- **Management:** supportive: ABCs. Correct low BP, hypoxia, acidosis, IV fluids, CCU/ITU monitoring. If <1–2 h and >10 tablets consider lavage ± **Activated charcoal** 50 g PO/NG if >10 tablets. Manage seizures with IV **Lorazepam** 2–4 mg or **Diazepam** 5–10 mg. *Avoid phenytoin which may be arrhythmogenic.* Monitor ECG: QRS >140 msec, long QT, VT, TdP, VF, heart block in CCU/ITU. IV MgSO₄ for TdP. Coma may persist 1–2 d and wake up with agitation/hallucinations.
- **VT:** CCU bed, overdrive pacing/IV **MgSO₄/lidocaine**. If QRS >120 msec or low BP or arrhythmias give 50 ml 8.4% **NaHCO₃** IV over 20 min and repeat if needed, aiming for pH of 7.50–7.55. Alkalosis raises protein binding, stabilises arrhythmias, high BP. TCA highly protein bound so haemodialysis not useful. Psychiatry assessment. Final: **IV glucagon**, inotropes for persisting low BP. Cardiac arrest: prolonged resuscitation. **Intralipid emulsion** 'lipid rescue' as TCAs are lipid-soluble.

14.34   Theophylline toxicity

- **Aetiology:** for asthma/COPD. Narrow therapeutic window. Inhibits phosphodiesterase with elevated cAMP and adrenergic stimulation.
- **Clinical:** nausea, severe vomiting, abdominal pain, raised HR, seizures.
- **Investigations:** ABG: metabolic acidosis. Low K, phosphate, Mg. Low/high Ca, hyperglycaemia. Check levels: range 10–20 mcg/ml, toxic levels >20 mcg/ml. ECG and telemetry: all arrhythmias, AF/atrial flutter/SVT/VT/VF.
- **Management:** stop any oral or IV theophyllines. ABC, give O₂ as per BTS guidelines. Manage seizures: **Lorazepam** 2–4 mg IV (▶Section 11.16). (May need ITU). Limit absorption: multidose activated charcoal (MDAC) is important to help elimination of theophylline. Gastric lavage if <1 h of a significant amount or sustained-release preparation. WBI may be considered. Manage hypokalaemia: cautious correction of low K. Arrhythmias: consider beta-blockers (C/I for asthma/COPD) or disopyramide.

14.35   Body packers ('mules')

- **About:** a normal AXR does not rule out body packing, a non-contrast abdominopelvic CT scan must be performed to confirm/refute the diagnosis. Drugs usually wrapped in some latex condom, balloon or finger of a latex glove. Nowadays more sophisticated with multilayered latex. May be 1–200 found. Usually heroin and cocaine but also amphetamine, Ecstasy and marijuana. Each packet holds 3–15 g of the drug. Total carried may be 1 kg. Each packet of heroin, cocaine or amphetamine contains a potentially life-threatening dose of the drug.
- **Clinical:** heroin OD causes coma, miosis, respiratory depression, apnoea and is treatable. Cocaine and amphetamine OD with pupil dilatation, diaphoresis, tachycardia, hypertension, seizure and coma, MI, VF, symptoms of small bowel obstruction or perforation.
- **Classification** (I, II, III are radiolucent, IV is radiopaque): type I: loosely packed cocaine covered by two to four layers of condoms or other latex-like material; this type has the highest risk for leakage/rupture. Type II: tightly packed cocaine powder or paste covered in multiple layers of tubular latex. Type III: tightly packed cocaine powder or paste covered by aluminium foil. Type IV: dense cocaine paste is placed into a device, condensed and hardened and packaged in tough tubular latex covered with coloured paraffin or fibreglass. Least likely to cause problems.
- **Investigations:** FBC, U&E, LFT, ECG. Usually but not always seen on abdominal X-ray or by abdominal USS. CT AP Hounsfield unit cocaine = 219 heroin = 520 opium = 165–200.
- **Management:** endoscopy avoided with risk of perforation of packages. If there are symptoms suggesting perforation or obstruction then urgent surgery is advocated. Total/whole bowel irrigation with PEG may be given. Laxatives (avoid oil-based laxatives). Close observation and detection and management of any related drug toxicities. Cocaine overdose is fatal in 60%. Follow local policies regarding involvement of police.
- **References:** Kelly *et al.* (2007) Contemporary management of drug packers. *World J Emerg Surg*, 2:9. Pinto *et al.* (2014) Radiological and practical aspects of body packing. *Br J Radiol*, 87:20130500.

14.36 Cannabis toxicity

- **About:** from plant *Cannabis sativa*. IV usage more toxic. Smoked (effects within 10–20 min) or ingested (effects 1–2 h) or IV.
- **Clinical:** euphoria/psychosis, drowsiness, visual distortions, HTN, raised HR. Low BP, AKI, watery diarrhoea, pulmonary oedema, DIC.
- **Investigations:** urine toxicology: positive for several days. U&E: AKI.
- **Management:** ABC. **Diazepam** 5–20 mg IV for aggression. Start IV NS at 250 ml/h for low BP. Serious poisoning rare. Resolves quickly.

14.37 Sulfonylurea toxicity

- **Examples:** gliclazide, glipizide (short-acting), chlorpropamide (long-acting).
- **Clinical:** mild to severe hypoglycaemia. Short-acting drugs less harmful.
- **Investigations:** U&E, LFT. Low glucose (confirm lab glucose).
- **Management:** 10% glucose infusion with **Octreotide** 50 mcg IV. **NaHCO$_3$** to alkalinise the urine reduces the half-life of chlorpropamide.

14.38 Methaemoglobinaemia

- **Aetiology:** methaemoglobin (MetHb) unable to bind O_2 as iron in Fe^{3+} state.
- **Causes:** dapsone, primaquine and other drugs, nitrites. Can be inherited.
- **Clinical:** blue breathless patient, chocolate-coloured blood.
- **Investigations:** low SpO_2 usually 85% with a normal PaO_2.
- **Management:** high MetHb level on ABG. If >30% then **Methylthioninium** (methylene blue) 1–2 mg/kg over 5 min. May be repeated after 30–60 min.

14.39 Phenobarbital toxicity

- **Clinical:** sedation, coma, low HR and low BP.
- **Investigations:** CT head if unsure of cause of coma.
- **Management:** ABC, supportive care. Urinary alkalinisation to pH 7.5–8 and **multiple doses of activated charcoal** can enhance the elimination.

14.40 Carbamazepine toxicity

- **About:** enzyme inducer. Toxicity with enzyme inhibitors.
- **Clinical:** drowsy, ataxia, confusion, nystagmus, TEN/SJS.
- **Investigations:** ECG: arrhythmias.
- **Management:** ABC, supportive, repeat dosing of activated charcoal. WBI is important. Haemoperfusion if end-organ toxicity becomes evident. Serious harm very rare. WBI requires 1.5–2 L/h (20–30 ml/min) of PEG. NaHCO$_3$ if QRS >100 msec carbamazepine toxicity and sodium channel blockade.

14.41 Lead, arsenic, mercury, thallium toxicity

- **Toxic metals:** lead, mercury, and cadmium. Other metals, e.g. iron, used in physiology but may be toxic in excess. Some, e.g. radioactive metals like polonium, are toxic due to emitting particles. Acute toxicity usually industrial. Take expert help. Similar clinically to lead.

- **Clinical:** mixed picture of nausea, vomiting, dehydration, abdominal pain, hepatotoxicity, pancreatitis, seizure, Fanconi syndrome, acute encephalopathy, neuropathies, e.g. foot drop, gout in suspicious setting. Thallium: painful sensory neuropathy and alopecia. Arsenic: clinical signs of pancytopenia.
- **Investigations:** FBC: (lead) anaemia and basophilic stippling on blood film. U&E, AKI/ATN, ECG, metabolic acidosis. LFTs, amylase, lactate. If suspicious measure whole blood lead in lead-free tube. Urine spot test for arsenic and 24 h urine collection for total arsenic excretion.
- **Management:** lead, mercury, arsenic, thallium. Remove source. WBI with PEG may help. Chelation therapy (IV EDTA). Chelating agents – BAL (British anti-Lewisite) or DMSA (2,3-dimethylenediaminetetracetic acid) on expert advice. Thallium needs Prussian Blue. Arsenic may need dialysis and BAL.

14.42 Nitrous oxide/laughing gas toxicity

- **About:** nitrous oxide (N_2O), commonly known as 'laughing gas', increasingly used as a recreational drug.
- **Aetiology:** prolonged use of nitrous oxide causes functional inactivation of vitamin B12 with myelopathy, sensorimotor peripheral neuropathy.
- **Clinical:** relaxation, calmness, giggles, tinnitus, progressive limb weakness and ataxia with demyelinating features, anaemia, psychosis.
- **Investigations:** macrocytic megaloblastic anaemia, low B12, raised levels of homocysteine and/or methylmalonic acid.
- **Management:** give Vitamin B12 1 mg IM. Neurology may improve and sensation and gait improved. Pregnant women should not use nitrous oxide recreationally, because chronic use is also teratogenic and toxic to the fetus.

15 Frailty

15.1 Frailty and Clinical Frailty Score

- Frailty is related to the ageing process. It describes how our bodies gradually lose their buffer against disease and trauma. Frail patients are more vulnerable to trauma, illness and other challenges. They are at risk of falls, delirium and disability.
- Issues include sarcopenia, weakness as well as arthritis, poor eyesight, deafness and cognitive problems. Patients walk slower, have poorer physical reserve and tire easily. Patients may need advice on exercise programmes (for strength and balance), mobility aids, supportive footwear and home adaptations.
- Weight loss is a characteristic feature of frailty as muscles become thinner and weaker, which we call the sarcopenia aspect of frailty. Medications, especially secondary prevention, have often become more risk than benefit, e.g. BP meds. Review and stop polypharmacy. Adverse drug reactions (ADRs) account for 6.5% of hospital admissions for older people.
- Common culprit drugs for falls include nitrates, CCBs, ACEi/ARBs and diuretics, and for delirium (opiate analgesia; benzodiazepines). Benzodiazepines can harm older people with increased risk for falls and delirium, and they contribute to the fatigue state of frailty. Vitamin D and calcium can be helpful.
- There are various ways to assess frailty and the visual Rockwood Clinical Frailty Score (see *figure* below) is commonly used. A Grade of ≥5 usually signifies mild frailty.
- Even those living independently and driving have much less reserve to recover well from trauma or infection or a major operation. In many scenarios less is more, and avoidance of intervention where the risk and benefits scales are finely balanced is best if possible.

CLINICAL FRAILTY SCALE

1	VERY FIT	People who are robust, active, energetic and motivated. They tend to exercise regularly and are among the fittest for their age.
2	FIT	People who have no active disease symptoms but are less fit than category 1. Often, they exercise or are very active occasionally, e.g., seasonally.
3	MANAGING WELL	People whose medical problems are well controlled, even if occasionally symptomatic, but often are not regularly active beyond routine walking.
4	LIVING WITH VERY MILD FRAILTY	Previously "vulnerable," this category marks early transition from complete independence. While not dependent on others for daily help, often symptoms limit activities. A common complaint is being "slowed up" and/or being tired during the day.
5	LIVING WITH MILD FRAILTY	People who often have more evident slowing, and need help with high order instrumental activities of daily living (finances, transportation, heavy housework). Typically, mild frailty progressively impairs shopping and walking outside alone, meal preparation, medications and begins to restrict light housework.
6	LIVING WITH MODERATE FRAILTY	People who need help with all outside activities and with keeping house. Inside, they often have problems with stairs and need help with bathing and might need minimal assistance (cuing, standby) with dressing.
7	LIVING WITH SEVERE FRAILTY	Completely dependent for personal care, from whatever cause (physical or cognitive). Even so, they seem stable and not at high risk of dying (within ~6 months).
8	LIVING WITH VERY SEVERE FRAILTY	Completely dependent for personal care and approaching end of life. Typically, they could not recover even from a minor illness.
9	TERMINALLY ILL	Approaching the end of life. This category applies to people with a life expectancy <6 months, who are not otherwise living with severe frailty. (Many terminally ill people can still exercise until very close to death.)

SCORING FRAILTY IN PEOPLE WITH DEMENTIA

The degree of frailty generally corresponds to the degree of dementia. Common symptoms in mild dementia include forgetting the details of a recent event, though still remembering the event itself, repeating the same question/story and social withdrawal.

In moderate dementia, recent memory is very impaired, even though they seemingly can remember their past life events well. They can do personal care with prompting.

In severe dementia, they cannot do personal care without help.

In very severe dementia they are often bedfast. Many are virtually mute.

DALHOUSIE UNIVERSITY

Clinical Frailty Scale ©2005–2020 Rockwood, Version 2.0 (EN). All rights reserved. For permission: www.geriatricmedicineresearch.ca Rockwood K et al. A global clinical measure of fitness and frailty in elderly people. CMAJ 2005;173:489–495.

Rockwood Clinical Frailty Scale. Reproduced with permission from Dalhousie University.

15.2 Falls and silver trauma

- **About:** seen mainly in older population. The price of our bipedal upright posture is the risk of falls. A fall is defined as inadvertently coming to rest on the ground or other lower level without TLOC (temporary loss of consciousness) (otherwise the issue is syncope) and other than paralysis, epileptic seizure, excess alcohol intake. The cause may be unknown if there was a head injury or amnesia post fall.
- **Information:** try to get as much information and witness statements. It may be due to walking on an uneven surface, slips on snow and ice or trips on a rug or the cat. A patient letting themselves slowly to the ground is a fall. Falls without syncope can be for a variety of reasons: awareness and some degree of self-protection are intact so injuries may be less severe.
- **Causes** are usually related to poor gait, be they musculoskeletal or neurological or sensory – neuropathy or blindness as well as medication and acute illnesses, e.g. UTI and most are often multifactorial. Frequent fallers are those with ≥2 in a 6-month period.
- **Prevention:** we can prevent falls by simply not allowing patients to walk, but the immobility and cost in terms of reduced independence and function and quality of life is very high. We need to aim to prevent falls and learn to reduce falls risk (it can never be eliminated) where possible. Anyone can fall but in most cases it is the frail elderly and so is a well-developed geriatric specialty.
- The risk of falls can cause huge loss of confidence and fear of falling over (FOFO) which can be doubly disabling. Falls themselves can cause significant trauma especially fractures, e.g. neck of femur, wrist, forearm, vertebral, femur, pelvis, humerus as well as head injury and SDH and even ruptured spleens.
- Post fall all patients need a top to toe trauma assessment and radiology/CT head where fractures or head injury suspected. May need to involve silver trauma and orthopaedics team.
- Taking referral/answering bleep: how is the patient now? Observations? Why and how did the fall happen? Any head or other injury? If so, what is GCS? Any bony pain: hip, back pain, wrist, etc.? What were the events of fall: low BP, chest pain, breathless, confusion?
- Wards have policies to reduce falls – ensure these are in place and being adhered to. Most are reported on Datix for audit. The most effective fall prevention strategies involve multidisciplinary interventions targeting identified risk factors.

On arrival (assess those >65 for silver trauma)

- A BP of 110 mmHg in an older hypertensive person may be significant and suggest bleed, sepsis etc.
- Anticoagulation is a red flag in all older trauma patients – SDH, bleed into pelvis, haemothorax, GI bleeds, retroperitoneal.
- Easy to miss trauma – SDH may take time to enlarge and cause neurology, pelvic fracture missed until walked or rib fractures until moved.
- In most patients it is a fall from own height, with the head and thorax and hip/pelvis being the commonest body areas injured.
- **Review all information:** see GP, ambulance and ED notes, review observations and medication. Mechanical fall, i.e. simple trip with clear consciousness. Medical fall – patient unwell or presyncopal or faint or hypoglycaemia or confused prior? Assess any obvious injury: fracture or head injury and arrange imaging as needed. Colle's fractures suggest consciousness and outstretched hand. Analgesia and orthopaedic review for fracture. CT head if any persisting neurology. General examination

especially for low BP. Neurological observations if head injury or seizure occurred. Document findings – anticoagulants increase risk of SDH and haematomas. ECG and telemetry and regular observations best on CCU if any suggestion of arrhythmia or vascular cause.

- **Secondary trauma:** exclude SDH, ICH, ruptured spleen, fractures. Non-displaced hip fracture may be missed and not all have classical leg shortening and external rotation. Repeat exams may be needed. Pain may not be noted until attempts to mobilise. Initial trauma surveys can miss things so have a low threshold to repeat examination and imaging if there is evidence or suspicion of possible problems. Do not get distracted by the secondary trauma and so forget about the primary cause of syncope. Special attention to those needing frequent toileting and those with delirium.
- **Practical environmental steps to reducing falls risk.** Frames surrounding toilets and raised toilet seats. Availability of chairs of varying heights to suit patients with different heights. Access to walking aids out of hours to ensure safe mobility and transfers. Chair raisers to suit the height of patients. Supply of approved slippers for patients. Bars along walls to assist and support those patients who are frail in walking independently. Access to appropriate bed rails to support patients who may be at risk of rolling or slipping out of bed.
- **Needs therapy assessment:** occupational therapy and physiotherapy can often do a comprehensive assessment of footwear, gait, safety awareness, home environment and help give a plan to reduce falls risk. For some, rehabilitation may help and nutrition is important in others. Loss of muscle bulk can be helped with enrolling in exercise programmes incorporating gait and balance training. Others may need walking aids and other devices to reduce risk. Syncope-inducing medications stopped. Those at risk of fractures with osteoporosis may be started on bisphosphonate + calcium and vitamin D. Other issues may be correcting vision, e.g. cataract removal or new glasses may help or avoid wearing wrong glasses when doing stairs. A very holistic but forensic approach is needed. A home visit may help to identify and manage hazards and risks. Stairs are risky – consider additional stair rail, assisted supervised usage, stairlift or downstairs living.
- **Long term:** may consider referral to localised falls clinic. Discussing falls risk realistically with patient and family key. For those with possible syncope further tests such as tilt table or telemetry may be considered. Pacing may be helpful with cardioinhibitory syncope.

15.3 ▸ Proximal femoral fracture in older patients

- **About:** not uncommon in older population who may be confused and delirious. Screen any older patient who falls. Mortality 10% in first month.
- **Aetiology:** trauma, osteoporosis, females, pathological – tumour.
- **Clinical:** pain in the hip following fall, shortened and externally rotated. Pain on mobilising, bruising, agitation, delirium. Check skin integrity and detail comorbidities.
- **Investigations:** FBC, U&E, Ca, LFTs, INR if on warfarin, CXR, ECG – any medical cause of fall. AP pelvis and lateral X-ray hip and orthopaedic review. MRI preferred or CT pelvis if unsure. Fractures may be intracapsular or extracapsular. CT head if any associated head trauma or neurology.
- **Management:** is based on multidisciplinary working – surgeons, geriatricians, nurses, therapists. Identify and manage both the cause of the fall and any

comorbidities such as anaemia, anticoagulation, volume depletion, electrolyte imbalance, uncontrolled diabetes, uncontrolled heart failure, correctable cardiac arrhythmia or ischaemia, acute chest infection, exacerbation of chronic chest conditions, so as not to delay surgery. Ensure analgesia (paracetamol ± codeine), hydration, nutrition, skin care. Thromboprophylaxis.

- **Surgical management:** schedule hip fracture surgery on a planned trauma list same day if possible. Perform replacement arthroplasty (hemiarthroplasty or total hip replacement) in patients with a displaced intracapsular fracture. Offer total hip replacements to those with a displaced intracapsular fracture who were able to walk independently out of doors with no more than the use of a stick, who are not cognitively impaired and are medically fit for anaesthesia and the procedure. Use extramedullary implants such as a sliding hip screw in preference to an intramedullary nail in patients with trochanteric fractures above and including the lesser trochanter. Surgery and fixation or total hip replacement improves pain control and mobility and outcome compared with non-operative approach. Mobilise day after surgery. Transfuse any bleeding. Adequate analgesia but avoid opiate/codeine toxicity. Operate on patients with the aim to allow them to fully weight bear (without restriction) in the immediate post-operative period. In high risk patients, e.g. end-stage dementia, a non-operative approach may be justified. Long-term convalescence.
- **Analgesia:** analgesic step ladder. Consider a fascia iliaca compartment block: a single bolus of local anaesthetic is injected into this potential space. Best anaesthetic option in this patient because it reduces the need for opioids. It can also provide more than 12 hours of analgesia. You should consult a clinician who is skilled in performing the regional block.
- **Complications:** avascular necrosis, pneumonia, skin lesions, anaemia, hyponatraemia, SIADH, UTI.
- **Reference:** NICE (2011) CG124: Hip fracture: management.

15.4 ▶ Fractured pubic ramus in older patients

- **About:** pelvic fractures range in severity from low energy, relatively benign injuries to life-threatening, unstable fractures. Those at the more benign end often come to medicine for management of pain and rehabilitation. They must first be reviewed by those specialised in trauma and orthopaedics to exclude other injuries. Fractures of pubic rami with insignificant or minimal trauma can be a presentation of osteoporosis. They are common in the older generation and often missed. A fracture of a pubic ramus is the commonest fracture of the pelvis. They are stable fractures and managed conservatively.
- **Risks:** dementia, delirium, osteoporosis.
- **Investigations:** FBC, U&E, Ca, plain X-ray, ECG, CT may be useful.
- **Management:** patients require adequate analgesia and mobilisation as tolerated. VTE is a risk, as is continence and loss of confidence, and these patients may need prolonged rehabilitation, and many will end up in placement. Be careful with those on anticoagulation as pelvic bleeds can be severe and the Hb can drop. Consider Ca/vitamin D and bisphosphonate. Falls assessment. Such a fracture has been shown to reduce long-term survival.

15.5 ▶ Rib fractures in older patients

- **About:** commonly seen as part of silver 'old age' trauma. The naïve may try to admit medical but really needs good trauma specialist care and access to post op type analgesia, e.g epidural/PCA on a trauma surgical ward.
- **Complications:** lung contusions, lacerations to liver, kidneys and spleen, pneumonia, pneumothorax and/or haemothorax, flail chest. Flail chest: at least 2 fractures per rib in at least 2 adjacent ribs are needed to produce a flail segment. Flail segments cause paradoxical inspiratory movements, compromise breathing and may be life-threatening. Pulmonary complications often only become evident 48–72 h after the injury.
- **Higher risk:** bilateral or >2 fractures, first rib, flail segments, lung contusions, additional injuries, anticoagulants, hypoxia, chronic lung disease.
- **Clinical:** fall and chest wall pain. Breathless. Pyrexia. Unable to cough due to pain. Anticoagulation may increase risk of haemothorax.
- **Investigations:** ABG to exclude respiratory failure, CXR, CT scan chest.
- **Management:** ABC, humidified O_2, analgesia. Treat in the trauma pathways. May need to move to trauma centre. Paracetamol/Codeine/Morphine. Assess pain score. Lidocaine patches. May need IV Morphine PCA. Gabapentin. Consider serratus anterior or paravertebral block/catheter or rib fixation and pain team.
- Saline nebulisers 10 ml 4-hourly. Salbutamol nebuliser may help. Respiratory therapy. Goal is to enable coughing and deep breathing to reduce atelectasis and pneumonia and hypoxia: "Please take a long, slow, deep breath in, ideally through your nose. Hold your breath for 2–3 seconds. Breathe out gently, like a sigh. Repeat this technique for 3–5 breaths approximately every hour".
- Consider a low threshold for CPAP/NIV or mechanical ventilation as they develop respiratory fatigue from poor chest wall mechanics in order to prevent morbidity associated with sudden respiratory decompensation.

15.6 ▶ Accidental hypothermia

- **About:** drop in core body temp below 35°C. Elderly at highest risk. Core temperature <32°C is moderate, <28°C is severe. Ask why – did hypoxia or cardiac arrest precede hypothermia? With cardiac arrest do not stop resuscitation until patients are warm and 'dead'.
- **Aetiology:** body heat from basal metabolic rate and muscle activity. Heat lost by conduction, convection and evaporation. Hypothalamus manages temperature. Core set at $37 \pm 0.5°C$. Peripheral vasoconstriction and shivering are normal response.
- **Risks:** falls, stroke, sepsis, confusion, hypothyroidism, patient with dementia and wandering. Alcohol, phenothiazines, immersion in water. Suicide attempt. Those in cold water may do better than those in warm water.

Classification (measure rectal temperature)
- **Hypothermia I:** conscious, shivering, core 35–32°C – warm area, warm clothing, warm sweet drinks, and active movement where possible.
- **Hypothermia II:** impaired consciousness, not shivering, core 32–28°C. Needs cardiac monitoring, rest to avoid arrhythmias, horizontal position and immobilisation, full-body insulation, active external and minimally invasive rewarming techniques (warm environment; chemical, electrical, or forced-air

heating packs or blankets; warm parenteral fluids). IV NS warmed to 43.0°C. Warm peritoneal lavage and dialysis.

- **Hypothermia III:** unconscious, not shivering, vital signs present. Core 28–24°C. Hypothermia II + manage airway. Consider transferring to a centre that offers ECMO or cardiopulmonary bypass if there is cardiac instability that is refractory to medical management.

- **Hypothermia IV:** no vital signs. Core <24°C. Hypothermia II + III plus CPR and up to three doses of Adrenaline (epinephrine) 1 mg IV or IO and defibrillation, with further dosing guided by clinical response; rewarming with ECMO or cardiopulmonary bypass (if available) or CPR with active external and alternative internal rewarming. Mechanical chest compression device may be used. Resuscitate until core temperature >32°C. Central line insertion should be cautious as arrhythmias occur easily.

- **Clinical:** mild ataxia, confusion and dehydration, low HR, low BP. AF common when temp <32°C. Confusion and lack of awareness so no attempt is made to reduce heat loss. Severe (<28°C) coma, absent pupillary responses and corneal reflex, cardiac standstill. Seen with stroke or falls patients incapacitated in a cold environment. Rectal probes inserted 15 cm but may be 0.5–1°C above core.

- **Investigation:** FBC: raised haematocrit and raised urea/creatinine from dehydration. U&E: raised K >10 mmol/L is not associated with survival and is considered a marker of hypoxia before cooling. Lactate and pH less reliable. Raised cardiac troponin if any ACS/MI. ECG: arrhythmias, e.g. CHB, AF, VT/VF, ectopics. The height of the Osborn/J wave is roughly proportional to the degree of hypothermia.

- **Blood gases:** metabolic acidosis, low HCO_3, raised lactate. TFT: raised TSH low T_4 as hypothyroidism can cause hypothermia. Cortisol/short synacthen: low threshold for suspecting hypoadrenalism. **Amylase:** raised in pancreatitis which may be subclinical. Toxicology screen: overdose, e.g. opiate, benzodiazepine. Carboxyhaemoglobin: carbon monoxide poisoning. **CT head:** if comatose or focal neurology.

- **Differential:** stroke or any brain injury – consider urgent CT. (Intentional?) drug overdose – alcohol, opiates, benzodiazepines, etc. Myxoedema coma, hypoglycaemia. (See Coma, ▶ Section 11.4).

- **Management:** ABCs and give O_2 as per BTS guidelines. Consider urinary catheter to detect oliguria/anuria. *Always use a low reading rectal thermometer.* Axillary, tympanic, and oral temperatures can all be misleading. Full monitoring and resuscitation facilities must be available as patient may develop VF and need defibrillation. Use warm blankets and warm drinks if able and not severe – beware excess vasodilation which can drop BP. Cardiac monitoring and repeated bloods in severe cases. **Get IV access** and give IV fluids warmed to 38–42°C and several litres of crystalloid may be needed due to cold diuresis and then vasodilation on warming which, if excessive with low BP, can be treated with **vasopressin**. Consider rarities of hypopituitary, hypoadrenalism and/or hypothyroidism. Consider IV **hydrocortisone**, IV **glucose, thiamine, naloxone**.

- **Reference:** Brown *et al.* (2012) Accidental hypothermia. *N Engl J Med*, 367:1930.

15.7 ▶ Polymyalgia rheumatica (PMR)

- **About:** PMR is a common acute inflammatory disease of older patients. A common indication for long-term steroid therapy. Watch out for symptoms of GCA. Suspected PMR + normal ESR/CRP needs secondary care review.

- **Aetiology:** cause unknown, genetic and environmental factors, disease susceptibility and severity. Possible mycoplasma, chlamydia pneumonia, and parvovirus B19 infections.
- **Clinical features:** age >50, duration >2 weeks, bilateral shoulder or pelvic girdle aching, or both, morning stiffness >45 min. Commonest age >65. Usually in northern Europeans. Clinical resolution with steroids is usually rapid and dramatic within hours/days and can help confirm diagnosis.
- **Differentials:** exclude mimicking conditions: infection, cancer, painful conditions OA, degenerative, peri-articular conditions of the shoulder, neck and hips, RA, inflammatory arthropathies, SLE, other rheumatic diseases and inflammatory myopathies, drug-induced myalgia (e.g. statins), pain syndromes (e.g. fibromyalgia). Hypothyroid, Parkinson's disease.
- **Investigations:** FBC, U&E, LFT, bone profile, ESR, CRP, plasma viscosity, dipstick urinalysis, immunoglobulins and electrophoresis (consider Bence Jones protein), TFTs, CK, rheumatoid factor, ANA, CXR (if prominent systemic symptoms).
- **Early referral to Rheumatology** if atypical features or features that increase likelihood of a non-PMR diagnosis, such as: patient <60 y, chronic onset (>2 weeks), lack of shoulder involvement, lack of inflammatory stiffness, red flag features: prominent systemic features, weight loss, night pain, neurological signs, peripheral arthritis or other features of CTD or muscle disease, normal or very high ESR/CRP. Atypical or prolonged response to steroids.
- **Management:** after counselling/explanation start **Prednisolone** 15 mg for 3 weeks, then 12.5 mg for 3 weeks, then 10 mg for 6 weeks, followed by reduction by 1 mg every 6 weeks. Early rapid improvement in symptoms is typical. A significant improvement in 1 week is likely to be PMR. If a less marked response consider giving **Prednisolone** 20 mg OD. If this fails then reconsider diagnosis and refer to Rheumatology. All steroids make people feel some degree better so you need a significant improvement. Usually 1–2 years of steroid treatment is needed. Bone protection (weekly bisphosphonate and calcium or vitamin D supplementation) should be co-prescribed with steroids therapy. Assess for steroid side-effects: weight gain, diabetes, osteoporosis, hypertension and lipid dysregulation.
- **Reference:** NICE (2021) CKS: *Polymyalgia rheumatica management.*

15.8 Abnormal gaits

- Walking a patient is an excellent test of neurological, cardiorespiratory and locomotor systems as well as cognition, vision and safety. Getting patients up to both examine and assess their ability and their safety for discharge is a key tool in acute medicine. Done on the post take round it can shorten length of stay. It starts rehabilitation.

Gait description
- **Hemiplegic:** flexed arm, extended straight leg. Circumduction gait.
- **Spastic diplegia:** scissors-type walking. Increased tone. Seen with MS, cerebral palsy.
- **Proximal myopathy:** waddling gait. Movement initiated by trunk to swing leg forward.
- **Parkinsonism:** flexed slow hesitant freezing gait. No arm movement. Associated signs.
- **Cerebellar:** unsteady ataxic, usually worse on one side unless central lesion. Nystagmus and other signs.

- **Dorsal column:** high stepping foot slapping. Falls with eyes closed. Sensory neuropathy.
- **Foot drop:** has to lift foot higher, may rotate pelvis.
- **Dyspraxic:** slow, small steps, unsteady. Small vessel stroke disease.
- **Antalgic:** painful slow usually hip pain.

15.9 ▶ DNACPR

- No one would think that BLS/ALS provides a dignified end to the long life of a frail elderly person. Generally patients are often not on cardiac monitors and in view of this unless there is a witnessed collapse the chance that you can provide good quality early CPR that will enable return to a life of quality is doubtful. There will be the occasional exception.
- One might get a ROSC but many die before discharge or go to a nursing home for all care and a lingering death from pneumonia. The chances of successful resuscitation are even less at home. If there is no DNACPR in place then medico-legally one is obliged to initiate resuscitation. Therefore it is important to discuss it. CPR is regarded as a medical intervention like an operation or medication.
- If the medical view is that CPR is not appropriate and we should allow a natural death then it is important that we explain that if they are found one day with no pulse and not breathing that outcomes are poor and we would not then be offering resuscitation. I then manage the patient's or family's reaction. I always state, however, if they do have a pulse and are breathing and unwell we will provide standard care.
- Most patients >80 have seen enough of life and death to accept this. Others may need more explanation. Others will insist on CPR. The aim is to complete a DNACPR form which the patient takes home with them which will direct healthcare/ paramedics to avoid CPR. If they are adamant that they want CPR then they will simply refuse the form. In that case further decisions can be reviewed in the future as the need arises.
- I do emphasise that it is a medical decision, but the law and simple ethics does not allow us to complete a form without discussion with the patient and/or their lasting power of attorney for health or equivalent or someone important to them if they lack capacity. Without informing the patient, family or those important to the patient the form cannot be completed.
- For many families in particular it is a relief when the medical team make the decision rather than it being foisted onto a family who are distressed and have little knowledge or experience on the issue. A small number don't want to discuss death. Communication is key. This has been clearly stipulated legally to include ringing relatives at 3 am if needed. It is about the patient's 'right to life'. You must inform and discuss and explain. It is good to get consensus if possible.
- If no one is contactable and time is short despite reasonable attempts and the patient lacks capacity then share the decision with the team, e.g. senior nursing staff or colleagues – at least a phone call. Always consult others. If death is imminent and the family or patient insist on CPR then document it and seek a second opinion to support your view. It remains a medical call.
- **New guidance:** *Decisions relating to CPR* from BMA/RCN/UK Resuscitation Council (2016) 3rd ed. (1st revision) states that "if the healthcare team is as certain that a person is dying of an underlying disease or catastrophic event and CPR would not start the heart and breathing for a sustained period then CPR should not be

attempted". This is not the default position and is for extreme time-critical situations and family should always be consulted about the healthcare decision. It is illegal for doctors to sign a DNACPR form without attempting dialogue with patient, family or the wider healthcare team.

15.10 End of life care

- This is one of the most challenging aspects of current medicine when the increasing expectations of contemporary medical practice come up against the realities of the human condition. Medicine is fundamentally about care, adding quality to life and reducing suffering. We must strive to prolong life but not to prolong an unpleasant death.
- Withdrawal of medical care and supportive management often happens at a time when discussions with the patient are not possible. It is important to involve close family. Keep them informed at all stages. It is difficult and input from colleagues can be helpful and reassuring when decisions are difficult. Strategies to involve the patient and close family in discussing end of life care much earlier need to be promoted to optimise such care.
- If the patient has a well-defined terminal illness then the natural history of the disease will be helpful. In some the natural history is less clear, such as stroke or sepsis complicating mild dementia. However, be cautious especially with acute deteriorations which may have simple remedies, e.g. UTI, hypoglycaemia, opiate toxicity and it can be reasonable to trial therapy for 24–48 h. Many malignancies and advanced dementia and other neurodegenerative diseases, heart failure and often chronic lung disease are terminal illnesses with high morbidity and mortality. Some patients are dying due to a multitude of age-related issues which lead to frailty, weight loss, immobility and becoming progressively bed-bound and often succumbing to chest infections.
- Before an end of life discussion, make sure you are completely up to date on the patient's letters and notes. Get the GP patient record if possible. Be well briefed before you talk to family. When you do make sure you get the right family – record names of those involved in discussions, it is always best to find out first what they know because they may have additional information for you or tell you things not recorded. Discover what they have been told. What are their expectations? Some issues have been discussed in the NICE end of life guidance (2015) on which the following is based. EOL decisions on new frail older patients should be avoided based on a snapshot initial assessment which may not reflect the true state, but on sequential assessments over several days.
- **Recognising when a person may be in the last days of life:** it can be difficult to be certain that a person is dying. Experienced clinical judgment is needed to manage any uncertainty. If dying, assess person's physiological, psychological, social and spiritual needs, current clinical signs and symptoms, medical history and the clinical context, including underlying diagnoses, the person's goals and wishes and views of those important to the person about future care.
- **Monitor for clinical changes:** agitation, Cheyne–Stokes breathing, deterioration in level of consciousness, mottled skin, noisy respiratory secretions and progressive weight loss, increasing fatigue and loss of appetite. Observe reduced communication, deteriorating mobility or performance status, or social withdrawal. Improvements could indicate that the person may be stabilising or recovering.

- **Investigations:** avoid if unlikely to affect care in the last few days of life unless there is a clinical need to do so with clear benefits.
- **Multidisciplinary:** interprofessional discussions and information sharing is key and issues discussed. Monitor at least every 24 h and update the person's care plan. Include a second/senior opinion when there is uncertainty about optimal management.
- **Communication is key:** with family, other staff and when possible with the patient. Establish the communication needs and expectations of people who may be entering their last days of life. Ask if they would like a person important to them to be present when making decisions about their care. Assess their current level of understanding that they may be nearing death. Assess cognitive status and if they have any specific speech, language or other communication needs. How much information would they like to have about their prognosis? Respect cultural, religious, social or spiritual needs or preferences.
- **Consent:** healthcare professionals caring for adults at the end of life need to take into consideration the person's current mental capacity to communicate and actively participate in their end of life care.
- **Information:** provide where possible information about prognosis (unless they do not wish to be informed), explaining any uncertainty and how this will be managed, but avoiding false optimism. Discuss fears and anxieties, and invite questions about their care in the last days of life. Offer further discussions. Discuss any advanced decisions or wishes. Ensure well documented. Discuss any personal goals and wishes, preferred care setting, current and anticipated care needs, including: preferences for symptom management and needs for care after death, if any are specified. Ensure appropriate revisions and updates as time passes. If it is not possible to meet the wishes of a dying person explain the reason why to the person and those important to them.
- **Maintaining hydration:** support the dying person to drink if they wish to and are able to. Address any difficulties. Offer frequent care of the mouth and lips to the dying person as part of standard care, with cleaning of teeth or dentures, if they would like. Offer frequent sips of fluid. Monitor hydration status. Assess if appropriate or desirable to start clinically assisted hydration, respecting the person's wishes and preferences. It may give some symptom relief. It may, however, cause problems – overload, local oedema, pain and may prolong life or extend the dying process. Discuss with the dying person or those important to them before starting clinically assisted hydration. Factors to consider are culture, religious beliefs, wishes, their level of consciousness, ability to swallow, evidence of thirst, risk of pulmonary oedema and the possibility of even temporary recovery. Consider a trial of hydration if there is belief that it may help and keep under review. In all of these actions involve the multidisciplinary team. If unsure of correct plan then get input from a colleague or the palliative care team.
- **Reference:** NICE (2015) NG31: Care of dying adults in the last days of life.

Palliative care drugs

- Review symptoms at least every 24 h and adjust and record accordingly. Syringe driver useful as needle can be placed subcutaneously especially when unconscious, dysphagia, vomiting, confused. All IV or SC drugs to be given by a standard calibrated syringe pump. Consult local guidance.

Pain and dyspnoea management: see *BNF*

- **Morphine** is the most important drug for controlling pain and breathlessness. It is given 5–10 mg every 4 h (low dose 2.5 mg if opiate-naïve, renal dysfunction). Lower doses given for dyspnoea. Increase dose as needed until pain relieved or side-effects substantial. Often may be given as Morphine 10 mg in syringe driver over 24 h in opiate-naïve patients with an anti-emetic. Longer-acting oral **Morphine** can be given 12 hourly. Morphine 30 mg PO = Morphine 15 mg SC = Diamorphine 10 mg SC.
- **Oxycodone:** can also be used if morphine not tolerated. Given as Oxycodone 6.6 mg = Morphine 10 mg PO = Morphine 5 mg IV.
- **Fentanyl:** if significant renal impairment transdermal fentanyl recommended as 72 h patches. The initial dose **Fentanyl** '12' patch = Morphine 30 mg OD.
- **Buprenorphine patches** can be given and there is a table in the *BNF* showing dose equivalence. Starting dose is **Buprenorphine** '5' patch.
- **Breakthrough pain** give 1/10th to 1/6th of the daily dose.

Others

- **Capillary bleeding:** Tranexamic acid 1 g TDS PO. Gauze soaked in tranexamic acid 100 mg/ml or adrenaline/epinephrine solution 1 mg/ml (1 in 1000) can be applied to the affected area. Vitamin K where it is deficient.
- **Constipation:** often an opioid and/or disease side-effect. Consider **co-danthramer** or **lactulose** solution with a **senna** preparation.
- **Anxiety:** treat pain and support. Consider Diazepam or IM/SC Midazolam which can be given as syringe driver.
- **Seizures:** Levetiracetam and Midazolam.
- **Nausea and vomiting: Haloperidol** 1–1.5 mg SC PRN 4 h up to 10 mg/d. Ongoing need haloperidol infusion 5 mg SC over 24 h. **Levomepromazine** 6 mg every 2 h PO. Give levomepromazine 12.5–50 mg/24 h by syringe driver. **Cyclizine** 50 mg 8 h PO/SC. Cyclizine 150 mg/d by infusion if needed. Alternative: Ondansetron 8 mg PO/ IV BD (may need laxative).
- **Bowel obstruction:** Hyoscine butylbromide 60–120 mg/24 h SC. Octreotide can reduce bowel secretions.

Considerations in the dying patient

- Reduce or stop non-essential usual primary and secondary prevention medications, e.g. statin, aspirin, antihypertensives, etc. Retain only drugs for symptom control, e.g. a diuretic to avoid pulmonary oedema if fluid intake continues. Judge each case individually.
- Stop inappropriate investigations. Remove cardiac monitors and O_2 sats and stop blood tests. Stop EWS-type observations. Monitor for pain, agitation, distress, skin lesions, bowels, bladder, nausea, vomiting and manage those.
- Stop IV or SC fluids if these are futile treatments because they tend only to prolong death rather than life. Oral fluids and mouth care for care and symptom support as part of EOL care.
- Ensure DNACPR and any escalation policy is completed and has been communicated to the nursing staff. Ensure family are aware and up to date on the status of the patient. Any religious or spiritual needs or cultural expectations of care of the body after death which will be handled by the bereavement office.

- Ensure death certification and any referral to coroner is done as early as possible after death and liaise with the bereavement office. GP should be made aware through local arrangements rather than reading local obituary columns.

6 Cs of end of life care
- Communication with patient and family and GP and others as appropriate.
- Consent – involving the patient in determining their care.
- Compassionate care at all times.
- Control of symptoms – see below.
- Culture – respect religious and cultural views and expectations.
- Clear documentation of plan and discussions and handovers.

15.11 Managing pressure sores and ulcers

- Elderly adults at high risk usually have multiple risk factors and should be assessed **within 6 h of admission** by nursing teams and then daily during inpatient stay (e.g. limited mobility, nutritional deficiency, inability to reposition themselves, significant cognitive impairment).
- Encourage high risk adults to change their position frequently at least every 4 h. Offer a nutritional assessment if intake is inadequate.

Grade
- **Category I:** non-blanchable redness of intact skin usually over a bony prominence. May be painful, firmer, or softer, or warmer or cooler than adjacent tissue.
- **Category II:** partial thickness skin loss or blister. Shallow open ulcer with a red/pink wound bed, without slough.
- **Category III:** full thickness skin loss (fat visible), bone, tendon, muscle are not exposed.
- **Category IV:** full thickness tissue loss (muscle/bone visible).

Assessment
- Document the surface area and depth of all pressure ulcers in adults (transparency tracing or a photograph). Use **high-specification foam mattresses.** If not sufficient to redistribute pressure, consider the use of a dynamic support surface. Assess the seating needs of adults who have a pressure ulcer who are sitting for prolonged periods. High specification foam or equivalent for those who use a wheelchair or sit for prolonged periods and who have a pressure ulcer. Consider debridement if necrotic tissue and tolerated. Consider systemic antibiotics if there is clinical evidence of systemic sepsis, spreading cellulitis or underlying osteomyelitis. Take local antimicrobial advice. Try to develop strategies for heel ulcers to offset pressure.
- **Reference:** NICE (2014) CG179: Pressure ulcers: prevention and management.

15.12 Rehabilitation, function and discharge

- Rehabilitation is an active process in which an attempt is made to improve a patient's level of functional ability to manage their own personal needs – eating, washing, dressing, transferring, toileting, mobility, shopping, working and independence. One needs an 'acute rehabable pathology', e.g. acute stroke, UTI, infection, fracture, where the natural processes of healing and repair will deliver gains in strength, dexterity, cognition, etc., that therapists can exploit to regain natural functional return to live as independent a life as possible. Pathologies such as progressive cancer and dementia or simply ageing respond poorly to rehabilitation. Rehabilitation requires a patient who is willing to cooperate and focus on the tasks. The clinician can start the process with simply encouraging sitting out of bed and activity because, to paraphrase a wise orthopod, "Bed rest is rehabilitation for the coffin".

- Getting a patient out of bed on Day 1 if appropriate will reduce length of stay, reduce risk of VTE, enable more normal bowel and bladder function and normal eating and drinking. Transfers are an important concept to describe the process by which we, in our daily lives, move our bottoms from one surface to another. In the most dependent this may be by hoist or, in those with some abilities, using aids such as rota stands, boards and other devices. A patient who can transfer their weight from a bed to a chair to a toilet has a better life than simply being bed-bound and hoisted. It is wise to get patients up and walking before discharging them. Walking is a very good screening test of cognition, vision, sensation, cardiovascular, respiratory and other neurological functions. If unsafe then ask why and involve therapy. Patients, especially older ones, often need a functional assessment prior to discharge – can they toilet, wash and feed themselves, are they safe in a kitchen, who does the shopping, access to toilet, can they manage stairs? Consider these things and involve family early.
- Before discharge simple knowledge like getting care packages back in place is key. Does the patient live in a ground floor flat with easy access or a house with 2 flights of stairs to the bedroom/bathroom? Is there a ground floor toilet? All of this can be key. Before discharge visualise your patient's day. How do they get out of bed, wash and dress, prepare a meal, eat, shop, etc.?
- A quick call to the next of kin can be hugely time-saving and allow a more realistic plan. How long does rehabilitation continue? – as long as it is continuing to deliver real and meaningful improvements in function that will improve quality of life. Stop rehabilitation if goals are constantly missed and build as much quality into the patient's world around their functional status, using equipment, carers, family support and optimising the environment. The key steps are to try to improve the patient and, once optimal, change the environment around them if needed. A good holistic clinician should be able to imagine life beyond hospital.

15.13 ▶ Acute delirium/confusion

- **<u>Taking referral/answering bleep:</u>** what is patient doing and how long for? How were they yesterday? Is it new? Age, why is patient in hospital? Check set of observations. AMTS.
- **<u>On arrival:</u>** see notes, review observations and medication. Confusion in new admissions with poor cognitive reserve is common and may suggest some serious issues and poorer prognosis. Is this confusion on a background of milder confusion or normality? Is this confusion, psychosis or dysphasia? Is this delirium or dementia, or dementia with delirium?

The confusion assessment method (CAM)

- **A: Acute onset and fluctuating course:** is there evidence of an acute change in mental status from baseline? Does abnormal behaviour come and go? Fluctuate during the day? Increase/decrease in severity?
- **B: Inattention:** does the patient have difficulty focusing attention? Are they easily distracted? Do they have difficulty keeping track of what is said?

- **C: Disorganised thinking:** is the patient's thinking disorganised, incoherent? Does the patient have rambling speech/irrelevant conversation? Unpredictable switching of subjects? Unclear or illogical flow of ideas?
- **D: Altered level of consciousness:** alert, vigilant, lethargic, stuporous, comatose? CAM method: delirium = A + B + either or both C and D (Inouye *et al.*).

General assessment
- Comprehensive clinical assessment from head to toe, drug history and corroborating history as possible. Work through common causes, e.g. infection (chest/urine), metabolic (low Na), malignancy (high Ca), drugs, e.g. codeine.
- Establish baseline. Use and record answers to the mental test score (AMTS) or some standard questions in terms of cognition, recall, orientation to time and place, speech, comprehension and attention span.
- The abbreviated MTS or the more complex mini mental state examination. Any recording of cognition is useful. The main issues are when nothing is recorded.

Abbreviated mental test score

- What is your age? (1 point)
- What is the time to the nearest hour? (1 point)
- Memory test, e.g. ask to remember an address. Then test at end (1 point)
- What is the year? (1 point)
- Name the hospital or location where you are situated (1 point)
- Can you recognise two people (doctor, nurse, home help, etc.)? (1 point)
- What is your DOB? (day and month sufficient) (1 point)
- In what year did World War II begin? (1 point)
- Name the present monarch/prime minister/president (1 point)
- Count backwards from 20 to 1 (1 point)

Causes of confusion/delirium
- **General sepsis:** examine chest and CXR, sats for pneumonia. Check urine for UTI, check lactate/WCC. U&E for sepsis. Intra-abdominal sepsis, skin sepsis. Assess temp, WCC, CRP. CXR. Check urine, stool and treat empirically.
- **Drugs: always examine drug chart and GP drugs:** illicit and prescribed drugs: cocaine, heroin, amphetamine; codeine, opiates (may be a patch), tramadol, morphine, L-dopa, alcohol, large dose steroids, anticholinergics.
- **Hypoglycaemia:** check capillary blood glucose. Suspect if on hypoglycaemic diabetic meds.
- **Occult head injury:** was there head trauma which has been missed by emergency department? Is a CT needed? Look for bumps and abrasions and cuts. Blood in ear canal.
- **CNS infections:** obtunded, neck stiffness, rash. Meningitis (a common cause in elderly), encephalitis. Consider CT to exclude SOL/abscess and urgent LP and treatment. ▶Section 11.11.
- **Delirium tremens:** agitated delirium with acute alcohol withdrawal. **Pabrinex** IV paired vials TDS for 1–2 d.
- **Wernicke's encephalopathy:** eye signs, delirium, ataxia, B1 deficiency. Often alcoholics, also hyperemesis, malnutrition. Give **Pabrinex.**
- **Acute stroke:** dysphasia often misinterpreted as confusion. Delirium vs. dysphasia. The dysphasic patient cannot follow simple tasks – close eyes, touch nose, touch left ear. Even the most confused patient can. Is there right-sided weakness, hemianopia? ▶Section 11.19.

- **Acute pain:** elderly person and acute urinary retention, or fractured neck of femur, or acute abdomen, or MI. Agitated. Incoherent.
- **Cardiac:** ACS/silent MI in elderly, diabetes. Pericarditis, fast AF, low BP.
- **Hypoxia:** check ABG, CXR, COPD, CO poisoning. Look for CO_2 retention.
- **Drug withdrawal:** alcohol, benzodiazepines, opiates, antidepressants.
- **Acute psychosis:** schizophrenia or other mental health disorder. Hyperactive, agitated, delusions, psychotic.
- **Metabolic:** low or high Na, liver failure, renal failure, myxoedema madness, apathetic thyrotoxicosis, high Ca, Addison's disease, pituitary failure, SIADH, porphyria.
- **Vitamin:** suspect if malnourished, alcoholic, hyperemesis, give Pabrinex, B12 deficiency with pernicious anaemia and other causes. Pellagra.
- **Malaria:** travel or endemic area send thick/thin films. Treat if real possibility. Also consider other tropical disease if recent travel. HIV conversion.
- **Autoimmune/limbic encephalitis:** autoimmune which may or may not be paraneoplastic. NMDA receptor antibody encephalitis, voltage-gated potassium channel-complex antibody-associated limbic encephalitis (VGKC-LE). MRI FLAIR shows medial temporal signal changes. Cancers – lung, breast, testis, lymphoma, teratoma, thymoma. Treatment: remove tumour and/or immune modulation with varying success.
- **Steroid-responsive encephalopathy associated with autoimmune thyroiditis (SREAT): F>M.** Psychosis, seizures. tremor, myoclonus, stroke mimic. Normal MRI. High CSF protein. Abnormal TFTs. Positive antithyroid peroxidase antibodies (anti-TPO, antithyroid microsomal antibodies, anti-M) and antithyroglobulin antibodies. Responds to steroids.
- **Structural brain pathology:** abscess, stroke, SAH, encephalitis, meningitis, tumour, hydrocephalus, CJD; CT/MRI scan helpful. Consider LP.
- **Seizure/NCSE:** EEG, CT/MRI/LP. Treat. ▶Sections 11.15 and 11.16.
- **Malignancy:** high Ca, liver metastases, brain metastases, paraneoplastic.
- **Inflammatory disease:** any acute inflammatory illness or flare-up. Neurosarcoidosis, Behçet's disease, etc.
- **Encephalitis:** infectious – usually HSV infection, also HIV, Murray Valley and Japanese encephalitis can be seen in epidemics. Take expert advice. Send CSF and viral and PCR. ▶Section 11.8.
- **Creutzfeldt–Jakob:** can progress over weeks. Myoclonus a useful clue. CSF to Edinburgh Prion Unit for real-time quaking induced conversion (RT-QuIC) is 92% sensitive and 100% specific for sporadic CJD. Rapid, older. Variant – younger, slower, ataxia. MRI changes. EEG changes are late. Palliation.

Reversible and non-reversible dementias
- **Progressive dementias:** Alzheimer's, vascular, Lewy body, frontotemporal, alcoholic, Huntington's disease, CJD, Pick's disease, Parkinson's disease, HIV, SSPE, PML.
- **Reversible 'pseudodementias':** B12/folate/thiamine/thyroxine deficiency, SDH, normal pressure hydrocephalus (NPH), operable tumour (e.g. meningioma), depression.

Investigations
- **Blood:** glucose, FBC, ESR, U&E. Calcium, B12 and folate. TFTs. Urinalysis.
  ABG: hypoxia, hypercarbia, CO-Hb level.

- **CXR:** tumour, infection, hypoxia. **ECG:** silent MI, AF.
- **CT head:** look for SDH, abscess, stroke, tumour, oedema, etc.
- **Lumbar puncture:** meningitis/encephalitis/SAH. CSF removed in NPH done to see if improvement in walking but controversial.
- **EEG:** focal seizure or non-convulsive status or encephalopathy.
- **Infections:** HIV test, malaria thin and thick films, LP.
- **Rare:** thyroid antibodies, NMDA receptor antibody, VGKC-LE.
- **Measure ammonia:** high with hepatic encephalopathy, drugs such as valproate and some chemotherapy can cause an ammonia encephalopathy.
- **MRI:** can help if encephalitis or inflammation or stroke or malignancy or other structural lesions are suspected.

Management

- **Supportive:** manage anxiety, keep lights on, calm, friendly reassurance, and involve familiar people or family. Work through potential causes as listed above. May need sedation or even full sedation and airway management for a CT brain. Balance risks vs. benefits.
- **Sedation (avoid IV):** when patient at risk of harm to themselves. Last resort. Not for convenience. Go slow. **Lorazepam** 1–4 mg PO/IM can be tried or **Haloperidol** 0.5–2 mg PO/IM/SC (low doses 0.5–2 mg in elderly) are useful but avoid if at risk of seizure. Get help if risk of over-sedation and airway management. Low threshold for a CT head is needed. Avoid haloperidol in Lewy body dementia.
- **Antibiotics/Aciclovir:** treat if suspicion for bacterial meningitis (ceftriaxone + amoxicillin) and HSV encephalitis (Aciclovir). Get LP if possible.
- **Give Pabrinex** IV paired vials TDS for 1–2 d prior to IV glucose.
- **Stop opiates.** Remove any opiate pain patch and give naloxone.
- **Give Lorazepam** 1–2 mg IM if non-convulsive status suspected. Get EEG.
- **Reference:** Inouye *et al.* (1990) Clarifying confusion: the confusion assessment method. A new method for detection of delirium. *Ann Intern Med*, 113:941.

15.14 Dementias

- **About:** a global loss of brain function, of memory, personality, decision-making, speech, walking, eating. Eventual weight loss and frailty. Some can coexist – AD and vascular.
- **Definition:** acquired and persistent compromise in multiple cognitive domains that is severe enough to interfere with everyday functioning. Insidious and progressive decline.
- **Clinical:** history is vital of >6 months of cognitive decline supported by formal testing and compatible imaging and testing. Delirium can muddy the waters in hospital so the diagnosis is preferred post discharge via memory assessment clinic. Support with assessments such as MMSE, the MoCA, AMTS. These help grade into mild/moderate and severe.
- **Acute issues:** the main query is whether any decline is disease progression and unlikely to reverse or disease plus other pathologies and that must be weighed up and balanced on the evidence found.
- **Investigations:** FBC, U&E, LFTs, glucose, B12, TFT, ECG. EEG and CSF not usually needed. CT/MRI to exclude SOL and see atrophy. Syphilis serology, HIV test as needed.

Causes of dementia

- **Alzheimer dementia (AD):** commonest. 5–10% of age >70. Extracellular amyloid (tau) plaques and intracellular neurofibrillary tangles. Progressive short-term memories. Remembers distant events not recent ones. Then visuospatial and language affected. Increasing immobility. Ends up bed-bound, akinetic and mute. Death from infection and frailty. Most sporadic, rarely genetic. Risk: trisomy 21, low educational attainment, head injury. MRI: atrophy of hippocampus and medial temporal lobes. Treat with cholinesterase inhibitors, memantine. Carers support with ADLs.
- **Vascular dementia:** step-wise progressive decline of cognition in a patient with stroke disease. Dyspraxic gait, incontinence. May be associated with AD. Risks – HTN, smoker, lipids. CT/MRI severe white matter disease. Cholinesterase inhibitors may help.
- **Lewy body dementia:** age >70. Dementia with hallucinations, parkinsonism, REM sleep disorder. MRI may show hippocampal atrophy. Trial of Madopar for parkinsonism and cholinesterase inhibitors for cognition.
- **Frontotemporal dementia:** manifest as altered behaviour with disinhibition and rigid thinking. Others with primary progressive aphasia. Alien limb phenomenon. Seen in those aged 40–60. Gross atrophy of frontal and temporal lobes seen on MRI. Treat with SSRI, neuroleptics.
- **Normal pressure hydrocephalus:** reduced cognition, dementia, dyspraxic gait, urinary incontinence. Falls, confusion. CT/MRI degree of hydrocephalus is out of proportion to any expected ventriculomegaly due to simple atrophy. T2 FLAIR shows periventricular hyperintensity. LP and CSF removal of 30–50 ml of CSF can result in improved gait and mentation but very subjective and false positives and negatives. Needs expert review to decide need for shunting. Improvement with CSF removal does not guarantee improvement with shunting.
- **HIV dementia:** gradual onset of dementia. Need low threshold for detection and testing. Atrophy on MRI. Check HIV and CD4. Consider HAART.
- **Creutzfeldt–Jakob disease: sporadic form:** middle-aged, rapid decline, myoclonic jerks, typical EEG and MRI findings as progresses. Elevated CSF protein 14-3-3. A newer test that detects the specific marker for sporadic CJD, the prion protein (PrPCJD), by means of real-time quaking induced conversion (RT-QuIC) testing of CSF has a sensitivity of 80–90%. Call Edinburgh reference lab before taking sample.

15.15 Parkinson's disease

- **About:** chronic neurodegenerative disease with both motor and non-motor manifestations. Predominantly affects older patients but younger patients can be affected. First known description James Parkinson in 1817.
- **Prevalence:** 1.6/1000 population. Incidence rises with age. Males > females. Not all those with tremor and stiffness have IPD. Many other causes of parkinsonism especially drug-induced and vascular and genetic causes. Always review diagnoses. Best clinicians are wrong 1 in 4. Sometimes it takes months or years to diagnose Parkinson's disease with certainty.
- **Aetiology:** premature loss of 30–70% of melanin-containing dopaminergic neurons in the substantia nigra of the midbrain with disruption of local circuits. Deposition of alpha synuclein which become misfolded and build up and form as Lewy bodies which are found in the substantia nigra in midbrain.

- **Braak's hypothesis:** disease starts in peripheral autonomic system and olfactory bulb and dorsal nucleus of vagus and proceeds up to involve cortex. The disease has often been present years before diagnosis. Levodopa converted to dopamine.
- **Different forms:** juvenile age <21 y usually associated with a Parkin gene mutation. Early onset 21–50 and late onset >60.
- **Acute issues:** the main query is whether any decline is disease progression and unlikely to reverse, or disease plus other pathologies and that must be weighed up and balanced on the evidence found.

Clinical diagnosis

- **Step 1.** Diagnosis of parkinsonian syndrome: bradykinesia + one of the following: muscular rigidity (lead-pipe or cogwheel) OR 4–6 Hz rest (pill rolling) tremor OR postural instability not due to other cause.
- **Step 2.** Exclusion criteria for Parkinson's disease: repeated strokes with stepwise progression of parkinsonian features OR a history of repeated head injury OR definite encephalitis OR oculogyric crises or neuroleptic treatment at onset of symptoms OR >1 affected relative OR sustained remission OR strictly unilateral features after 3 years OR supranuclear gaze palsy or cerebellar signs OR early severe autonomic involvement OR early severe dementia with disturbances of memory, language, and praxis OR Babinski sign OR cerebral tumour or communication hydrocephalus on CT/MRI OR no response to large doses of levodopa in absence of malabsorption or MPTP exposure.
- **Step 3.** Supportive prospective positive criteria for Parkinson's disease: ≥3 required for diagnosis of definite Parkinson's disease in combination with step 1 of unilateral onset OR rest tremor present OR progressive disorder OR persistent asymmetry affecting side of onset most OR excellent response (70–100%) to LD OR severe LD-induced chorea OR LD response for 5+ years OR clinical course of 10+ years.

Signs and symptoms and functional loss

- Difficulty turning in bed, walks slow flexed posture, loss of arm swing, festinant gait, frozen shoulder, constipation, watch stops as arm movements not sufficient to keep it going, 'Rolex sign'. Difficult dressing, buttons, fine motor skills. Unable to stir food or wipe. Instability and falls. Increased isolation and dependence. Freezes walking through doorways.
- Non-motor problems: early: anosmia (no smell), constipation, autonomic dysfunction sweats, REM sleep disorder, depression, cognitive and behavioural issues, sialorrhoea, seborrheic dermatitis, dementia.

Investigations

- FBC, U&E, CRP, screen for Wilson's disease in young adults (treatable).
- MRI brain to exclude other diagnoses, especially stroke disease.
- SPECT ligand binds dopamine. Dopamine transporter scan (DaTscan). Shows reduced uptake/asymmetry. Use only where differential is essential tremor. Does not help differentiate IPD from vascular or other causes of parkinsonism.

Management

- Review every 6 months to access diagnosis and progression and response to treatment. Balance dosing and effect. Too little medications is no use. Too much leads after several years to dyskinesias. If motor symptoms affect activities of daily life, then consider a dopamine agonist (DA) in younger patients or levodopa (LD) in older. No evidence that medication slows/delays disease progression. Management is multi-professional. OT/PT/SALT can help in managing symptoms and providing advice, therapy if needed and equipment. PD nurses can help with invaluable advice and monitoring and support. Exercise can improve quality of life.

- **Avoid/stop:** dopamine blockers such as neuroleptics haloperidol, chlorpromazine, metoclopramide. Avoid tetrabenazine and methyldopa.
- **Uncertainty:** mild early disease a watch and wait strategy is fine. Diagnosis clinical. Main differential in elderly is vascular/stroke, drug-induced, essential tremor and slowness of frailty. Diagnosis/meds need regular review. Trial Madopar 62.5 mg TDS for 5 d and double dose and reassess. Consider setting realistic functional goals ADLS.
- **Monoamine oxidase type B (MAOB) inhibitors:** rasagiline 1 mg OD. Selegiline rarely used. Prevents dopamine breakdown. Give with LD.
- **Levodopa (LD) with peripheral decarboxylase inhibitor:** 1st-line in older (>65). LD is always given with a peripheral decarboxylase inhibitor. Centrally converted to dopamine. This reduces side-effects and dose needed. There are two formulations, co-careldopa and Madopar; same efficacy. Short half-life so must be dosed several times a day. Start with either preparation at 12.5/50 mg (12.5 of DCI + 50 mg LD) 3/d spaced out and increase gradually. Dyskinesias seen with doses over 500 mg/d. Patients may prefer to be 'on' with dyskinesias rather than 'off' and frozen with none. Controlled release formulations available which are given BD (Sinemet/ Caramet CR). Side-effects: nausea, orthostatic hypotension.
- **Dopamine agonists:** used often in younger (age <65) as single agent. May also be added to levodopa (LD). Acts on dopamine receptors. Fewer side-effects than LD and less efficacy. Used in mild–moderate disease. Ergotamine agonists avoided as caused heart and lung fibrosis. Consider ropinirole or pramipexole or rotigotine which comes as a patch. Start **Ropinirole** 250 mcg TDS. Max dose 9–16 mg/d. **Pramipexole** 88 mcg TDS max 3.3 mg/d. Side-effects include hallucinations, sleepiness.
- **Catechol-O-methyltransferase (COMT) inhibitors** given with L-dopa and carboxylase inhibitor entacapone. Called Stalevo with LD+DCI. Alternative **Opicapone** 50 mg OD bedtime.
- **Amantadine:** used nowadays for dyskinesias which limits adding more LD.
- **Anticholinergics:** original treatment for tremor with PD. Benefits offset by worsened cognition, hallucinations, constipation, dry mouth, and impaired urination. Avoided generally, especially in older patients.

Specialist care

- **Deep brain stimulation:** stimulating electrodes placed stereotactically into the deep structures of the brain. Electrodes connected to battery-powered implanted pulse generator. It reduces motor fluctuations in advanced IPD. Targets globus pallidus interna or subthalamic nucleus. Dose of dopaminergic drugs can be reduced. Mimics effect of levodopa without dyskinesia. Helps tremor, rigidity and bradykinesia. Consider if full medical therapy not controlling symptoms or excess side-effects.
- **Levodopa-carbidopa intestinal gel (LCIG):** new delivery system. Leads to reduced motor fluctuations/dyskinesias. It is a gel that contains LD (2000 mg) and carbidopa (200 mg). Known as Duodopa. Given as a continuous infusion using a portable pump via PEJ tube. Single cassette contains a single day's treatment. Licensed for advanced LD-responsive PD with severe motor fluctuations and hyper-/ dyskinesia when available combinations of medicinal products are unsatisfactory. Expensive.
- **Apomorphine:** DA less used as rotigotine can be given to those who cannot take enteral medications. Given by syringe drive. Specialist use.

Problem-solving

- **Off symptoms:** consider change increase/spread dose frequency and amount. Consider COMT inhibitor. **Opicapone** 50 mg ON.
- **Constipation:** bulking agents, ensure hydration, mobility.
- **Daytime sleepiness:** consider modafinil (specialist).
- **Sialorrhoea:** sweets, chew gum. Oral anticholinergic meds dry mouth. Scopolamine patch. 1% atropine eye drops taken as 1–2 drops under the tongue per day to dry the mouth. *Botulinum* toxin to salivary glands.
- **Anxiety/depression:** consider psychology and antidepressant. Consider citalopram, sertraline, fluoxetine, venlafaxine, mirtazapine.
- **REM sleep disorder:** consider clonazepam or melatonin to treat RBD if a medicines review has addressed possible pharmacological causes.
- **Low libido/erectile dysfunction:** counselling support, sildenafil.
- **Nausea/vomiting:** domperidone is anti-emetic of choice.
- **Impulse control disorders:** levodopa or dopamine agonist medication is associated with impulse control disorders. Patients indulge in pathological gambling, binge eating and hypersexuality. Inform patients and carers so that it can be recognised, understood and managed.
- **Unable to turn in bed:** bed levers, low friction silk sheets.
- **Swallowing issues:** chin tuck. SALT review. PEG in selected cases.
- **Unable to take usual meds:** do not stop anti-parkinsonian medication abruptly. Causes acute akinesia or neuroleptic malignant syndrome. Consider dispersible meds via NG or rotigotine patch.
- **Dementia:** cognitive support. Rivastigmine and memantine.

End-stage PD life expectancy 6–12 months

- Severe motor symptoms and complications. Falls, dyskinesias. Frailty.
- Cognitive decline, spends most of time in bed/chair.
- Weight loss, dysphagia, speech issues, low BMI.
- Focus is on palliation and advanced care planning.

Prognostic markers

- More benign course: early onset, tremor predominant, female sex.
- Rapid course: male, late onset, postural instability, rigidity or bradykinesia as presenting issue, dementia, poor response to levodopa, comorbidities.

Hospital admission

- It is vitally important that anti-PD medications continue uninterrupted. Drugs should be written up as usual with correct timings. Abrupt stopping can lead to a neuroleptic malignant syndrome as well as distress and freezing. If NG tube, then usually drugs can be given in dispersible forms. If an NG tube is not possible then consider **Rotigotine** patches. Take specialist advice if unsure.
- There is an excellent online resource at www.pdmedcalc.co.uk which will calculate the dose depending on the medication being taken.

15.16 Wernicke's encephalopathy

- **About:** Wernicke's encephalopathy is a degenerative brain disorder caused by the lack of thiamine (vitamin B1).
- **Causes:** may result from an alcohol-based diet which is low in thiamine, dietary deficiencies, AIDS, surgery, anorexia, prolonged vomiting – hyperemesis gravidarum, eating disorders, or the effects of chemotherapy.
- **Pathology:** damage to mammillary bodies, dorsomedial nuclei of the thalamus and adjacent grey matter. If glucose is administered, the remaining thiamine in the mammillary bodies is consumed, leading to irreversible damage.
- **Clinical:** anorexia, cachexia, worsening cognition, altered gait and nystagmus, ophthalmoplegia, ataxia, confusion. Untreated is irreversible with Korsakoff's syndrome with short-term memory loss and confabulation.
- **Differential:** cognitive issues common in chronic drinkers – dementia, falls and head injuries and assaults and brain injuries, SDH.
- **Investigations:** do not defer treatment for tests. Raised plasma pyruvate and reduced red cell transketolase. MRI scan may show changes. CT at least to exclude SDH and other causes of neurology in drinkers.
- **Management:** prevent with dietary advice for alcoholics. **Pabrinex IV ×2** TDS for 2–3 days. **Longer if high suspicion.** Long-term **Thiamine** 100 mg OD PO. Abstention from alcohol. Manage specific causes with feeding and dietetics.

16 Pregnancy/postpartum

16.1 General issues

- The call to the obstetric unit for medical issues can be intimidating to even the most accomplished doctor. This is a collection of a few basic facts and principles to help you. As ever, if unsure of what you are doing then get help. This is to deal mainly with acute and on-call questions. Pregnancy is covered within resuscitation, asthma and DVT/pulmonary embolism and headache sections.
- **Higher risk:** black ethnic background, *in vitro* fertilisation (IVF) resulting in the current pregnancy.
- *High risk patients for VTE will receive prophylaxis during pregnancy until at least 6 weeks postpartum. Do not stop it without expert guidance.*

General principles

- Most women in pregnancy are healthy. Those with known or anticipated medical disorders require expert care. The obstetric team liaise with medical specialists as needed. Communication is key.
- Medical disorders are those caused by the pregnancy or pre-existing ones exacerbated by the pregnancy, e.g. heart disease, asthma, immune disorders, clotting disorders, epilepsy.
- It is important to involve senior members of the obstetric team when making any significant management plans that can affect the pregnancy.
- Be aware that detected mental health issues should be flagged up.

Altered physiology

- Increased heart rate + 10–20 bpm particularly in third trimester.
- Lowered BP by 10–15 mmHg by 20 weeks, but normal by term.
- No change respiratory rate (RR). RR >20 breaths/min is abnormal.
- No change oxygen saturation or temperature.
- Systolic flow murmurs may be heard – get ECG, CXR, echo if unsure.

Altered lab tests

- FBC: Hb (105–140 g/L); WBC (6–16 × 10^9/L).
- Renal function: measure creatinine but eGFR better guide.
- Alkaline phosphatase × 3–4 from placenta especially 3rd trimester.
- Troponin high with pre-eclampsia, PE, myocarditis, arrhythmias and sepsis.
- D-dimer not useful, raised. CK is lower in pregnancy.
- TFT variable so use local gestation-specific ranges.

ECG changes that are normal in pregnancy

- Sinus tachycardia 15° LAD due to diaphragmatic elevation.
- T wave changes – commonly T wave inversion in lead III and aVF.
- Non-specific ST changes, e.g. depression, small Q waves.
- Holter monitor SVT and ventricular ectopics are more common.

Respiratory

- CXR: vascular markings, raised diaphragm due to gravid uterus, flattened left hemidiaphragm. Peak expiratory flow rate (PEFR) is unchanged.

- ABG: mild, fully compensated respiratory alkalosis is normal during pregnancy.
- Suspected PE and a normal CXR, a perfusion lung scan is preferred to CTPA because the radiation dose to maternal lung and breast tissue is lower.

Chest pain in pregnancy

- Red flags for chest pain requiring opioids. Pain to arm, shoulder, back or jaw. Sudden onset, tearing or exertional chest pain. Look for haemoptysis, breathlessness.
- Chest pain with syncope or abnormal neurology. Chest pain and abnormal observations. Usually causes of chest pain are PE, ACS, aortic dissection and musculoskeletal pain.
- There is increased risk of PE and dissection. PE is commoner in the postpartum phase when prophylaxis should be continued for at least 6 weeks in high-risk patients. Aortic dissection is commoner in the 3rd trimester. A CTPA may diagnose both but a simple lung perfusion scan will miss a dissection so be wary. Pneumomediastinum is a rare diagnosis that may be seen with protracted vomiting in the first trimester.

Palpitations in pregnancy

- Palpitations are a common physiological symptom during pregnancy. SVT is common. Treat with vagotonic manoeuvres, adenosine, calcium channel blockers and β-blockers. If needed, consider DC cardioversion with fetal monitoring and anaesthetic input.
- Always consider causes such as hypovolaemia, anaemia, thyrotoxicosis, phaeochromocytoma and even a pulmonary embolism. Each case needs a full assessment.
- Red flags are a family history of sudden cardiac death or structural heart disease or previous cardiac surgery or associated syncope or chest pain or persistent and severe tachycardias. These may warrant cardiological assessment and monitoring and echocardiography.

Breathlessness in pregnancy

- Breathlessness is common, affecting up to 75% of women and may commence in early pregnancy often described as an 'air hunger', worse at rest or talking and relieved by mild exertion. Usual causes of breathlessness – asthma, pneumothorax, pneumonia, Covid, etc. PE is a significant risk through pregnancy and postpartum.
- Another specific diagnosis is heart failure due to peripartum cardiomyopathy can occur in the third trimester or postpartum. Pre-existing and undiagnosed heart disease, e.g. mitral stenosis, may deteriorate from the second trimester onwards.
- Red flags would be sudden-onset breathlessness, orthopnoea, breathless with chest pain or syncope, respiratory rate >20/min, low O_2 <94% at rest or on exertion, breathless with associated tachycardia.

Headache and stroke in pregnancy

- **Migraine** often reduces in pregnancy. If it follows its classic pattern from before pregnancy that is reassuring. If it does not, have a low threshold for scanning. NSAIDs are safe to take up to 32 weeks gestation for migraine.
- **Red flags** are headaches that are of sudden onset or thunderclap or worst headache ever suggesting SAH. A headache that takes longer than usual to resolve or persists for >48 h needs further assessment. Headache with fever, seizures, focal neurology, photophobia, diplopia needs assessment or one where patients need excessive use of opioids.

- **Posterior reversible encephalopathy syndrome** (PRES) can present with headache in the third trimester (▶Sections 16.6 and 11.40).
- **Reversible cerebral vasoconstriction syndrome** (▶Section 11.41).
- **Cerebral vein thrombosis** most commonly in the 3rd trimester and postpartum. Needs assessed and anticoagulated. Infarcts with oedema and bleeding on CT/CTV.
- **Meningitis/encephalitis:** *Streptococcus pneumoniae* and *Listeria monocytogenes* are more common during pregnancy.
- **Pre-eclampsia:** seen in 3rd trimester only and postpartum. BP >140/90 mmHg. Urinary protein: creatinine ratio (PCR) >50: refer to obstetric team.
- **Idiopathic intracranial hypertension:** worsens as weight increases. Acetazolamide is safe.
- **Stroke:** no contraindication to thrombolysis, thrombectomy or stenting during pregnancy for acute ischaemic stroke. Refer stroke team. Liaise with obstetrics.
- **Investigations:** discuss with Radiology. CT may be done with CTA/CTV if needed. Discuss. MRI is the most useful modality and non-contrast studies may be enough to diagnose stroke and vasoconstriction and PRES. Gadolinium is contraindicated.

Mental health issues

- Mental illness can occur in pregnancy from long-standing issues or *de novo* problems such as postpartum psychosis and bipolar affective disorder. Can occur during and in postpartum period. Suicide is a significant cause of postpartum mortality and needs risk assessed. Anxiety and depression are also common. Specialist perinatal psychiatric services have expertise in this area for women who experience symptoms during this time.
- Red flags in those with psychiatric complaints are a recent significant change in mental state or emergence of new symptoms. New thoughts or acts of violent self-harm. New and persistent expressions of incompetence as a mother or estrangement from the baby.

Medical advice on managing pregnant patients

- There are two (or sometimes more) patients.
- Give folate prior to conception and in the 1st trimester.
- Tachypnoea or raised HR must not be ignored.
- A pink venous cannula is useless in a sick pregnant patient.
- Ectopic pregnancy can be atypical, e.g. 'fainting, D&V'.
- Ultrasound, CT head and chest are fine (discuss if pelvis needs imaged).
- MRI is safe in pregnancy but gadolinium contrast should be avoided.
- CXR is initial test for the breathlessness (1 day background shield fetus).
- Lung perfusion scan preferred to CTPA for PE but CTPA is higher yield/shows other diagnoses. Take expert advice.
- Avoid prescribing in 1st trimester unless proven safety.
- Avoid NSAIDs, ACEi, ARBs, trimethoprim, warfarin.
- For anticoagulation use LMWH or IV heparin.
- Consider diagnosing PE by diagnosing a DVT first if leg symptoms.
- For hyperemesis give thiamine (give Pabrinex) at risk of Wernicke's.
- You can use salbutamol, steroids and magnesium for asthma.
- Use magnesium for preventing eclamptic seizures.
- Accidental magnesium overdose can be fatal. Give IV **calcium gluconate.**

- **Reference:** RCP (2019) Acute care toolkit 15: Managing acute medical problems in pregnancy. www.rcplondon.ac.uk/guidelines-policy/acute-care-toolkit-15-managing-acute-medical-problems-pregnancy

16.2 Resuscitation in pregnancy

Call 'Maternal Cardiac Arrest team' Obstetric team and Paediatrics and 100% oxygen. Continue CPR and if uterus is palpable above the umbilicus consider immediate resuscitative caesarean section.

- **About:** resuscitation of a pregnant woman is an infrequent event. Follow usual guidance and start quality CPR. Occurs in 1 in 30,000 late pregnancies. Modifications to systematic ABCDE approach during maternal collapse.
- **NB:** if >20 weeks consider a peri-mortem caesarean (resuscitative hysterotomy) to save the mother and baby. It must be done within 5 min of the cardiac arrest.
- **Possible causes:** bleeding coagulopathy, DIC, sepsis, acute MI, concealed haemorrhage – placental abruption, ectopic pregnancy, rupture or dissection of aneurysms, pulmonary embolus (thrombolysis if life-threatening PE), amniotic fluid embolism (immediate caesarean), anaesthetic complication, known or new cardiac disease, HTN, pre-eclampsia/eclampsia, placenta abruptio/placenta praevia. Discuss an urgent management plan for these if ROSC – most are obstetric.

Procedure (get Obstetrics/Anaesthetics/Paediatrics)

- Left lateral uterine displacement should be used to minimise aortocaval compression and maximise cardiac output after 20 weeks gestation.
- IV access above diaphragm. Give O_2 target 94–98%.
- Give IV fluid bolus if there is hypotension/hypovolaemia.
- Preoxygenate 100% O_2 before intubation as more rapid onset of hypoxaemia.
- Positioning for CPR, chest tubes, defibrillator pads higher on the chest wall.
- Assess if any drugs have been taken and reverse if possible.
- Cardioversion and defibrillation will not harm the fetus.
- Consider therapeutic hypothermia in a comatose patient with ROSC.
- For an Rh-negative woman who has vaginal bleeding after trauma, administer Rh immunoglobulin (RhoGAM): a 50-mcg dose in the 1st trimester and a 300-mcg dose in the 2nd or 3rd trimester.
- Fetal monitor for any pregnant woman >24 weeks gestation who suffers trauma to the abdomen and continue to monitor for 4–6 h.
- If patient has been given excess magnesium sulfate suspect Mg *toxicity*, give 10 ml IV 10% **Calcium gluconate.**
- Give **Tranexamic acid** 1g IV for postpartum haemorrhage.
- Consider early tracheal intubation by a skilled operator. Find and treat reversible causes (e.g. haemorrhage). Focused ultrasound by a skilled operator can be used to identify reversible causes and may also be used to assess if a fetal heart rate is present. Consider extracorporeal CPR (ECPR) as a rescue therapy if ALS measures are failing.

Procedure for a peri-mortem caesarean (resuscitative hysterotomy)

- Perform within 4 min of resuscitation; if unsuccessful, deliver the fetus by emergency hysterotomy aiming for delivery within 5 min of collapse.

- No time for gown/hat/mask or to wash your hands surgically. Don gloves and an apron. Clean the skin then incise from the umbilicus to the pubic bone vertically. If you're used to can do horizontal (Pfannenstiel) incision. Avoid urinary bladder which is close to the lower segment of the uterus. The bladder will probably be full, but don't waste time with a catheter.
- Use any big surgical sterile swabs to help you grip, and to control bleeding – count them in if possible. After your incision, you should be able to spot the uterus, and deliver the fetus.
- Exposing, or delivering, the uterus is only done where there is bleeding from the broad ligament and in an arrest situation there shouldn't be much bleeding – if there is you would definitely need an obstetric consultant to assist.
- Once baby delivered if the placenta won't come out easily, leave it *in situ* and wait for obstetric assistance – it may be a placenta accreta, and pulling it out will make things worse! Continue to resuscitate your patient and resuscitate the neonate too if applicable.

References
- www.rcemlearning.co.uk/foamed/cardiac-arrest-in-the-pregnant-patient/
- UK Resus Council (2021) Special circumstances guidelines.

16.3 ▶ Pharmacology in pregnancy

- **Sources of prescribing advice in UK:** *BNF* or your local equivalent. The UK Teratology Information Service (www.uktis.org) has phone support and there is also BUMPS (best use of medicines in pregnancy – www.medicinesinpregnancy.org) and also www.toxbase.org.
- **Known or potential teratogens to stop/avoid:** ACEi, ARBs, NSAIDs, statins, cigarette smoking, cocaine, warfarin, fluconazole, isotretinoin (Accutane), lithium, misoprostol, penicillamine, tetracyclines, doxycycline, thalidomide, valproic acid, cyclophosphamide, mycophenolate, sirolimus.
- **Some possible teratogens:** alcohol binge drinking, carbamazepine, colchicine, disulfiram, ergotamine, glucocorticoids (benefits often outweigh risks), lead, metronidazole, primidone, quinine (suicidal doses), streptomycin, vitamin A (high doses), zidovudine (AZT).
- **Drugs to avoid when breastfeeding:** chloramphenicol, metronidazole, nitrofurantoin and sulphonamides (haemolysis with G6PD deficiency), tetracycline (stains teeth and bones), lithium, antineoplastics and immunosuppressants, psychotropic drugs (relative).
- **Drugs which can be used acutely in pregnancy:** heparin and LMWH, ampicillin, cephalosporins, clindamycin, erythromycin, gentamicin, paracetamol (acetaminophen), folate, pyridoxine, thyroxine, steroids, salbutamol, aspirin, magnesium, anticholinergic inhalers, theophyllines, lorazepam, diazepam, phenytoin. Give usual doses of GTN, IV nitrates, furosemide, morphine, calcium blocker, mechanical support, e.g. IABP, LVAD, digoxin, beta-blockers.

Choosing meds: check all drugs in the *BNF* if pregnant/breastfeeding
- **Antibiotics:** avoid trimethoprim, tetracyclines.
- **Anti-emetics:** cyclizine, metoclopramide.
- **Analgesia:** paracetamol safe; avoid NSAIDs in 3rd trimester.
- **Opiates:** risk of withdrawal in the baby. Breastfed babies have developed sedation, respiratory depression and bradycardia.

- **Blood pressure/heart failure:** avoid ACEi and ARBs.
- **Anti-arrhythmic agents:** adenosine, β-blockers, flecainide and verapamil are all safe if needed.
- **Anticoagulants:** LMWH used in pregnancy. Avoid Warfarin as teratogenic unless exceptional circumstances under expert supervision. Lack of evidence to support the use of DOACs in pregnancy and in breastfeeding.
- **Anti-epileptic agents:** Sodium valproate contraindicated. For status epilepticus, IV lorazepam or benzodiazepines or levetiracetam safe.
- **Bronchodilators:** all safe. Steroids: safe.

16.4 Amniotic fluid embolism

- **About:** amniotic fluid (fetal cells, hair or other debris) enters maternal circulation with cardiac arrest or shock. At birth or <30 min postpartum.
- **Aetiology:** fetal squamous cells found in the maternal pulmonary circulation. These are also found in well patients. Possibly complement activation.
- **Clinical:** dyspnoeic, low BP, hypoxia, cough, seizures, arrest. Coagulopathy, haemorrhage. Resembles anaphylaxis.
- **Investigations: ABG:** type 1 RF. **CXR:** pulmonary oedema. **ECG:** non-specific. **Coagulation** screen: coagulopathy.
- **Management:** as per cardiac arrest (see ▶ Section 1.2 and Section 16.2). CPR, ABCs, intubate and ventilate. Manage with IV fluids for low BP. Invasive monitoring and exclude alternative diagnoses. Manage any coagulopathy. Haemodialysis with plasmapheresis for AKI. Steroids if immune-mediated mechanism suspected.

16.5 Hypertension in pregnancy

- HTN in pregnancy is associated with raised perinatal mortality, preterm birth, low birthweight. Pre-eclampsia and gestational hypertension come on later in pregnancy, often 3rd trimester. Pre-existing HTN can be discovered at initial contact in 1st trimester. Avoid ACEi/ARB drugs in pregnancy.

HTN in pregnancy (BP >140/90 mmHg, 2 readings seated 6 h apart)
- Gestational (pregnancy induced) HTN (new onset but minimal proteinuria).
- Pre-eclampsia and eclampsia (new hypertension with proteinuria).
- Chronic hypertension (renal disease, primary/essential hypertension).
- Pre-eclampsia superimposed on chronic hypertension.

Severity
- Mild: DBP 90–99 mmHg and SBP 140–149 mmHg.
- Moderate: DBP 100–109 mmHg and SBP 150–159 mmHg.
- Severe: DBP >110 mmHg and SBP >160 mmHg.

Safe drugs
- Labetalol, nifedipine, amlodipine, methyldopa, doxazosin.

16.6 Pre-eclampsia and eclampsia

- **About:** 5% of pregnancies >20 weeks to 6 weeks postpartum. Maternal mortality is 5%. 43% of maternal deaths due to pulmonary oedema.
- **Aetiology:** poorly understood vasospastic uteroplacental disorder.

- **Pre-eclampsia:** 2 of 3: BP >140/90 mmHg, proteinuria >300 mg/24 h and oedema. Severe PET = PET + end organ damage. BP >160/110 mmHg.
- **Eclampsia:** generalised seizures in patient with pre-eclampsia, hypertension and proteinuria. Aspirin 75 mg reduces pre-eclampsia in high-risk women.
- **Hypertension:** severe: BP ≥160/110 mmHg; moderate: BP between 150/100 and 159/109 mmHg; mild: BP between 140/90 and 149/99 mmHg.
- **Risk factors:** moderate risk factors: 1st pregnancy, age >40, pregnancy interval >10 years, high BMI, family history of pre-eclampsia, multiple pregnancy. High risk factors (give Aspirin 75 mg OD from 12 weeks): HTN during previous pregnancy, CKD, APL, T1DM, T2DM, chronic HTN.

Clinical

- **Pre-eclampsia (PET):** severe headache, severe pain just below ribs, epigastric or hypochondrial (hepatic congestion/liver capsule stretching). Is baby moving normally (fetal wellbeing)? Visual problems such as blurring or vomiting, flashing before eyes, sudden swelling of face, hands or feet. Disorientated, hyperreflexia, clonus, stroke and cerebral oedema.
- **Severe pre-eclampsia:** severe headache, visual problems, papilloedema, clonus >3 beats. Liver tenderness.
- **Eclampsia:** generalised tonic–clonic seizures 60+ sec preceded by facial twitching. Muscle contraction. May be coma and period of hyperventilation.

Complications

- **Stroke:** ischaemic/haemorrhagic/venous thrombosis and SAH.
- **PRES:** seizures/cortical blindness, brain oedema (see ▶ Section 11.40).
- **HELLP:** plt <100 × 10⁹/L, haemolysis (high LDH), high LFTs. Fatal in 2%.
- **AKI** (acute cortical or tubular necrosis): fall in GFR, elevated creatinine, urea. Oliguria, proteinuria >5 g/24 h. Others: fetal growth retardation, fetal death, placental abruption, ARDS, hepatic infarction, DIC.

Investigations

- **FBC:** plt count <100 (HELLP syndrome). Anaemia due to microangiopathic haemolysis (schistocytes, burr cells) or usual haemodilution of pregnancy.
- **U&E:** AKI: renal dysfunction (late), raised urate in eclampsia.
- **LFTs:** raised AST/ALT, mild: increase LDH or bilirubin. Low haptoglobin levels with haemolysis.
- **Clotting:** (not routinely if platelets >100 × 10⁹/L).
- **MSU:** to exclude UTI as cause of protein.
- **CT head:** post seizure to exclude haemorrhage or other pathology. Patients can develop vasogenic brain oedema and PRES. Supportive management. Seen as part of pre-eclampsia.
- **Fetal assessment:** fetal HR, USS for growth, CTGs. Maternal: cervical assessment (depending on gestation).

Prevention

- **Aspirin** 75 mg (81 mg in US) started at 12 weeks reduces risk of PET. Gives reductions in PET, preterm delivery and serious outcomes.
- **Start Aspirin in those at high risk:** hypertensive disease during a previous pregnancy, CKD, SLE or APLS, type 1 or type 2 diabetes, chronic hypertension.

Management (involve obstetrics immediately)

- **Antihypertensives considered safe in pregnancy:** can use methyldopa, labetalol, clonidine, prazosin, doxazosin, nifedipine. Diuretics avoided.
- **PET:** mild BP consider **Labetalol** 200 mg PO and monitor closely to keep BP <150/80–100 mmHg. In more severe cases, e.g. SBP >170 mmHg then consider **Labetalol** 20–40 mg IV bolus and IV infusion. **Hydralazine** slow IV 5–10 mg diluted in 10 ml NS Nifedipine 10 mg oral tablet PO.
- **Eclampsia seizures:** get help. Left lateral positioning, and continuous fetal heart rate monitoring is needed, Airway management, **Oxygen,** IV access. Check NEWS, ECG, CBG, U&E. Give **Magnesium sulfate** 4 g IV slowly over 10 min via syringe driver. Consider 2–3 g/h maintenance, for seizure prophylaxis. Alternative **Lorazepam** 2–4 mg IV. If side-effects to Mg occur give 10 ml 10% **Calcium gluconate** IV. Once stabilised then delivery. BP >160/110 mmHg **Hydralazine** slow IV 5–10 mg diluted in 10 ml or **Labetalol** 20–40 mg IV. If the fetus is less than 34 weeks of gestation, **Corticosteroids** are given. In those with severe pre-eclampsia, delivery should not be delayed for fetal lung maturation or administration of corticosteroids. Vaginal delivery preferred. **Magnesium** is continued for 24 h postpartum.
- **Posterior reversible encephalopathy syndrome:** ▶See Section 11.40.
- **Gestational hypertension:** avoid ACEi, ARBs. Aspirin 75 mg from 12 weeks. Ensure underlying causes excluded, consider α-methyldopa, hydralazine, labetalol and nifedipine (avoid sublingual as it can cause sudden low BP). Diuretics are not contraindicated but are generally avoided.
- Chronic hypertension: stop ACEi, ARBs. Switch to safer drugs in pregnancy. Give Aspirin 75mg or 81 mg from 12 weeks.
- **Reference:** NICE (2019) NG133: *Hypertension in pregnancy.*

16.7 ▶ HELLP syndrome/pre-eclampsia

- **About:** haemolysis, elevated LFTs, low platelets. Usually 2+ weeks up to 6 weeks postpartum. Part of PET / pre-eclampsia spectrum (see above).
- **Definition:** (1) BP >140/90 mmHg/proteinuria/oedema; (2) haemolysis, raised LFTs, low platelets.
- **Clinical:** often well, raised BP may not be present. Epigastric pain, N&V, jaundice. No liver failure. Eclampsia with seizures or coma.
- **Investigations:** FBC: low Hb, plt <100 × 10^9/L, WCC normal. Raised LDH >600 U/L (haemolysis). Smear: schistocytes and burr cells. LFT: raised AST, raised GGT. Liver USS normal. Urate normal. PT normal. Proteinuria >300 mg/24 h. Urine dipstick >1+.
- **Management:** vaginal delivery if >34th gestational week or fetal/maternal conditions deteriorate. High maternal/perinatal morbidity mortality rates.
- **Hepatic infarct haematoma and rupture:** seen with HELLP, AFLP, TTP, HUS or pre-eclampsia. Subcapsular haemorrhage with hepatic rupture with death of mother and fetus. Fever, shock, RUQ pain, haemoperitoneum. CT infarct left lobe. Rupture seen more in HELLP. Best managed surgically by a trauma team as liver lacerations. Prompt delivery and ITU care.

16.8 ▶ Diabetes in pregnancy

- **Target BM:** fasting glucose <5.3 mmol/L. 1 h glucose <7.8 mmol/L. 2 h glucose <6.4 mmol/L. Test urgently for ketonaemia if diabetic or unwell, exclude DKA.

- Reducing HbA1c level towards 48 mmol/mol (6.5%) is likely to reduce congenital malformations in baby.
- Avoid pregnancy if HbA1c level >86 mmol/mol (10%) because of the associated risks. Use isophane or long-acting insulins. Avoid ACEi, ARBs, stop statins.

16.9 ▶ Liver disease in pregnancy

- Liver disease is rare in pregnancy. The liver or spleen is not usually palpable. AST, ALT, GGT, bilirubin, LDH, PT, PTT are normal. ALP, WBC, fibrinogen, caeruloplasmin, alpha and beta globulins, AFP are elevated. Alkaline phosphatase ×3–4 from placenta especially 3rd trimester.
- There are reduced levels of Hb, albumin, gamma-globulins, uric acid, urea, total protein, and antithrombin III. Management of liver disease in pregnancy requires collaboration between obstetricians and hepatologists.
- Use the gestational age of the pregnancy as the best guide to the differential diagnosis of liver disease in the pregnant woman.

Liver disease by trimester

- **All stages:** will be pre-existing disease which may only be detected at pregnancy. Needs general liver assessment as any other patient. Look for viral, autoimmune and drug-induced hepatitis. Take expert hepatology and obstetric advice.
- **First trimester:** hyperemesis gravidarum high AST (<1000 U). Nausea, vomiting, weight loss, nutritional deficiency. Give Pabrinex if concerned.
- **Second/third trimester: pre-eclampsia/eclampsia** with hypertension, oedema, proteinuria, neurological deficits (headaches, seizures, coma) OR **intrahepatic cholestasis of pregnancy** with pruritus, jaundice, fatigue, abdominal pain, steatorrhoea.
- **Third trimester: acute fatty liver of pregnancy** (AFLP). Nausea, vomiting, abdominal pain, fatigue, jaundice OR **HELLP** syndrome of haemolysis, elevated liver tests, and low platelets. Abdominal pain, nausea, vomiting, oedema, hypertension, proteinuria.
- **Postpartum:** acute fatty liver of pregnancy, HELLP syndrome, Budd–Chiari syndrome.

Particular conditions

- **Budd–Chiari syndrome:** cause of acute liver failure related to prothrombotic. Needs USS. Seen any time. May need transplant.
- **Wilson's disease:** continue penicillamine.
- **Autoimmune liver disease:** continue azathioprine.
- **Ascites:** treat with amiloride rather than spironolactone.

16.10 ▶ Obstetric cholestasis

- **About:** usually seen 2nd trimester and may cause jaundice. Common if Asian/Chilean origin. Risk of prematurity and stillbirth.
- **Clinical:** jaundice. Severe pruritus (no rash) worse at night, palms and soles.
- **Investigations:** raised AST <1000U. ALP ×4. Biopsy: cholestasis.
- **Management:** check LFTs every 1–2 weeks. If worsening escalate and consider other diagnosis. Check postnatal resolution of pruritus and LFTs. Topical emollients are safe. **Ursodeoxycholic acid** 250 mg BD improves pruritus and liver function. Treat to bring bile acids below 40 μmol/L. If PT prolonged then vitamin K is

indicated. Long-term risk of gallstones, cholecystitis, pancreatitis, diarrhoea, steatorrhoea. Recurs in subsequent pregnancies.

16.11 Hyperemesis gravidarum

- **About:** 1st trimester. Commoner multi-fetal pregnancies/hydatidiform mole.
- **Clinical:** severe N&V. Retching can lead to oesophageal tear and pneumomediastinum. Malnourishment to severe thiamine deficiency.
- **Investigations:** elevated AST but <1000 U.
- **Management:** allow to rest with NBM until improving. Anti-emetics (metoclopramide) can be given, IV fluids. Small frequent meals. Resolves by week 20, rarely can persist. Management supportive, fluids, nutrition, thiamine. Give IV Pabrinex if any concerns. Rarely TPN is needed. Home IV fluids can supplement oral.

16.12 Acute fatty liver of pregnancy (AFLP)

- **NB:** AFLP is a very rare and serious condition. It occurs in about 1 in 20,000 pregnancies and is more common in first pregnancies, male babies and twins. Serious condition can lead to acute liver and renal failure and even death.
- **About:** Causes acute liver failure unlike HELLP. Potentially lethal in 3rd trimester. Seen 1 in 20,000, death 1.8%. Mitochondrial cytopathy.
- **Risks:** male fetus, homozygous fetal LCHAD deficiency in baby.
- **Clinical:** 3rd trimester jaundice, malaise, abdominal pain, nausea and upper GI bleed. AKI with oliguria, uraemia, hypoglycaemic episodes. Fulminant liver failure: jaundice, encephalopathy, coagulopathy. Pancreatitis.
- **Diagnostic criteria:** need >5 of: (1) Vomiting; (2) Abdominal pain; (3) Encephalopathy; (4) Bilirubin >14; (5) Glucose <4 mmol/L (72 mg/dl); (6) Urate >340; (7) WCC >11; (8) Ascites/bright liver US; (9) AST/ALT >42; (10) Creatinine >150 µmol/L; (11) PT >14 s; (12) Microvesicular steatosis on biopsy.
- **Investigations:** FBC, U&E: anaemia, AKI, raised urate. LFTs: conjugated hyperbilirubinaemia, raised AST, raised ALT, raised PT. Clotting: look for DIC: raised PT, low fibrinogen, low antithrombin levels. Amylase increased if pancreatitis. USS/CT abdomen may be normal or show increased echogenicity. Biopsy usually not done due to coagulopathy. Hepatitis viral serology and other differentials. Differential: HELLP, viral, drug/toxin-Induced hepatitis.
- **Management:** supportive care and immediate vaginal (preferred) delivery of the fetus. Manage acute liver failure – discuss with tertiary centre. Manage cerebral oedema and raised ICP, hepatic encephalopathy, manage infection with antibiotics. Vitamin K.

16.13 Gallstones

- **About:** pregnancy increases biliary sludge and gallstones which may resolve after delivery. If possible, acute cholecystitis is best managed medically in the 1st and 3rd trimesters, when the risk of premature delivery prompted by surgery is greater than in the second trimester.
- **Management:** USS and choledocholithiasis can be managed with diagnostic and therapeutic ERCP (shield fetus and restrict fluoroscopy time) which may be necessary in the management of symptomatic common bile duct stones leading to cholecystitis or pancreatitis.

16.14 Chronic liver disease in pregnancy

- **About:** chronic hepatitis B/C, autoimmune hepatitis, Wilson's disease, PBC, cirrhosis present throughout the pregnancy, variable course from patient to patient. PBC compatible with normal pregnancy.
- **Primary sclerosing cholangitis** pregnancy rare but monitor closely. AIH: fetal death is seen. Use of azathioprine may be harmful. Wilson's disease – higher risk of fetal loss. Trientine may be teratogenic. Take expert advice.
- **Portal hypertension** leads to increased risk of variceal bleeding, liver failure and encephalopathy, jaundice, splenic artery aneurysm. Varices can enlarge. Screen pregnant women with cirrhosis for varices from 2nd trimester and start on beta-blockers if indicated. Avoid vasopressin.

16.15 Acute viral liver disease in pregnancy

- **About:** take expert advice. Acute viral infection – HSV, CMV, HEV. HSV infection – IV aciclovir, thus not requiring early delivery. The natural course of acute hepatitis A or B is not altered in the pregnant woman, and interruption of the pregnancy or early delivery is not indicated.
- **Acute hepatitis A:** can occur during pregnancy but has no effect on the fetus.
- **Acute hepatitis B:** immunoglobulin/vaccination given to the fetus at birth prevents transmission of hepatitis B to the fetus if the mother is infected. In the 2nd or 3rd trimester may pose a risk for transmission to the baby, and immunisation with hepatitis B immunoglobulin (HBIG) and hepatitis B vaccine at birth is advocated.
- **Chronic hepatitis B or C** requires no therapy in pregnancy but poses a risk of transmission to the offspring. Take advice. HCV 1% risk of vertical transmission.
- **Hepatitis E** may lead to acute liver failure much more commonly in pregnancy.
- **References:** Lee & Brady (2009) Liver disease in pregnancy. *World J Gastroenterol*, 15:897. Riely (1999) Liver disease in the pregnant patient. *Am J Gastroenterol*, 94:1728.

16.16 Pulmonary embolism and pregnancy

- **About:** PE is a leading cause of pregnancy-related death usually due to extensive iliac vein thrombosis. Risks extend from early pregnancy to 4–6 weeks postpartum. ▶Section 4.17.
- **Clinical:** difficult if signs subtle because signs and symptoms resemble physiological changes of pregnancy. The tests are imperfect and must be gauged with clinical findings.
- D-**dimer** is often mildly elevated and so a raised value must be corroborated with other investigations. Involve senior obstetricians, radiologists and respiratory team urgently if patient compromised or peri-arrest. If clinically likely **treat as such with LMWH or IV heparin** whilst tests awaited.
- **The RCOG** published a Green top guideline (GTG37b) in 2015 detailing who should get VTE prophylaxis during and after pregnancy. High-risk women should be considered for prophylactic **LMWH from 28 weeks and will usually require prophylactic LMWH for 6 weeks post-natal with a risk reassessment.** Risks include obesity (BMI >30), age >35, parity ≥3, smoker, gross varicose veins, current pre-eclampsia, immobility, e.g. paraplegia, family history of unprovoked or oestrogenic-provoked VTE in 1st-degree relative, low-risk thrombophilia, multiple

pregnancy, IVF/assisted reproduction. Consult with Obstetrics/Haematology to advise on VTE prophylaxis.

- **Investigations:** you should do a CXR. It is appropriate and may identify and rule out other pathology (PTX, effusion, consolidation, pneumonia, cancer) and involves a tiny radiation dose and the fetus can be shielded.
- **USS Doppler of leg veins for a DVT** if any lower limb symptoms (ask radiologist to screen from calf veins to inferior vena caval bifurcation as there are often large pelvic thrombi) will indicate a need for anticoagulation without radiation.
- **Echocardiogram** may show right heart changes in PE in compromised patient.
- **VQ scan:** perfusion (Q) only part may be used. **CTPA may be considered,** especially where there has been preceding lung disease or where aortic dissection is in the differential. The theoretical concern is CTPA irradiating pregnant breast tissue with long-term breast cancer risks, but misdiagnosis kills mother and fetus and the radiation risk is small compared with the risk of misdiagnosis and not treating. If there is diagnostic suspicion and Q scan and echo/Doppler equivocal/unhelpful then CTPA. CTPA may be preferred if aortic dissection which is seen in pregnancy also considered. It is a diagnosis to be made before anticoagulation.

> **Standard treatment is LMWH. Warfarin is contraindicated. IV heparin preferred if imminent delivery being contemplated and should be stopped 4–6 h before.**

- In extreme situations thrombolysis, and catheter and surgical embolectomy have been performed. Take local expert advice because protocols vary. Manage with obstetric input at all stages. After delivery warfarin can be started and is safe in breastfeeding. Continue anticoagulation for at least 6–12 weeks post-delivery.

16.17 ▶ Acute severe asthma in pregnancy

- **Pregnancy:** treat very actively as in non-pregnant. Asthma can kill mother and child. Real risk is under-treatment.
- **In pregnancy:** asthma in 1/3 improves, 1/3 worsens and 1/3 no change. Always continue medications to ensure good asthma control.
- **Uncontrolled asthma** is associated with many maternal and fetal complications, including hyperemesis, hypertension, pre-eclampsia, vaginal haemorrhage, complicated labour, fetal growth restriction, preterm birth, increased perinatal mortality and neonatal hypoxia.
- **Must stop smoking.** Take anti-asthma drugs (safe to use in pregnancy and during breastfeeding). Give standard therapy as needed. Leukotriene antagonists may be continued in women who have demonstrated significant improvement in asthma control with these agents prior to pregnancy not achievable with other medications.
- **In labour:** if anaesthesia is required, regional blockade is preferable to general anaesthesia. Prostaglandin E2 may safely be used for labour inductions. However, use prostaglandin F2α with extreme caution in women with asthma because of the risk of inducing bronchoconstriction. Women receiving steroid tablets at a dose exceeding **prednisolone** 7.5 mg/d for more than 2 weeks prior to delivery should receive parenteral **hydrocortisone** 100 mg 6–8 hourly during labour.

16.18 Status epilepticus in pregnancy

- **About:** women with epilepsy should be delivered in a consultant-led maternity unit and one-to-one midwifery care given during labour. Low threshold for epidural anaesthesia. Anti-epilepsy drug meds should be continued during labour and post-natally with neurology input. An elective caesarean section should be considered if there have been frequent tonic–clonic or prolonged complex partial seizures towards the end of pregnancy. Valproate is avoided as an anticonvulsant in pregnancy. All women should be given folate 5 mg OD.
- **Status epilepticus** (see ▶Sections 11.15 and 11.16) (exclude eclampsia, BP, urine, platelets, LFTs and get obstetric help to assess mother/fetus): establish the ABCs, and check vital signs, including oxygenation. Maternal airway and O_2 should be maintained at all times. Intraosseous or venous access should be in SVC distribution. If seizures associated with eclampsia then use IV $MgSO_4$. If seizure persists give **Lorazepam** 2–4 mg IV or **diazepam** as per usual protocol. Consider **levetiracetam** IV. Check laboratory findings, including electrolytes, anti-epilepsy drug levels, glucose, and toxicology screen. If signs of fetal distress consider urgent delivery.
- **Juvenile myoclonic epilepsy:** 1st-line are valproate and lamotrigine. However, in fertile females valproate avoided due to fears of teratogenicity and side-effects.
- **Delivery should be expedited following a seizure during labour,** and neonatal expertise should be available. Consider CT to exclude intracranial pathology if fits are atypical or symptoms or signs suggest new pathology or worsening baseline pathology.
- **Causes of** *de novo* **fit in pregnancy:** idiopathic, low Na, low glucose, CVT, eclampsia, RCVS, sagittal vein thrombosis, autoimmune encephalitis, APL, infarction, ICH, TTP, amniotic fluid embolism, gestational epilepsy, alcohol withdrawal, brain tumour, SAH, vasculitis and other causes.
- **Pregnancy/eclampsia:** ABC, **Magnesium sulfate** 4 g (16 mmol) in 100 ml NS over 20 min and then 1 g/h for 24 h in addition to **lorazepam** and get obstetric help. If seizures continue then load with anticonvulsant. Choice will depend if patient already taking anti-epilepsy drug. Neurology consult.

16.19 Cardiac disease in pregnancy

- **About:** pregnancy is a cardiac stress test with increased cardiac output at week 20. Therefore subclinical disease, e.g. mitral stenosis may present acutely.
- **Main issue nowadays** is maternal congenital heart disease especially in those with Eisenmenger's syndrome. There is a drop in SVR with pregnancy so in those with R–L shunts this favours increased right to left shunting and so reduced pulmonary oxygenation of blood which can worsen cyanosis and hypoxia. Patients may also develop a peripartum cardiomyopathy and present with heart failure and arrhythmias. Aortic dissection is a cause of dissection in and just after pregnancy.
- **Management:** LMWH in those at enhanced risk of VTE. The optimal delivery is vaginal with appropriate anaesthetic support and low dose epidural. Oxytocin is generally avoided. General postpartum complications are badly tolerated in those with Eisenmenger's. Those with murmurs or known cardiac disease must be managed during pregnancy by specialists. Those with LV impairment and failure may need urgent cardiology review for possible angiography and revascularisation or balloon pump or LVAD. Some may need surgery.

16.20 Inflammatory bowel disease and pregnancy

- **About:** IBD if inactive does not affect fertility. Complications such as fetal loss and infertility are seen in active disease. Good effective treatment is therefore important. IBD should be well controlled prior to trying for pregnancy.
- **Drugs:** aminosalicylates, steroids and azathioprine may be used and do not affect conception or pregnancy. Methotrexate is contraindicated at conception in both partners and in pregnancy. Mycophenolate and ciclosporin are also avoided.

16.21 Acute kidney injury in pregnancy

Causes
- Pre-renal sepsis/hypovolaemia/dehydration/postpartum haemorrhage.
- Renal toxicity NSAIDs, pre-eclampsia, HELLP, HUS, TTP, acute fatty liver, AIN, post-renal obstruction or ureteric damage during delivery.
- See AKI, ▶ Section 10.4.

16.22 Infections in pregnancy

- **Antibiotics:** usual treatment depending on the causal organism and sensitivities. Penicillin, cephalosporins and macrolides such as erythromycin are all safe. Avoid tetracyclines.
- **Viral infections:** varicella zoster pneumonia is common and often severe during pregnancy. High fetal and maternal mortality rate. Presents as pneumonia, after the vesicular rash up to 1 week before. Diagnose clinically or PCR. Can cause an interstitial pneumonitis with a characteristic nodular appearance on CXR. Admit for supportive care and treatment with IV **Aciclovir** for 10 d.
- **Tuberculosis:** African and Asian women. Untreated TB is associated with premature delivery and low birthweight. Transmission to the fetus is unusual. If TB confirmed treat with antituberculosis meds as benefits outweigh risks. Look for HIV. Refer for treatment.
- **UTI:** increased incidence. Treat asymptomatic bacteriuria to prevent ascending renal tract infection. Pyelonephritis is more common. It can trigger premature labour.

17 Oncology

Introduction

20% of new cancers present following an emergency admission and are associated with poor one-year survival. Any patient with a suspected new cancer diagnosis should be referred to the site specialist cancer team.

17.1 Malignancy-related hypercalcaemia

- **About:** seen 44% of malignancies. Moderate 12–14 mg/dl or 3–3.5 mmol/L; severe >14 mg/dl or 3.5 mmol/L. See ▶ Section 5.5.
- **Causes:** lung, breast, solid tumours. Myeloma, acute leukaemias, lymphomas.
- **Aetiology: PTH-related peptide** increases renal calcium reabsorption. Osteolytic hypercalcaemia due to primary or secondary bone lesions.
- **Clinical:** dehydration, vomiting, anorexia. Signs of underlying malignancy.
- **Investigations:** FBC, AKI, high Ca, PTH, ECG short QT, PTH-related peptide, CXR. Serum immunoglobulins, Bence Jones protein, skeletal survey.

Management

- ABC and fluid resuscitation. If moderate 3–3.5 severe >3.5 mmol/L admit. Rehydrate with 4–6 L 0.9% saline over 24 h. Caution if elderly/ heart failure.
- **Bisphosphonates:** once rehydrated check calcium and renal function before **Zoledronic acid** 4 mg in 50 ml 0.9% saline over 15 min is the standard dose. **Pamidronate** 60–90 mg over 4 h is an alternative. Bisphosphonates begin to work within 48 h. Usually normalises within 5 d. If poor response repeat after 5 d. Osteonecrosis of the jaw seems uncommon when bisphosphonates/denosumab used as a one-off dose.
- **Furosemide** may help lower calcium but only if euvolaemic/hypervolaemic. Stop calcium/vit D supplements.
- **Denosumab** 120 mg SC weekly may be considered if bisphosphonates fail. Liaise with their oncologist or palliative care specialist if uncertainty about ongoing management. Osteonecrosis of the jaw seems uncommon when bisphosphonates/denosumab used as a one-off dose.
- **Palliation:** early recognition of dying and appropriate end of life care is important where appropriate. DNACPR discussions.
- **References:** Nifosì (2016) Hematologic emergencies. *Open Journal of Internal Medicine*, 6:83–92.

17.2 Tumour lysis syndrome

- **About:** lymphomas/leukaemias (high LDH high risk of AKI).
- **Aetiology:** high WCC, bulky, chemosensitive tumours. Cell death releases large quantities of nucleic acids, phosphate, potassium, raised LDH and urate. Caused by chemotherapy or steroids.
- **Chemotherapy:** acute leukaemias (ALL, AML, APML, CLL/CML with blast crisis). High-grade NHL, Burkitt's lymphoma. Breast, SCLC, sarcomas.
- **Clinical:** lethargy, nausea, vomiting. Tingling (low Ca), seizure, arrhythmias.
- **Investigations:** FBC, U&E: AKI raised creatinine, uric acid, LDH, phosphate, K. Low Ca. High CRP suggest infection, inflammation or malignancy. ECG and

telemetry to detect effects of high K. Raised lactate, ABG: anion gap metabolic acidosis. Coagulation screen: can develop DIC.

- **Management:** pre-hydration with IV fluids for good diuresis. Consider diuretics to increase urine. Central line if needed (4–5 L per day). ECG monitor for hyperkalaemia which is main concern. Hypocalcaemia can occur. Be ready to treat. Check K/Ca/Mg/phosphate/creatinine 2–3 times daily for 48–72 h after treatment and manage high K, low Ca. High uric acid: reduce with **Allopurinol** 300 mg TDS (reduce if CKD/AKI) or **rasburicase** before treatment. Those with renal impairment may need dialysis prior to treatment. Urinary alkalinisation with $NaHCO_3$ to maintain a urine pH >7.0 can help clearance of uric acid.
- **Reference:** Nifosì (2016) Hematologic emergencies. *Open Journal of Internal Medicine*, 6:83–92.

17.3 ▶ Hyperviscosity syndrome

- **About:** increased plasma viscosity due to increased cells (red and white cells) or large proteins, e.g. immunoglobulins.
- **Causes:** Waldenström's (IgM), myeloma (IgM, IgA, IgG3, light chains), IgM paraproteins. Leukaemias (WCC >100), myeloproliferative diseases, polycythaemia vera, thrombocytosis. Eisenmenger's syndrome.
- **Clinical:** visual disturbances, bleeding (GI bleeds, mucous membranes, epistaxis, retinal haemorrhage), neurological manifestations, e.g. stroke/TIA, vertigo and hearing loss.
- **Investigations:** FBC, U&Es, LFT, ESR, Ca. PPE: monoclonal band, urinary Bence Jones protein. CT brain: if stroke/TIA, CXR: if breathless.
- **Management:** ABC, IV access and good hydration, treat infection. Acutely may consider phlebotomy with simultaneous infusion of isovolaemic fluid for RBC/WCC excess. **Plasma exchange** is the gold standard treatment.

17.4 ▶ Brain tumour

- **About:** primary or more commonly secondary metastatic. Some grow slowly over years, some very rapid. Histology can help plan treatment. Refer to MDT.
- **Causes:** primary: often single but primary CNS lymphoma often multifocal. Metastatic: single or multiple (×10 times commoner than primary). Most are intradural. Leptomeningeal disease with adenocarcinomas.
- **Risks: primary brain:** radiation, HIV/AIDS, genetics – von Hippel–Lindau disease, tuberous sclerosis, Li–Fraumeni syndrome and neurofibromatosis. **Secondary:** smoker + lung cancer, breast lumps, skin melanoma, renal mass, haematuria, etc.
- **Differential:** stroke, abscess, encephalitis, inflammatory, infection, PML.
- **Clinical:** seizures, morning headache, vomiting, raised ICP, papilloedema, cognitive, behavioural changes. Focal neurology depends on tumour location: cerebellar signs, hemianopia, personality change. May present as stroke, e.g. with subcortical hypodensity or with a haemorrhage. Leptomeningeal spread more insidious with cranial nerve palsies, headache.
- **Clinical signs of an extracranial primary malignancy:** lung: weight loss, cough, hoarseness, Horner's syndrome. Breast lump, Paget's disease of nipple, localised nodes. Testicular mass. Haematuria, renal mass: renal cell tumour. Anaemia: gastrointestinal primary. Skin pigmentation: look for melanoma.

Investigations

- **Bloods:** FBC: anaemia from GI malignancy, U&E, LFT, Ca, ALP: liver metastases. Tumour markers.
- **CT brain + contrast:** usually a well demarcated hypodense lesion with ring enhancement often sited at grey–white matter border, or within the dura ± vasogenic oedema. In adults most supratentorial with a minority in the posterior fossa. Look for hydrocephalus. Melanomas, renal cell carcinomas, lung tumours and choriocarcinomas tend to bleed.
- **MRI head + gadolinium:** FLAIR, T1/T2 with contrast can confirm lesion.
- **CXR:** lung tumour or lung metastases.
- **CT chest abdomen pelvis** for primary malignancy. **PET scan:** specialist use only.
- **Brain biopsy:** to confirm histology at open craniotomy or CT-guided stereotactic techniques. **LP:** generally avoided especially with a large SOL and oedema and risk of brain herniation.

Causes

- **Metastatic tumours** (64/100,000 p.a.): lung, renal cell cancer, colonic tumour. Melanoma, breast cancer, testicular tumours/choriocarcinoma.
- **Primary tumours** (10 per 100,000 p.a.): **Gliomas:** Grade IV: glioblastoma multiforme is aggressive (high grade), Grade III: anaplastic astrocytomas (high grade), Grade II: astrocytoma, Grade I: pilocytic. Oligodendrogliomas: anaplastic oligodendroglioma (high grade). **Ependymal:** lining of ventricles: anaplastic ependymoma (high grade). **Others:** medulloblastomas (posterior fossa in children), meningiomas (falx, sphenoid, skull base, resection usual), pituitary tumours, craniopharyngiomas, vestibular schwannomas, CNS lymphoma: HIV, deep in brain, cause seizures, multiple.

Management

- Depends on age, morbidities, performance status, nature of the tumour, size, location, responsiveness to surgery, chemotherapy or radiotherapy and patient choice. Determine primary if possible – for some metastatic tumours the primary cannot be found. **Care is coordinated through local neuro-oncology MDT so ensure referral made.** Involves oncology, neuroradiologists, neurosurgeons, palliative care and specialist nurses.
- **Steroids:** symptoms of raised ICP and oedema usually **Dexamethasone** 8–16 mg/d PO or IV + PPI. Then dose can be titrated down as needed. Avoid steroids after 2 pm as will cause insomnia. Avoid steroids where lymphoma is suspected when it is preferable to do a brain biopsy first. If falling GCS: consider IV mannitol. See ▶ Section 11.4.
- **Acute obstructive hydrocephalus.** Discuss with neurosurgeons if external ventricular drainage appropriate. Mannitol if decompensating.
- **Seizures:** consider phenytoin or levetiracetam PO/IV if seizure activity.
- **Neurosurgery:** some tumours can be removed and survival improved, e.g. meningioma, pituitary, solitary lesions. More difficult if brainstem or language (eloquent areas) or sensorimotor areas or basal ganglia. Palliative surgical resection or debulking of the primary or secondary tumour.
- **Whole brain radiotherapy:** 30 Gy in 10 fractions in 2 weeks. Usually for low grade tumours. But no improved survival; may cause cognitive decline.
- **Chemotherapy:** primary cerebral lymphoma or small cell lung cancer, NHL and germ cell tumours combined with radiotherapy. Median prognosis is 6 months and depends on primary.

- **Palliation:** early recognition of dying and appropriate end of life care is important where appropriate. DNACPR discussions.

17.5 Febrile neutropenia

- **About:** temp >38°C with signs or symptoms of sepsis + neutrophil count <0.5 × 10^9/L. Mortality significant once neutrophil count <0.5 × 10^9/L. Those on steroids/NSAIDs/immunosuppression and elderly may not mount a febrile response. Pyrexia due to cytarabine, lymphomas, renal carcinoma.
- **Microbiology:** Bacterial/fungal infections. Gram-positives via indwelling lines. Invasive *Aspergillus* and *Candida*. Gram-negatives from bowel.
- **Causes of neutropenia:** bone marrow suppression 1–2 weeks post chemotherapy is commonest. Carbimazole or propylthiouracil cause agranulocytosis, infection. Idiosyncratic drug reaction (check all new drugs): azathioprine and allopurinol. Malignant bone marrow infiltration, SLE, RA, splenic sequestration. Benign ethnic neutropenia is seen in those of African and Middle Eastern descent.
- **Clinical:** patient may be septic but no fever. Usually temp >37.5°C, diarrhoea, malaise. Sore throat, cough, sputum, dysuria, low BP, raised HR, oliguria, rigors after flushing a central line. Inspect mouth, skin and perineum for infection. Defer rectal exam until antibiotics given. Look for other infections, e.g. herpes zoster. Look for tenderness or erythema around cannula/central line sites. Chronic neutropenia causes chronic sinusitis and mouth ulcers.
- **Investigations: FBC**, blood film, U&Es, LFTs and ESR, CRP. Lactate. Urine dipstick and culture. Culture Hickman lines, blood, urine, sputum, stool. Baseline CXR in all especially if any chest signs or symptoms. Additional: folate, B12, iron and ferritin, LFTs, ANA, dsDNA, RF, TFTs. CT chest/abdomen and pelvis or USS: abdominal candidiasis and other infections. Viral infection suspected: HSV or VZV – send glass slide touched against opened lesion and allowed to air dry. Transport in a slide carrier (vesicular skin lesion kit). Swabs and blood for viral PCR and send serum (clotted blood) for IgG and IgM. Send EDTA blood for CMV PCR. Fungal infection suspected: EDTA blood for *Aspergillus* and *Candida* PCR.

Management

- **ABC** and high flow O$_2$ if shocked and fluid resuscitate as for sepsis. Isolate and reverse barrier nursing and good handwashing. Admit, observe, take blood cultures. Manage sepsis; ▶Section 2.21. Do not remove central venous access devices as part of the initial empiric management of suspected neutropenic sepsis – take advice first. Temperature control with tepid sponging and **Paracetamol** 1 g PO QDS or NSAIDs can be used (check renal function).
- **Antimicrobials:** don't wait for blood results; once FN is suspected administer immediate empirical antibiotics. Liaise with microbiology if needed. If no penicillin allergy **Tazocin** 4.5 g TDS IV + IV **gentamicin** to all patients with suspected neutropenic sepsis. Non-severe penicillin allergy **Meropenem** 1 g TDS IV. Severe penicillin allergy: IV **Vancomycin** + **Gentamicin** + **Metronidazole** 500 mg TDS. If fever persists and central line *in situ* add IV **Vancomycin** 1–1.5 g BD for suspected line sepsis to cover MRSA or coagulase-negative staphylococcal sepsis. Review after 48–72 h and if patient stable, cultures negative, and neutrophil count >1.0 then consider discharge with a 5-d course of **Ciprofloxacin** 750 mg BD and **Co-amoxiclav** 625 mg TDS PO and advise on safety-netting. Take ongoing specialist advice. Persisting symptoms may lead to consideration of **amphotericin** IV based

on microbiological advice. Consider **co-trimoxazole** if pneumocystis considered. Oral **aciclovir** and oral **fluconazole** for prophylaxis may be indicated depending on local policies. If there is evidence of active HSV or VZV infection, then give **Aciclovir** 5 mg/kg 8 h IV for HSV and 10 mg/kg 8 h IV for VZV infection.

* **Colony-stimulating growth factors** (G-CSF, GM-CSF) may be considered in cytotoxic therapy-induced neutropenia. Discuss with haematologist.
* **Autoimmune neutropenia** may require steroids, high dose IVIg and G-CSF – arrange urgent haematological assessment.
* **Reference:** Christie NHS Foundation Trust (2021) Clinical guidance for the management of sepsis (neutropenic sepsis).

17.6 Malignant superior vena caval obstruction

* **Causes: malignancy:** mediastinal tumours, lung cancer, metastases, NHL, Hodgkin's lymphoma, testicular, breast, thrombosis from malignancy. **Non-malignant:** mediastinal fibrosis: histoplasmosis, TB, sarcoid. Thrombosis: central line/pacemaker/ICD leads. Compression from thoracic aortic aneurysms. Behçet's disease, fibrosis from radiation.
* **Clinical:** breathless, facial oedema, headache, sensation of fullness. Cough, haemoptysis, weight loss, dilated veins upper chest and neck. Horner's syndrome, clubbing, hoarseness. Phrenic nerve palsy with raised hemidiaphragm. Lymphadenopathy, testicular mass, hepatosplenomegaly. Cerebral or laryngeal oedema suggests a poor prognosis. Raised SVC pressure can even lead to oesophageal varices and bleeding. Pemberton's sign: mediastinal mass occludes thoracic outlet. If arms raised above head >1 min with facial flushing, distended veins, stridor, raised JVP.
* **Investigations:** FBC, U&Es, LFT, ESR, CRP, Ca, CXR: mass, hilar lymphadenopathy, TB. CTPA defines tumour extent, site of occlusion, stenosis and extent of any thrombus. SVCO can be an incidental finding. May need bronchoscopy, sputum cytology, staging and biopsies. CT head for oedema/metastases.
* **Management:** O_2 as per BTS guidelines. Airways management, remove any central venous lines if cause. Ensure restricting clothing is loosened and upper arms are supported on pillows. SVCO requires histological diagnosis for decision of optimal treatment. Few patients will require immediate intervention.
* **Dexamethasone** 8–16 mg/d in divided doses with a PPI. Give all doses before 2 pm. Take advice where lymphoma suspected. Based on CTPA findings consider referral for endovascular stenting, thrombectomy, thrombolysis and anticoagulation if the patient's condition permits. Refer if appropriate for **endovascular stenting** for an extrinsic compressive cause and helps non-malignant/fibrotic causes but improved venous return can lead to pulmonary oedema. **Anticoagulation:** if thrombosis may need anticoagulation at least for VTE prophylaxis. Full anticoagulation if the obstruction is thrombotic. Systemic anti-cancer therapy (SACT) and radiotherapy for small cell lung cancer (SCLC) if patient's condition permits. Get advice from Acute Oncology and/or the Respiratory team.
* **Palliation:** early recognition of dying and appropriate symptom management and end of life care is important where appropriate.
* **Reference:** Scottish Palliative Care Guidelines (2019).

17.7 Severe nausea and vomiting

- **About:** may be single cause or multifactorial.
- **Causes to screen for:** constipation/bowel obstruction, dehydration and uraemia. Check I/O, opiates, chemotherapy, radiotherapy, brain tumour and raised ICP, oesophageal obstruction, gastric outlet or small or large bowel obstruction.
- **Investigations:** FBC, U&E, amylase, Ca, glucose, CT head, CXR, AXR/CT.
- **Management:** IV fluids – rehydration. Hold any chemotherapy/biological therapies until senior advice is taken. Look for and treat cause. Anti-emetic: **Metoclopramide** 10 mg PO/IV 6h, **Ondansetron** 8 mg PO/IV BD (needs laxative), **Cyclizine** 150 mg/d via a syringe driver or **Levomepromazine** 2.5–5 mg by SC BD as needed or 5–15mg in 24 h by continuous subcutaneous infusion. Others: **Dexamethasone** 4–8 mg PO 12 h V, **Haloperidol** 0.5–2 mg PO 8 h.

17.8 Malignant spinal cord/cauda compression

- **About:** malignant spinal cord compression (MSCC) of the spinal cord or cauda equina. Back pain + malignancy warrants urgent assessment to detect and treat cord/cauda compression preventing loss of motor/sensation/sphincters.
- **Aetiology:** lesion usually extradural compressing dural sac and the cord/cauda in the canal. May be preceding canal stenosis. Vulnerable to compression. Malignancy, prolapsed disc, haematomas, AVM. Compression causes oedema, venous congestion and demyelination. Oedema makes it worse. Eventually cord infarcts. Cord (UMN) ends L1, cauda (LMN). Cord UMN, cauda LMN.
- **Levels:** 70% thoracic, 20% lumbosacral and 10% cervical.
- **Cancers:** lung, prostate, breast, renal cell, myeloma, colorectal, lymphoma. Primary tumours: ependymomas, astrocytomas, haemangioblastomas.
- **Clinical:** known malignancy or new presentation. Progressive worsening back pain. Cord: sensory level, spastic often asymmetrical weakness below (increased tone, upgoing plantar, clonus), loss of sphincters, autonomic dysfunction if high cord. Cauda: motor weakness is LMN and may be asymmetrical with reduced/absent reflex, reduced tone, plantars downgoing or absent. Sensory loss over saddle area, genitals, perianal. Flaccid anal sphincter. Localised tenderness can localise lesion, radicular pain.
- **Investigation:** bloods: FBC, U&Es, ESR, Ca, PSA, CRP, CXR, LDH, myeloma screen. MRI scan of entire spine ± gadolinium within 24 h: 25% have multiple lesions. If MRI not available or contraindicated, then CT spine imaging. Abdominal CT: to help find primary if unknown. Histology: if unknown cancer then obtaining histology is of paramount importance. Plain films may show bony changes, e.g. 'erosion of pedicle', 'bone lesions'. Bladder scan: retention >150 ml may suggest neurological damage.
- **Management:** nurse patient flat. Give **Dexamethasone** 10–16 mg PO stat + PPI then daily in divided doses before 2 pm. Get imaging of whole spine MRI. Take oncology advice before steroids if suspicion of lymphoma. Liaise early and closely with acute oncology, radiology and spinal surgery teams. Until stability of spine known, patient have spinal precautions lie flat with neutral spine alignment. 'Log rolling' when required for pressure relief and toileting. Manage pain, manage bowels and catheterise bladder if needed. VTE assessment. Malignant spinal cord compression median survival is now 6 months.

- Discuss with oncology/haem/surgeons. MRI within 24 h. See spinal instability neoplastic score (SINS). Referral to Spinal Team: surgery may be considered if single compressive lesion, unknown primary or other areas to biopsy, radio-resistant tumour, progressions despite radiotherapy, bone compression or vertebral collapse in a patient with good performance status. If there are none of these, but there are spinal metastases, then radiation without surgery may be considered. Emergency radiotherapy (same day) for those with radiosensitive tumours such as lymphoma, myeloma, small cell lung cancer, seminoma, neuroblastoma and Ewing's sarcoma. If a patient has complete paraplegia with loss of sphincter control for >48 h, then any treatment is unlikely to improve functional outcomes. Radiotherapy can help the pain, e.g. in breast, prostate, myeloma but may take time. Surgeons prefer not to operate post-radiotherapy as wound healing is impaired.
- **Ongoing management:** review steroid dose and side-effects. Review pain control, need for a catheter (if appropriate). VTE assessment and prophylaxis.
- **Palliation:** early recognition of dying and appropriate end of life care is essential where appropriate. DNACPR discussions.
- **Reference:** Macdonald *et al.* (2019) Malignant spinal cord compression. *J R Coll Physicians Edinb*, 49:151.

17.9 ▶ Systemic anti-cancer treatment

Introduction
- Always withhold oral anti-cancer drugs in the event of toxicity and seek advice from acute oncology; this includes IV pumps.
- **Cytotoxic drugs:** these are given in 3–4 week 'cycles' and cause nausea and vomiting within 1–3 d. Sometimes 'delayed' within 7 d. Febrile neutropenia typically 7–14 d post chemotherapy.
- **5FU/capecitabine:** can cause coronary artery spasm and arrhythmias with treatment and severe diarrhoea after.
- **Tyrosine kinase inhibitors** e.g. sunitinib, erlotinib (delivered as daily oral and continuous) can cause rash, cardiac problems and long QT.
- **Monoclonal antibodies:** cetuximab, rituximab, trastazumab can cause hypersensitivity and rashes.

Management
- **Severe diarrhoea:** fluids, exclude *Clostridioides difficile*, loperamide.
- **Nausea/vomiting:** review anti-emetics, fluids, give drugs subcutaneously.
- **Brain metastases seizures, altered personality:** dexamethasone, head CT.
- **Hypercalcaemia confusion, dehydration:** fluids, bisphosphonates.
- **Reference:** RCP (2015) Acute care toolkit 7: Acute oncology on the acute medical unit.

17.10 ▶ Malignancy of unknown origin (MUO)

- **Introduction:** challenging patients to manage appropriately. They should receive early oncology opinion as to fitness for treatment and thus minimise unnecessary investigations. Suspected newly diagnosed cancer patients should be referred to the site-specific team immediately with the option of early discharge and fast-track outpatient slot.

- **Assessment:** needs a detailed history, examination, routine bloods and a chest X-ray are regarded as a minimum standard of investigation in the acute setting. All other investigations should be symptom- and patient-fitness led. Aim to try to discharge for outpatient investigations where possible.
- **Reference:** RCP (2015) Acute care toolkit 7: Acute oncology on the acute medical unit.

18 Miscellaneous

18.1 Malignant hyperpyrexia

- **About:** previous uneventful anaesthesia does not preclude malignant hyperpyrexia. Usually precipitated by drugs in those genetically susceptible.
- **Aetiology:** autosomal dominant 1 in 20,000. Genetic defect, e.g. ryanodine receptor on 19q13. Rises in cell calcium, causes rigidity and rhabdomyolysis.
- **Causes:** inhalational agents (not nitrous oxide): halothane, methoxyflurane.
- **Clinical:** onset <1 h of drug administration. Masseter muscle spasm an early sign. Hyperpyrexia >40°C, raised HR, muscle stiffness. Monitor end-tidal CO_2 is early, sensitive and specific sign of malignant hyperpyrexia.
- **Investigation:** FBC: high WCC. High glucose. Coagulation: monitor for DIC. U&E: raised K. AKI: dehydration/myoglobinuria, high CK, phosphate.
- **Complications:** AKI/rhabdomyolysis, arrhythmias, raised K, lactic acidosis.
- **Management:** ABC, high FiO_2 initially and then O_2 as per BTS guidelines and reassess after ABG. Telemetry for raised K. Try cooling and allow heat loss. Tepid sponging, fans, avoid paracetamol/salicylates. Genetic counselling as familial. Acute anaesthetic management: stop causative drug immediately and stop surgery if possible. Do not waste time securing another anaesthetic machine, use an Ambu bag and an O_2 cylinder initially. Hyperventilate the patient with 100% O_2 at 10 L/min via a clean breathing circuit. Otherwise maintain anaesthesia with IV agents such as propofol until surgery is completed. Cooling management – cool IV fluids and ice packs. **Dantrolene** 1 mg/kg bolus then repeat doses of 1 mg/kg (max 10 mg/kg) until the HR, rise in CO_2 production and pyrexia start to subside.

18.2 Acute rhabdomyolysis

- **About:** muscle damage can lead to AKI. Damage to striated muscle can lead to myoglobinuria. Plasma Mb levels exceed protein binding. Precipitates in the tubules can lead to AKI, renal vasoconstriction and direct nephrotoxicity.
- **Causes:** trauma/crush injuries, high voltage electrical injury, near-drowning. Falls and lying on floor for prolonged periods, severe exercise. Neuroleptic malignant syndrome (NMS), malignant hyperthermia. Cocaine/heroin use, amphetamines, ketamine, LSD. Generalised seizures, alcohol, methanol, ethylene glycol, carbon monoxide. Ischaemic limb with muscle necrosis, polymyositis, viral myositis – influenza. HIV, Coxsackie, echovirus, statins ± fibrates, hypo-/hyperthyroidism. Snake bites with action of phospholipases, compartment syndrome. Muscle genetic disorders – carnitine deficiency, caffeine, aspirin. Low K, hypophosphataemia, DKA/HHS. McArdle's disease.
- **Clinical:** muscle pain and weakness. Muscles hard and tender especially when crush injury. Dark urine – burgundy coloured or dark tea. Cause may be apparent, e.g. trauma. Evidence of trauma or falls or prolonged immobility. Family history might suggest genetic cause. Drug history – neuroleptics. Fever, increased tone, neuroleptic malignant syndrome.
- **Investigations:** FBC: raised WCC. U&E: raised urea, raised creatinine. Tissue damage: raised K, raised CK, raised urate, raised myoglobin, phosphate, myoglobinuria.

ABG: metabolic acidosis. Coagulation screen: DIC. MRI detects muscle damage. ECG and raised cardiac troponin if myocardial injury suspected. MI/myocarditis can raise CKMB.

- **Complications:** raised K, hypovolaemic shock, AKI. DIC, sepsis, death.

Management

- ABCs, IV fluids, watch and treat high K. Risk of AKI low if CK <15,000–20,000 units/L. CK >60,000 units/L is predictive of AKI and death.
- **Early hydration** (even prior to hospitalisation) with NS. Goal is a good diuresis (200–300 ml/h). Carefully monitor for fluid overload, particularly in elderly/CCF. **Furosemide** can enhance diuresis if overloaded.
- **Alkalinisation of urine:** enhances myoglobin solubility. Target urine pH >6.5 with IV NaHCO$_3$ where CK >6000. Can lead to hypocalcaemia, with tetany and seizures.
- **Dialysis** in AKI or refractory hyperkalaemia or fluid overload.
- **Mannitol** 200 ml of 20% (20 g/100 ml) IV over 30–60 min and can be repeated to enhance diuresis, renal vasodilator and free radical scavenger.
- **Treat DIC:** see ▶ Section 8.3.
- **Bromocriptine/dantrolene** if neuroleptic malignant syndrome.
- **Compartment syndrome:** surgical fasciotomy. **Limb ischaemia:** vascular review.

18.3 ▶ Painful leg

- **Taking referral/answering bleep:** painful since when? Was there trauma or fall? Is patient mobile on it? Any redness, shortened and externally rotated? Is there a pyrexia? Normal observations? Why is patient in hospital? Are they on anticoagulants – ?haematoma.

Differentials

- **Necrotising fasciitis:** hard woody feeling, intense pain, gas bubbles below skin, margin which is moving. Needs urgent antibiotics and surgical review.
- **Acute ischaemic limb:** mottled, pale, painful, pulseless, perishing with cold. A vascular emergency.
- **Trauma – soft tissue injury – bruising and swelling.** Rest, ice, elevate. Severe trauma can cause rhabdomyolysis and compartment syndrome. Follow appropriate criteria, e.g. Ottawa guidance for ankle pain. Bony tenderness needs X-ray for fracture. In older patient assume any patient with leg pain warrants exclusion of pelvic/hip fracture or long bone fracture as clinical signs can be reduced and difficult in confused/dementia patients.
- **Deep vein thrombosis:** warm, dilated veins, swollen, calf tender, raised D-dimers. Important diagnosis as can rapidly kill if missed and untreated. If suspected treat immediately.
- **Compartment syndrome:** post trauma or fracture or ischaemic limb needs fasciotomy. Distal ischaemia and reduced pulses. Surgical emergency.
- **Haematoma:** trauma ± excessive anticoagulants and muscle haematoma. Check clotting. Reverse all anticoagulation. See ▶ Sections 8.8–8.12.
- **Inflammation:** acute gout or pseudogout or septic arthritis: red-hot joint, effusion. Aspirate.
- **Osteomyelitis:** acute or chronic bony pain, sickle cell. Soft tissue infection, e.g. diabetic foot.
- **Sciatica:** pain radiating down leg. Limited straight leg raising.

- **Cellulitis:** warm red tender leg starting distally and moving proximally. Bilateral cellulitis is unusual. Florid red legs may be chronic and cool to the touch. Check for diabetes and skin infection entry points. Emollients for dry skin. Antibiotics for confirmed cellulitis.
- **Rheumatoid arthritis:** can affect the knee as a tender warm joint with synovial thickening and may have an effusion. Rarely acutely inflamed. Patient has clinical features of rheumatoid arthritis. Check ESR/CRP and serology. Aspirate knee if joint sepsis suspected.
- **Lymphoedema:** unilateral swollen leg may be painful. Look for evidence of malignancy if new. Check nodes at groin. Pyoderma gangrenosum – may be seen with bowel disease and presents as a painful non-healing violaceous rash with ulceration. Dermatological referral.
- **Paget's disease:** bone pain, warm, deformed. Older males. Raised ALP. Plain X-ray changes. Bone scan increased uptake. Consider new bisphosphonates.
- **On arrival:** check general observations, EWS and review notes. Examine legs: front and back for tenderness, red – possible cellulitis. Tender muscles: suspect rhabdomyolysis – check CK and statin usage or other causes. Recent trauma/ischaemia and pain – compartment syndrome which will need urgent surgical decompression. Recent fall – even something trivial can cause a fracture. Fractured neck of femurs have few signs if undisplaced. Check for pubic bone fracture. Any doubts X-ray. Acute gout can cause a painful large toe – check urate. Tender erythematous. Calf – always consider DVT and D-dimer may help but may need USS leg veins. Start **LMWH** treatment whilst you get Doppler if DVT suspected.

18.4 Acute limb ischaemia

- **About:** early action may preserve life and limb, either thrombotic occlusion or embolic. Acute on chronic limb ischaemia. Rarely severe venous thrombosis can lead to ischaemia.
- **Aetiology: thrombotic/stenosis:** HTN, smoking, diabetes, male, age, cholesterol. **Embolic** AF is a common embolic source. On heparin? HITT– check for falling platelets. LV thrombus from MI, cardiac murmurs, aortic aneurysm.
- **Buerger's disease:** young heavy smokers. North Africa. Rare also arteritis.
- **Clinical:** limb is pale, painful, pulseless, paraesthesia, perishing with cold. May be background of shortening claudication distance. Leriche syndrome with associated buttock pain and impotence. Coexisting vasculopathies – stroke, TIA, MI. Embolic is sudden and complete onset over minutes; thrombosis is incomplete over hours/days. May have bruits.
- **Investigation:** FBC: WCC, platelets (low platelets with HITT). Coagulation screen. U&E: AKI: hyperkalaemia, glucose, troponin. CXR: cardiomegaly. ECG: AF, MI. Doppler ultrasound: can give evidence of flow and flow rates. Angiography: evidence of thrombus.
- **Ankle/brachial BP:** ABPI 0.6–0.9 with claudication. Resting ischaemia with ABPI 0.3–0.6. Tissue loss if <0.3.

Management
- **ABC,** O_2 resuscitation. Surgical review. IV access and start 1 L NS.
- **Analgesia: Morphine** 5 mg IV + **Cyclizine** 50 mg IV.
- **Vascular surgical review:** embolism is acute and sudden and a clinical diagnosis and needs embolectomy and anticoagulation. Thrombosis is less acute and may

need medical treatment, bypass or thrombolysis. Those who are very frail with a mottled white leg with skin petechiae and hard painful muscles may need amputation or palliation. Consider comorbidities. If an acute white cold leg in a patient with good performance status without advanced changes, then vascular surgeons need to decide whether to preserve the limb or not via embolectomy, angioplasty or bypass. Compartment syndrome may require fasciotomies to be done. Warfarin may be considered post-operatively.

- **Heparinisation/thrombolysis/embolectomy:** consider heparin 5000 units IV bolus and then 1000 units/h with APTT 2–2.5. Embolectomy can be done under local anaesthesia.
- **Long-term:** smoking prevention, control vascular risks, statin.
- **Amputation:** indicated if all options are futile. Must be done at a level high/proximal enough to allow for stump healing to sustain a prosthesis.
- **Sympathectomy:** percutaneous lumbar sympathectomy under CT guidance.
- **Gabapentin for ongoing pain can be helpful.**
- **Severe venous thrombosis:** leg ischaemia: elevation, consider thrombolysis – discuss with interventional radiologists, heparin and analgesia.
- **Complications:** death, limb loss, ARDS, pneumonia, sepsis, rhabdomyolysis, high K, DIC, AKI.

18.5   Abdominal aortic aneurysm (AAA)

- **About:** 'triple A' is an increased aortic diameter >50% and therefore >3 cm. Those >5.5 cm need surgical repair, the rest are monitored. They begin below the renal arteries and extend down as far as the iliac arteries. Mortality of elective surgery is 6% and emergency surgery 50%.
- **Aetiology:** chronic inflammatory process with loss of smooth muscle. May be a genetic basis leading to a weakness in the wall. Reduced elastin and collagen is seen. May be a factor. Can be fusiform or saccular. Wall tension increases with radius so increasing risk of rupture.
- **Risk factors:** smoking, increasing age, male ×5, increased height and BMI. Connective tissue disorders. Family history is a risk factor. Others for rupture: female ×3, smoking, low FEV_1.
- **Clinical:** think AAA if abdominal/back pain + low BP and/or a pulsatile expansile mass. An aortoenteral fistula may cause an upper GI bleed (fistula between the AAA and the 4th part of duodenum). Distal clot embolisation leading to limb ischaemia.
- **Investigations:** FBC, U&E, amylase, LFTs, group and cross-match 6+ units. USS abdomen – identifies and measures AAA. Can see mural thrombus – this may be done in ED as a focused assessment with sonography, and if the aorta appears dilated (>3 cm) in an unstable patient then assume leaking AAA and resuscitate and call vascular surgeons. Any bleeding is retroperitoneal. Emergency CT scan which can aid the decision for surgery.
- **Acute management:** ABC and urgent resuscitation if needed. Get good IV access fast. Group and cross-match 6–8 units. Fast bleep vascular surgeons. Emergency repair has grim prognosis. Abdominal muscles contract splints aneurysm. This is reversed with anaesthesia with subsequent low BP. Laparotomy and aorta cross-clamped above the leak. Mortality and complications including MI, renal failure, coagulopathy are common.

- **Elective repair:** no survival benefits for operating with stable AAA <5.5 cm. Operate elective surgery AAA >5.5 cm 10% 1-year risk of rupture. Midline incision, aorta cross-clamped, heparinised. Dacron graft used. Trouser graft if iliacs included enclosed in aneurysmal sac.
- **Endovascular aneurysm repair** (EVAR) can repair the aneurysm by endovascular stenting which avoids a laparotomy and cross-clamping can be done on selective cases via the femoral artery.

18.6 Envenomation (snakes, scorpions, spiders)

- **About:** venomous creatures, such as some snakes, scorpions, spiders and marine animals, inject sufficient venom by a bite or a sting into a prey item or perceived predator to cause deleterious local and/or systemic effects.
- **Effects:** localised pain, swelling, blistering, bleeding and necrosis, or minimal local effects and/or major systemic effects which may include one or more of neurotoxic paralysis, neuroexcitatory effects, rhabdomyolysis, coagulopathy and haemorrhage, AKI, pulmonary oedema, shock, or cardiovascular collapse.
- **Geography: UK** there are only 3 indigenous snakes and most are harmless. The adder (grey or reddish-brown, with a dark zig-zag shaped stripe) is the only venomous snake (grass snakes and smooth snakes are not). **Europe:** European adder. **South America:** rattlesnake. **Africa:** black-necked spitting cobra, **India:** common Indian cobra, monocled cobra, Russell's viper, green pit viper, saw-scaled viper.
- **Clinical:** flaccid paralysis (some snakes, some ticks, cone snails, octopus). Excitatory: autonomic (scorpions, spiders, jellyfish). Cardiotoxic: some snakes, jellyfish, scorpions. Coagulopathy. Nephrotoxic. There are various local syndromic presentations which can help diagnosis.
- **Investigations:** inspect urine – haematuria may suggest coagulopathy. Dark urine: rhabdomyolysis. **20-minute whole-blood clotting test** showing no clot suggests coagulopathy.
- **Management:** in UK call 999 and attend ED. Do not go near the snake, or try to catch or kill it. Do not try to suck or cut the poison (venom) out of the bite. Do not tie anything tightly round the part of the body where the bite is. Do not take aspirin or ibuprofen, as they can make bleeding worse. Stay calm, most snake bites in the UK are not serious and can be treated. Keep the part of your body that was bitten as still as you can. Lie in the recovery position if you can. Take paracetamol for any pain. Try to remember the colour and pattern of the snake to tell the doctor. Remove any jewellery and loosen clothes near the bite in case it swells. Tetanus and assess if needs antivenom. Will need a period of observation.
- **Generally outside UK:** needs local expert help and antivenom where available for the snake suspected.
- **Severe reaction:** ABC. Oxygen. Supportive and symptomatic care is essential. Get patient to hospital immediately. Delaying onset of severe envenomation (keep still, immobilise limb) so allowing time for supportive and definitive treatment. **Antivenom** is specific immunoglobulin to the venom. It is only available for some major venomous species. It can cause an allergic response. Be ready to manage any anaphylaxis.

18.7 Decompression sickness / Caisson disease

- **About:** diving 10 m underwater increases pressure by 1 atm. On decompression nitrogen bubbles can form which can cause microvascular damage. Uncommon for dives <10 m deep. Can be seen following multiple dives. Divers should avoid flying for 24 hours after their last dive.
- **Clinical:** malaise and headache to paraesthesia, lymphoedema, rash, joint pain and ataxia, paralysis and altered mental status. Myelinated tracts of brain and thoracic cord most likely affected.
- **Management:** ABC, keep patient horizontal. Give 100% O_2 to flush out nitrogen. If possible, chamber recompression is the gold standard therapy. Transport may need low altitude helicopter transport. Often this is not an option, especially in a critically unwell patient. Patients should be kept horizontal. Give 1 L NS. Analgesia should be avoided. Do not give NSAIDs. The Divers Alert Network can be contacted for international advice and support.

18.8 Immersion pulmonary oedema

- **About:** affects divers and surface swimmers, particularly in the swim stage of triathlons. Initial thought to be drowning but management different.
- **Aetiology:** immersion results in exposure to hydrostatic pressure which can cause altered cardiac function and alveolar oedema.
- **Risks:** overhydration, overexertion, heart disease, hypertension and cold water. Snorkel or scuba equipment.
- **Clinical:** dyspnoea, haemoptysis, frothy sputum, within 10 minutes of starting swimming, and of variable onset with diving.
- **Management:** ABC, remove from water. Warm patient. Sit up. 100% O_2 and treat with nitrates, diuretics and CPAP. Recurrence rates are around 30%.

18.9 Acute mountain sickness/high altitude cerebral oedema and pulmonary oedema

- **About:** hypoxia causes cerebral vasodilation and raised intracranial venous volume and an increase in CSF production. There is impaired gas exchange.
- **Clinical:** symptoms start within 4 hours of ascent above 2500 m within the prior 4 days. Can be mild to severe. Those with cerebral oedema can have reduced GCS. Some develop pulmonary oedema with cough and dyspnoea.
- **Investigations:** CXR shows pulmonary oedema.
- **Management:** descent if symptoms persist or become severe. Rest, simple analgesia. Resolves after 1–3 days at a stable altitude but may recur with further ascent. Some may develop high altitude cerebral oedema (HACE) or pulmonary oedema and need oxygen and descent, or portable hyperbaric chambers is essential. Give **Acetazolamide** 250 mg TDS for treatment and lower doses as prophylaxis. **Dexamethasone** 8 mg may be used. **Nifedipine** (60 mg modified release divided into 2–3 doses) is also recommended for high altitude pulmonary oedema.

18.10 Drowning

- **About:** in-water rescue is not recommended for untrained individuals – remember 'Reach, Throw, Row, Don't Go'.
- **Risk:** alcohol, male, youth, elderly, seizures, mental illness, cardiac disease, coldness. Cold water <6°C may be protective.
- **Aetiology:** cold water stimulates hyperventilation and hypocapnia and blackouts and water in larynx/pharynx causes laryngospasm with hypoxia and then larynx relaxes, and water enters lungs. Leads to hypoxia, acidosis. In some, water entry into lungs is minimal ('dry' drowning).
- **Investigations:** ABG, CXR, FBC, U&E, CT head/neck if injury suspected. Lactate. Troponin. Echo.
- **Complications:** ARDS, hypoxic brain injury.
- **Management:** ABC, O_2, CPAP, ECMO. BLS/ALS. Slowly rewarm patient. ALS until patient has been rewarmed (if hypothermic) and persisting asystole. Mortality in cardiac arrest is 93%. For those who have had a near drowning experience, if they are now asymptomatic, with no respiratory compromise, a normal CXR and normal ABG they can be discharged home after 6–8 h of observation.

19 Dermatology

19.1 Important medical causes of rashes

- **About:** there are several rashes which must be diagnosed because early treatment may be life-saving:

Life-threatening rashes not to be missed

- **Severe sepsis:** a mottled rash or meningococcal rash, cyanosis.
- **Anaphylaxis:** the spreading urticaria and erythema that may suggest anaphylaxis along with wheeze, hypotension. ▶Section 2.18.
- **Meningococcaemia:** non-blanching purpuric rash with possible sepsis and meningitis. ▶Sections 2.21 and 11.10.
- **Necrotising fasciitis:** rapidly advancing all-consuming, painful, red, which spreads in hours. The slower advancing red, hot, tender cellulitis or erysipelas which can result in systemic sepsis. ▶Section 19.6.
- **Toxic epidermal necrolysis/Stevens–Johnson syndrome:** ▶Section 19.2.
- **Drug rash with eosinophilia and systemic symptoms:** ▶Section 19.7.
- **Toxic shock syndrome** (TSS): ▶Section 2.19.
- **Rocky Mountain spotted fever:** ▶Section 9.6.

19.2 Toxic epidermal necrolysis/Stevens–Johnson syndrome

- **About:** involves skin as well as mucous membranes – mouth, genitals, vagina, eyes. SJS involves <10% skin. TEN involves >30% of skin. Those with 10–30% have mixed picture. **NB:** stop all possible culprit drugs. Management largely supportive. Mortality 30%.
- **Aetiology:** immune-driven by drug. Detachment/necrosis of the epidermis.
- **Causes:** sulphonamides, cephalosporins, antibiotics, anticonvulsants, NSAIDs, cocaine, nevirapine, mirtazapine. Commoner with HIV and in slow drug acetylators. Viral or *Mycoplasma pneumoniae* infections. Genetic testing for Han Chinese who may develop SJS due to carbamazepine and allopurinol. If no drug or other found cause prognosis is worse.
- **Clinical:** preceding flu-like illness with myalgia, fever in recent days. Milder: erythema, target lesions, blistering on skin and oral/genital mucosa. Spreading tender erythema and confluent blistering rash followed by loss of sheets of epidermis. Pain may be severe. Involves skin and oral/genital mucosa and eye. Detachment of the skin and mucosal epidermis. Progressive exfoliation. Recovery may lead to scarring, altered pigmentation and loss of sweating. Positive Nikolsky sign when lateral pressure to the epidermal surface slips upper layers away from lower. TEN proceeds over hours. Emergency.
- **Differential: staphylococcal** scalded skin syndrome (seen in children and mucosa spared). Toxic shock syndrome, phototoxic skin reactions. Drug reaction with eosinophilia.
- **Prognostic severity factors use ScoreTen:** age >40 years +1, HR >120 +1, cancer/haem malignancy +1. Body surface area >10% +1, urea >10 mmol/L +1, HCO_3^- <20 mmol/L +1. Blood glucose level >14 mmol/L +1. Sum scores. Mortality rates: 0–1 = 3%, 2 = 12%, 3 = 35%, 4 = 58%, ≥5 = 90%.

- **Investigations:** FBC, U&Es, LFT, CRP, glucose, Mg, phosphate, *Mycoplasma* serology. Blood cultures, urine culture, CXR if febrile. Skin biopsy: necrotic keratinocytes with full thickness epithelial necrosis and sheets of epidermal detachment helps differentiate from staphylococcal scalded skin syndrome.
- **Management:** ABC check for airways involvement. New evidence suggests Steroids and Etanercept may improve outcomes and should be considered. IVIG has also been used. Take specialist advice. Stop all possible causative drugs or all drugs if possible. Venous cannula in non-lesional skin. Monitor fluid balance carefully. Encourage oral fluids. If unable to maintain nutrition, then NG tube feeding. Urinary catheter if needed. Skin >10% then transfer to burns unit or ITU. MDT with dermatology/plastics/ITU to determine care. Strict barrier nursing to prevent nosocomial. Pressure-relieving mattress. Room at 25–28°C. Swab for bacteria and fungi. Systemic antibiotics only if signs of infection. Clean wounds with warm sterile water/saline or antimicrobial **chlorhexidine** (1 in 5000). Apply 50/50 paraffin to whole epidermis. Decompress blisters by piercing and expression or aspiration of contents. Apply non-adherent dressings. Ophthalmology review and eye care to avoid scarring. VTE prophylaxis assessment. Avoid the drug in the future.
- **Reference:** Creamer *et al.* (2016) U.K. guidelines for the management of Stevens-Johnson syndrome/toxic epidermal necrolysis 2016. *Br J Dermatol*, 174:1194. & *J Plast Reconstr Aesthet Surg*, 69:e119.

19.3 ▶ Soft tissue infections: cellulitis/erysipelas

- **About:** beware over-treating chronic bilateral usually cold or warm tender red legs. It's possible, but unusual, for cellulitis to be symmetrical. May be chronic changes. Examine all cases yourself. Unwrap bandages. Look at CRP. Emollients can soften dry eczematous legs.
- **Organism:** most due to β-haemolytic streptococci. Often slow to respond to therapy or may worsen initially due to toxins produced by group A strep. and other local tissue factors. Less common *Staph. aureus* and MRSA.
- **Clinical:** subcutaneous skin infection. Red, very painful swelling often of a limb. Pyrexia and malaise. Inguinal nodes. Look for the point of entry – dry cracked skin between toes, insect bite, trauma. Look at heels, back of legs.
- **Diagnosis:** erysipelas is more superficial than cellulitis and is typically more raised and demarcated but may have systemic symptoms of fever, malaise. Treat the same.

Antibiotic management

- **Mild–moderate cellulitis:** non-severe – afebrile and systemically well and no osteomyelitis. Give **Flucloxacillin** 500 mg QDS PO for 7–14 d. If penicillin-allergic, then **Clarithromycin** 500 mg BD IV/PO for 7–14 d.
- **Severe cellulitis: Flucloxacillin** 1–2 g QDS IV/PO until clinical improvement, no sepsis and tolerating oral intake then switch to oral therapy. Outpatients consider **Ceftriaxone** 2 g IV OD. Penicillin allergy **Teicoplanin** 6 mg/kg IV BD × 3 loading doses then 6 mg/kg OD.
- **Orbital cellulitis (serious infection):** has various causes and may be associated with serious complications including visual loss. Prompt diagnosis and proper management are essential. Unless very mild needs admission and CT + contrast and monitor function and IV antibiotic therapy. **Co-amoxiclav** 1.2 g TDS IV or treat as

severe cellulitis as above. Fungal infection requires IV antifungal therapy along with surgical debridement.

- **Soft tissue infection and MRSA positive:** consider **Vancomycin** 1–1.5 g BD or **Teicoplanin** 6 mg/kg IV BD × 3 loading doses then 6 mg/kg OD.
- **Leg ulcers, pressure sores:** treat with antibiotics only if demarcated cellulitis or systemic infection observed. Refer to the cellulitis guidelines above. Wound cleaning and skin. Discuss with tissue viability specialist.
- **Following clean surgery:** *mild/moderate*: **Flucloxacillin** PO/IV doses as for cellulitis. *Severe*: **Benzylpenicillin** 1.2–2.4 g QDS + **Flucloxacillin** 1 g QDS IV.
- **Impetigo:** *mild*: **Mupirocin** 2% ointment 8 h or **Fusidic acid** 2% cream TDS. *Moderate*: **Flucloxacillin** 500 mg QDS PO.
- **Erysipelas:** *mild*: **Amoxicillin** 500 mg TDS PO. *Severe*: **Benzylpenicillin** 1.2–2.4 g QDS IV.
- **Periodontal abscess/dental infections: Amoxicillin** 500 mg TDS PO + **Metronidazole** 400 mg TDS PO. Alternatively **Co-amoxiclav** 1.2 g TDS IV. Should be accompanied by drainage and removal of source of infection. Maxillofacial/dental referral.

19.4 Erythroderma (exfoliative dermatitis)

- **About:** several causes. Determine underlying cause but 25% are idiopathic. Males > females. Intense redness of skin due to inflammatory skin disease.
- **Causes:** dermatitis (atopic, contact and seborrhoeic types). Drug reaction. Psoriasis after withdrawal of steroids. Pityriasis rubra pilaris. Cutaneous T-cell lymphoma (Sézary syndrome), idiopathic. HIV infection, toxic shock syndrome.
- **Clinical:** warm red intolerable itch. Eyelid swelling. Scaling at days 2–6. Thick skin on scalp and hands. Hair and nail changes and loss. Heat/fluid loss. Hypothermia, lymphadenopathy. Fluid/electrolyte imbalance. Capillary leak syndrome may cause cutaneous oedema and acute lung injury.
- **Differential** (see causes): cellulitis, cutaneous T-cell lymphoma. Stevens–Johnson syndrome, toxic epidermal necrolysis, toxic shock syndrome.
- **Investigations:** FBC: raised WCC. U&Es: AKI, raised CRP, ESR. LFTs: low albumin. Skin biopsy may be required. Increased serum IgE.
- **Management:** stop unnecessary medications. Bed rest, keep warm, bland emollients. Monitor I/O and replace. Wet wraps, emollients and mild topical steroids. Systemic steroids can make things worse so take advice. Systemic steroids avoided in severe pustular psoriasis and staphylococcal scalded skin syndrome. Consider HDU care and close monitoring for those with capillary leak syndrome. Retinoids are 1st-line for severe pustular psoriasis. Antibiotics for any bacterial infection. Take dermatology advice.

19.5 Animal/human bites

- **Animal/human bites: Co-amoxiclav** 625 mg PO – 1.2 g TDS IV if severe. Pen allergy **Doxycycline** 100 mg BD PO + **Metronidazole** 400 mg TDS PO. Also dog/cat saliva: *Capnocytophaga canimorsus* and *Pasteurella multocida*.
- **Human bites also** consider HBV, HIV and tetanus. Review at 24 h especially if near a joint.

19.6   Necrotising fasciitis

- **About: medical and** surgical emergency. Minutes matter. Rapid and lethal. Early diagnosis can save life/limb. Polymicrobial 75%. Can present to ED, Surgery, Urology, T&O, Medicine. Infection moves rapidly through the subcutaneous layer and the fascial plane.
- **Microbiology:** spontaneous usually caused by *Strep. pyogenes* Group A Strep (GAS). Post penetrating injury mixed aerobic/anaerobic bacterial infection. Rare form tropical/subtropical/marine exposure due to *Aeromonas hydrophila* and *Vibrio vulnificus*.
- **Risks:** diabetics, alcoholism, chronic liver disease, IVDU, PVD. Mild trauma, malignancy, immunosuppression, TB.
- **Clinical:** severe localised pain and erythema, myalgia, malaise, fever. Crepitus and surgical emphysema from gas-forming bacteria in the soft tissue. Blistering and 'wood-like' hardening. Mark out limits of erythema.
- **Differential:** severe cellulitis, deep haematoma, pyoderma gangrenosum.
- **Investigations:** FBC: raised WCC, ESR, CRP. U&Es: AKI, high K.
- **Plain X-ray** of affected area may show gas in soft tissues.
- **MRI/CT:** infection. Do not delay for imaging if clinical suspicion high.
- **Needle aspirate:** at edge of lesion and Gram stain can help. Finger test: suspected area infiltrated with local anaesthesia and a 2 cm incision is made in the skin down to the deep fascia. Bleeding should be evident. A lack of bleeding suggests affected area. May just see dirty fluid. Explore deeper.
- **Score:** assess risk indicators for NF (**LRINEC**) score; see MDCalc.
- **Management:** ABC, high flow/hyperbaric O_2. IV fluids (needs may be high with capillary leak) and immediate antibiotics and surgical consult.
- **Broad spectrum antibiotics: Flucloxacillin** IV 2 g 6 h, **Clindamycin** 900 mg TDS – as well as antimicrobial effect it is a potent suppressor of bacterial toxin synthesis. Also give **Benzylpenicillin** 2.4 g QDS and **Gentamicin** IV and **Metronidazole** 500 mg TDS. Liaise closely with microbiology. *Aeromonas hydrophila* and *Vibrio vulnificus* consider **Ceftazidime** or **Ciprofloxacin** with **Doxycycline.**
- **Surgery is key:** needs early and aggressive surgical debridement of necrotic tissue until healthy viable (bleeding) tissue is reached. Amputation may be needed following extensive debridement. Later reconstructive surgery.
- **ITU/burns unit:** complications include AKI, sepsis, limb loss, toxic shock, so no time to delay. Early senior escalation.

19.7   Drug reaction with eosinophilia and systemic symptoms (DRESS)

- **About:** drug hypersensitivity syndrome within 2 weeks of starting drug.
- **Causes:** carbamazepine, phenobarbital, phenytoin, allopurinol, olanzapine and the sulphonamide group of antibiotics. Genetic predisposition.
- **Clinical:** rash, facial swelling, enlarged lymph nodes. Associated with fever.
- **Complications:** hepatitis, AKI, myositis, uveitis, meningoencephalitis.
- **Management:** stop all medications. Dressing, topical steroids, oral antihistamines. Urgent Dermatology advice. Avoid drugs in future. Ciclosporin may be useful.

19.8 Pyoderma gangrenosum

- **About:** autoinflammatory disorders known as neutrophilic dermatoses.
- **Clues:** they may have IBD (UC>CD), RA, myeloma, MGUS, leukaemia, lymphoma, PBC. Idiopathic in 20%.
- **Clinical:** patient usually unwell. Single/multiple ulcers with violaceous borders anywhere from face to limbs. Commoner on anterior legs. Trauma makes it worse (pathergy). Pain out of proportion to that expected of typical arterial/venous ulcer. May also have erythema nodosum.
- **Investigations:** FBC, U&E, CRP, ESR, Ca. Lesion biopsy.
- **Management:** treat cause. Consider topical steroids or 0.1% tacrolimus ointment. May need oral steroids and ciclosporin. Anti-TNF drugs. Advise patients to avoid trauma which can set off new lesions.

19.9 Other important skin conditions

- **Erythema multiforme:** erythematous tender target lesions usually on palms, arms and legs and mucosa. Causes are HSV, EBV, sulphonamides, anticonvulsants, *Mycoplasma* infection, SLE, PAN, HIV, WG, carcinoma, lymphoma. Can help with diagnosis of systemic disease.
- **Lupus pernio:** reddish-brown dermal papules on the face and elsewhere. Consider sarcoid – may have CXR changes or raised calcium.
- **Erythema nodosum:** red roundish raised nodules seen on the shins. Streptococcal infection, TB, sarcoid, IBD, penicillin, etc.
- **Scabies:** mites burrow into stratum corneum and cause pruritus (worse at night) and serpiginous burrows (lines) often between fingers and toes. Dry eczematous rash. May be seen in care homes. Treat with permethrin cream, washing/drying all clothing/bedding, treat close contacts. More severe form Norwegian scabies.

20 General management

20.1 Enteral feeding

- **Screening adults:** the MUST tool is a five-step screening tool to identify those who are malnourished, at risk of malnutrition (undernutrition), or obese. It also includes management guidelines which can be used to develop a care plan. See risk calculator at www.bapen.org.uk.

- **Before** commencing nutrition always consider the risks of *re-feeding syndrome* and screen the patient. Enteral feeding is used where there is a functioning GI tract but some physical reason (e.g. acute stroke or MND, or facial or ENT surgery) that prevents normal swallowing. The enteral route is always preferable to the parenteral route if possible. It is important to note that directly feeding the stomach does not necessarily prevent aspiration as gastric contents can reflux and enter the lungs if there are poor protective reflexes and an inability to cough.

- **Nasogastric tube:** commonly used but uncomfortable and can cause nasal trauma. Easily dislodged and only used as a temporary feeding measure for up to several weeks. If there is a clearly defined time for which swallowing will not be possible then best to replace with better option. Where outcome is unpredictable and survival unsure it may be used for several weeks, e.g. acute stroke. It is important that these are placed properly and local guidelines followed.

- **Never events:** NG tubes can be accidentally placed in bronchi and feed given – this is regarded as a never event; see ▶ Section 21.8. To show the tip is in gastric lumen an aspirate is obtained and checked for <pH 4 and if any doubt a CXR should show the NG tube in the **midline in the thorax and then passing down below the diaphragm.** Usual distance from nose to oesophageal junction is about 40 cm.

- **Percutaneous endoscopic gastrostomy (PEG):** medium- to long-term need for ongoing enteral feeding. There is no decrease in risk of aspiration pneumonia with placement of gastric or post-pyloric feeding tube and there might be increased risk. There is no evidence that PEG feeding improves nutritional markers or decreases the risk for pressure ulcer formation or improves healing of ulcers in a demented patient. PEG tubes do not appear to contribute to comfort at the end of life. Performed by gastroenterologists at endoscopy and involves a puncture from abdominal surface through to the gastric lumen. Risks are real and include infection, peritonitis, sepsis, haemorrhage and displacement and the risks of sedation. Other intra-abdominal organs can be punctured. A fibrous fistulous tract forms over about 10–14 days, after which replacement of any tube can be undertaken.

- **Percutaneous endoscopic jejunostomy (PEJ):** same as a PEG but tube advanced beyond pylorus.

- **Radiologically inserted gastrostomy:** ideal where there is a medium- to long-term need for ongoing enteral feeding and the patient, for whatever reason, does not tolerate endoscopy. Performed by radiologists under fluoroscopy and involves a puncture from abdominal surface through to the gastric lumen. Complications and principles similar to PEG.

- **Needle catheter jejunostomy:** fine catheter inserted into jejunum at laparotomy and brought externally through a puncture in the abdominal wall.

- **Enteral feeding regimen:** with a simple polymeric diet consisting of protein and fat and carbohydrate containing essential minerals and vitamins. In those with small bowel disease a more elemental diet may be given such that proteins are given more as amino acids and fats as medium chain triglycerides.

20.2 Parenteral feeding

- **Assess for risk of re-feeding syndrome.** Parenteral route really only used where the GI tract is non-functional. Higher risk of complications than enteral feeding, particularly sepsis. In terms of feeding it is much less physiological. Not usually considered when needed for <1 week. Several routes.
- **Peripheral venous line:** used with low osmolality feeding as it soon causes thrombophlebitis. The lines are 20 cm in length and can be used for up to 5 days.
- **Peripherally inserted central catheter (PICC):** a 60 cm catheter inserted in the antecubital fossa. The distal end lies within central veins. Hyperosmolar solutions may be used. Thrombophlebitis is less. These can last up to a month and may be inserted before a central venous line is considered.
- **Central venous line:** feeding via jugular/subclavian or femoral line using a silicone catheter. The infraclavicular subclavian route is often preferred and is most practical. A skin tunnel is usually created. The complications are the same as those of inserting any central line here and include infection, haemorrhage, arterial puncture and pneumothorax. Catheter-related sepsis should always be considered if any signs of infection. This will require IV antibiotics and removal of the line.
- **Different preparations** of feed are given depending if central or peripheral access, but all attempt to give about 3 L of feed over 24 h containing between 1700 and 2250 calories with sufficient protein, glucose, lipid, electrolytes, vitamins, water, and fat-soluble and trace elements. Steroid and heparin and insulin may also be given. The feeds are usually prepared by pharmacy in liaison with the dietitian and intensivists. These patients are normally on the HDU/ITU or surgical wards.
- **Parenteral feeding:** requires frequent monitoring and daily U&Es and glucose, and 2–3 times per week FBC, LFTs, Ca, P, Mg, Zn and glycerides. Monitor nutritional status. Any signs of sepsis requires FBC, CRP, blood cultures and assessment for chest or UTI. Take advice from seniors and microbiology as to management of the catheter. If that is the presumed or proven source then it will need to be removed.

Nutritional support and feeding regimens

Needs	Information	Comment
Water	Usually 2–3 L/d	Increased if other losses, e.g. urinary, GI, fistulas
Energy	1750–2400 kcal/d	Titrated to needs
Protein	10–15 g/d of nitrogen in about 90 g of protein	More in severely catabolic states, e.g. burns
Minerals	Na 100 mmol/d, K 60–90 mmol/day, Ca, Mg	Increased K needed with some GI losses
Trace elements	Selenium, iodide, fluoride, iron, zinc, manganese and chromium	Increased for enteral as uptake not 100%
Vitamins	Give all fat and water soluble as per minimal daily requirements (not covered here)	Increased for enteral as uptake not 100%. Vitamin K added to parenteral feeds

20.3 Re-feeding syndrome

- **About:** potential fatal metabolic consequence of rapidly providing calories enterally or parenterally to severely malnourished patients.
- **Physiology:** feeding leads cellular metabolism to switch from catabolism to anabolism. Insulin is released and causes glycogen, fat and protein synthesis and cellular uptake of potassium, phosphate and magnesium as well as water causing low phosphate, magnesium and potassium.
- **At-risk patients have one or more of the following:** BMI <16 kg/m^2, unintentional weight loss >15% in the past 3–6 months, little or no nutritional intake for >10 d, low levels of potassium, phosphate or magnesium before feeding. Or the patient has two or more of the following: BMI <18.5, unintentional weight loss >10% in the past 3–6 months, little or no nutritional intake for >5 d, history of alcohol misuse or drugs, including insulin, chemotherapy, antacids or diuretics.
- **Management:** re-feeding should be started at a low level of energy replacement. Vitamin supplementation should also be started with re-feeding and continued for at least 10 d. Bloods should be checked and dietetic input needed.
- **Reference:** NICE (2006) CG32: Nutritional support for adults.

20.4 Pain management

- Successfully managing pain requires some knowledge of analgesia. Become familiar with a core group of medications. The team looking after a patient should certainly work with the hospital pain team. The perception of pain is multifactorial and often subjective and personal and varies with cause, depression, fears as to causation and control, and often cultural and social issues.
- Some patients are stoical and will accept mild to occasional moderate pain if explained without recourse to analgesia. Others will want all discomfort minimised. All effective analgesics carry side-effects and these need to be weighed up with their usage. Paracetamol within normal dose range is probably the safest but only appropriate as a single agent for mild pain but can be combined with stronger medications.
- Pain is feared by patients and the experience will vary between those with post-operative pain and those with pain related to a chronic disease or malignancy. Pain control must be appropriate and proportionate. Be aware of the WHO analgesic ladder which you ascend, but manage pain based on severity. Don't forget to consider specific management of fear, anxiety and depression which may well be pain multipliers. Anxiety may be based on mistaken fears which can be addressed. Addiction to opioids when used for pain control is very rare indeed.

WHO pain ladder

- **Mild: Paracetamol** 1 g IV/PO 6–8 hourly if not controlled then step up. SE: liver/renal failure with overdose. Avoid in liver failure.
- **Moderate: Paracetamol** 1 g 6–8 hourly + **Codeine** 30–60 mg 6–8 hourly or **Ibuprofen** 400 mg 8 hourly. **Voltarol** (**diclofenac**) 50 mg 8 h or slow release 75 mg (max 150 mg daily) PO/PR in 2–3 divided doses. **Voltarol** 100 mg suppository PR. Caution with NSAIDs in those with impaired renal function as can cause AKI. **Tramadol** 50–100 mg 4–6 hourly is another possibility; even mild opiates can cause delirium in the elderly.

- **Severe:** strong opioid, e.g. **morphine** 5 mg 4 hourly PO and then calculate the daily requirement and give as a long-acting agent, e.g. **morphine** if pain is ongoing or likely to worsen. Others include IV or SC **diamorphine** ± non-opioid, ± adjuvant.

Managing specific pain syndromes

- NB: Have a low threshold to convert to **Oxycodone** 5 mg every 4–6 hours for acute severe pain when there is evidence of renal failure.
- **Acute MI/ACS: GTN, Nitrates, Diamorphine** 2.5–5 mg or **Morphine** 5–10 mg IV and anti-emetic. ECG and assessment + IV **Ondansetron** 4 mg.
- **Acute abdomen:** IV **Morphine** 5–10 mg + IV **Cyclizine** 50 mg or IV **Ondansetron** 4 mg.
- **Bone fracture:** IV **Morphine** 5–10 mg + IV **Cyclizine** 50 mg or IV **Ondansetron** 4 mg.
- **Bone pain, inflammation pain:** NSAIDs, e.g. **Diclofenac** 50 mg 8 h or **Ibuprofen** 400–600 mg 8 h. Bisphosphonates can help in some forms of bone pain, e.g. myeloma, Paget's disease, especially with high Ca. Try IV **Pamidronate** or **Zoledronate**.
- **Headache of malignancy:** dexamethasone, radiotherapy, codeine.
- **Ischaemic pain:** NSAIDs, ketamine, morphine.
- **Liver metastases:** steroids.
- **Localised pain:** analgesic infiltration, e.g. lidocaine or nerve root blocks.
- **Metastatic bone disease:** osteolytic metastases and bone pain with breast cancer or myeloma. Bisphosphonates, e.g. **Pamidronate** 60–90 mg IV every 4 weeks, NSAIDs, morphine.
- **Neuropathic pain:** gabapentin, amitriptyline often given at night, pregabalin, steroids and radiotherapy may be useful in malignancy-related neuropathic pain, shingles, trigeminal neuralgia.
- **Non-specific:** (e.g. back pain): TENS machine, acupuncture.
- **Renal colic:** consider **Voltarol** 50 mg TDS PO/PR or **Diclofenac** 75 mg OD PO/PR. A second dose can be given after a minimum of 30 min if necessary. Alternative is **Morphine** 5–10 mg IV + cyclizine 50 mg IV.

Using opiates and other analgesics

- When prescribing opiates the **drug, dose and frequency and route of administration** should be written clearly. If it is as part of a prescription, then the dose must also be spelt out. When pain is expected to be temporary, e.g. post-op or for some other reason, it is wise to time limit the drug so that it is reviewed days or weeks later, so that it does not continue indefinitely if not required.
- Weak opiates are often effective both short- and long-term. However, with dehydration and renal failure they can become toxic, especially in the elderly, and caution must be taken. Always consider codeine as a cause of reduced awareness and delirium and coma and consider a trial of **naloxone** if unclear. Side-effects are constipation, and a laxative should be added. They may also cause nausea and vomiting and are often combined with an anti-emetic. **Diamorphine** in reasonable concentrations can be given along with metoclopramide, cyclizine or haloperidol in a syringe driver. Myoclonus may also be seen.
- Strong opiates include **morphine, diamorphine** and fentanyl. They should be commenced at low starting doses: **Morphine** 5 mg every 4–6 h which can be given orally or IM or IV or SC. **Diamorphine** 2.5 mg can be given parenterally only. Both should be increased as needed and titrated to pain.

- **Fentanyl** is often used transdermally and may be preferred with renal dysfunction and when there are difficulties with oral formulations. However, at times it may accumulate and lead to confusion and coma and the patch should be removed and analgesia needs assessed. With oral medications there is a simple feedback loop. If the medication causes coma then no more medications are taken and the patient recovers until able to swallow the next dose. With parenteral and transdermal routes this pseudo-safety feedback loop does not exist and extra care must be taken.
- **Morphine** comes as either a faster-acting immediate release formulation which works in minutes and covers about 4 h. Can be started as **Oramorph** 5 mg 4–6 hourly. Once **morphine** need is estimated a longer-acting once-daily controlled release formulation can be used. Additional immediate release morphine should be available for breakthrough pain. Patient dose varies with tolerance and renal function and patients may take anywhere from 10 to 5000 mg of **morphine** per day. Pethidine is sometimes used but has a very short $t_{1/2}$.

Opiate equivalence doses
- Morphine 10 mg PO = Morphine 5 mg IM/IV/SC = Diamorphine 3 mg IM/IV/SC = Codeine 100 mg PO = Dihydrocodeine 100 mg PO = Tramadol 100 mg PO = Oxycodone 7 mg PO.
- Great care must be taken – doses shown are for 24 h. For medications just for 4–6 h, these need to be divided into their individual dose.

Non-steroidal anti-inflammatory drugs
- Very useful for acute and chronic pain management, but chronic usage can lead to peptic ulcer disease and renal impairment. Avoided in CKD, or PUD, or low platelets, or bleeding, or in acute illness, as can precipitate AKI. If there is dyspepsia then adding a PPI may be useful. Side-effects limit usage in the elderly. Consider **ibuprofen** and **diclofenac.**
- **Neuropathic pain:** most anticonvulsants and TCAs have action against neuropathic pain. Examples include gabapentin, amitriptyline and carbamazepine. Specialists may use pregabalin, ketamine.

20.5 Venous thromboembolism prevention
- Screen all for their risk of DVT/PE and manage according to NICE guidance with mechanical or pharmacological agents after risk assessment.
- Avoid pharmacological VTE prophylaxis if the patient has a risk factor for bleeding and the risk of bleeding outweighs the risk of VTE.

Patients who are at increased risk of VTE
- Medical or surgical or trauma patients.
- Mobility reduced for 3+ days or expected to have ongoing reduced mobility relative to normal state plus any VTE risk factor (see below).
- If total anaesthetic + surgical time >90 min or if surgery involves pelvis or lower limb and total anaesthetic + surgical time >60 min.
- If acute surgical admission with inflammatory or intra-abdominal condition.
- Significant reduction in mobility or any VTE risk factor present (see below).

VTE risk factors

- Active cancer or cancer treatment or obesity (BMI >30 kg/m²).
- Age >60 years, critical care admission, dehydration, known thrombophilias.
- One or more significant medical comorbidities (e.g. heart disease, metabolic, endocrine, respiratory, acute infectious diseases; inflammatory conditions).
- Personal history or 1st-degree relative with a history of VTE.
- HRT or oestrogen-containing contraceptive therapy.
- Varicose veins with phlebitis.

Patients who are at risk of bleeding

- History of bleeding, acquired bleeding disorders.
- Concurrent use of anticoagulants (such as warfarin with INR >2).
- LP/epidural/spinal anaesthesia <4 h ago or expected within the next 12 h.
- Acute stroke or uncontrolled systolic hypertension (>230/120 mmHg).
- Thrombocytopenia (platelets <75 × 10⁹/L). See ▶Section 8.4.
- Untreated bleeding disorders (haemophilia or von Willebrand's disease).

Choice of method

- **Mechanical VTE prophylaxis:** anti-embolism stockings (thigh or knee length), foot impulse devices, intermittent pneumatic compression devices (thigh or knee length).
- **Pharmacological VTE prophylaxis:** most Trusts use LMWH; however, doses need to be adjusted if there is renal failure. Alternatives include fondaparinux. Dabigatran, rivaroxaban and apixaban have been used in elective hip and knee surgery. Follow local policies.
- **Stroke patients:** there is no fixed standard and practices vary between centres. Compression devices are recommended for the first 30 days. Some centres use LMWH, in some patients with severe disability and at high risk of VTE even in haemorrhagic strokes. LMWH may still be considered after the acute period. Follow local guidance. Balance against risks of haemorrhage.
- **Pregnancy or up to 6 weeks postpartum:** VTE prophylaxis if undergoing caesarean section or if any of the following risk factors: expected to have significantly reduced mobility for ≥3 days; active cancer or cancer treatment; age >35 years; critical care admission, dehydration, excess blood loss or blood transfusion; known thrombophilias; obesity (pre-pregnancy or early pregnancy BMI >30 kg/m²); significant medical comorbidity (such as heart disease, metabolic, endocrine or respiratory pathologies, acute infectious diseases or inflammatory conditions); personal history or 1st-degree relative with history of VTE; pregnancy-related risk factor, including ovarian hyperstimulation, hyperemesis gravidarum, multiple pregnancy, pre-eclampsia; varicose veins with phlebitis.
- **References:** NICE (2010) CG92: Venous thromboembolism: reducing the risk. RCOG (2015) GTG37a: *Reducing the risk of venous thromboembolism during pregnancy and the puerperium.*

20.6 ▶ Duties of a doctor

- Good advice is given by the GMC. Doctors need to be satisfied that they have consent from a patient, or other valid authority, before undertaking any examination or investigation, providing treatment, or involving patients in teaching and research. The GMC has very useful guidance on the duties of a doctor. Patients must be able to trust doctors. To justify that trust you must show respect for human life and you must: always make the care of your patient your first concern and protect and promote the health of patients and the public. Provide a good standard of practice and care. Keep your professional knowledge and skills up to date. Recognise and work within the limits of your competence. Work with colleagues in the ways that best serve patients' interests.

- Treat patients as individuals and respect their dignity: treat patients politely and considerately. Respect patients' right to confidentiality. Work in partnership with patients: listen to them and respond to their concerns and preferences. Give patients the information they want or need in a way they can understand. Respect patients' right to reach decisions with you about their treatment and care. Support patients in caring for themselves to improve and maintain their health. Be honest and open and act with integrity. Act without delay if you have good reason to believe that you or a colleague may be putting patients at risk. Never discriminate unfairly against patients or colleagues. Never abuse your patients' trust in you or the public's trust in the profession. You are personally accountable for your professional practice and must always be prepared to justify your decisions and actions.
- **Reference:** General Medical Council (2014) *Good Medical Practice*.

20.7 ▶ Medical errors and harm

- 'To err is human' is true. We all make errors, the question is how we prevent errors, especially those that can cause patient harm, and what we do when we realise that an error has occurred. Errors by definition are unintentional. Health systems are complex, interconnected and multitasking, with lots of competing priorities, and different levels of knowledge and experience.
- One of the commonest sources of error is with medication. Avoid writing up drugs on rounds, sit down and do it later when not distracted. Always examine the drug chart as well as the patient on all hospital rounds. It is impossible here to go into the complete list of medical errors, but there are a list of events which should 'never occur'. These are called **'never events' and are listed below.**
- When clinical errors result in clinical harm, alert your consultant immediately. Immediately reduce any possible further harm done. Take advice. Be honest about errors with everyone involved – the patient, their family, others in the team, your boss. Document everything, fully. Say sorry when things have gone wrong. That one word may make trouble simply disappear. It may be difficult to say it, but say it.
- Sorry does not in itself admit blame or liability. Once you start to focus on an error the responsibility rarely lands on one set of shoulders. There may be educational and training issues, work issues, responsibility issues. Most errors occur as several events conspired to happen together and a mistake that would have been caught any day was able to perpetuate itself through until real harm had occurred.
- It has become clear that a simple blame culture does little to perpetuate change and improve things. In many cases, but not all, the error could have happened to most of us and the only differentiating factor has been bad luck. Many systems seem set up to allow failure and blaming a scapegoat is, sadly, still a part of healthcare culture which we must try to change.

20.8 ▶ The duty of candour

- The principle of the duty of candour is that care organisations have a general duty to act in an open and transparent way in relation to care provided to patients.
- Organisations will have to ensure they have systems in place to capture notifiable safety incidents and processes to inform the patient and provide support. A 'notifiable safety incident' means any unintended or unexpected incident that occurred in respect of a service user during the provision of a regulated activity that, in the reasonable opinion of a healthcare professional, could result in, or appears to have resulted in:
  - (a) the death of the service user, where the death relates directly to the incident rather than to the natural course of the service user's illness or underlying condition, or
  - (b) moderate or severe harm, or prolonged psychological harm.
- The Organisation must, as soon as possible after becoming aware that a notifiable safety incident has occurred, inform the patient (or their representative) and provide reasonable support to him/her in relation to the incident. This is followed by written notification of the incident with an apology and details of further enquiries into the incident that are to be undertaken.
- Provide support to the patient to ensure that the patient understands the discussions (this may include providing emotional support). Keep a written record of all discussions and correspondence. The consultant must be involved and will be key in ensuring this is done.

20.9 ▶ NHS never events

- The NHS has defined a list of never events. Systems and practices should be enabled to prevent these. All need thorough investigation.
- **Surgical:** wrong site surgery, wrong implant or prosthesis, retained foreign object post-procedure.
- **Medication:** mis-selection of a strong potassium-containing solution, wrong route of administration of medication, overdose of insulin due to abbreviations or incorrect device, overdose of methotrexate for non-cancer treatment, mis-selection of high strength midazolam during conscious sedation.
- **Mental health:** failure to install functional collapsible shower or curtain rails.
- **General:** falls from poorly restricted windows, chest or neck entrapment in bedrails, transfusion/transplantation of ABO-incompatible blood components or organs, misplaced naso- or oro-gastric tubes, scalding of patients.

20.10 ▶ Risk management and risk register

- Acute medicine clinicians should play a fundamental role in risk management. All NHS organisations should have a risk management framework, which provides assurance to the Board that appropriate processes are in place to manage corporate and operational risks effectively; recommending procedures for the effective identification, prioritisation, treatment and management of risks to minimise or maximise the effect of an uncertain event or set of events on the delivery of objectives; ensuring a cohesive approach to the governance of risk; identifying risk management resources; and establishing risk management as an integral part of the NHS culture.

- Risks to patient safety and care should be identified and the risk mitigated against. All risks should have a risk owner and an action owner who mitigates the risk and updates those involved on the progress of this. Risks are assessed using a score of 1–5 for harm if it occurs and a score of 1–5 in terms of likelihood, and a resultant product value obtained. Risks over a certain value are escalated for further action. Risks and issues often get confused and a useful way of remembering the difference is: *risks* are things that might happen and stop us achieving objectives, e.g. safe surgery, or otherwise impact on the success of the organisation; *issues* are things that have happened, were not planned and require management action.
- Each Trust has a risk register which should contain as a minimum a risk reference; risk owner, risk description, ratings of likelihood and impact (for both current and after actions), risk proximity, action plans, action owner for each action, and completion date for each action.

20.11 ▶ Admitting and discharging patients safely

- Beds are always tight. You can only admit if you discharge other patients. Discharging patients safely is a skill developed through knowledge and experience. Patients should only be admitted if there is no alternative.
- Determining if someone is medically ready is really a decision for the registrar or above unless it has been anticipated and a criteria-based plan made.
- Before admitting a person ask why: is being onsite going to mitigate some anticipated risk, what is the natural history here, what are the risks? Often there are social and medical reasons. Is admission to a busy, noisy potentially infectious assessment area in the patient's best interest? A patient getting 1:1 care at home may be safer than 1:10 care in hospital.
- Hospitals are sources of new infections, strange environments that will cause significant new cognitive challenges leading to falls and overmedication of elderly patients, with insomnia from their agitated neighbours.
- Your hospital should have same-day clinics that can do blood tests, monitor symptoms and continue investigations. Patients should not have to sleep in hospital to have an urgent test done – this is irrational and uneconomical.
- Admission means packages of care are terminated which can be time-consuming to reinstate. Many expect an oasis of peace, quiet and relaxation but this is just not possible on a busy acute assessment unit.
- In terms of hospital admission there is often an 'illusion of safety'. Patients are often placed overnight onto busy wards far from the doctors on take with 2 trained nurses and a healthcare assistant serving 25 or more patients. The patient may be in a side room.
- If the patient develops a problem it may take time for them to raise help (if the call buzzer is out of reach perhaps) and even longer for the nurse to alert the medical team in another part of the hospital and have them attend.
- The medical team have to prioritise their ill patients in the emergency department with ward patients and this adds to delays. In some instances it is better to let stable, mobile and able patients go home, where they will have 1:1 care from a sensible spouse or carers who can call 999 and have an emergency ambulance attending within minutes, providing very solid basic medical care if the need arises. This is obviously not appropriate for those with a STEMI or acute severe asthma, but for some patients with less severe conditions it certainly bears consideration.

- So when sending patients home with their particular illness you need to have a sensible understanding of the natural history of the disease and its expected behaviour. I ask myself – what is the most reasonable worst-case scenario and can I mitigate against it in any way?
- Before you do a discharge check that the patient wants to go home. Make sure they know to come back via 999 if there are any problems – make this very clear to the patient and it helps if family support this. Ensure that you have documented a thorough assessment, including what you have told the patient, and make sure all are happy and agree. Do not do this if the patient is sick and lives very distant from the hospital or is alone or has cognitive or mental health issues, or there is a lack of family support or a general reluctance for the plan.
- The most fundamental question is 'did I put the welfare of the patient first?' In difficult cases it is very reasonable to take senior advice or a rapid second opinion from a fellow clinician who agrees plan in best interests.

20.12 Self-discharge

- An informed competent patient should be able to refuse admission with no prejudice to ongoing care. Patients can absolutely decline what we consider best care. Is there a second-best way, ambulatory care or a rapid outpatient clinic? Is sleeping in the hospital really needed? If that is the only way to rapidly access a service then you need to think how to change your services.
- Hospitals are not prisons and patients with capacity (they have capacity until proven otherwise) have a right to leave at any time. It would be good if they told us why and even told us they were going but some will just go. Most of the time it is frustrating but harmless.
- Doctors have a duty of care, sometimes patients who have ongoing needs do decide to leave. It is important to define why they need to stay – are they at risk of arrhythmias or do they need urgent tests? Try to find out why – can the patient leave and do whatever they deem important and come back? The need to leave may be entirely understandable and so try to be reasonable and flexible in your approach but do negotiate a reasonable level of cooperation and ensure that you document any risks which you have informed them of.
- If you feel there is significant risk of harm but the patient has the capacity to appreciate this, then document conversations and advice given and quickly take senior advice. It would be wise to ring the GP then or next morning who may call and visit the patient. There may be a change of heart. Families can often help but you need patient consent.
- Most hospitals have a standard form for self-discharge, but even if the patient refuses to cooperate then medical and nursing staff should record contemporaneous notes over what was said and what happened and all advice given.
- Tell them to come back if they get worse or change their mind even though that may mean via A&E. **Always do a discharge letter to document the events and keep in it any advice and make sure the GP is made aware.**
- Problems arise when you suspect that there is impaired capacity. If you are worried that the patient is non-capacitous due to acute delirium (alcohol withdrawal, sepsis, hypoxia, etc.) or has chronic problems (e.g. dementia) then take senior advice. You will need to consider Deprivation of Liberty Safeguards (DoLS). One may need to

restrain the patient in such a case, either passively by stalling or very occasionally physically or with sedation, but this should be done with senior (preferably consultant) advice and using hospital staff or even the police if needed, usually under common law initially and must only ever be done in the best interests of the patient. If a septic delirious patient leaves and dies you may be blamed for your inaction and have to answer in a coroner's court.

- If the patient does leave and you have not been able to restrain them then involve hospital security and police. It is not your role to physically restrain patients unless you have training in this. Be seen to be doing all possible to protect the patient. The care of the patient must always be your main focus.

20.13   Suicidal patients

- Suicidal patients who perhaps came in with an overdose should not be allowed to discharge against advice without senior involvement. Involve psychiatry. Take senior advice immediately. If they go you should involve police. Involve the GP. It is rare but it does happen that overdose patients leave the hospital and finish their lives by some other means. You must act.
- All patients admitted with an attempted suicide must be seen by the psychiatry team or equivalent prior to discharge. Senior advice must be taken if there is any attempt to abscond or self-discharge, or if they leave the premises which will usually mean police involvement. These are some of the risk factors for those who go on to die by suicide. Note that most people who die by suicide have seen a doctor in the preceding month.

Factors to screen for increasing suicide risk

- History of depression and substance abuse or borderline personality disorder.
- Age >45 years, living alone. Puerperal, chronic painful illness.
- Gender: men try more lethal means, women try more often.
- Marital status: never married, divorced, widowed, recently separated.
- Extensive and detailed plans or plans using highly lethal means.
- Family history of suicide, still expressing a wish to die, recent job loss.
- Recent loss of loved one or the anniversary of the loss.
- Previous suicide attempts – this is one of the best predictors.
- Gay/lesbian youth, Caucasian youth, impulsive or reckless behaviour.

Assessment

- **Ask about suicidal ideation:** where concerned, always ask patients about suicide and their intentions. Do they feel life is worth living? Have they thought of ending it? Most patients will discuss. It is very rare, but the person committed to suicide will say whatever gets them out of hospital. Older, single men with financial worries and job loss are one group of concern and you should take experienced advice regardless of what they say.
- **Management:** check your local policy, but anyone with a suicide attempt or suicidal ideation should have a psychiatric evaluation before discharge. Patients may even try to self-discharge. Get immediate help from psychiatry and take senior advice.

20.14 Common law and Mental Health Act

- When the patient is unconscious or lacks capacity, common law allows the doctor to act in the patient's best interests. This may enable urgent detention against the patient's will to allow further assessment and treatment when a delay would result in immediate potential harm to the patient, and where there is no time for a more measured approach to be used.
- In the Emergency Department common law is used. It allows life-saving surgery or sedation and detention to give IV antibiotics for confusion due to sepsis, meningitis or to treat hypoglycaemia, etc. When time is available then admit patient and use the MHA.

Mental Health Act (MHA)

- **Section 5(2):** allows a ward doctor to detain a patient for a mental health assessment on ward for 72 h; form H1 is completed and the duty psychiatry team should be informed. The patient should have a mental health assessment at earliest opportunity. Seek support from on-call psychiatry and the appropriate consultant. It is sometimes called a 'holding power'. During the 72 h the person would be assessed for Section 2 or 3.
- **Section 5(4):** nursing staff can use this to detain a patient if a doctor is not available and this is valid for up to 6 h. Complete form H2. If the doctor/approved clinician has not arrived within 4 h the duty consultant should be contacted by the clinical team leader/senior nurse on call and should attend.
- The MHA does not allow you to treat physical conditions against a patient's will but only the mental health issues, unless the physical cause is the cause of the mental issues. However, you may consider doing so if capacity is uncertain and you have the defence of patient's best interests. Take advice. Otherwise the Mental Capacity Act 2005 is used.

20.15 Mental capacity

- An assessment of capacity is decision- and time-specific. Patients are only lacking capacity for the particular question asked. Assume capacity to make the decision in question until proven otherwise. The Mental Capacity Act Code of Practice describes a test of capacity you can use to decide whether a person is able to make that decision.
- An assessment that a person lacks capacity to make a decision must never be based simply on their age or their appearance, assumptions about their condition or any aspect of their behaviour. The risks and benefits should be discussed in detail to satisfy the questions below.
- In many cases the loss of capacity is partial, it may also be temporary and it may change over time. It can be useful to repeat the assessment on a 'better' day. There are several things to consider when assessing if a person can make a decision.
- There are 2 clear stages to the mental capacity assessment. Any assessment should begin with stage 1 and only proceed to stage 2 if the first stage is met. Each stage is set out as a question to be answered as follows:

The importance of the statutory principles

- A person must be assumed to have capacity unless it is established that they lack capacity.

- A person is not to be treated as unable to make a decision unless all practicable steps to help him to do so have been taken without success.
- A person is not to be treated as unable to make a decision merely because he makes an unwise decision.

Stage 1: Is there the presence of an impairment or disturbance?

- Does the person have an impairment of, or disturbance in the functioning of the mind or brain? Such states may be permanent or temporary as well as diagnosed or undiagnosed.

Stage 2: If so then perform a 4-point functional test of capacity

Does the impairment or disturbance mean that the person is unable to make the specific decision when they need to? This requires an assessment. The functional test consists of 4 elements, each of which you must test the person's ability in. They are:

- The ability to **understand** information about the decision (the 'relevant' information);
- Ability to **retain** the information long enough to make the decision;
- Ability to **use, or 'weigh up'** the information as part of the decision-making process; and
- The ability to **communicate** their decision through any means.

20.16 Opiate addicts

- **Note:** do not initiate methadone or buprenorphine treatment without senior advice or without arranging continuation of treatment on discharge with addiction services.
- **About:** usual GMC responsibilities for doctors apply and a non-judgmental approach should be followed. The clinician must treat the drug misuser but should determine the impact of their drug misuse on other individuals, especially dependent children, and child protection policies followed. Heroin users are the largest single group. Opiate substitution prevents people dropping out of treatment, suppresses illicit use of heroin, reduces crime, reduces the risk of infections and death.
- **Complications:** addicts have increased risk of viral hepatitis, bacterial endocarditis, HIV, tuberculosis, septicaemia, pneumonia, deep vein thrombosis, pulmonary emboli, abscesses and dental disease. Assaults and violence, falls and trauma. Only in exceptional circumstances should the decision be made to offer substitute medication without specialist advice being sought, e.g. a drug misuser presenting with opioid withdrawal in late pregnancy, a patient with serious concomitant physical or psychiatric illness where withdrawal is complicating the clinical problems, someone who is opioid-dependent and demonstrating withdrawal. Indeed, in such circumstances it is vital that the doctor fulfils their responsibilities by ensuring adequate assessment and appropriate management that facilitates the retention of the patient in treatment.
- **Treat any emergency or acute problem first.** Take history including dosage, route of administration, time last used, and check for injecting sites. Take appropriate screen for opiate drugs to confirm/deny. **Assessment:** general examination, including IV sites, local and systemic sequelae of injecting. Urinalysis for illicit drugs (with consent) should be undertaken. In pregnancy, prescribing should be supervised by a specialist in maternity management.

- **Clinical:** look for evidence of **opiate withdrawal syndrome:** drug craving, anxiety, drug seeking (6 h), yawning, sweating, running nose, lacrimation (8 h), dilated pupils, goose skin, tremors, hot/cold flushes, aching bones/muscles, loss of appetite, abdominal cramps and irritability (12 h), insomnia, hypertension, N&V, diarrhoea, febrile, fetal position. Opiate-dependent individuals undergoing opiate withdrawal syndrome may present to relieve the distressing symptoms of opiate withdrawal whilst in hospital. Do not give in to undue pressure to prescribe immediately. Take time to assess the patient. But they may not, if experiencing withdrawal symptoms, be able to cooperate with staff. Look for objective signs of opioid withdrawal. A negative urine test for opioids makes addiction unlikely.
- **Prescribing (take senior advice first – SpR and above):** do not feel pressurised to prescribe. Methadone and buprenorphine are both approved for the treatment and prevention of withdrawals from opioids but this must only be prescribed following liaison with the community drug team. Methadone is preferred. Optimal doses for most people lie between 40 and 120 mg, but will depend upon size, gender, age, other health problems and metabolic clearance rates. Same care as in prescribing any opiate.

Advice
- Do not give methadone if heroin taken in past 8 h or methadone in past 24 h.
- Do not give more than 10 mg (methadone mixture 1 mg/1 ml) as an initial dose to patients not receiving a methadone prescription in the community.
- Do not exceed more than 40 mg of methadone in the first 24 h period.
- Do not give methadone to a patient intoxicated with opioids/other drugs including alcohol.
- Treat opioid overdose with standard resuscitation techniques and with the use of naloxone. Naloxone is given 0.4–2.0 mg parenterally (IV/IM/SC) and this can be repeated after every 5 min, up to a maximum dose of 10 mg. The half-life of naloxone is much shorter than methadone and other opioids.
- **Managing opiate withdrawal:** may need **Loperamide** (diarrhoea) 4 mg stat followed by 2 mg after each loose stool (max 16 mg daily), **Metoclopramide** (N&V) 10 mg TDS or **Prochlorperazine** 5 mg TDS oral or 12.5 mg IM BD. **Mebeverine** (stomach cramps) 135 mg TDS, **Diazepam** (agitation/anxiety) 5–10 mg TDS, **Zopiclone** (insomnia) 7.5 mg nocte, **NSAIDs**, paracetamol.

20.17 ▶ Driving and disease

- The law is quite clear. If a patient has a condition that impairs their ability and makes them unsafe to drive then the doctor has a duty to inform the patient and *the patient is legally obliged to inform and follow the advice of the DVLA* (Driver and Vehicle Licensing Agency).
- Ultimately it is the DVLA who will determine if the patient can retain their driving licence. All driving advice given (or advice not to drive) should be documented in the notes. Licences are normally issued valid until age 70 years unless restricted to a shorter duration for medical reasons as indicated above. There is no upper limit but after age 70 renewal is necessary every 3 years.
- All licence applications require a medical self-declaration by the applicant. This guidance is for a private car or motorcycle. **For those with a licence to drive a bus, coach or lorry, all must inform the DVLA because there are more stringent restrictions**. See the DVLA website (dvla.gov.uk) for more information

and in particular for the DVLA document entitled 'Fitness to drive', which can be obtained online. If you have any concerns you can ring the DVLA medical advisors. When assessing a patient, consider if they would be in full control of the car at all times, e.g. can they do an emergency stop? For borderline cases there are driver assessment centres. Car modifications can allow a disabled patient to drive to the necessary standard. Advise the patient to also inform their car insurers.

- Group 1 licences are normally valid until 70 years of age (the 'til 70 licence) unless restricted to a shorter duration for medical reasons. There is no upper age limit to licensing, but after age 70 renewal is required every 3 years.
- Group 2 licences expire at age 45 and they will need to have a D4 medical examination. Drivers above the age of 45 will need to renew their driving licence every 5 years and will need to have a D4 medical examination each time they renew. Once a Group 2 driver reaches the age of 65, they need to renew their licence and have a D4 medical examination every year.

Guidance (but always check latest information from DVLA)
- Always check the DVLA website (dvla.gov.uk) as specific advice changes at times. Online pdf 'Assessing fitness to drive – a guide for medical professionals'. Ultimately it is up to the DVLA to decide so advice where unclear is for patient to self-refer to the DVLA who will decide.
- They will send the named consultant a questionnaire form to complete. Motorists belong to one or both classes of **Group 1 Private car drivers and Group 2 Coach, lorry, bus drivers, with more severe restrictions.**

Quick guide (see online and refer to DVLA if unsure)
- **TIA:** Group 1: can drive >28 days. Group 2: can drive >1 year.
- **Multiple TIA:** Group 1: can drive >3 months. Group 2: can drive >1 year.
- **Stroke no deficits:** as for TIA. **Stroke with deficits:** refer DVLA.
- **First ever seizure:** Group 1: can drive 6 months after last seizure. Group 2: 5 years seizure-free. **Epilepsy:** Group 1: can drive 12 months after last seizure. Group 2: 10 years seizure-free.
- **Unexplained TLOC:** Group 1: restricted for 6 months. Group 2: restricted for 12 months. Concerns if structural heart disease or abnormal EEG. Refer DVLA.
- **Pacemaker, PCI, AICD**, post procedure: see guidance.
- **Diabetes and insulin/hypoglycaemics:** Group 1: need to be aware of hypos. Two or more hypos needing help of another person in past 12 months is a bar to driving – inform DVLA. Group 2: full hypo awareness; regular monitoring; one episode of hypo needing help in past 12 months stop driving and inform DVLA.
- **Reference:** www.gov.uk/government/collections/assessing-fitness-to-drive-guide-for-medical-professionals.

20.18 Roles and responsibilities after death

Introduction
- The diagnosis of death has been formalised by the Academy of Medical Royal Colleges (2008) paper *A code of practice for the diagnosis and confirmation of death* which should be read. The definition of death should be regarded as *the irreversible loss of the capacity for consciousness, combined with irreversible loss of the capacity to breathe.* This may be secondary to a wide range of underlying problems in the body, for example, cardiac arrest. The irreversible cessation of brainstem function,

whether due to intra-/extracranial events will produce this clinical state and therefore irreversible loss of function of the brainstem equates with the death of the individual and allows the diagnosis of death.

- Loss of the capacity for consciousness does not equal death. Patients in the vegetative state have also lost this capacity. Those declared dead by virtue of irreversible cessation of brainstem function do not breathe unaided. This also means that even if the body of the deceased remains on respiratory support, the loss of integrated biological function will inevitably lead to deterioration and organ necrosis within a short time.

Diagnosing death

- During the day or when on call you may well be called to see patients who have died to 'certify them' as dead. These are usually patients who have had unsuccessful attempts at resuscitation or who have died and who are not for resuscitation. In some, such as those on care plans for the dying and palliation, the death will have been expected, in others it may not have been.
- Diagnosing death is rarely an urgent request but one should seek to certify as soon as convenient so that the patient can be moved off the ward to the morgue. Check that family have been informed – they will rarely need to speak to a doctor unless the death is entirely unexpected. If you do have to speak to the family then it is best to set aside some time and find a convenient space to talk to them, preferably with nursing staff to hand. Any contentious issues should be escalated to the responsible consultant to liaise with the family in normal hours.
- **In practice, attend the patient and listen and auscultate the chest for 5 min** to show absence of continued cardiorespiratory arrest, the absence of the pupillary responses to light, of the corneal reflexes, and of any motor response to supra-orbital pressure, should be confirmed and the time of death is recorded as the time at which these criteria are fulfilled. Document your findings and ensure accurately timed and dated and signed and GMC number. Additional comments, e.g. RIP and religious comments are not needed.
- **Nurses:** the nurses prepare the body which usually involves closing eyes and mouth. Pumps and syringe drivers are removed but the actual lines are left *in situ*. Orifices are packed with cotton wool. The patient is wrapped in a sheet. The porters will usually come with a special trolley to bring the patient to the mortuary. Often the nurses will close the curtains on adjacent beds whilst this occurs.

Brainstem death

- Mainly an ITU issue in ventilated patients in whom withdrawal of support is being considered. Reversible causes of persisting unconsciousness must be excluded. There should be no doubt as to the cause of irreversible brain damage, so when the cause is unclear brainstem testing cannot be undertaken. One must try to exclude any potentially reversible causes of coma – exclude depressant drugs – narcotics, hypnotics and tranquillisers. Consider hypothermia, renal or hepatic failure.
- Time may be allowed for drug excretion. Naloxone and flumazenil given as indicated. Body temperature should be >34°C before testing. Glucose and electrolytes should be normalised. K <2 mmol/L or Na >160 mmol/L or <115 mmol/L and Mg and phosphate should be corrected. Hypothyroidism and Addison's disease should be treated. Neuromuscular blockers stopped. In a trauma patient C-spine should be imaged to exclude high-cord lesion causing apnoea.

Testing for absence of brainstem reflexes

- Needs a consultant and a doctor registered for at least 5 years.
- Pupils are fixed and do not respond to sharp changes in light intensity. No corneal reflex.
- Absent oculo-vestibular reflexes – no eye movements with slow injection of 50 ml of ice-cold water over 1 min into each external auditory meatus in turn.
- No motor responses within the cranial nerve distribution can be elicited by adequate stimulation of any somatic area.
- No motor response can be elicited within the cranial nerve or somatic distribution in response to supra-orbital pressure.
- No cough reflex response to bronchial stimulation by a suction catheter placed down the trachea to the carina, or gag response to stimulation of the posterior pharynx with a spatula.
- Hypercarbia – apnoea test.

20.19   Death certification

- Even if you are the person who certified the patient as deceased you cannot do the death certificate unless you personally attended the patient within the past 14 d. Prompt and accurate certification of death is essential. The death certificate provides legal evidence of the fact and cause of death, which has legal and statistical importance and enables the death to be formally registered. Only then can the family make arrangements for cremation/burial of the body.
- As a new doctor the 'Bereavement office' will be calling on your services frequently and it is wise to work well with them. They have little flexibility and the death certificate should be done as soon as is reasonably possible – you are required by law to do so. Death certification can be done by an F1 or above, but it is important that you take advice from senior members of the team. You are legally responsible for the delivery of the death certificate to the registrar, but the bereavement office staff will often do this and usually it is the family who bring it to the registrar.

Information requested as part of death certification

- **Patient's age at death:** work it out from the notes and check it is correct.
- **Place of death:** record the precise place of death (e.g. typically the name of the hospital and ward or the address of a private house or, for deaths elsewhere, the locality). It is particularly important that the relative or other person responsible for registering the death is directed to the Registrar of Births and Deaths for the sub-district where the death occurred, unless (from 1st April 1977) they have decided to make a declaration of the details to be registered before another registrar.
- **When last seen alive by me:** record the date when you last saw the deceased alive, irrespective of whether any other medical practitioner saw the person alive subsequently.
- **Information from post-mortem:** you should indicate whether the information you give about the cause of death takes account of a post-mortem. Such information can be valuable for epidemiological purposes. If a post-mortem has been done, circle option 1. If information may be available later, do not delay the issue of your certificate, circle option 2 and tick statement B on the reverse of the certificate. The registrar will then send you a form for return to the Registrar General

giving the results of the post-mortem. If a post-mortem is not being held, circle option 3.

- **Seen after death** (only one option can be circled): you should indicate, by circling option a, b or c, whether you or another medical practitioner saw the deceased after death.
- **NB:** ask the bereavement office staff to check your work – it can save you lots of problems if there are issues or simple mistakes or typographical errors.

When to refer a death to the coroner

You should refer when any of the following occur. In hospital the bereavement office staff will usually assist with this. You may speak to the coroner or their officer who will advise. Occasionally the staff may ask for a written referral which is faxed over. Follow local policy.

- The cause of death is unknown or it cannot readily be certified as being due to natural causes.
- The deceased was not attended by the doctor during his last illness or was not seen within 14 days or viewed after death.
- There are any suspicious circumstances or history of violence.
- The death may be linked to an accident (whenever it occurred).
- There is any question of self-neglect or neglect by others.
- The death has occurred or the illness arisen during or shortly after detention in police or prison custody (includes voluntary attendance at a police station).
- The deceased was detained under the Mental Health Act.
- The death is linked with an abortion.
- The death might have been contributed to by the actions of the deceased (such as a history of drug or solvent abuse, self-injury or overdose).
- Death could be due to industrial disease or related to the deceased's employment.
- The death occurred during an operation or before full recovery from the effects of an anaesthetic or was in any way related to the anaesthetic (in any event a death within 24 h should normally be referred).
- Death related to a medical procedure or treatment whether invasive or not.
- The death may be due to lack of medical care.
- There are any other unusual or disturbing features to the case.
- Death within 24 h of admission to hospital (unless admission was purely for terminal care).
- It may be wise to report any death where there is an allegation of medical mismanagement or care issues.

Cause of death

- This section of the certificate is divided into Parts I and II. Part I is used to show the immediate cause of death and any underlying cause or causes. Part II should be used for any significant condition or disease that contributed to the death but which is not part of the sequence leading directly to death. State the cause or causes of death accurately to the best of your knowledge and belief. It is wise to take senior advice routinely especially if unsure or any doubts. **Underlying cause of death:** consider the main causal sequence of conditions leading to death. State the disease or condition that led directly to death on the first line [I(a)] and work your way back until you reach the underlying cause of death, which initiated the chain of events leading ultimately to death. **The lowermost completed line in Part I**

should therefore contain the underlying cause of death. Sometimes there are apparently two distinct conditions leading to death. If there is no way of choosing between them, they should be entered on the same line indicating in brackets that they are joint causes of death, e.g. ischaemic heart disease and chronic bronchitis. 'Smoking' may be included if accompanied by a medical cause of death.

- Do not use the following as the single sole cause of death, e.g. *asphyxia, debility, respiratory arrest, asthenia, exhaustion, shock, brain failure, heart failure, syncope, cachexia, hepatic failure, uraemia, cardiac arrest, hepatorenal failure, vagal inhibition, cardiac failure, kidney failure, vasovagal attack, coma, renal failure, ventricular failure, liver failure.* These are clinical syndromes which need pathological explanation as to why they occurred. Old age or senility, although acceptable, should not be used as the only cause of death in Part I unless a more specific cause of death cannot be given and the deceased was aged ≥70. **Part II:** should be used when one or more conditions have contributed to death but are not part of the main causal sequence leading to death. It should not be used to list all conditions present at death. In some cases you can put an interval as to the diagnosis of each in hours, days, months or years before the death occurred. In Part I and II, you should give information about clinical interventions, procedures or drugs that may have led to adverse effects, e.g. warfarin-induced bleeds, etc.

Example of acceptable entries
- I(a): cerebral metastases, I(b): squamous cell lung cancer, I(c): smoking.
- I(a): respiratory failure, I(b): lobar pneumonia, I(c): squamous cell lung cancer. II: Type 2 diabetes mellitus.
- **Employment-related death:** if you believe that the death may have been due to (or contributed to by) the employment undertaken at any time by the deceased, you should indicate this. Tick the appropriate box on the front of the certificate and then report it to the coroner.
- **Sign the form:** you must sign the certificate and add your qualifications, address and the date. It would greatly assist the registrar if you could also PRINT YOUR NAME IN CAPITAL LETTERS. If the death occurred in hospital, the name of the consultant who was responsible for the care of the patient must also be given. Have you remembered your signature, notice to informant, counterfoil? Even now I always get bereavement office staff to check through what I have done. They might spot simple errors, which could cause problems for the family in getting the patient registered. It is so easy to get a date wrong and this can halt a funeral or a cremation ceremony. The bereavement office staff are experts and will help to prevent any problems.

20.20 Surgical referrals and problems

- Some surgical emergencies are included here in this text. This is to remind the physician that surgical patients can get into the medical take and surgical patients have medical problems and it is not uncommon for surgeons not to take 'surgical' patients, especially if no operative intervention is foreseen. They need identifying and referral. They may benefit from medical optimisation. If it is thought that an urgent surgical procedure is needed then keep patient fasted as they may need anaesthesia.
- Manage fluid and electrolytes and give adequate analgesia. Issues may include decisions on managing/reversing antithrombotic therapy, correcting electrolytes, etc. and detecting and fixing critical unresolved medical issues and pointing

out critical issues and priorities in older patients with multiple pathologies and polypharmacy.

- Increasing evidence shows physicians can add value to perioperative surgical care, especially that involving older patients. Fitness for surgery is an anaesthetic/surgical issue.
- **It is not your job to deem fitness for surgery but only to optimise medically and ensure anaesthetists and surgeons are aware of your findings especially when they would increase surgical and perioperative risks. It may be useful to explain that frailty might greatly increase risks of a poor outcome.**
- Sometimes your role will be seeing the whole patient and identifying major issues suggesting medical and possibly surgical futility and communicating this to all. As ever take senior advice if unsure.

20.21 ▶ Drains and tubes

- **Chest drains:** inserted into 4/5th intercostal pleural space to drain the pleural space of air and fluid. End inserted into water drain to ensure one-way movement of fluid/air. Inserted into the pleural space to allow removal of air or fluid. Can be thin (20 Fr) for air and in children to thick tubes (40 Fr) for blood or viscous pleural fluid in adults. Placed in the safe triangle (see ▶ Section 4.12 on pneumothorax) in 4/5th intercostal spaces in the anterior axillary or mid-axillary line. Connected to underwater one-way seal. Fluid and air can exit but not enter. Inspiration compresses the space and pleural contents should exit unless there is a leak and air continues to fill the space.
- Used for pneumothorax, haemothorax often as an emergency, or for a persistent/large pleural effusion. They are also commonly placed at the end of thoracic surgeries to allow for appropriate re-expansion of the lung tissue. A CXR should be obtained after any chest tube insertion to ensure appropriate placement. There is a radio-opaque line on the drain which should be checked. Ensure all holes lie within chest. Respiration should cause fluid to swing and shows tube is patent and working. If air bubbles are seen in a PTX patient, then this suggests an air leak which may take a few days. Persisting leak needs specialist review. A CXR should be done for any change clinically, especially if there is a suspected blocked tube which may need to be removed and reinserted. Drains inserted for effusion can be removed when daily output <100–200 ml/d.
- **Closed suction drains:** used post-op where fluid collection and risk of infection. Kept until output <20 ml/d. The output may be blood, bile, urine or pus/exudate depending on the site and each needs a specific management of cause.
- **Gastro/jejunostomy:** can be used to give feed or to decompress a distended upper GI tract, e.g. due to distal obstruction. **Jejunostomy tubes** are used exclusively for feeding and are usually placed to lie distal to the ligament of Treitz. Where suction is needed, keep <60 mmHg.

21 Procedures

21.1 Checks before any procedure

- The content here is to refresh memories and reinforce points to users who have been conventionally trained and are competent in these procedures. Do not perform a procedure in which you have not been trained. Get supervision if you are not competent. Generally, get written consent unless dire emergency. Most invasive procedures should not take place out of hours except in an emergency.
- In terms of procedures, be aware that the only way to avoid complications is not to do any. Before you undertake a therapeutic procedure ask will it improve circumstances (e.g. a chest drain) or a diagnostic procedure (e.g. central line placement to measure CVP/pulmonary artery pressures), consider whether the procedure will change management significantly; can you get the information elsewhere?
- Complications will happen and you can make a patient even worse, so ensure that the emergency procedure was valid and vital and could someone support or supervise you, or be doing it? Procedures are time-consuming and this time might be better spent doing other things.

Questions before any procedure
1. Is it the right patient?
2. Is it the right procedure?
3. Is it the right (or left) side?
4. Have I the right to do it, i.e. has informed consent been obtained?
5. Is the patient anticoagulated or have a coagulopathy?
6. Is this the right time: can it wait until working hours?
7. Am I the right person to do this (should someone more skilled do it or supervise me)?

21.2 Venepuncture

- Equipment: sharps bin, cannula, sterile bung and micropore tape (check for known allergies). Non-sterile gloves (check for latex allergy), alcoholic wipe 2% chlorhexidine (Clinell), tourniquet, dressing (sterile), cotton wool (sterile), trolley, syringe (10 ml), flushing agent (NS for injection).

Technique
- Introduce self, explain procedure and get verbal consent. Make sure that the cannula used is appropriate for indication. Choose vein and apply tourniquet above vein. Prepare skin at the selected insertion site with a med swab, wait 30 sec to allow the area to dry. Do not re-palpate the vein or touch the skin. Remove the needle guard and inspect the cannula for any faults. Hold the patient's hand/wrist/forearm using the thumb, to keep the skin taut. Do not contaminate the site. Place the needle tip several mm distal to the proposed site for cannulation, with the bevel facing up and elevate the angle of the cannula to 15–25° and insert the cannula into the skin (fragile veins require a lower angle of insertion). Once the vein has been located with the needle, lower the angle for insertion. Look for back flow of blood into the cannula chamber, unless the vein is small in which case this may be delayed. Hold the cannula steady relative to the vein whilst withdrawing the needle slightly and then slowly advance the cannula.

- If there is any sign of swelling, haematoma, pain or resistance the vein wall may be ruptured. If so, release tourniquet or you will cause a haematoma. Remove cannula. Apply pressure with cotton wool. Otherwise, when flashback is seen along the length of the cannula the investigator or delegated person will advance the cannula until it is fully inserted into the vein. Release the skin tension and the tourniquet. Apply gloved digital pressure to the distal end of the cannula to prevent blood spillage. Remove the introducer needle and discard into an appropriate yellow sharps container.
- Now secure a sterile bung to the end of the cannula. Secure the cannula to the patient using a sterile dressing. Flush the cannula with a minimum of 2 ml of IV NS for injection and cap off. Check the patient feels no discomfort, and observe the cannula site for signs of swelling or redness. Ensure that you complete cannula chart and any accompanying documentation. If you fail then try again, but if you have tried several times with no success either get some help or come back to the task later. If it is an emergency then get help urgently.
- You cannot resuscitate a patient successfully without IV access. If you have found the cannula is intra-arterial (pulsatile, high pressure, bright red blood) then remove cannula and apply pressure over the site for 10+ min until haemostasis. Check distal pulses. Take senior advice if pulseless or distal ischaemia.

21.3 ▶ Chest drain insertion

- **Introduction:** ask the 'right' questions (▶ Section 21.1): note the use of ultrasound-guided insertion is associated with lower complication rates. Incorrect placement of a chest drain can lead to significant morbidity and even mortality. Follow local guidance. Do not attempt unless trained.
- **Indications:** (1) Pneumothorax: not all require a chest drain (see ▶ Section 4.12). The differential diagnosis between a PTX and a bulla requires careful radiological assessment including CT. (2) Pleural fluid: malignant pleural effusion, simple pleural effusions in ventilated patients, empyema and complicated parapneumonic pleural effusion, traumatic PTX or haemopneumothorax. (3) Postoperative: e.g. thoracotomy, oesophageal surgery, cardiothoracic surgery. The urgency of insertion will depend on the indication and degree of physiological derangement that is being caused by the substance to be drained.
- **Procedure to insert a chest drain:** only to be done by trained or supervised persons. Done well there are 3% early complications and 8% late complications. Training reduces complications.
- **Potential complications:** incorrect placement with drain outside the pleura, in the fissure, tube kinked. Injury to intercostal vessels. Trocar must not be used as risk of spearing heart, liver and other organs. *Excessive bleeding risk*: ensure no coagulopathy – clotting screen and platelets if unsure.
- **Equipment:** aseptic pack with sterile drapes, iodine or equivalent solution. Gauze, scalpel, 2/0 silk and curved needle, 5 and 10 ml syringes. Orange and green needles, sterile gloves, chest drain (Seldinger or 'trocar' type). Chest drain bottle or bag with flutter valve.

Methods

- **Pre-procedure: informed consent** obtained and documented unless dire emergency. Check identity of the patient and the site of insertion of the chest drain. Confirm the clinical signs (percuss the chest and listen) and review the latest CXR and clinical indications. As ever, all equipment needed to insert a chest drain should be available before commencing the procedure.

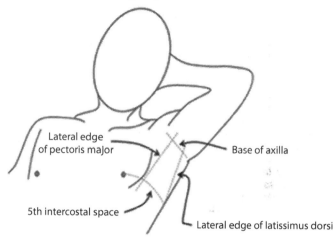

- **Patient positioning:** as comfortable as possible because the procedure may be prolonged. Much will depend on the clinical state of the patient. If possible patient lying back at 45° with the arm on the side used flopped behind head to open up rib spaces (see figure above). Alternatively, fatigued patient may lean forward resting on some pillows on a table, as long as access to the axilla is preserved.
- Occasionally the procedure is done with a patient lying on their side with the affected side uppermost. In a trauma situation, or ITU, an emergency drain insertion is more likely to be performed whilst the patient is supine.
- **Premedication:** analgesia should be considered – **morphine** 5 mg IM with cyclizine or **midazolam** 1–5 mg IV if not hypoventilating with appropriate monitoring (pulse oximetry) and resuscitation equipment immediately available. 100% O_2 should be given to all PTX patients if appropriate as it helps resolution. **Aseptic technique:** full aseptic precautions (washed hands, gloves, gown, antiseptic preparation for the insertion site and adequate sterile field) in order to avoid wound site infection or secondary empyema.

Choice of chest drain

- Sizes 10–36 ch. drains may be inserted via direct surgical incision (thoracostomy) or using the Seldinger technique with guide wire and dilator system. Spontaneous PTX and non-viscous effusions can be drained with relatively small-calibre drains via Seldinger method. Better tolerated with less discomfort, but traumatic pneumothoraces, haemothoraces and empyemas may need larger drains, typically 26F and above.
- **Inserting the drain:** most commonly placed in 5th intercostal space (ICS) in the mid-axillary line – the lowest axillary hair is useful marker where present. Area known as the *safe triangle* with anterior border of latissimus dorsi, the lateral border of the pectoralis major, a line superior to the horizontal level of the nipple and an apex below the axilla as shown above. Any other placement should be discussed with a chest physician. In an apical PTX, placement in the 2nd ICS can

be considered but is difficult to maintain. A specific position (identified with CT or ultrasound) may also be required for a loculated effusion.

- **Seldinger chest tube technique:** infiltrate with up to 10 ml of 1% lignocaine along the intended track. Remove catheter, dilator, introducer wire and introducer needle from pack and insert introducer needle into the thoracic cavity into the chosen site. Withdraw air with a syringe to confirm placement. Now thread introducer wire through needle lumen into the chest. Whilst holding wire tip and then base, remove needle leaving introducer wire running into chest. Thread dilator over introducer wire, and advance into chest, dilating a track for catheter. Remove dilator. Thread tube over the wire fully into chest ensuring side holes lie within chest cavity. Remove wire. Suture catheter in place. Attach catheter to drainage unit. *Obtain post-procedure chest X-ray.*

- **Rigid chest tube insertion:** infiltrate with 10–15 ml of 1% lignocaine along the intended track, make a 3–4 cm incision through skin and subcutaneous tissues between the 4th and 5th ribs, parallel to the rib margins. Continue incision through the intercostal muscles, and right down to the pleura and use dissecting forceps to bluntly dissect down to the pleura and then insert through the pleura and open the jaws widely, again parallel to the direction of the ribs. This will create a PTX if not locally present and allows the lung to fall away from the chest wall somewhat. Insert gloved sterile finger through your incision and into the thoracic cavity. Make sure you are feeling lung (or empty space) and not liver or spleen. Grasp end of chest tube with the forceps (convex angle facing down towards ribs), and insert chest tube through the hole you have made in the pleura. After tube has entered thoracic cavity, remove forceps and manually advance the tube. Clamp distal tube end with forceps and suture and tape tube in place and attach tube to drainage. *NEVER EVER USE A TROCAR TO INSERT DRAIN.* Obtain post-procedure chest X-ray for placement; tube may need to be advanced or withdrawn slightly. Need to be a bit firm but gentle. The chest tube should be placed in the pleural cavity; significant force should never be used as this risks sudden chest penetration and damage to essential intrathoracic structures. The operator should ensure controlled spreading of the intercostal muscles on the superior surface of the ribs to avoid injury to the intercostal vessels and nerves that run below the inferior border of the ribs. **The drainage system:** connect to an underwater seal drainage system. This employs positive expiratory pressure and gravity to drain the pleural space. Tube is submerged at least 2 cm below water of the reservoir/collection chamber. Underwater seal acts as a one-way valve to expel air from the pleural space. Keep collection chamber below the patient at all times or air will re-accumulate in the pleural space. **Large pleural effusions:** drained in stages. Rapid shifts in pleural pressures and re-expansion can cause re-expansion pulmonary oedema, a serious complication. A limit of 1–1.5 L of fluid should be drained before the tube is clamped. If the patient starts to cough or complains of chest pain before this point is reached, drainage should be stopped and may be resumed a few hours later. **Portable valve systems** can be used for patients with ongoing air leaks or fluid drainage and these use a one-way flutter valve which is generally lower resistance to drainage than with conventional underwater seal units. Ambulatory systems exist. **Securing the chest drain:** secure with 1/0 silk suture anchored to the skin and the drain with a suitable non-slip knot technique. This should prevent excessive travel of the drain in and out of the chest wall. The skin incision can be closed each side of the chest tube usually with one 2/0 silk suture each side. Nylon/Ethilon can be used but is more difficult to tie. Tie sutures securely. Purse string sutures should be avoided because they convert a linear wound into a circular wound which can be painful and leave an unsightly scar. **Dressings:** purpose-designed dressings should be used, i.e. *Drainfix* for small-bore drains and *Mefix* for large-bore drains. Excessive dressings restrict chest wall movement or cause moisture collection. Dressings should allow site inspection. Drain connections should not be covered. A tag of adhesive dressing tape can support the tube and protect it against being pulled out. Patient should be aware to look after the drain and keep the underwater bottle below the chest, avoid compressing the tube by sitting or lying on it and avoid tension on the tube. **Analgesia:** ensure regular analgesia is prescribed whilst the chest drain is in place. Dressings should be changed daily for the following reasons: to enable the insertion site to be monitored for signs of infection (swab if any signs of infection), as well as to monitor for surgical emphysema, to ensure the chest drain remains well placed, and the anchor suture is intact. **Monitoring/recording:** fluid in tube should swing with respiration due to changes in intra-pleural pressure. Fluid should rise on inspiration and fall on expiration. Bubbling and swinging are both dependent on an intact underwater seal and so can only be picked up if the drain tube extends below the water level in the bottle. Ask patient to take deep breaths and cough and assess. Absence of swinging suggests drain is occluded or is no longer in the pleural space. Try flushing the drain and if no success obtain a chest X-ray to determine the underlying cause. Bubbling in the underwater seal fluid chamber generally indicates an ongoing air leak which may be continuous, present on one phase of spontaneous ventilation, or only on coughing. Persistent bubbling throughout the respiratory cycle may indicate a continuing broncho-pleural air leak. Faulty connections and entrained air through the skin incision should also be assessed. If drain inserted for a fluid collection, e.g. effusion or empyema, then record volume and nature of the drain fluid recording. Drains inserted just for fluid should not bubble so the presence of this feature is abnormal and should be recorded. Any abnormal signs or complications should be referred for medical review. **Bleeding** from a drain inserted for drainage of a haemothorax (± PTX) needs urgent medical review. With fractured ribs most bleeding is from the intercostal vessels, which slows down as the lung reinflates. However, continued bleeding into the drain bottle is indicative of pathology that may need thoracic surgical intervention. After thoracic trauma, >1500 ml of blood into the bottle initially or continued bleeding of >200 ml/h requires discussion with the thoracic surgeons. Small-bore drains should be flushed regularly with NS; the flush should be prescribed on the Treatment Sheet and carried out by appropriately trained personnel. Full respiratory and cardiovascular observations should be carried out and documented. **Clamping chest drains:** chest tubes for PTX should not be clamped. Exceptions to this may be when the drainage bottle requires replacement or when testing the system for air leaks. Clamping a pleural drain in the presence of a continuing air leak may result in a tension PTX or possibly worsening surgical emphysema. If a chest tube is clamped it should be under the direct supervision of a respiratory physician or surgeon on a ward with experienced nursing staff. A patient with a clamped tube should not leave the specialist ward environment. Instructions should be left that if the patient becomes breathless or develops surgical emphysema, the chest tube must be unclamped immediately and the medical team alerted. In cases of PTX there is no evidence that clamping a chest drain at the time of removal is beneficial. Drains for fluid drainage can be clamped or closed to control drainage rate as necessary.

Changing the drain bottle

- When changing the drain bottle because it is full, temporary clamping of the drainage tube may be necessary to prevent entry of air into the pleural cavity. It is acceptable to clamp the tube between thumb and forefinger. This has the advantage of removing the risk of inadvertently leaving the tube clamped. Local policy should be followed with regard to asepsis and infection control. Suction: a patient who is free from pain and who can cough will generate a much higher pleural pressure differential than can safely be produced with suction. If a patient cannot re-inflate his own lung or a persistent air leak is preventing re-inflation, high volume, low-pressure thoracic suction in the range of 3–5 kPa (approximately 30–50 cmH$_2$O) should be used. Prescription of suction is a medical responsibility. Purpose-made low grade suction units (max 30 kPa) should be used when applying to a chest drain. Standard high volume, high-pressure suction units should not be used because of the ease with which they may lead to air stealing and hypoxaemia, the perpetuation of persistent air leaks, and possible damage to lung tissue caused by it becoming trapped in the catheter. Suction that is not working properly or is turned off without disconnecting from the drain bottle is the equivalent of a clamped drain, so when suction is no longer needed it should be disconnected from the drainage bottle. The use of suction may cause continuous bubbling from the tube; movement/swinging of fluid in the tube may not be visible. Mobility: if appropriate, patients should be encouraged to walk around. If the drain is on suction the patient will be restricted to the bedside. Exercise to prevent complications such as a frozen shoulder or deep venous thrombosis is essential, as are deep breathing exercises to aid re-expansion of the lung. Removal of the chest drain: removal of the chest drain depends on reason for insertion and clinical progress. Give adequate analgesia before removal of the chest drain. As for insertion, an aseptic technique should be used for removal and the chest drain and drainage kit disposed of appropriately. When the tube is ready to be removed, the patient should be asked to perform a Valsalva manoeuvre (to raise the pleural pressure and prevent air entering the pleural cavity) or, if that is not possible, then deep inspiration and the tube withdrawn quickly. The previously placed suture is then tied to close the hole. The operator should be able to tie sutures securely. The wound site should be checked, condition documented and an appropriate dressing applied. An X-ray should be performed following removal of the chest drain to ensure resolution. Surgical emphysema is the abnormal presence of air within the subcutaneous tissues with the 'Michelin man' type appearance, which may cause upper airways respiratory compromise. Its presence suggests that the drain is inadequate (too small gauge) to deal with size of air leak or occluded or misplaced. Applying suction, inserting a second drain or a larger-bore tube, can improve drainage. Worsening surgical emphysema is uncomfortable, interferes with clinical examination of the patient and, at its worst, may track up to the neck and face, potentially causing airway compromise.

21.4 Central venous line insertion

- **Introduction:** ask the 'right' questions (▶ Section 21.1). Possible sites: internal jugular vein, subclavian vein, femoral vein. Femoral vein is often avoided as risk of infection, but studies show no significant difference with other sites. Generally, however, neck veins are preferred.

- **Indications:** (1) Measurement of CVP, drug administration, TPN, **amiodarone,** etc. (2) Administering IV fluids when peripheral access poor (poor way to give fluids quickly). (3) Insertion of Swan–Ganz catheter to measure pulmonary wedge pressures. (4) Insertion of a pacing wire, pre-operative, e.g. CABG in theatre.
- **Equipment:** central line pack, sterile drapes, sterile gloves. 5–10 ml lidocaine 1–2%, iodine or equivalent, central line. 2 × 10 ml of saline/heparin flush, scalpel, 2–3 × 5–10 ml syringe. Green and blue needles and 100 ml bag NS.
- **Risks:** skill and luck and experience of the operator can vary as can body habitus and ease of access. Complications higher for emergency vs. elective insertion. Risks include infectious, mechanical and thrombotic complications. Obtain chest X-ray (subclavian/internal jugular) to confirm placement and to assess for complications. Infection. Strict asepsis – hand washing, gown and gloves for all cases. Preferably in appropriate area where a sterile field can be maintained, e.g. anaesthetic room or ITU or CCU procedure room. Avoid attempts in a dimly lit general ward – those days have long gone. Catheter infections due to local site infection or via haematogenous seeding of the catheter. Use chlorhexidine skin antisepsis, selection of an optimal catheter site. Ensure daily review of the need for the catheter or removal.

Contraindications to central venous line insertion

- Severe uncorrected coagulopathy: INR >1.6, platelets <50 × 10^9/L (relative contraindication). Femoral or internal jugular site is preferred with a coagulopathy because vessels can be directly compressed in the event of serious haemorrhage which may be arterial.
- There is NO safe route. Consider delaying procedure to correct coagulopathy or thrombocytopenia.
- Infected skin over the entry site, thrombosis of target vein, those unlikely to tolerate PTX or lower risk approaches to internal jugular or femoral sites may be preferred.

Potential complications of central venous line insertions

- Arterial puncture when the associated artery lies close (apply pressure and wait 5–10 min), haematoma, PTX, tension PTX, haemothorax. Arrhythmia, localised and systemic infection.
- Thrombotic complications: risk of venous thrombosis and embolism. Thrombosis can occur first day after cannulation. Lowest risk for thrombosis is the subclavian vein. Early removal of the catheter decreases the risk of catheter-related thrombosis.

General procedure

- Patient must be head down tilt when cannulating neck veins and head up when cannulating femoral vein to prevent air embolism. Raise bed to suitable level for yourself. Head down tilt can compromise breathless patients. Telemetry for arrhythmias. Monitor O$_2$ saturation.
- Wash hands, asepsis. Cleanse a 15–20 cm^2 or larger area with povidone–iodine solution. Usually the right side is preferred due to more direct line to the atrium, reduces injuring the thoracic duct, is easier in the right-handed operator, and dome of lung and pleura are lower than on left. Drape the patient with the paper/plastic drape with centre cutout provided. Estimate the length of catheter to be placed to end up with tip above right atrium. Using the blue needle, make a weal under the skin at the desired spot, and anaesthetise the subcutaneous tissue. Using the green needle, anaesthetise deeper.

- Always withdraw the plunger before injecting to detect if you are in the vein or artery to avoid intravascular injection of 1–2% **lidocaine.** Open the pack and place the guide wire, dilator, catheter and scalpel on the sterile drape for easy reach when needed.
- **Ultrasound guidance:** ultrasonography accurately locates the target vein, suggests venous pressure and the presence of intravascular thrombus and is strongly recommended. When using ultrasound guidance, enlist an assistant either to handle the probe or to remove it when it is no longer needed. The vein and artery appear circular and black on the ultrasound image; the vein is much more compressible when gentle pressure is applied to the skin via the probe. The needle appears echogenic and can be followed into the image of the vein. Most useful in internal jugular attempts.
- Using the 18-gauge finder needle (largest needle in the kit) and a small syringe, enter the skin at the top of the jugular triangle. Gradually advance the needle, always gently pulling back on the plunger as you progress. Look for a flashback of dark blood which indicates entrance into the vein. *Bright red or pulsatile flow should suggest carotid artery puncture. Withdraw needle and apply pressure for about 10 min before proceeding.* You can pierce the needle through the vein without blood, gradually withdraw; you may still get into the vein as you may have collapsed it on the way in.
- Once in the vessel, hold the needle steady and remove the syringe, holding a thumb over it, to prevent bleeding and reduce risk of embolism, and thread in the **j-tipped guide wire.** It should be a smooth process and if resistance is felt NEVER force it. Guide wire over-insertion can be dangerous. The wire needs to be advanced only far enough to maintain reliable control of the tract from the skin surface to the intravascular space.
- Watch monitor as guide wire is advanced. Ventricular ectopy indicates over-insertion and the guide wire must be withdrawn a few cm. Holding the guide wire, remove needle from skin. Make a small nick with the number 11 blade where wire enters skin with the cutting edge away from the wire. Advance dilator over guide wire with a twisting motion; there will be resistance.
- Remove dilator, holding guide wire and having some gauze 4 × 4 in your hand to apply pressure to a site that will now bleed after dilation. Place catheter over guide wire; it should advance easily. Hold guide wire at skin entrance and feed it back through distal port of central line (brown cap). When wire comes out, grab it at the end and finish advancing catheter. Remove guide wire and flush line through all 3 ports. Ensure all ports are closed.
- Now suture catheter in place via flange with holes. If >1–2 cm of catheter is exposed due to length, either suture the catheter down or use the snap-on flange provided in the kit. Apply a clear dressing.
- Get a chest X-ray to evaluate for line placement and complication. The tip of the catheter should be at the junction of the SVC and right atrium on chest X-ray film. New data would suggest that this is 2 cm below the superior right cardiac silhouette, which is made up by the right atrial appendage.

Internal jugular vein (IJV) cannulation

- **Visualise landmarks:** locate the triangle formed by heads of sternocleidomastoid and the clavicle. Entry point is apex. IJV runs deep to the sternocleidomastoid muscle. USS is highly recommended for locating and cannulating and makes procedure safer and reduces carotid cannulation. The vein's compressibility is visible. Place patient in head down position to prevent air embolism. In obese patients where the landmarks are not discernible, a reasonable rule of thumb is to go three finger breadths lateral from the tracheal midline, and three finger breadths up from the clavicle. Some suggest that patients turn head away from side whilst others suggest keep head in neutral midline position.

- As the head rotates away from neutral, there is an increase in both the overlap and proximity of the IJV and carotid artery which increases the risk of carotid puncture. Some advocate the use of a small-gauge pilot needle to locate the internal jugular vein and an innovative technique to then stabilise it. This small-gauge pilot needle may be particularly useful when patients have coagulopathy or when ultrasonography is not available. Palpate for the carotid impulse and make sure you are lateral to this. Insert the needle at the apex of the triangle and the needle should point down towards same side nipple with needle at 30° to horizontal. The vein is usually <1.5 cm below surface.

Subclavian vein cannulation

- Complications such as pneumothorax higher and so this must be carried out by experienced operators only. Benefits are more comfort for longer-term catheterisation than alternative sites and so can be used for dialysis or feeding. The adult subclavian vein is approximately 3–4 cm long and 1–2 cm in diameter and is a continuation of the axillary vein at the lateral border of the first rib which it crosses over and passes in front of the anterior scalene muscle. The anterior scalene muscle is approximately 10–15 mm thick and separates the subclavian vein from the subclavian artery, which runs behind. The vein continues behind medial third of clavicle where it is immobilised by small attachments to the rib and clavicle. At the medial border of the anterior scalene muscle and behind subscapularis joint, the subclavian unites with the internal jugular to form the innominate/brachiocephalic vein. The large thoracic duct on the left, and smaller lymphatic duct on the right, enter the superior margin of subclavian vein near internal jugular junction.
- **Technique:** head down position, well hydrated if possible. USS role is limited as vein lies behind clavicle. Keep patient's head in neutral position, though some teach to turn head away. Anaesthetise locally with lidocaine down to the periosteum of the clavicle. Locate subclavian vein with a 22-gauge needle and pass introducer needle parallel to retrace path. Ensure that the needle is kept very shallow to skin at no more than 10–15° from horizontal. Generally the needle is advanced medially from an entry point 1 cm below junction of middle and medial one-third of clavicle towards the posterior superior angle of the clavicle (the suprasternal notch). Advance needle aspirating. The subclavian artery, lung and brachial plexus are all posterior to subclavian vein; if the vein is not cannulated, at least the other structures will not be hit. Once cannulated use a Seldinger technique as described above. The risk of PTX is 5%. Incidence of damage to the subclavian artery <5%. Direct pressure cannot be applied to enable haemostasis. Ensure post procedure CXR to check position of the line and to exclude PTX.

Femoral vein cannulation

- The femoral vein can be used for central access. It can allow the patient to sit up slightly. The fear of infection is greater at this site but not borne out in studies. It is a useful site in patients with SVC obstruction. The femoral vein is the continuation of the popliteal vein and accompanies the femoral artery in the femoral triangle. The vein ends medial to the artery at the inguinal ligament, where it becomes the external iliac vein. Relations: nerve, artery, vein and Y fronts – NAVY. USS can be useful to enable cannulation.

- **Technique:** extend the leg and abduct slightly at the hip. Adopt full asepsis. Locate the femoral artery, keep a finger on the artery and introduce a needle attached to a 10 ml syringe at 45°, 1.5 cm medial to the femoral artery pulsation, 2 cm below the inguinal ligament. Slowly advance the needle towards the head and posteriorly while gently withdrawing the plunger. When a free flow of blood appears, follow the Seldinger approach, as detailed previously. Potential complications include wound sepsis and septicaemia, deep vein thrombosis, femoral nerve or arterial damage, haematoma, arteriovenous fistula. It is certainly an easier site to control any coagulopathy as pressure can be applied.

Peripherally inserted central catheter

- It is a silicone rubber tube, which is placed in the antecubital fossa of the arm (the elbow crease) with the tip of the catheter lying in the superior vena cava. Check on post procedure that the tip is above the carina and so not in the right atrium.
- Uses: lack of peripheral access, infusion of inotropes, infusions of vesicant, irritant, parenteral nutrition or hyperosmolar solutions, long-term (>10 d) venous access required.
- Insertion is into one of the following upper limb veins in order of referred. Basilic, brachial, cephalic veins. PICC lines are described by their gauge, number of lumen, and if they are valved (no clamp) or open-ended (with clamp). The indications for different line types vary between centres. Whenever TPN is used a dedicated lumen must be used.

21.5 Lumbar puncture

- **Introduction:** ask the 'right' questions (▶ Section 21.1).
- **Contraindications:** incipient brain herniation syndrome suggested by seizures, GCS <13, focal CNS signs (including ocular palsies), papilloedema, pupillary dilation, impaired eye movements, coma and low HR and rising BP, older patients, HIV, recent head trauma (CT headfirst). Coagulopathy, anticoagulants, warfarin, heparins, DOACs, platelets <50 × 10^9/L. Spina bifida or skin appearances of spina bifida occulta or deformities, local infection or pressure sore, severe cardiorespiratory compromise.
- **Complications:** coning due to brain herniation, epidural haematoma with root or cauda equina compression, SAH, infection (e.g. meningitis), low pressure headache, backache, nerve palsies (e.g. diplopia from cranial nerve VI), lumbosacral nerve palsies (extremely rare), dermoid formation.
- **Preventing post-LP headache:** replacement of stylet before removal of needle otherwise leaves 'dural hole open', direction of bevel, number of puncture attempts, non-cutting needle, and smaller size of the spinal needle.
- **Patient advice:** consent patient. Risk headache and infection. May experience a sharp shoot of pain down one leg and if this happens they should let the operator know and that it does not mean something has gone wrong. LP is done below end of spinal cord (L1) where the canal contains lower nerve roots. Pain can result if needle touches a nerve root. Give the patient a copy of patient information sheet.
- **Preparation:** know what samples need to be sent. Have relevant tubes. Inform microbiologist/lab of intended procedure. Ensure you have all equipment including manometer. Any focal signs or suggestions of coma which could suggest raised ICP, then get a CT first to exclude SOL or dilated third ventricles, midline shift, etc.

- *Patient positioning is key to success*: patient is best positioned lying comfortably on their side, at the edge of the bed with a pillow between knees, back flexed, with the spine horizontal and perpendicular to the couch throughout its entire length. Keep chin as close to the patellae as possible in a fetal-like position. Knees and ankles should be symmetrical and together. Good positioning and patient cooperation increase the chance of success.
- *Skin preparation*: prepare a wide sterile area. For skin preparation use **chlorhexidine or iodine aqueous solution.** It is important to use good technique for sterilising, starting in the centre and wiping in circular motion to outside of area. *Position of LP site*: cord ends lower margin of L1. Needle is usually introduced at L3/4 interspace at level of the tips of the iliac crests. If unsuccessful at this level try L2/3.
- **Procedure:** local anaesthetic: the skin and deeper tissues of the needle track are infiltrated. Use up to 5 ml of 2% lidocaine which should be infiltrated into the skin with a blue needle, waiting for it to take effect and then infiltrating deeper with a green needle. Continually aspirate with the syringe before injecting to ensure not in blood vessel or even CSF (e.g. in thin patient). Allow time for this to be effective. LP needle insertion: use a sharp disposable fine LP needle (e.g. gauge 22 or smaller) with a stylet in position; introduce through the skin and advance through the space between the two spinous processes. The top of the bevel should always be parallel to the back (e.g. for a patient horizontal on their side, the bevel will point to the ceiling). The needle point needs to be directed slightly forwards (anteriorly).
- Insert to a depth of 4–7 cm; firm resistance which gives way as the ligamentum flavum is reached. Beyond this there is a slight give as the needle punctures the dura. The stylet is removed and clear CSF will drip out of the needle if this has been correctly positioned. If no fluid appears or bone is encountered, it is probable that the needle is not in the correct position. The stylet should be reinserted, the needle partially withdrawn and then advanced with a slightly different angle aiming for the umbilicus. Once in position and CSF is obtained, the stylet should be placed in the centre of the sterile trolley and kept sterile as it will need to be reinserted prior to taking the LP needle out at the end of the examination.
- *Failure*: commonest causes of failure are that the needle is not in the midline, the patient's back is not perpendicular to the bed (e.g. twisted at shoulders, or legs not together) or is at too great an angle with the skin. NB: if unsuccessful after 2–3 attempts, take more senior advice before giving up, or ask another more experienced doctor to try. If that is unsuccessful, X-ray screening may be used or contact a friendly anaesthetist.
- If LP is to evaluate presence of xanthochromia, then further attempts need to be performed at this time and not delayed by more than 2–4 h, otherwise altered blood may be found as a consequence of the 'bloody' traumatic tap and the test becomes unhelpful if xanthochromia is found. Measure opening pressure: ensure familiarity with the 3-way tap. Measure and record CSF pressure (normal <20 cmH$_2$O) using manometry and the patient lying horizontally. Sample collection: take 4 tubes and fill each with 3–5 ml (up to 40–50 ml CSF can be safely removed). Label all bottles carefully. Number them 1 to 4 in the order they were filled.
- **Routine samples:** CSF for Gram stain, microscopy and sensitivity, protein, paired sugar (blood + CSF fluoride bottles), cytology sent when indicated at least 10 ml, oligoclonal bands if demyelination suspected and also send serum sample. CSF + serum glucose important in bacterial/fungal meningitis – the CSF sugar is usually <2 mmol/L or <40% blood glucose level. Microscopy and culture: Gram stained and examined routinely for bacteria, also stains for fungi, cryptosporidium or acid-fast bacilli as requested.

- **Xanthochromia:** send 3 sequential samples for red cell count. If SAH suspected and CT negative do not perform until 12 h from headache have elapsed. Time is required to convert haemoglobin to bilirubin (xanthochromia). Bloody tap if significant RBCs; as a guide about 10 white cells/7000 red cells would normally be expected.
- **Other CSF samples:** CSF lactate: in bacterial and TB meningitis the CSF lactate >3.3 mmol/L. Lactate samples need to go the lab on ice. Inform the lab first. TB PCR can also be checked but false positives may sometimes be seen. Latex agglutination can detect *Haemophilus influenzae* B, *Strep. pneumoniae* and *Neisseria meningitidis* in >75% of affected patients. Encephalitis: samples are sent for viral PCR (e.g. HSV, VZV, CMV, etc.). ACE levels: neurosarcoid. VDRL: suspected neurosyphilis.
- **Finishing the LP:** replace the sterile stylet before removing the LP needle to reduce post-LP headache. Remove iodine with saline-soaked gauze to prevent skin rashes or burns. Lying supine for a short period usually advocated. Hydration is sensible but does not prevent headache.
- **Post-LP low pressure headache** is a known complication and can be mild to severe and always occurs soon after sitting or standing – it should completely disappear on lying flat (or significantly diminish if patient already had headache prior to LP). Whilst this may settle, if it continues then the longer that treatment is delayed, the less chance of success. Analgesics are to be avoided as they may perpetuate headache. Oral caffeine does not prevent post-LP headache. An infusion of IV caffeine is the most appropriate 1st-line management of post-LP headache (e.g. **caffeine** 500 mg in 500 ml NS over 2 h). Persisting low pressure pain: consider blood patch – ask anaesthetists who are experienced at this.

21.6 ▶ Abdominal paracentesis

- **Introduction:** ask the 'right' questions (▶Section 21.1). Indications: relieve ascites due to cirrhosis or malignancy – primary ovarian, colon, stomach, pancreas, lung and breast cancers, but it can also be associated with primary liver or peritoneal cancers. A diagnostic paracentesis should be performed in all cirrhotic patients with ascites who have signs and symptoms of peritoneal infection, including the development of encephalopathy, renal impairment, or peripheral leucocytosis without a precipitating factor to exclude spontaneous bacterial peritonitis (SBP).
- **Side-effects:** local haemorrhage, infection and may precipitate hepatorenal syndrome.
- **Relative contraindications:** coagulopathy (INR >2.0 reverse, seek advice), pregnancy, localised cellulitis, low platelets (<50), bowel obstruction.
- **Equipment:** gauze swabs, sterile dressing pack, sterile gloves, iodine or equivalent. Green and blue needles, several 5–10 ml syringes, lignocaine 1–2%. Ascitic drain and bag, adhesive dressings.
- **Investigations:** serum ascites–albumin gradient (SA–AG) >11 g/L: cirrhosis, cardiac failure, nephrotic syndrome. SA–AG <11 g/L: malignancy, TB, pancreatitis. SBP: neutrophil count of >250 cells/mm^3 empiric antibiotic therapy should be started. Check ascitic amylase if pancreatic disease suspected.
- **Procedure:** obtain consent. Ask patient to micturate first. With ascites when lying supine the fluid is lowest and air-filled bowel floats to the surface. The flanks are dull and fluid-filled. The safest place to go is right or left inguinal fossa just 2 cm above and medial to anterior superior iliac spine. Others suggest 2 fingerbreadths below the umbilicus in the midline. Wash hands and prepare field with iodine. Ensure sterile field and sterile gloves. Identify chosen spot. For a simple diagnostic

aspiration, e.g. to detect SBP, a green needle is sufficient with appropriate asepsis. On insertion avoid inferior epigastric arteries which run in a pair just a few centimetres lateral of the midline. Apply local anaesthetic down to the point at which you can freely aspirate ascitic fluid.

- Remove needle and pierce skin with scalpel. Insert paracentesis catheter (Bonanno catheter) in a Z-shaped pathway at 45°, aspirating via syringe. The tip is pig-tailed. Withdraw introducer whilst advancing the drain. *Patients with portal hypertensive ascites usually receive 100 ml 20% human albumin solution (20 g of albumin) for each 2–3 L ascites drained*. Volume replacement is not routinely required for malignant ascites unless the patient shows low BP during drainage. May be reasonable to simply give 250 ml NS colloid fluid challenge if required.
- Send fluid for urgent cell count, microscopy, culture and sensitivity, LDH, protein and cytology. Remove drain after 6 h if cirrhosis as there is a high risk of peritonitis. Drains for malignant effusions may be left in for longer but the risk of peritonitis still exists. If SBP then consider IV **Co-amoxiclav** or **Tazocin.**

21.7 ▶ Arterial blood gas

- **Introduction:** check radial/ulnar pulses. If absent consider femoral artery.
- **Arterial blood gas kit:** 1 ml vented, pre-heparinised usually with dry lithium heparin plastic syringe. One orange or blue needle (longer needles are required for brachial and femoral artery puncture). Needle guard to prevent accidental needlestick injuries. Vent cap (for evacuation of air bubble), one biohazard-labelled plastic bag. Two 1 × 1 sterile gauze, alcohol prep pad, specimen/patient label, iodine pad. One adhesive bandage, lab form, ice.
- **Contraindications:** no absolute contraindications, mostly just extra precautions and hazards. Avoid dialysis AV shunt; mastectomy – use opposite side. Anticoagulant therapy – hold pressure on puncture site longer than normal.
- **Preparation:** introduce yourself and explain what is ordered and get informed consent. Patient cooperation helps. Check patient ID, ask patient their name, check patient ID wristband. ***Choose artery:*** select site and palpate the right and left radial arterial pulses and visualise the course of the artery. Pick strongest pulse. Radial artery is always the first choice and should be used because it provides collateral circulation. If radial pulse weak on right, move to left; if pulse on left weak, then try brachial. Brachial used as alternative site and femoral is the last choice in normal situations. Always have a fallback plan. ***Check Allen test*** using radials. In a conscious and cooperative patient simply compress ulnar and radial arteries at wrist to obliterate pulse and have patient clench and release fist until hand blanches. With radial still compressed, release pressure on ulnar artery and watch for pinkness to return. It should pink up within 10–15 sec. If patient unconscious then compress ulnar and radials and elevate hand above head, squeeze hard and release ulnar and lower hand below heart. Palpate left and right radial arteries noting maximal pulse. The one with the stronger pulse will be your site of entry.
- **Procedure:** wash hands, put on gloves. Connect needle to syringe ensuring needle kept sterile and eject excess heparin and air bubbles. If using syringe with liquid heparin pull back syringe plunger to at least 1 cm^3 to give room for blood to fill syringe when puncture is made (NEVER recap needle). Stabilise the wrist in the position that gives maximal pulse (hyper-extended, using a rolled-up towel if necessary) and clean chosen area with an alcohol and/or iodine wipe. Secure needle to syringe and remove cap from needle. Pierce the skin at puncture site

aiming proximally and keep needle angle constant and bevel of needle up, or into the arterial flow (bevel faces the heart) and slowly advance in one plane. When the artery is punctured, blood will enter the syringe flashback. Slowly allow blood to fill syringe. If no blood appears, remove, change needles, and start again. Upon removal of the needle, hold pressure on the puncture site for at least 5 min. Pressure may need to be held longer (>5 min) if the patient is on anticoagulant therapy. ***Post puncture procedure*:** remove any air bubbles from sample and cap syringe and dispose of needle in sharps container. Roll syringe to mix heparin with sample and immediately try to lower temperature and metabolism of sample by immersing in ice and ensure rapid delivery to lab. *On lab request form indicate*: FiO_2, patient temperature and ventilator parameters. ***Post procedure*:** check for bleeding, movement of fingers and tingling sensation, pulse distal to puncture. If radial pulse not palpable consider an urgent vascular opinion.

- **Complications:** arterial spasm: may occur secondary to pain or anxiety. Reassure patient; explain procedure and purpose. Haematoma: leakage of blood into tissue. You possibly didn't press hard enough and long enough. Ensure using small diameter needle. Ensure proper technique in holding site for 5 min post puncture. Haemorrhage: patient receiving anticoagulant therapy or patients with known blood coagulation disorders. Two minutes after pressure is released inspect site for bleeding, oozing or seepage of blood; continue pressure until bleeding ceases. A longer compression time is necessary. Other very rare: laceration of artery, sepsis, infection/inflammation adjacent to puncture site. Avoid sites indicating presence of infection or inflammation. Discuss with vascular surgeons any possible vascular injury. Failure: consider using femoral artery.

21.8 Nasogastric tube insertion

- **Introduction:** ask the 'right' questions (▶ Section 21.1). Contraindications (or take expert advice): ENT abnormalities or infections. Suspected oesophageal stricture or pouch. Recent oesophagectomy or upper GI surgery. Recent suspected or known fractures of the base of the skull. Oesophageal varices, oesophageal perforation or oesophageal surgery. Risk of aspiration, suspected atrial–oesophageal fistula. Thrombolysed patient – delay NG insertion certainly after stroke thrombolysis.

Procedure

- NG tubes are long polyurethane or silicone tubes passed via the nose and oesophagus into the stomach. Deaths may occur due to feeding tubes displaced into the lungs causing gastric aspiration. NG tubes are most commonly inserted by nurses who are often the local experts. Sometimes done by doctors, e.g. anaesthetists in theatre. The main indications are: feeding in those, for example, with neurological disease or other cause of impaired swallowing (e.g. stroke); aspirating gastric contents (e.g. obstructed patient) which decompresses the stomach and so prevents vomiting and possible aspiration. Nasojejunal tubes are longer versions of NG tubes. They are inserted under endoscopic guidance to lie further in the jejunum and may be useful in feeding patients with pancreatitis. *Obtain consent* – verbal consent is usually sufficient. Explain the insertion procedure, together with the reasons why the tube is necessary. In some patients actions will need to be done in best interests as consent cannot be communicated.
- **Preparation:** after washing hands, prepare a trolley including gloves, local anaesthetic jelly or spray, a 60 ml syringe, pH strip, kidney tray, sticky tape and

a bag to collect secretions. Determine length of NG tube to insert by external measurement from the tip of the nose to a point halfway between the xiphoid and the umbilicus distance. Usually 40–60+ cm. Better to have too long than too short – don't want the tip in the lower oesophagus. The patient should sit up. An appropriately sized tube is chosen and the tip is lubricated by smearing aqua gel or local anaesthetic gel. Anaesthetic gel is a drug so if it is used it must be prescribed, and precautions taken such as checking for allergies. The wider nostril is chosen and the tube slid down along the floor of the nasal cavity. The head should not be tilted back. Patients often gag when the tube reaches the pharynx. Asking them to swallow their saliva or a small amount of water may help to direct the tube into the oesophagus. Once in the oesophagus, it may be easy to push into the stomach. The correct intragastric position is then verified (see below). The tube is fixed to the nose/forehead using adhesive tapes. The stomach is decompressed by attaching the 60 ml syringe and aspirating its contents. Blocked tubes can be flushed open with saline or air.

- **Verifying correct intragastric positioning:** there are two recommended ways of confirming the tube position. These are by **pH test and X-ray.** Other methods can be inaccurate and should not be used. **(1) Measuring pH:** the NG tube is aspirated and the contents are checked using pH paper, not litmus paper. It is recommended that it is safe to feed adult patients only if the pH is <5.5. Note that taking proton pump inhibitors or H_2 receptor antagonists may alter the pH. Similarly, intake of milk can neutralise the acid. **(2) Chest X-ray:** when in doubt it is best practice to use X-ray to check the tube's location. Patients who have swallowing problems, confused patients and those in ICU should all be given an X-ray to verify the tube's intragastric position. This involves taking a chest X-ray including the upper half of the abdomen. The tip of the tube can be seen as a white radio-opaque line and should be below the diaphragm on the left side. **Syringe test:** do not use! This test is mentioned here for historic interest only. Also known as the whoosh test, it has been shown to be an unreliable method of checking tube placement, and the NPSA has said that it *must no longer be used*. **Repeated confirmation of position:** correct intragastric positioning should be confirmed at least daily and immediately after initial placement. Before each daily feed – need to wait 1 h before testing pH. Following vomiting/coughing. Decreased O_2 saturation. If the tube is dislodged or the patient complains of discomfort. Never insert the guide wire while the NG tube is in the patient.
- **Complications:** misplaced tube and delivery of feed directly into lungs causing pneumonia/pneumonitis. Gastric possibly overfeeding with vomiting also leading to pulmonary aspiration pneumonia. Nasal trauma and local mucosal damage when NG inserted roughly or in for a prolonged time. Use lubricants. Gagging or vomiting, therefore suction should always be ready to use.

22 Laboratory values

22.1 Clinical chemistry values

Blood gases (breathing air at sea level)
Blood H+ 35–45 nmol/L

pH	7.36–7.44
PaO_2	11.3–12.6 kPa
$PaCO_2$	4.7–6.0 kPa
Base excess	± 2 mmol/L
Carboxyhaemoglobin	non-smoker <2%, smoker 3–15%

Serum values

Na	137–144 mmol/L
K	3.5–4.9 mmol/L
Cl	95–107 mmol/L
HCO_3	20–28 mmol/L
Anion gap	12–16 mmol/L
Urea	2.5–7.5 mmol/L
Creatinine	60–110 µmol/L
Ca	2.2–2.6 mmol/L
Phosphate	0.8–1.4 mmol/L
Serum total protein	61–76 g/L

Liver values

Albumin	37–49 g/L
Total bilirubin	1–22 µmol/L
Conjugated bilirubin	0–3.4 µmol/L
ALT	5–35 units/L
AST	1–31 units/L
ALP	45–105 units/L (>14 years)
GGT	4–35 units/L (<50 units/L in males)
LDH	10–250 units/L

Cardiac biomarkers

CK	(males) 24–195 units/L; (females) 24–170 units/L

Others

Cu	12–26 µmol/L
Caeruloplasmin	200–350 mg/L
Al	0–10 mcg/L
Mg	0.75–1.05 mmol/L
Zn	6–25 µmol/L
Urate	(males) 0.23–0.46 mmol/L; (females) 0.19–0.36 mmol/L
Plasma lactate	0.6–1.8 mmol/L
Plasma ammonia	12–55 µmol/L
Serum ACE	25–82 units /L

Fasting plasma glucose	3.0–6.0 mmol/L
HbA1c	3.8–6.4%
Fructosamine	<285 µmol/L
Serum amylase	60–180 units/L
Plasma osmolality	278–305 mOsm/kg

Lipids and lipoproteins: assess overall lifetime risk

Serum cholesterol	<5.2 mmol/L
Serum LDL cholesterol	<3.36 mmol/L
Serum HDL cholesterol	>0.55 mmol/L
Fasting serum TG	0.45–1.69 mmol/L

Serum tumour markers

α-fetoprotein	<10 kunits/L
Carcinoembryonic antigen	<10 mcg/L
Neuron-specific enolase	<12 mcg/L
Prostate-specific antigen	(males >40) <4 mcg/L; (males <40) <2 mcg/L
hCG	<5 units/L
CA125	<35 units/ml
CA19–9	<33 units/ml

Cerebrospinal fluid

Opening pressure	50–180 mmH$_2$O
Total protein	0.15–0.45 g/L
Albumin	0.066–0.442 g/L
Chloride	116–122 mmol/L
Glucose	3.3–4.4 mmol/L
CSF lactate	1–2 mmol/L
Cell count	lymphocytes 60–70%; monocytes 30–50%; neutrophils: none
IgG/ALB	<0.26
IgG index	<0.88

Urine

Albumin/creatinine ratio (untimed specimen)	(males) <3.5 mg/mmol; (females) <2.5 mg/mmol
GFR	70–140 ml/min
Total protein	<0.2 g/24 h
Albumin	<30 mg/24 h
Ca	2.5–7.5 mmol/24 h
Urobilinogen	1.7–5.9 µmol/24 h
Coproporphyrin	<300 nmol/24 h
Uroporphyrin	6–24 nmol/24 h
Δ-aminolevulinate	8–53 µmol/24 h
5-hydroxyindoleacetic acid	10–47 µmol/24 h
Osmolality	350–1000 mOsmol/kg

22.2 Haematology values

Full blood count

Haemoglobin	(males) 13.0–18.0 g/dl; (females) 11.5–16.5 g/dl
Haematocrit	(males) 0.40–0.52; (females) 0.36–0.47
MCV	80–96 fL
MCH	28–32 pg
MCHC	32–35 g/dl
White cell count	4–11 × 10^9/L
White cell differential	(× 10^9/L)
∘ neutrophils	1.5–7
∘ lymphocytes	1.5–4
∘ monocytes	0–0.8
∘ eosinophils	0.04–0.4
∘ basophils	0–0.1
∘ platelet count	150–400
∘ reticulocyte count	25–85 OR 0.5–2.4%
ESR	males <50 y: ESR <15 mm/h
	females <50 y: ESR <20 mm/h
	males >50 y: ESR <20 mm/h
	females >50 y: ESR <30 mm/h
Plasma viscosity	1.50–1.72 mPa/sec

Coagulation screen

Prothrombin time	11.5–15.5 sec
INR	<1.4
APTT	30–40 sec
Fibrinogen	1.8–5.4 g/L
Bleeding time	3–8 min

Coagulation factors

Factors II, V, VII, VIII, IX, X, XI, XII	50–150 IU/dl
Factor V Leiden, vWF	45–150 IU/dl
vWF antigen	50–150 IU/dl
Protein C	0–135 IU/dl
Protein S	80–120 IU/dl
Antithrombin III	80–120 IU/dl
Activated protein C resistance	2.12–4.0
Fibrin degradation products	<100 mg/L
D-dimer screen	<0.5 mg/L or 0.50 µg/ml or 500 ng/ml. Check units. Age adjust if over 50. Age-adjusted upper limit = patient age/50 × usual upper limit; e.g. age 75 is 0.75 mg/L.

Haematinics

Serum iron	12–30 µmol/L
Serum iron-binding capacity	45–75 µmol/L
Serum ferritin	15–300 mcg/L

Serum transferrin	2.0–4.0 g/L
Serum B12	160–760 ng/L
Serum haptoglobin	0.13–1.63 g/L
Serum folate	2.0–11.0 mcg/L
Red cell folate	160–640 mcg/L

Haemoglobin electrophoresis

Haemoglobin A	>95%
Haemoglobin A2	2–3%
Haemoglobin F	<2%

23 Drugs (use with *BNF*)

23.1 Prescribing and side-effects abbreviations

Route
IM = intramuscular
IO = intraosseous
IV = intravenous
PO = oral
SC = subcutaneous

Frequency
OD = once per day (no time specified)
OM = once in the morning
ON = once at night
BD = twice per day (12 h)
TDS/TID = three times per day (every 8 h)
QDS/QID = four times per day (every 6 h)

Code for side-effects
APX = anaphylaxis
C = constipation
D = diarrhoea, F = fever
H = headache, N = nausea
R = rash, SEIZ = seizures
V = vomiting

Drug calculations
1 g = 1000 mg
0.1 g = 100 mg
1 mg = 1000 mcg (microgram)
0.1 mg = 100 mcg
1 L = 1000 ml
e.g. digoxin 0.125 mg = 125 mcg

Digoxin is almost always prescribed in microgram (mcg) and an equivalent dose in milligrams is 1000× times the dose and lethal. Microgram should be written in full – the symbol µg must never be used in a prescription.

23.2 Antibiotic prescribing advice

Principles of antimicrobial prescribing
- Do not start antimicrobial therapy unless there is clear evidence of infection.
- Take a thorough drug allergy history.
- Initiate prompt effective antibiotic treatment within ONE hour of diagnosis (or as soon as possible) if severe sepsis or life-threatening infections.
- Avoid inappropriate use of broad-spectrum antibiotics and once the agent is identified, switch to a targeted narrow-spectrum agent.
- Obtain cultures prior to commencing therapy (but do not delay therapy).
- Check previous microbiology results and history of MRSA/ESBL/CPE/*Clostridioides difficile*.
- Comply with local antimicrobial prescribing guidance.
- Document clinical indication (and disease severity if appropriate), drug name, dose and route on drug card and in clinical notes.
- Include a review/stop date or duration on the prescription.
- Document the exact indication on the drug chart (rather than stating long-term prophylaxis) for clinical prophylaxis.
- Encourage oral antimicrobials whenever possible.
- Use IV antimicrobials in serious infections or unable to take oral medication.
- After 48–72 h of IV therapy review the patient and consider switching to oral medication.

- A 5-day course should suffice for uncomplicated infections.
- Review antimicrobials and clinical progress on a daily basis in the light of current microbiology results.

Standard TOTAL duration IV + oral (days)

- Infective exac. of COPD 5–7; pneumonia, uncomplicated 5, severe 7–10.
- UTI, uncomplicated 3; pyelonephritis 14; cellulitis 10–14.
- Meningitis: *Neisseria meningitidis* 7; *Streptococcus pneumoniae* 14; *Haemophilus influenzae* 10.

Penicillin allergy

- Penicillins can be life-saving antimicrobials and patients should not be labelled 'penicillin-allergic' without careful consideration. Nausea, vomiting or diarrhoea alone do not constitute an allergic reaction and are not a contraindication for penicillin use. Anaphylaxis related to histamine release occurs about 30–60 min after administration of a penicillin; symptoms may include erythema or pruritus, angioedema, low BP or shock, urticaria, wheezing, rhinitis. Patients with a history of immediate hypersensitivity/anaphylaxis to penicillin should NOT receive a cephalosporin. History taking is key.
- **Meropenem** is an alternative to penicillin for some severe infections. If there is a history of an anaphylactic reaction, or an accelerated allergic reaction DO NOT prescribe these drugs. Please discuss alternative antibiotics with a microbiologist. Remember, penicillins (and cephalosporins) can also be nephrotoxic (as they can induce an interstitial nephritis).
- **Definite penicillin allergy:** avoid amoxicillin, Augmentin (co-amoxiclav), benzylpenicillin (penicillin G), flucloxacillin, phenoxymethylpenicillin (penicillin V), piperacillin/tazobactam (Tazocin), pivmecillinam, temocillin.
- **WARNING:** this is a quick look-up guide for drugs with which you should be familiar and in no way replaces the *BNF*. All drugs should be checked in the *BNF* for safety of use in pregnancy, breastfeeding and renal and liver failure. Allergy is such an obvious contraindication that it is not mentioned. All allergies should be documented.

23.3 ▶ Important drug interactions and metabolism

- **Enzyme inducers:** reduce drug efficacy with treatment failure: barbiturates, carbamazepine, chronic alcohol, phenytoin, rifampicin, inhaled anaesthetics.
- **Enzyme inhibitors:** increase toxicity: amiodarone, cimetidine, ciprofloxacin, acute alcohol, erythromycin, ketoconazole, fluconazole, metronidazole.
- **Allopurinol and azathioprine:** allopurinol slows the metabolism of azathioprine, increasing levels of 6-MCP resulting in serious blood dyscrasias.
- **Digoxin and quinidine:** increase concentrations of digoxin.
- **Sildenafil/isosorbide mononitrate:** cause dramatic drops in BP.
- **Potassium chloride, spironolactone, amiloride, ACEi:** severe hyperkalaemia.
- **Theophylline and ciprofloxacin:** theophylline toxicity.
- **Warfarin/DOAC and NSAID, aspirin, clopidogrel:** increased bleed risk despite no change in INR; expert assessment for combination therapy.
- **Omeprazole, lansoprazole and clopidogrel:** decrease efficacy of clopidogrel; consider pantoprazole or H_2 blocker instead of PPI.
- **Amiodarone and levofloxacin, azithromycin, clarithromycin, erythromycin, antihistamines, antidepressants:** increased QTc and TdP.

- **Carbamazepine or digoxin AND clarithromycin, erythromycin:** increased carbamazepine or digoxin toxicity.
- **Amiodarone and simvastatin:** increased statin side-effects, e.g. rhabdomyolysis and myopathy; try fluvastatin, rosuvastatin, or pravastatin.
- **Simvastatin and amlodipine, or verapamil or diltiazem** (inhibit simvastatin metabolism): with these drugs the maximum dose of simvastatin is now 20 mg; higher doses are 'off-label'. Consider atorvastatin.
- **IV verapamil and IV dantrolene:** potential risk of VF.

23.4 Potentially fatal drug errors

- Excessive opiate dosing due to unfamiliar or agents with similar names.
- Getting decimal place wrong ×10 dose error.
- Giving drug when there is a clear history of allergy.
- IV potassium infusion too concentrated or too fast (max is 20 mmol/h).
- Setting pumps wrong, e.g. 100 ml/h rather than 10 ml/h.
- Giving allopurinol + azathioprine.
- Omitting insulin after failing to recognise diabetes.
- Prescribing methotrexate daily instead of weekly.
- Giving drugs by wrong route in ITU, e.g. intra-arterial or into CSF; check where the line goes as IV doses into CSF can be fatal or an artery can lose a limb.
- Not monitoring INR. Not detecting hypoglycaemia.

23.5 Prescribing warfarin

- **About:** it inhibits synthesis of K-dependent coagulation factors II, VII, IX, and X and natural anticoagulants protein C and protein S. Involved in multiple interactions: varying genetic metabolism, drugs, alcohol, and vitamin K intake affects efficacy. Requires frequent monitoring via INR. Takes at least 72 h to be therapeutic. Give LMWH or UFH cover until therapeutic range achieved.
- **Dosing regimen and duration:** always ask your senior if unsure – what is target range and what is duration and make sure documented in notes and discharge/clinic letter.
- **Target INR:** is 2.0–3.0 for almost all indications, though mechanical heart valves can get 2.5–3.5. Bleeding is the most significant problem and significant bleeding is seen in 3–5% per annum. Risk increases markedly after INR of 3.0 and even more so after INR >4.5. Skin necrosis is a rare but significant complication. Warfarin use is avoided in pregnancy especially in first trimester.
- **Drugs that INCREASE INR:** broad-spectrum antibiotics kill vitamin K-forming bacteria leading to increased bleeding effect. Others: fibrates, thyroxine, amiodarone, fluconazole, cephalosporins, cimetidine, ethanol, fluvastatin, HMG-CoA reductase inhibitors, lovastatin, isoniazid, macrolides (clarithromycin, erythromycin), metronidazole, quinolones (ciprofloxacin), tricyclic antidepressants.
- **Drugs that DECREASE INR:** barbiturates, carbamazepine, colestyramine, cigarette smoking, St John's wort, vitamin K corticosteroids, oral contraceptives, phenytoin, primidone, rifampicin, broccoli and green vegetables. **Indications:** DVT, PE, cerebral venous thrombosis, cardiac: AF, PAF, metal valves, LV thrombus, axillary vein thrombosis, antiphospholipid syndrome.
- **Duration:** calf DVT 3/12, proximal DVT 6/12, PE 6/12, tissue heart valve 3/12. Target INR: most are 2.5 except recurrent embolic events consider 2.5–3.5. Mechanical

prosthetic valves are often 2.5–3.5 with target = 3.0, but dependent on the type of valve replacement used; take specialist advice.

- **Warfarin contraindicated (relative and absolute):** pregnancy, bleeding, GI blood loss, haematuria, anaemia due to possible blood loss, haemorrhagic stroke, frequent falls, imminent need for surgery, safe compliance issues, excess alcohol intake or severe liver disease, high **HAS-BLED** or **ORBIT** score.
- **Side-effects:** bleeding anywhere – brain, gut, renal, spine, soft tissue. Bleed risk increases dramatically with INR >3.0. Risk highest in those new on warfarin in the first 3 months of treatment. Alopecia, skin necrosis, urticaria, anorexia, GI upset, liver disease and pancreatitis.
- **Starting warfarin safely:** informed consent for patient and clearly document target range and duration. Explain drug/food interactions – need to check INR if new interacting drugs. Where anticoagulation not urgent, such as AF, then go slow with 3 mg OD and check INR Day 5. This should avoid the hypercoagulable state due to falls in protein C seen with rapid initiation. More rapid loading with 5–10 mg OD for DVT/PE or metal valve or other thrombosis with cover of LMWH (enoxaparin 1.5 mg/kg/d) until therapeutic INR check Day 2 and after. Follow-up with anticoagulation service. If INR stable then testing can be extended to every 2 weeks and then to every 4–6 weeks.
- **Follow-up:** ensure there is definite follow-up through an anticoagulation clinic to manage the warfarin. Make sure all referrals to anticoagulation clinic have been done. Nowadays if there is a rush to anticoagulate non-rheumatic AF, consider dabigatran or rivaroxaban or apixaban, which can be started immediately and are active within a few hours.
- **Tablets:** warfarin 0.5 mg white, 1 mg brown, 3 mg blue, 5 mg pink.

23.6   Corticosteroids

- **Indications – anti-inflammatory or to replace intrinsic steroid production:** *asthma, COPD, cord compression, cerebral oedema, PMR, temporal arteritis, RA, SLE, ulcerative colitis, adrenal replacement.*
- Prolonged or repeated courses for more than 3 months, or 3–4 courses per year; consider adding some bone protection, e.g. **calcium 1 g/d and vitamin D 800 units/d.**
- **SE:** short-term: agitation, insomnia (avoid in evenings if non-urgent), agitation, psychosis; long term: weight gain, hyperglycaemia, fluid retention, raised WCC, raised infection risk, osteoporosis + fracture risk, high BP, diabetes, cataracts. Prolonged courses need bone protection with vitamin D and calcium. Consider need for PPI. Where possible the steroids are often switched to a steroid-sparing agent.

Steroid equivalent doses: dose equivalent to 5 mg of prednisolone

- Betamethasone 750 mcg
- Cortisone acetate 25 mg
- Dexamethasone 750 mcg
- Hydrocortisone 20 mg
- Methylprednisolone 4 mg
- Prednisone 5 mg
- Triamcinolone 4 mg.

Index